ACTIVATION, METABOLISM AND PERFUSION OF THE HEART

DEVELOPMENTS IN CARDIOVASCULAR MEDICINE

Recent volumes

Perry HM, ed: Lifelong management of hypertension. 1983. ISBN 0-89838-582-2.
Jaffe EA, ed: Biology of endothelial cells. 1984. ISBN 0-89838-587-3.
Surawicz B, Reddy CP, Prystowsky EN, eds: Tachycardias. 1984. ISBN 0-89838-588-1.
Spencer MP, ed: Cardiac Doppler diagnosis. 1983. ISBN 0-89838-591-1.
Villarreal H, Sambhi MP, eds: Topics in pathophysiology of hypertension. 1984. ISBN 0-89838-595-4.
Messerli FH, ed: Cardiovascular disease in the elderly. 1984. ISBN 0-89838-596-2.
Simoons ML, Reiber JHC, eds: Nuclear imaging in clinical cardiology. 1984. ISBN 0-89838-599-7.
Ter Keurs HEDJ, Schipperheyn JJ, eds: Cardiac left ventricular hypertrophy. 1983. ISBN 0-89838-612-8.
Sperelakis N, ed: Physiology and pathophysiology of the heart. 1984. ISBN 0-89838-615-2.
Messerli FH, ed: Kidney in essential hypertension. 1984. ISBN 0-89838-616-0.
Sambhi MP, ed: Fundamental fault in hypertension. 1984. ISBN 0-89838-638-1.
Marchesi C, ed: Ambulatory monitoring: Cardiovascular system and allied applications. 1984. ISBN 0-89838-642-X.
Kupper W, MacAlpin RN, Bleifeld W, eds: Coronary tone in ischemic heart disease. 1984. ISBN 0-89838-646-2.
Sperelakis N, Caulfield JB, eds: Calcium antagonists: Mechanisms of action on cardiac muscle and vascular smooth muscle. 1984. ISBN 0-89838-655-1.
Godfraind T, Herman AS, Wellens D, eds: Calcium entry blockers in cardiovascular and cerebral dysfunctions. 1984. ISBN 0-89838-658-6.
Morganroth J, Moore EN, eds: Interventions in the acute phase of myocardial infarction. 1984. ISBN 0-89838-659-4.
Abel FL, Newman WH, eds: Functional aspects of the normal, hypertrophied, and failing heart. 1984. ISBN 0-89838-665-9.
Sideman S, Beyar R, eds: Simulation and imaging of the cardiac system. 1985. ISBN 0-89838-687-X.
Van der Wall E, Lie KI, eds: Recent views on hypertrophic cardiomyopathy. 1985. ISBN 0-89838-694-2.
Beamish RE, Singal PK, Dhalla NS, eds: Stress and heart disease. 1985. ISBN 0-89838-709-4.
Beamish RE, Panagio V, Dhalla NS, eds: Pathogenesis of stress-induced heart disease. 1985. ISBN 0-89838-710-8.
Morganroth J, Moore EN, eds: Cardiac arrhythmias. 1985. ISBN 0-89838-716-7.
Mathes E, ed: Secondary prevention in coronary artery disease and myocardial infarction. 1985. ISBN 0-89838-736-1.
Lowell Stone H, Weglicki WB, eds: Pathology of cardiovascular injury. 1985. ISBN 0-89838-743-4.
Meyer J, Erbel R, Rupprecht HJ, eds: Improvement of myocardial perfusion. 1985. ISBN 0-89838-748-5.
Reiber JHC, Serruys PW, Slager CJ: Quantitative coronary and left ventricular cineangiography. 1986. ISBN 0-89838-760-4.
Fagard RH, Bekaert IE, eds: Sports cardiology. 1986. ISBN 0-89838-782-5.
Reiber JHC, Serruys PW, eds: State of the art in quantitative coronary arteriography. 1986. ISBN 0-89838-804-X.
Roelandt J, ed: Color Doppler Flow Imaging. 1986. ISBN 0-89838-806-6.
Van der Wall EE, ed: Noninvasive imaging of cardiac metabolism. 1986. ISBN 0-89838-812-0.
Liebman J, Plonsey R, Rudy Y, eds: Pediatric and fundamental electrocardiography. 1986. ISBN 0-89838-815-5.
Hilger HH, Hombach V, Rashkind WJ, eds: Invasive cardiovascular therapy. 1987. ISBN 0-89838-818-X
Serruys PW, Meester GT, eds: Coronary angioplasty: a controlled model for ischemia. 1986. ISBN 0-89838-819-8.
Tooke JE, Smaje LH: Clinical investigation of the microcirculation. 1986. ISBN 0-89838-819-8.
Van Dam RTh, Van Oosterom A, eds: Electrocardiographic body surface mapping. 1986. ISBN 0-89838-834-1.
Spencer MP, ed: Ultrasonic diagnosis of cerebrovascular disease. 1987. ISBN 0-89838-836-8.
Legato MJ, ed: The stressed heart. 1987. ISBN 0-89838-849-X.
Roelandt J, ed: Digital techniques in echocardiography. 1987. ISBN 0-89838-861-9.
Sideman S, Beyar R, eds: Activation, metabolism and perfusion of the heart. 1987. ISBN 0-89838-871-6.

ACTIVATION, METABOLISM AND PERFUSION OF THE HEART

Simulation and experimental models

edited by

S. SIDEMAN, D.Sc.
Professor of Chemical Engineering and R.J. Matas / Winnipeg Professor of Biomedical Engineering

R. BEYAR, M.D., D.Sc.
Senior Lecturer Department of Biomedical Engineering Technion Israel Institute of Technology, Haifa, Israel 3200

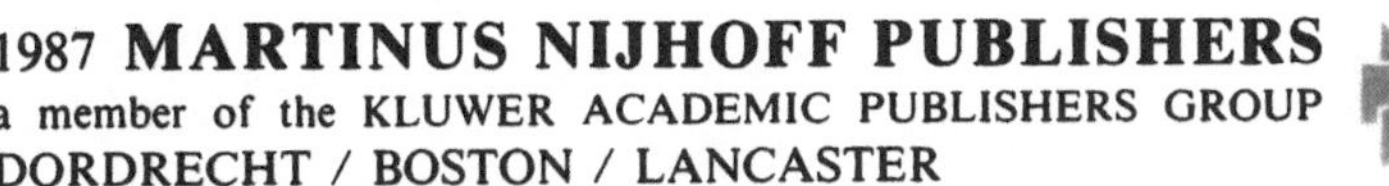
1987 **MARTINUS NIJHOFF PUBLISHERS**
a member of the KLUWER ACADEMIC PUBLISHERS GROUP
DORDRECHT / BOSTON / LANCASTER

Distributors

for the United States and Canada: Kluwer Academic Publishers, P.O. Box 358, Accord Station, Hingham, MA 02018-0358, USA
for the UK and Ireland: Kluwer Academic Publishers, MTP Press Limited, Falcon House, Queen Square, Lancaster LA1 1RN, UK
for all other countries: Kluwer Academic Publishers Group, Distribution Center, P.O. Box 322, 3300 AH Dordrecht, The Netherlands

Library of Congress Cataloging in Publication Data

Activation, perfusion, and metabolism of the heart.

(Developments in cardiovascular medicine)
Proceedings of the 3rd Henry Goldberg Workshop, Mar. 31-Apr. 2, 1986; organized jointly by Technion, Israel Institute of Technology, Haifa, Israel and Rutgers State University of New Jersey, Piscataway, N.J. USA.
Includes index.
1. Heart--Congresses. 2. Heart--Diseases--Congresses. I. Sideman, S. II. Beyar, Rafael. III. Henry Goldberg Workshop (3rd : 1986 : Rutgers University) IV. Tekhniyon, Makhon tekhnologi le-Yiśra'el. V. Rutgers University. [DNLM: 1. Cardiovascular System--physiology--congresses. 2. Cardiovascular System--physiopathology--congresses. 3. Models, Cardiovascular--congresses. W1 DE997VME / WG 202 A188 1986]
QP111.2.A28 1987 612'.17 87-1721

ISBN-13: 978-94-010-7987-7 e-ISBN-13: 978-94-009-3313-2
DOI: 10.1007/978-94-009-3313-2

To those close and dear
whose love kindled the
fires of inspiration and
whose devotion and trust
made it all possible.

To our parents, wives and
children who, each in his
own way, encouraged unfail-
ingly and never ruffled
the wings of dedication.

To our students and colleagues
whose hard work and ingenuity
build a reality from dreams
and made it all worthwhile.

To the memory of
those who are gone,
to the nameless ones
yet to be born . . .

One humble offering in the endless
search for knowledge.

Proceedings of the 3rd Henry Goldberg International Workshop
on simulation and modeling of the cardiac system,
31 March–2 April 1986, organized jointly by Technion,
Israel Institute of Technology, Haifa, Israel
and Rutgers State University of New Jersey, Piscataway, NJ, USA

Scientific Advisory Committee

Prof. E. Sonnenblick, M.D.
Albert Einstein College of Medicine, Bronx, NY, USA (Chairman)

Prof. E.O. Feigl, M.D., Ph.D.
University of Washington, Seattle, WA, USA

Prof. H. Neufeld, M.D.
H. Shiba Hospital, Tel-Hashomer, Israel

Prof. K. Sagawa, M.D., D.Sc.
Johns Hopkins University, Baltimore, MD, USA

Prof. M.L. Weisfeldt, M.D.
Johns Hopkins University Hospital, Baltimore, MD, USA

Organizing Committee

Dr R. Beyar, M.D., D.Sc. (Secretary).
Technion-ITT, Haifa, Israel, and Johns Hopkins University, Baltimore, MD, USA

Prof. J. Bassingthwaighte, M.D., Ph.D.
University of Washington, Seattle, WA, USA

Prof. R. Plonsey, Ph.D.
Duke University, Durham, NC, USA

Prof. E. Ritman, M.D. Ph.D.
Mayo Medical School, Rochester, MN, USA

Prof. Y. Rudy, Ph.D.
Case Western University, Cleveland, OH, USA

Prof. S. Sideman, D.Sc. (Chairman)
Technion-ITT, Haifa, Israel, and Rutgers State University, Piscataway, NJ, USA

Prof. W. Welkowitz, D.Sc. (Co-chairman)
Rutgers State University, Piscataway, NJ, USA

Contents

Contributors

Adam, D.
Department of Biomedical Engineering, The Julius Silver Institute of Biomedical Engineering, Technion, Israel Institute of Technology, Haifa 32000, Israel

Arts, T.
Department of Biophysics, University of Limburg, 6200 MD Maastricht, The Netherlands
co-author: R. S. Reneman

Azhari, A.
Departments of Biomedical Engineering and Chemical Engineering, Technion, Israel Institute of Technology, 32000 Haifa, Israel
co-authors: R. Beyar, E. Barta, U. Dinnar and S. Sideman

Barta, E.
Department of Biomedical Engineering, Technion, Israel Institute of Technology, 32000 Haifa, Israel
co-authors: S. Sideman, H. Adachi and R. Beyar

Bassingthwaighte, J.B.
Center for Bioengineering WD-12, University of Washington, Seattle, WA 98195, USA
co-authors: L. Noodleman, R.T. Eakin and R.B. King

Becker, L.C.
Division of Cardiology, Department of Medicine, The Johns Hopkins Hospital, 600 N. Wolfe Street, Baltimore, MD 21205, USA

Beyar, R
Department of Biomedical Engineering, Technion, Israel Institute of Technology, 32000 Haifa, Israel (on leave at Division of Cardiology, Department of Medicine, Johns Hopkins Medical Institutions, Baltimore, MD 21205, USA)
co-author: S. Sideman

Binah, O.
Department of Physiology and Biophysics, Falculty of Medicine and Rappaport Family Institute for Research in the Medical Sciences, Technion, Israel Institute of Technology, 32000 Haifa, Israel
co-authors: I. Rubinstein and Y. Sweed

Burkhoff, D.
Department of Biomedical Engineering, The Johns Hopkins University School of Medicine, 720 Rutland Ave, Traylor Building, Baltimore, MD 21205, USA
co-author: W.L. Maughan

Clark, J.W. Jr.
Department of Electrical Engineering, Rice University Houston, TX 77001, USA
co-author: C.R. Murphey

Dinnar, U.
Department of Biomedical Engineering, Technion, Israel Institute of Technology, 32000 Haifa, Israel

Downey, J.M.
Department of Physiology, University of South Alabama, Mobile, Alabama 36688, USA

Eng, C.
Department of Medicine, Physiology and Biophysics, Albert Einstein College of Medicine, Forchheimer Bldg. 715, 1300 Morris Park Avenue, Bronx, NY 10461, USA

Fabiato, A.
Department of Physiology, Medical College of Virginia, Richmond, VA 23298 USA
co-authors: A.Y.K. Wong and J.B. Bassingthwaighte

Gallagher, K.P.
Thoracic Surgery Research Lab., 3484 Kresge 1, Box 0548, University of Michigan, Ann Arbor, MI 48109, USA
co-authors: R.A. Gerren, A.J. Buda and W.R. Dunham

Hoffman, J.H.E.
Cardiovascular Research Institute, University of California, San Francisco, CA 94143, USA
co-authors: A.C. Hill, H. Mori, W. Husseini and M.B. Stevens

Horowitz, A.
Department of Biomedical Engineering, Technion, Israel Institute of Technology, 32000 Haifa, Israel
co-authors: Y. Lanir and M. Perl

Lab, M.J.
Department of Physiology, Charing Cross & Westminster Medical School, Fulham Palace Road, London W6 8RF, United Kingdom

Lammers, W.J.E.P.
Department of Physiology, University of Limburg, Maastricht, The Netherlands
co-authors: A.L. Wit and M.A. Allessie

Lanir, Y.
Department of Biomedical Engineering, Technion, Israel Institute of Technology, Haifa 32000, Israel
co-authors: A. Horowitz and M. Perl

LeJemtel, T.H.
Division of Cardiology, Department of Medicine, Albert Einstein College of Medicine, Bronx, NY 10461, USA

Li, J.K.-J.
Cardiovascular Research Laboratory, Department of Biomedical Engineering, Rutgers University, Piscataway, NJ 08854, USA

Little, W.C.
Division of Cardiology, Department of Medicine, Bowman Gray School of Medicine, Wake Forest University, 300 S. Hawthorne Road, Winston-Salem, NC 27103, USA
co-authors: R.C. Park and G.L. Freeman

Marban, E.
Department of Medicine, Cardiology Division, Johns Hopkins Medical Institutions, Baltimore, MD 21205, USA
co-authors: H. Kusuoka and M.L. Weisfeldt

Marcus, M.L.
Department of Medicine, Cardiovascular Center, University of Iowa Hospitals and Clinics, Iowa City, IA 52242, USA
co-authors: J.A. Rumberger, S.J. Reiter, A.J. Feiring, D.J. Skorton, S.M. Collins and W. Stanford

Mates, R.E.
Department of Mechanical and Aerospace Engineering, Medicine and Physiology, State University of New York at Buffalo, 462 Grider Street, NY 14215, USA

Maughan, W.L.
Division of Cardiology, Department of Medicine, The Johns Hopkins Hospital, Baltimore, MD 21205, USA
co-author: D. Burkhoff

Nordin, C.
Department of Medicine, Albert Einstein College of Medicine, 1300 Morris Park Avenue, Bronx, NY 10461, USA
co-author: R.S. Aronson

Palsson, B.
Department of Chemical Engineering, University of Michigan, Ann Arbor, MI 48109-2136, USA

Perl, M.
Department of Mechanical Engineering, Technion, Israel Institute of Technology, 32000 Haifa, Israel
co-author: A. Horowitz

Plonsey, R.
Department of Biomedical Engineering, Physiology and Pediatrics, Duke University, Durham, NC 27706, USA
co-author: R.C. Barr

Ritman, E.L.
Department of Physiology and Biophysics, Mayo Medical School, Rochester, MN 55905, USA
co-author: E.H. Hoffman

Rudy, Y.
Department of Biomedical Engineering, Case Western Reserve University, Cleveland, OH 44106, USA
co-author: W.-L. Quan

Sideman, S.
Department of Biomedical Engineering, Technion, Israel Institute of Technology, 32000 Haifa, Israel (on sabatical leave at Rutgers Medical School, Rutgers State University, Piscataway, NJ 08854, USA)

Sonnenblick, E.H.
Division of Cardiology, Department of Medicine, Albert Einstein College of Medicine, Bronx, NY 10461, USA
co-author: T.H. LeJemtel

Spaan, J.A.E.
Department of Physiology and Physiological Physics, State University of Leiden, The Netherlands
co-authors: P. Bruinsma, I. Vergroesen, J. Dankelman and H.G. Stassen

Spach, M.S.
Departments of Pediatrics and Physiology, Duke University Medical Center, Box 3090, Durham, NC 27710, USA
co-authors: P. Dolber and J.F. Heidlage

Sperelakis, N.
Department of Physiology and Biophysics, University of Cincinnati, College of Medicine, Cincinnati, OH 45267-0576, USA

Tyberg, J.V.
Faculty of Medicine, University of Calgary, 3330 Hospital Drive N.E., Calgary, Alberta, T2N 4N1 Canada

Vusse, G.J. van der
Center for Bioengineering, University of Washington, Seattle, WA 98195, USA
co-authors: F.W. Prinzen and R.S. Reneman

Weber, K.T.
Division of Cardiology, Michael Reese Hospital, University of Chicago, Chicago, IL, USA
co-author: J.S. Janicki

Weisfeldt, M.L.
Division of Cardiology, Department of Medicine, The Johns Hopkins Hospital, Clayton Heart Center, Baltimore, MD 21205, USA
co-authors: E. Marban and H. Kusuoka

Weiss, H.R.
Heart and Brain Circulation Laboratory, Department of Physiology and Biophysics, University of Medicine and Dentistry of New Jersey, Rutgers Medical School, Piscataway, NJ 08854, USA
co-author: G.J. Grover

Welkowitz, W.
Department of Biomedical Engineering, Rutgers Medical School, Piscataway, NJ 08855, USA
co-authors: J.K.-J. Li and J. Zelano

Winegrad, S.
Department of Physiology, School of Medicine, University of Pennsylvania, Philadelphia, PA 19104-6085, USA
co-authors: G. McClellan, L. Er Lin and S. Windling

Wit, A.L.
Department of Pharmacology, College of Physicians & Surgeons, Columbia University, NY 10032, USA
co-authors: W.J.E.P. Lammers and M.A. Allessie

Wong, A.Y.K.
Department of Physiology and Biophysics, Dalhousie University, Halifax, Nova Scotia, Canada

Yue, D.T.
Department of Biomedical Engineering, Traylor Building, The Johns Hopkins University School of Medicine, 720 Rutland Avenue, Baltimore, MD 21205, USA

Welcome

I'm very pleased to come here this morning to welcome you to this third Henry Goldberg Workshop. As President of this very large institution I see many different facets of University life, and one of the things that delights me most is to see the University as a window in the world of scholarship, looking far beyond its own limitations and even far byond this nation. The only true cooperation the world will ever know is that fashioned from the intellectual scientific scene. That is why it is such a great pleasure for me to welcome you distinguished scientists to our University. Not that I can understand all that you are saying.I sometimes suspect that the importance of a colloquium is measured by how little I understand the titles . . . I thank you again for coming here from all over the globe and I wish you a very successful meeting.

Prof. E. Bloustein
President, Rutgers State University of New Jersey

Greetings

It is a pleasure to share in the greetings of this group. The medical school usually witnesses other sciences moving in on our territory with some hesitation, as we both go after the same research dollars. However, we know that the only way science can advance is by the sharing. Some time ago somebody's wisdom separated the Medical School from Rutgers University and has given us separate administration. But, fortunately, there's been a countervailing wisdom that has made it possible for us to share any number of forums and the integration of activities between Rutgers University and the Medical School. This group here represents such a sharing. I'm sure you're going to have exciting three days. We are pleased to be recognized as being part of it and I wish you all successful and productive deliberations.

Prof. R. Reynolds
Dean, Rutgers Medical School and University of Medicine and Dentistry of New Jersey (UMDNJ)

I Bring you the greetings of Professor Josef Singer, President of Technion. He is sorry he is unable to be here today, and has asked me to represent him on this occasion. On behalf of the Technion I would like to convey greetings to the participants in this third Henry Goldberg Workshop on Simulation and Modeling of the Cardiac System. We at the Technion believe that one of the most important goals of science and technology is to improve the quality of life. This philosophy is reflected in all of our departments but is most vividly expressed in this interdisciplinary blend of science, technology and medicine, Biomedical Engineering. The Henry Goldberg Workshop which serves to exchange new ideas throughout the world significantly contributes to the advancement of scientific knowledge in Biomedical Engineering. This is the third meeting, the first in the United States, following two highly successful meetings at the Technion in Israel. I am sure that this gathering will continue the excellent tradition set by the previous meetings, and that the discussion and intellectual interaction which will take place here will greatly stimulate scientific progress. The principle aim of this workshop is to integrate the mechanical properties, electrical activation, coronary circulation and metabolic and energy balance in the heart in order to attain a better understanding and better correlation between the various functions of the heart. I hope that this will lead to new techniques which will replace the current invasive measurements with non-invasive ones, and thus lead to better health care. Again, Prof. Singer's and my own best wishes for meaningful and fruitful discussions.

Prof. U. Dinnar
Chairman, Department of Biomedical Engineering,
Technion, Israel Institute of Technology

I would like to convey the greetings of the College of Engineering. Our College is separate from University of Medicine and Dentistry of New Jersey (UMDNJ) which is represented by Dr Reynolds. We award about 600 bachelor's degrees, 100 master's degrees, and 20 Ph.D's each year in the Engineering disciplines, which makes us the largest engineering school in New Jersey, but only medium-sized by national standards. The department of Biomedical Engineering is a part of the College of Engineering, and offers M.S. and Ph.D. degrees. We feel that this department needs to continue the growth which has been remarkable in the past few years. This group is highly rated by our internal evaluation team as one of the top graduate programs in the University. It especially appropriate to have this meeting at Rutgers at this time when we are inaugurating the new Department replacing the old 'program' in Biomedical Engineering. And I thank you all for coming to join us in this effort. Good luck.

Prof. E. Dill
Dean, College of Engeneering,
Rutgers State University of New Jersey

Opening address

President Bloustein, Mr & Mrs Henry Goldberg, Dean Dill, Dean Reynolds, distinguished guests from around the world, Professors and students, ladies and gentlemen.

It is indeed a pleasure and a privilege to welcome you all to the 3rd Henry Goldberg Workshop. It is a pleasure to acknowledge the foresight of Mr Henry Goldberg. It is the 3rd Workshop which he, single-handedly, made possible and we look forward to seeing him in many more.

In view of the intensity of of research in the numerous aspects of the cardiovascular field, it seems important to develop an integrated view of the various interrelated, but independently studied, parameters affecting the cardiac function.

The cardiac simulation program, as boldly initiated some four years ago at the J. Silver Institute in the Technion IIT, Haifa, Israel, attempts to relate the cardiac system performance to the basic parameters which affect its characteristics, including fiber structure and architecture, muscle mechanics, material properties, cardiac hemodynamics, micro-circulation and myocardial perfusion, metabolism energetics and oxygen consumption, electrical activation rates and patterns, heart rates, natural and external controls etc., all under normal and pathological conditions. Hopefully this interdisciplinary approach will provide a better insight into the normal and pathophysiological characteristics of the heart.

The first HG Workshop, held at the Technion in Haifa in 1984, introduced the concept of interaction, emphasizing imaging in the clinical environment. The 2nd workshop, also in Haifa, in 1985, discussed imaging, mechanics, electrical activation, perfusion and metabolism with a slant towards the control aspects. Following the success of these workshops, the 3rd HG Workshop, held in the USA this time, continues the previous efforts to elucidate the interactions between the many parameters which affect cardiac performance by bringing together the leading experts and the outstanding scientists from the various cardiac disciplines. These gatherings, we hope, generate some new questions, provide a few answers and, most important,catalyze personal interactions and encourage continued scientific cooperation.

The central theme of the 3rd Henry Goldberg Workshop is the transformation of the microscale activation phenomena to macroscale activity and performance, inter-relating electrophysiology, metabolism, and perfusion to cardiac mechanics. Emphasis is also given to some promising attempts to model and simulate the mechanical and metabolical aspects of ischemia and infarction, as well as the complex formation of arrhythmias.

This meeting could not have occurred without the support of President J. Bloustein and Dean E. Dill of the College of Engineering of Rutgers University. We acknowledge with thanks the continuous support of Mr Julius Silver and the warm encouragement of Mrs Enid (Silver) Winslow which has given the backbone to this hard task. The love and trust of the late Mrs Pearl Milch, ex-president of the Women's Division of the American Technion Society, provided the physical means for our cardiac research center and encouraged us to embark on this project. Others who helped bring us here include the Presidents, Mrs R. Silbert, Mrs M. Leighton, Mrs R. Wallach and Mrs Flo Cohen, Executive Director of the same organization. The support of the British Technion Society, and, particularly, Mr Michael Kennedy-Leigh and Mr Sidney Korob of London are gratefully acknowledged. The outstanding cooperation and friendship of the various distinguisted scientists, including the participants in these present and past workshops, too many to be listed here, gave us the confidence to proceed in our efforts. Finally, again, our warmest thanks to Mr Henry Goldberg whose forsight and generosity enables us all to meet here today.

The 3rd HG Workshop is officially open.

Electrical activation and propagation

1. Use of computer simulations for combined experimental-theoretical study of anisotropic discontinuous propagation at a microscopic level in the cardiac muscle

M.S. SPACH, P. DOLBER and J.F. HEIDLAGE

Abstract

This paper presents combined experimental-theoretical results pertinent to anisotropic discontinuous propagation at a microscopic size scale (<200 μm). We first simulated how the transmembrane and extracellular potential waveforms, and their derivatives, are theoretically related to each other and to the sodium current and conductance in normal propagating action potentials and at the site of a collision or end of a one-dimensional cable. We then applied the relationships between the time derivatives of the extracellular waveforms and the underlying action potentials in an experimental analysis of anisotropic propagation at this small size scale in human atrial muscle bundles of different ages. At sites where the boundary effects alter the rate of rise of the action potential, the time course of the internal membrane variables (g_{Na} and I_{Na}) are changed in a way that alters the total open time of the sodium channels during depolarization. In turn, this predicts that the same concentration of sodium channel blocking drugs should have an anisotropic distribution in the depression of $\dot{V}_{max}$ and conduction velocity, a prediction confirmed with preliminary experiments. The extracellular waveforms changed from a smooth contour during transverse propagation in young preparations to complex polyphasic waveforms in the older preparations. The differences in the extracellular waveforms and their derivatives indicated that there was electrical uncoupling of the side-to-side connections between small groups of fibers with aging. These changes produced a prominent zigzag course of transverse propagation at a microscopic level which, in turn, accounted for the marked complexity of the extracellular waveforms. The electrophysiological consequence was an age-related decrease in the 'effective' transverse conduction velocities to the range of very slow conduction which makes it possible for reentry to occur in small regions of cardiac muscle with normal cellular electrophysiological properties.

Introduction

The basic mechanism underlying directional differences in excitability, conduction velocity, and safety factor that lead to circus movement reentry in cardiac muscle is generally attributed to a spatial difference in the refractory period as originally described by Mines [1] or to a depressed segment as described by Schmitt and Erlanger [2]. A departure from this classical mechanism of cardiac conduction disturbances was introduced several years ago by evidence that the anisotropic passive electrical properties of cardiac muscle affect the shape of the upstroke of the action potential dependent upon the direction of propagation with respect to the orientation of the fibers [3]. That is, slow upstrokes occur with fast longitudinal propagation and fast upstrokes with slow transverse propagation. At present, however, there is still no satisfactory model to account for these directionally dependent shape changes due to structural complexities that exist at a microscopic level nor is there information in any species about how anisotropic excitation spread occurs in cardiac muscle based on experimental measurements at this small size scale ($<200\,\mu m$).

Since we originally reported the occurrence of directional differences in the shape of the upstroke in anisotropic cardiac muscle and suggested the hypothesis of anisotropic discontinuous propagation [3], we have attempted to perform a step-by-step theoretical analysis of one-dimensional cable models to gain insight to the effects of the upstroke shape changes on the kinetics of the ionic depolarizing currents while, at the same time, we have attempted to develop improved experimental methods to learn how excitation spread in two dimensions occurs at a microscopic level.

The fundamental problem from the experimental viewpoint is that the measurements of propagating depolarization in cardiac muscle involve quantities, such as $\dot{V}_{max}$, that are not directly descriptive of the underlying mechanisms of propagation. Rather they are composite results that represent the interaction of multiple internal processes and factors such as ion channel conductance, cell geometry, cell interconnections, junctions of muscle bundles, and boundaries where propagation begins and ends. Direct study of ionic channels and other internal membrane mechanisms can be accomplished only with specialized experimental techniques, such as voltage clamp or single channel recordings, that attempt to separate these mechanisms. With an action potential the primary measurable quantity is V_m, the transmembrane potential, as a function of time or time and space. Thus, for cardiac action potentials, mechanisms must be inferred by reconstruction based on hypothetical ionic channel and transport mechanisms suggested by voltage clamp data.

In contrast to what appears to be the general consensus, we have found that it is simply not practical to use intracellular microelectrode recordings of action potentials to measure the details of excitation spread at a size scale varying between 10 to $200\,\mu m$. To resolve measurements at distances $10\,\mu m$ apart, the major difficulty encountered is that cellular damage is produced, thus altering the excitation sequence under study. Also, even for intracellular recordings made at sites quite close together, it is not clear which specific fiducial point should be picked during the upstroke if one is to resolve the difference in the times of excitation at sites several microns apart.

The need for combined experimental-theoretical analyses stems from the increasing evidence that the inhomogeneous and anisotropic distribution of the connections between fibers and bundles of fibers, in the past considered to be of minor importance in the propagation of depolarization, results in previously unrecognized propagation phenomenon, such as that of anisotropic discontinuous propagation [3, 4]. Based on these considerations, we have studied two-dimensional propagation at a microscopic size scale in human atrial muscle bundles. Not only did we encounter the changes in shape of the action potential upstroke with changes in the direction of propagation as found in animal species, but in preparations from older subjects the extracellular waveforms indicated that anisotropic propagation was considerably more complex during transverse propagation than we had encountered in animals preparations.

Extracellular (rather than intracellular) potential measurements with a microelectrode were required for the analysis at a microscopic level. The major problem was to resolve the location of the source of each deflection of the polyphasic extracellular potential waveforms we found in preparations with nonuniform anisotropic properties. Masuda and Paes de Garvalho [5] encountered a similar difficulty in their analysis of complex waveforms in the atrial region of the dog sinus node. They concluded 'it would seem impossible to ascertain a priori whether a given biphasic complex is generated by a small bundle near the electrode or a larger bundle further away'. However, we found that it is theoretically possible to determine the difference between the size of the source (bundle size) and the distance to the source by examining the first and second time derivatives of the extracellular waveforms, which reveal the fine details of the original waveforms.

In this paper, we summarize some of the computer simulations that have provided insight to changes in the kinetics of the sodium conductance secondary to propagation boundaries. We also demonstrate the theoretical predictions from simulations of the relationship between the first derivative of intracellular and extracellular potentials. We relate the results to differences found by age with respect to uniform and nonuniform anisotropic properties of atrial muscle bundles. The results show that the combined use of computer simulations and experimental measurements at a microscopic level provide a basis for predicting anisotropic effects of sodium channel blocking drugs (without having any knowledge of the cause of directional differences in the shape of the action potential) and for improved understanding of the origin of quite low conduction velocities during transverse propagation in preparations from older subjects.

Methods

Experiment

We wanted to study tissues in which the anisotropic electrical properties might vary depending on underlying structural differences while the fibers remain strictly parallel, thus making practical a combined experimental, theoretical, and structural analysis. We found human atrial pectinate muscle bundles to be the most suitable because all such bundles demonstrated anisotropic properties. After approval of investigational protocols by an institutional committee for guidelines for human research, atrial specimens were obtained at cardiac surgery in 37 subjects who had no clinical evidence of hemodynamic or electrophysiologic dysfunction of the right atrium.

Each specimen was immediately placed in cooled superfusate solution at 2–5° C, brought to the laboratory, and pinned to the floor of a tissue bath (4 cm × 5 cm) and maintained at a temperature of 35° C. The composition of the perfusate, in mM, was as follows: NaCl, 128; KCl, 4.69; $MgSO_4$, 1.18; NaH_2PO_4, 0.41; $NaHCO_3$, 20.1; $CaCl_2$, 2.23; and dextrose 11.1. The solutions were gassed in a reservoir with a mixture of 95% O_2–5% CO_2 and perfused through a cannula to produce a high flow rate along a 1-cm wide area on the surface of the preparation. To study the anisotropic effects of sodium channel blocking drugs quinidine gluconate was added to the perfusate in the reservoir to produce a final concentration of 5–10 μg/ml.

The development of the extracellular microelectrode measuring technique is described in a recent paper by Spach and Dolber [6]. To analyze propagating depolarization at the size scale of 200 μm or greater, we used extracellular electrodes made of flexible tungsten wire, 50 μm in diameter and insulated except at the tip. However, during transverse propagation in some preparations the diameter of this electrode was too large to obtain adequate resolution of the site of origin of each of the multiple deflections. Therefore, we used extracellular metal microelectrodes (Diamond Electro-Tech, Inc.) which were insulated except for an exposed tip of approximately 1 μm and which had a resistance of 1–2 megaohms. Intracellular potentials were recorded with conventional glass microelectrodes filled with 3 M KCl and having resistances between 10 and 20 megaohms.

A PDP-11/44 computer system controlled the rate and synchronized the pacing stimuli with the data recording. The outputs of the recording amplifiers were sampled at a rate between 20,000 and 50,000 per second (12-bit samples). Although sampling rates up to 40,000 per second were frequently necessary to reproduce complex waveforms accurately, we noted no change in shape when the sampling rate was increased above that value, even with the fastest upstrokes (400 V/sec) and with the most rapid deflections of complex extracellular waveforms.

To analyze the spread of excitation along the longitudinal and transverse axes of the fibers, the extracellular metal microelectrode was moved in steps of 10 μm to 50 μm, as determined by the micrometer of a micromanipulator. The position of the tip was documented from photographs made with a Nikon F250 35-mm camera through a dissecting microscope (effective resolution better than 5 μm). After the conclusion of each experiment, the measured waveforms stored digitally were redisplayed and photographed for initial analysis. Following selection of appropriate waveforms, the original digitized values were transferred to a HP9000 computer for detailed analysis and automatic plotting. The transmembrane potential V_m was obtained by subtracting the extracellular potential from the intracellular potential. The first time derivative of V_m and the first and second time derivatives of the extracellular waveforms were obtained numerically and the values plotted in time steps of 20, 25, or 50 μsec. To minimize the sensitivity of the derivatives to the slight noise in the original waveforms, we used established techniques for finding the derivatives of slightly smoothed data [7]. The effective conduction velocity was estimated by dividing the distance between two electrodes by the difference in time at which the maximum negative slope of the extracellular potential occurred at each electrode.

Theory

Although the physical laws governing the extracellular potentials generated by ionic currents are well known (see Lorente de Nó [8], Rosenfalck [9], we could find no information about the relation between the extracellular depolarization waveforms and their time derivatives near the current sources. Also, at the membrane surface it is important to know how the measurable quantities of the transmembrane and extracellular potential waveforms and their derivatives are related to each other, and, in turn, to the underlying nonmeasurable quantities of the sodium current and its conductance. We first examined the theoretical relationship between the potentials at the membrane surface and the internal membrane variables, the sodium conductance and current. Next, we performed computer simulations to determine how the extracellular potentials are related to their time derivatives as the measurement site is shifted away from the membrane surface of bundles of different sizes.

We simplified the problem as much as possible by using a single transient sodium current mechanism with the equivalent electrical circuit of a continuous cable. This conduction model would be representative either of propagation in a long thin cell or of plane-wave propagation in a two- or three-dimensional group of tightly coupled cells. A macroscopic rather than single channel current description was desired because propagated transmembrane and extracellular potentials are determined by the macroscopic membrane currents as a function of time and space. Thus, we consider that models in the form of the Hodgkin-Huxley equations [10] for the macroscopic Na^+ current were most appropriate for this study because of the small time scale they describe and fit. We chose the Ebihara-Johnson description [11] of the fast sodium current because it is based on voltage clamp data in cardiac muscle under normal conditions. Evidence, however, has been provided in single cardiac cells of deviation from the single inactivation component of the sodium current of the Hodgkin-Huxley equations; i.e., there can be a delayed slow inactivation component of the sodium conductance [12]. In view of the increasing use of Hodgkin-Huxley type models of the macroscopic fast sodium current, we believe it is important to note here why a delayed slow second inactivation state of the sodium conductance should not alter the interpretation of propagating action potentials that have a takeoff potential more negative than −60 mV (i.e., action potentials which are generated by the fast sodium current).

To describe the Na^+ current for studies of the action potential and propagation, a mechanistic model of the Na channels is desirable. However, there is no general agreement yet on a physical model of the sodium conductance mechanism [13]. Several empirical models of the Na-conductance mechanism are available, however, in the general form of the Hodgkin-Huxley mathematical description (see McAllister et al. [14], Beeler and Reuter [15], Ebihara and Johnson [11]). The Hodgkin-Huxley mathematical formulation [10] used in these models is based on voltage-clamp experimental protocols that result in a transient Na^+ current that lasts only a few milliseconds, i.e., a rapid rise to its peak (activation) followed by a short decay phase (inactivation) that is fit by a single exponential. Here, the fast Na^+ current is described as being caused by a transient Na conductance g_{Na}

$$g_{Na} = \bar{G}_{Na} m^3 h, \tag{1}$$

where $\bar{G}_{Na}$ is the maximum sodium conductance and m and h are the dimensionless activation and inactivation variables respectively. However, voltage clamp experiments in single cardiac cells [16, 17] have demonstrated the occurrence of I_{Na} inactivation with an initial fast decay for 5 to 7 msec followed by a much slower decay. In this case, the Na conductance is envisaged as the sum of two conductances [18], for example:

$$g_{Na} = \bar{G}_{Na} m^3 h_1 + \bar{G}_{Na} m^3 h_2, \tag{2}$$

where the first term describes the fast transient conductance and the second the slow conductance.

As reviewed by Meves [18], interpretation of the experimental results of delayed inactivation (h_2) are contradictory and the interpretation is not simple. For example, apparent differences in the kinetics of inactivation can be due, at least in part, to differences in the voltage clamp protocols [19]. Until simulations based on a mathematical description of I_{Na} with the kinetics of a slow component of inactivation show otherwise, the following points suggest that for simulating propagating depolarization in cardiac muscle (and nerve), the Hodgkin-Huxley mathematical formulation provides an appropriate description of the kinetics of the macroscopic sodium current:

1. In the single-cell experiments of Brown et al. [16], they found that two time constants (τ_{h1} and τ_{h2}) were required to describe their I_{Na} inactivation data where τ_{h2} was 3 to 4 times as long as τ_{h1}. However, they also found that the Hodgkin-Huxley m^3 (or m^4) kinetics fit their data during the activation phase of the sodium current. Thus, in this paper the computed relationships between the measurable quantities ($\dot{V}_{max}$ and $-d\Phi_e/dt_{max}$) and the non-measurable internal membrane variables (I_{Na} and g_{Na}) during the rapid phase of the upstroke should be valid.
2. In voltage clamp experiments, the Na conductance is small during the delayed phase of inactivation [18]. Additionally, in a propagating action potential the τ_{h2} component would occur at a time near the peak value of V_m; i.e., when the driving force for the Na current is smallest. Thus, the magnitude of Na^+ current should be quite small during the time of delayed inactivation if the τ_{h2} component is present in a propagating action potential.
3. When present, a delayed slow component of I_{Na} inactivation should have no effect during the upstroke of a propagating action potential because the delayed slow component would occur 5 to 20 msec after $\dot{V}_{max}$ and/or the peak of the upstroke (taking into account the lower temperature of the voltage clamp experiments). For example, when the time of delayed inactivation is matched with the upstrokes of the experimental action potentials of this or other papers, a slow I_{Na} inactivation component should occur during the initial repolarization phase of the action potential.

For propagation in one dimension along a uniform structure, the relationship between the transmembrane potential V_m and the net transmembrane current I_m is a function of time and space governed by the cable equation:

$$I_m = \frac{a}{2R_i}\frac{\partial^2 V_m}{\partial x^2} = C_m \frac{\partial V_m}{\partial t} + I_{ion}, \tag{3}$$

where a is the radius of the cylinder, R_i is the internal resistivity, and C_m is the membrane capacity. We approximated the ionic current I_{ion} (per unit area) during the depolarization phase of the cardiac action potential by the fast, transient sodium current in parallel with a constant leakage (repolarization) conductance:

$$I_{ion} = \bar{G}_{Na} m^3 h\,(V_m - V_{Na}) + g_L\,(V_m - V_L), \tag{4}$$

where the dimensionless activation and inactivation variables m and h were assumed to follow the kinetics described by Ebihara and Johnson [11]. g_L is a constant, and V_{Na} and V_L are the sodium and leak equilibrium potentials respectively. In an attempt to approximate the effective size of a small bundle of fibers, we assigned a value of 25 μm to the radius. Equation 3 was solved over a length of six resting space constants, and the transmembrane potential was computed at the midpoint of the cable where there was uniform propagation (i.e., no end effects).

The extracellular potential Φ_e at a point on the membrane surface and at varying distances from the surface was derived by the following equation for a one-dimensional cable, as described previously [20]:

$$\Phi_e(P, t_0) = \frac{aR_e}{2} \int_{-\infty}^{\infty} \frac{I_m(x, t_0)}{\sqrt{|a+d|^2 + |x' - x|^2}} dx, \qquad (5)$$

where a is the radius of the cylinder, R_e is the resistivity of the extracellular fluid, $I_m(x, t_o)$ is the net transmembrane current (Equation 3) at point x and time t_o, d is the perpendicular distance between site x at the membrane surface and the observation point P, and $(x' - x)$ is the distance along the cylinder between point x and point x'. We used a value of 150 Ω-cm for the extracellular resistivity of the fluid comprising the homogeneous volume conductor [21].

In bundles of different sizes the actual effective radius of the active tissue producing the extracellular potentials is not known. To approximate the effective size of different bundles (cables), we assigned values of 25, 75, 150 and 250 μm to the radius in Equation 5 (the assumption was that each large cable represented a compact group of synchronously firing small bundles).

The values were computed on the HP 9000 computer for detailed analysis and plotting of the theoretical waveforms. The first time derivatives were obtained numerically from the computed valves of g_{Na}, I_{Na}, and the transmembrane potential. The extracellular waveforms, along with their first and second time derivatives, were plotted for each time instant at 20 μsec intervals.

Results

To emphasize selective features of models pertinent to anisotropic discontinuous propagation, we present representative results obtained from computer simulations that use one-dimensional models and we test the theoretical results by experimental measurements of propagation at a microscopic size scale. That is, for the computed results to be meaningful, we have tried to adhere to the constraint that our theoretical results (or predictions based on the computed results) should be tested against the experimentally measured data.

Transmembrane potential and internal membrane variables

Simulation predictions

Uniform propagation was identified when there was constant velocity and constant shape of the V_m, g_{Na}, and I_{Na} waveforms at adjacent sites. This type of conduction occurred at all sites along the simulated cable except in regions where the action potential initiated, collided, and approached the sealed end of the cable. Figure 1 shows the time course and rate of change of V_m, I_{Na}, and g_{Na} at a site of uniform propagation and at a collision. Note that the collision had no effect on the foot of the action potential (Figure 1A); i.e., starting at the resting potential of -80 mV, the rate of rise of V_m was the same in both until V_m reached -50 mV. The action potentials differed, however, during the upper part of the upstroke after turn-on of the sodium current, $\dot{V}_{max}$ and peak V_m being greater at the collision than at the site of the uniform propagation. The increase in $\dot{V}_{max}$ at the collision was accompanied by a considerable decrease in peak I_{Na} (Figure 1B); this is the opposite of the classical monotonic relationship between $\dot{V}_{max}$ and the maximum sodium current when the upstroke is altered by interventions such as ischemia, drugs, and premature stimuli. Although the collision had little effect on the maximum value of the sodium conductance (Figure 1C), peak g_{Na} occurred earlier and the area of the g_{Na} curve was 14% less than normal.

In Figure 2, phase-plane plots of $\dot{V}_m$ vs V_m and of the trajectories of I_{Na} and g_{Na} as a function of V_m show that the shapes of the $\dot{V}_m$ curves as a function of V_m were the same until they reached the potential at which the sodium current appeared (-45 mV), then they diverged. After I_{Na} turn-on in the normal, $\dot{V}_m$ increased less rapidly as it approached $\dot{V}_{max}$ [22, 23], whereas at the collision site $\dot{V}_m$ increased more rapidly to $\dot{V}_{max}$.

Experimental confirmation

We attempted to determine if the above shape differences could be confirmed during a collision vs uniform propagation in a one-dimensional structure; i.e., in a functionally single Purkinje strand of a dog. Figure 3A shows the digital phase-plane plots of the depolarization phase of the action potential during uniform propagation and during a collision. During uniform propagation the ascending limb of the phase-plane plot fit a linear trajectory, indicating an exponential rise of the foot. When two action potentials were made to collide at the site of the impaled cell, the ascending limb did not fit a single exponential, rather the initial slope of the foot was the same as that during uniform propagation with a more rapid rise after the foot, just as predicted in the simulation shown in Figure 2A. We considered this theoretical and experimental result to be pertinent to the question of the cause of the directional shape differences in anisotropic cardiac muscle: could collisions at a microscopic level be the cause of the more rapid rise of the upstroke during transverse propagation in anisotropic ventricular and atrial muscle bundles? The model of Geselowitz and Miller [24] proposes that during

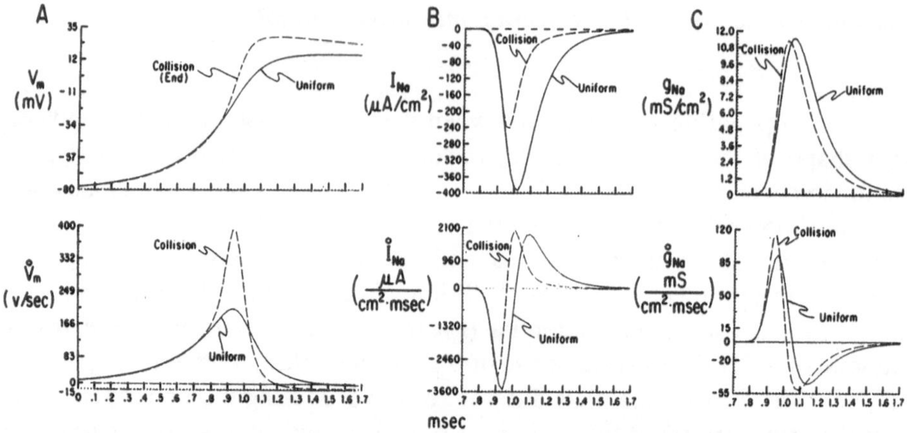

Figure 1. Computed transmembrane potential (A), sodium current (B), and the sodium conductance (C) at a site of uniform propagation and at a collision. The time course of V_m, I_{Na}, and g_{Na} is shown at the top and the first derivative of each variable is shown below. (Reproduced from IEEE Trans Biomed Eng BME 32: 743–755 (1985), by permission of The IEEE Engineering in Medicine and Biology Society.)

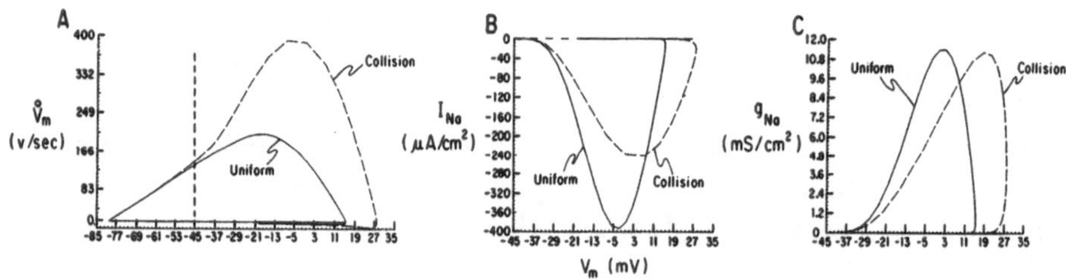

Figure 2. Computed phase-plane graphs of V_m and the trajectories of I_{Na} and g_{Na} as a function of V_m at a site of uniform propagation and at a collision. The plots are for the same action potentials of the previous figure. (Reproduced from IEEE Trans Biomed Eng BME 32: 743–755 (1985), by permission of The IEEE Engineering in Medicine and Biology Society.)

slow transverse propagation in anisotropic tissue 'each cell will be excited by colliding waves moving in opposite directions along the cell axis'. If so, a phase-plane plot of the upstroke of the action potential during transverse propagation in atrial or ventricular muscle should demonstrate an ascending limb that is not fit by a single exponential. Figure 3B shows a digital plot of the upstroke of a representative action potential in human atrial muscle during transverse propagation. Note that the ascending limb is well fit by a single exponential; i.e., there is no initial deviation as would be expected in a collision. Based on this experimental-theoretical test, we conclude that collisions do not account for the more rapid rate of rise of the action potential during slow transverse propagation as compared to the slower rate of rise during fast longitudinal propagation [3].

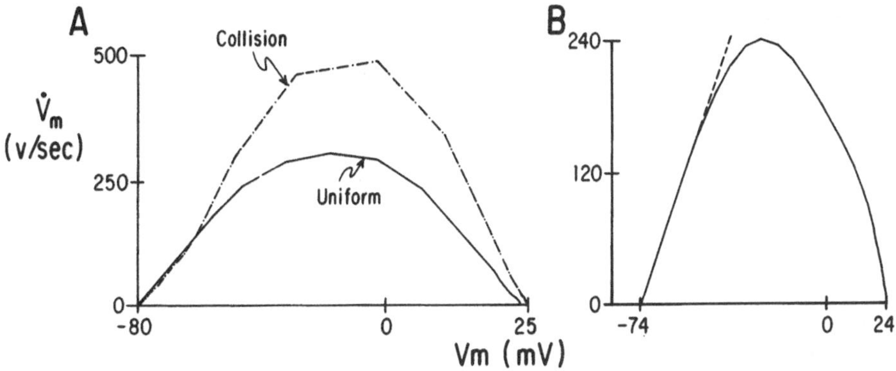

Figure 3. Experimental phase-plane graphs of $\dot{V}_m$ vs V_m for uniform propagation and a collision in a dog Purkinje strand (A) and (B) a similar graph for an action potential during propagation along the transverse axis of an atrial muscle bundle from a 33-year-old human subject. In Panel A, the foot of the action potential remained unchanged during a collision while $\dot{V}_{max}$ increased markedly, as predicted theoretically. Panel B illustrates that during transverse propagation in human atrial muscle that the ascending limb of the phase-plane plot fits a straight line; i.e., it is fit by a single exponential. (During longitudinal propagation, $\dot{V}_{max}$ for the same atrial cell was at the lower value of 135 mV.)

A further practical implication of the above theoretical results is that, without having any knowledge of the cause of the directional differences in the shape of the action potentials, it can be predicted that there should be an anisotropic effect of sodium-channel blocking drugs [25]. That is, during the more rapid rise of the action potential during slow transverse propagation, the kinetics of the sodium conductance should be altered by discontinuities so that the total open time of the Na^+ channels is changed. Since the uptake of Na^+-channel blocking drugs is dependent on the total Na^+ channel open time, the uptake of these drugs should have a nonhomogeneous distribution relative to the location of a cell when it is in a region of longitudinal vs transverse propagation. For example, these results predict that in anisotropic cardiac muscle, the relative depression of conduction by a given concentration of Na^+-channel blocking drug will be greater in a cell when propagation occurs in the longitudinal direction than in the transverse direction. This prediction arises from the fact that the shape and amplitude of depolarization of a cardiac action potential depend on the direction with respect to the orientation of the fibers (see [3]). The rate of rise and the amplitude of the upstroke is less with longitudinal than with transverse propagation, the same type of depolarization shape difference shown between uniform propagation and propagation at a collision site.

Our preliminary experimental results with superfusion of quinidine gluconate (5–10 μg/ml) show a greater relative decrease in $\dot{V}_{max}$ and conduction velocity in the longitudinal direction that in the transverse direction (unpublished results), as expected from the simulations. Also, with abrupt increases in stimulus rate, the time constant of drug blockade (predicted by an exponential decay of $\dot{V}_{max}$) is shorter in the transverse direction than in the longitudinal direction. These preliminary experimental results have considerable implication concerning new anisotropic mechanisms that are likely involved when drugs prevent of stop reentrant tachyarrhythmias, as well as when they enhance the occurrence of reentrant arrhythmias.

Time derivatives of extracellular potential waveforms near the sources

Simulation predictions

Figure 4 summarizes the computer simulations [25] that relate the extracellular and transmembrane potentials, and their derivatives, to each other and to the nonmeasurable internal membrane variables g_{Na} and I_{Na} for a uniformly propagating action potential. In Figure 4A (top), the asymmetric shape of the biphasic extracellular waveform with a more prominent minimum than maximum is accounted for by the asymmetry in the shape of depolarization of V_m. The lower row of Figure 4A shows the derivatives of the extracellular (above) and transmembrane (below) potentials. The maximum negative slope during the course of the biphasic extracellular waveform occurred at the same time as $\dot{V}_{max}$ of the transmembrane potential. Figure 4B (top) shows the computed temporal relation between $\dot{V}_m$ and the internal membrane variables. $\dot{V}_{max}$ occurred between the time of turn-on and the peak values of g_{Na} and I_{Na}. The computed derivatives of g_{Na} and I_{Na} (lower row), however, show that $\dot{V}_{max}$ coincided closely in time ($<20\,\mu$sec) with the maximum rate of increase of g_{Na} and I_{Na}. Therefore, both the negative peak of the first derivative of the extracellular potential and $\dot{V}_{max}$ of the transmembrane potential provide a marker for the instant of the maximum rate of increase of the sodium current and its conductance. Additional simulations [25] showed that the coincidence in time between $\dot{V}_{max}$ and the maximum negative slope of the extracellular potential waveform was unchanged for variations in the shapes of the waveforms with marked changes in the membrane properties and with propagation at sites where the transmembrane and extracellular potential waveforms were quite different and changed from site to site; e.g., at sites where Φ_c was entirely negative (where impulse conduction begins) and where Φ_c was largely positive (at collisions).

Experimental confirmation

A major practical significance of the above theoretical results is that the negative peak of the derivative of the extracellular waveform gives the same fiducial point as $\dot{V}_{max}$ of V_m and, thereby, it can be used to measure quite small differences in the timing of local excitation between points at a very small size scale. Thus, with the use of extracellular microelectrodes, it should be possible to map excitation at a microscopic size scale, at least to the practical limit of timing differences between sites 5–10 μm apart. To determine if the above relationships could be confirmed

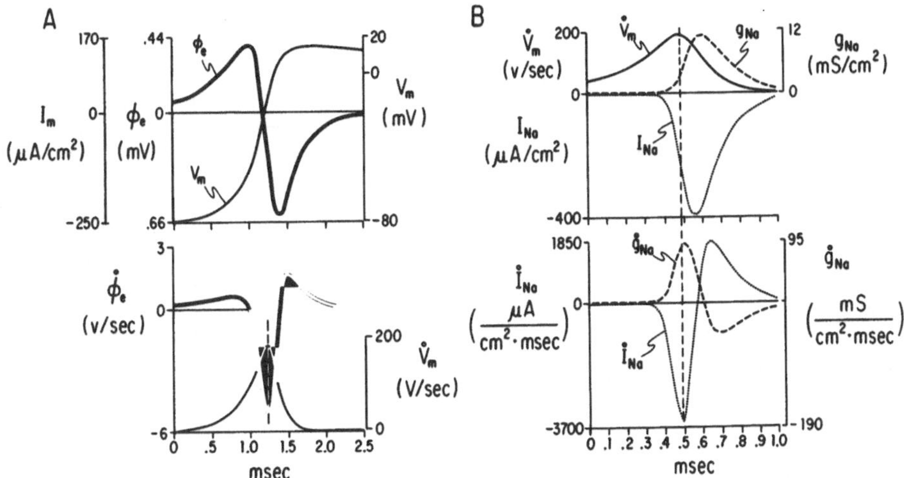

Figure 4. Theoretical predictions: simulations relating extracellular and transmembrane potentials, and their derivatives to each other and to the sodium current and conductance during uniform (normal) propagation. Panel A: computed extracellular and transmembrane potentials (top) and their first time derivatives (bottom) for a uniformly propagating action potential. The extracellular potential Φ_e was computed for a location at the surface of a cylinder with a radius of 25 μm. Panel B: computed temporal relationships between the first derivative of V_m and the nonmeasurable internal membrane variables I_{Na} and g_{Na}. The first time derivatives of I_{Na} and g_{Na} are shown below. (Reproduced from Circ Res 58: 356–371 (1986), by permission of the American Heart Association, Inc.)

experimentally for different shapes of the extracellular and transmembrane potential waveforms, we examined the measurable quantities V_m and Φ_e in human atrial bundles while the velocity was altered by 1. changing the direction of propagation and 2. initiating premature stimuli. A typical result is shown in Figure 5. In Figure 5A (1) the transmembrane potential rises faster and the amplitude is greater during slow (θ_T) propagation than during fast longitudinal (θ_L) propagation. The directionally dependent differences in shape were equally marked, or accentuated, when the action potential was initiated at less negative take-off potentials by early premature stimuli (Figure 5A (2)). However, the derivatives in each case (Figure 5B) confirmed the theoretical prediction that the maximum negative slope of the extracellular potential occurs at the same time as $\dot{V}_{max}$ of the transmembrane potential (time difference $<50\,\mu$sec).

Age-related differences in the anisotropic propagation properties

Preparations from children less than 15-years-old

Figure 6 shows the pattern of excitation spread and the waveforms of a preparation from a two-year-old male, a representative result obtained in atrial preparations from children. The major feature was characteristic uniform excita-

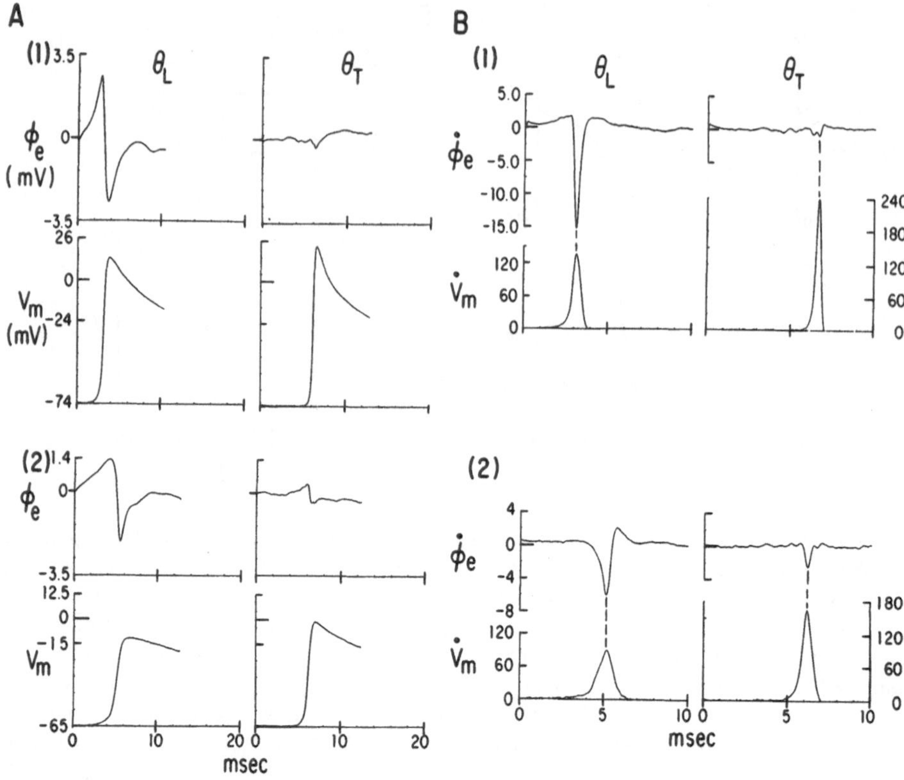

Figure 5. Experimental confirmation of theoretical predictions: measured temporal relationships between the derivatives of extracellular and transmembrane potentials. Panel A: V_m and Φ_e were changed by altering the direction of propagation from along the longitudinal axis of the fibers (θ_L) to a transverse direction (θ_T) and by initiating normal (1) and premature (2) action potentials. Panel B: first time derivatives of the original waveforms. The preparation was an atrial muscle bundle from a 43-year-old subject. (Reproduced from Circ Res 58: 356–371 (1986), by permission of the American Heart Association, Inc.)

tion spread. The associated extracellular waveforms maintained a smooth contour as the magnitude of the deflection decreased in association with the transition from fast longitudinal to slow transverse propagation. The derivatives of the waveforms also maintained a smooth contour in association with a decrease in the magnitude of the negative peak. Intracellular measurements demonstrated the expected directionally different shapes of the upstroke, as well as the coincidence in time of $-d\Phi_e/dt_{max}$ and $\dot{V}_{max}$ (arrows at bottom of Figure 6). In bundles from subjects one through fourteen years of age, the mean conduction velocity in the longitudinal (maximum) direction was 0.50 m/sec and the mean transverse (minimum) velocity was 0.11 m/sec, a θ_L/θ_T ratio of the means of 4.5.

We looked for evidence of local conduction delays at a microscopic level by measuring the instant of local excitation, taken as $-d\Phi_e/dt_{max}$ of the extracellular

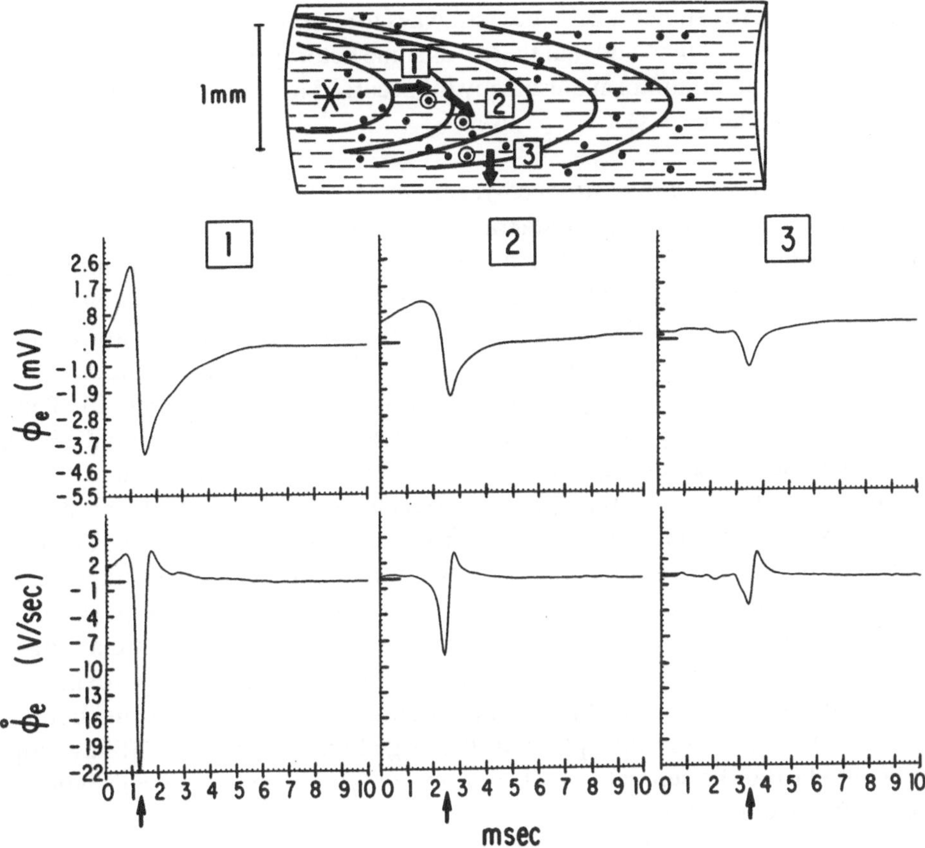

Figure 6. Representative pattern of excitation spread (top) and extracellular waveforms and the associated first time derivatives (bottom) from a representative atrial muscle bundle of a child. The isochrones are separated by 1 msec. The asterisk indicates the point at which propagation was initiated. The points on the outline of the preparation mark the locations of the extracellular recordings from which the activation map was constructed. The circled points indicate the three sites where the waveforms were measured: the accompanying arrows on the drawing of the preparation indicate the direction of propagation normal to the isochrones at each waveform site. The arrows at the bottom of each panel mark the times of $\dot{V}_{max}$ of the underlying action potentials. The preparation was from a two-year-old male. (Reproduced from Circ Res 58: 356–371 (1986), by permission of the American Heart Association, Inc.)

potential at sites 20 to 100 μm apart (less than a cell length), along the long axis of the fiber and at sites 10 to 20 μm apart (about a cell diameter) along an axis in the transverse direction. The waveforms and their derivatives maintained a smooth contour and there was a monotonic increase in the local excitation times without evidence of local delays in either direction.

The above results in young preparations, therefore, are consistent with an anisotropic propagation medium consisting of tightly coupled cells in both the longitudinal and transverse directions; i.e., the distribution of the sites of electrical coupling between fibers provides pathways for intracellular current flow in all directions. We hasten to add that there was some heterogeneity; often waveforms characteristic of nonuniform anisotropy [6] occurred near the junctions of major bundles (branching sites).

Preparations from subjects 40- to 65-years-old

A representative result of the older age group is shown for a preparation from a 42-year-old male in Figure 7. The major characteristic of excitation spread was the abrupt transition from fast longitudinal to slow transverse conduction. This is illustrated by the abrupt change in amplitude and shape of the extracellular waveforms and their derivatives at sites less than 60 μm apart in going from fast longitudinal propagation (Site 1) to slow transverse propagation (Site 2). There was a narrow zone of fast longitudinal propagation with most of the bundle being excited by slow transverse spread that was quite irregular in nature, as reflected by the complexity of the low amplitude extracellular waveforms and their derivatives. Note that with increasing distance from Site 1, there was a marked decrease in the amplitude of the large biphasic waveform and its derivative with virtually no change in the time of the deflection nor in that of the negative peak of the derivative. The multiple small deflections in the waveforms measured at Sites 2 and 3 had associated derivatives with multiple negative peaks at approximately the same time as those at Site 1, thus indicating that the small but definite irregularities in the terminal phase of the large biphasic waveform (Site 1, top) originated from the separate small adjacent bundles undergoing propagation in the transverse direction.

In bundles from the older subjects, the mean longitudinal velocity was 0.69 m/sec and the mean effective transverse velocity was 0.07 m/sec, a θ_L/θ_T ratio of the means of 9.8. Thus, the average longitudinal velocities were greater ($P<0.01$) and the average effective transverse velocities were lower ($P<0.01$) than the respective velocities of the preparations from the young subjects. We looked for conduction delays by measuring the instant of local depolarization, measured as $-d\Phi_e/dt_{max}$ at sites 10 to 100 μm apart, as done in the young preparations. In the zone of fast conduction along the long axis of the cells, there was a monotonic progressive increase in the excitation times without evidence of local jumps or delays (or changes in waveform shape). In the transverse direction in the zone of slow conduction, however, the pattern was quite complex with both delays and 'jumps' of the local excitation times.

The results in the older age group suggest an anisotropic propagation medium comprised of cells that are tightly coupled along the longitudinal axis of the fibers, but along the transverse axis there are recurrent areas in which side-to-side electrical coupling of adjacent groups of parallel fibers is absent. Thus, when compared to the tightly coupled medium with uniform anisotropic propagation of the young preparations, there is a progressive loss with age of side-to-side electrical coupling between groups of parallel oriented atrial fibers. Such a

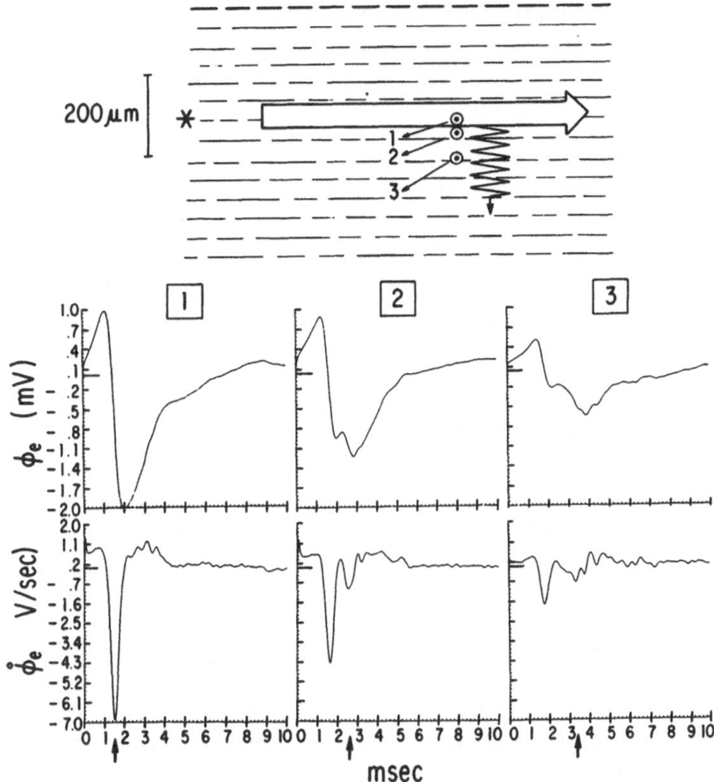

Figure 7. Representative pattern of excitation spread (top) and the extracellular waveforms and the associated first time derivatives (bottom) typical of atrial muscle bundles from older human subjects 40–65 years of age. The open arrow on the outline indicates the narrow region of fast propagation along the longitudinal axis of the fibers. The 'sawtooth' curve denotes the irregular zigzag course of excitation spread in a direction transverse to the long axis of the fibers. The arrows at the bottom mark the times of $\dot{V}_{max}$. The preparation was from a 42-year-old subject. (Reproduced from Circ Res 58: 356–371 (1986), by permission of the American Heart Association, Inc.)

medium would account for the uniform fast propagation without delays in the direction of low axial resistivity (the long axis of the fibers) in the presence of nonuniform slow propagation with delays along the axis of high axial resistivity (the transverse direction). The periodic absence of side-to-side electrical coupling between groups of fibers should also produce a zigzag course of transverse propagation. A significant zigzag component of excitation spread, in turn, would generate numerous deflections in the extracellular waveforms. Although not shown, additional measurements during transverse propagation often demonstrated local excitation times consistent with microscopic spread along the longitudinal axis of small groups of fibers (in either direction), a finding that did not occur in the uniform anisotropic preparations of the young subjects. Thus, we conclude that in changing from longitudinal to transverse propagation, the conduction velocity decreases not only because the effective axial resistance is greater but also because the conduction pathway, being quite irregular (zigzag), is longer.

Time derivatives of potential waveforms near the sources

Theoretical considerations

The above results at a microscopic level suggest that for different bundles the rapid spreading out of the ionic currents in extracellular space produces a complex relationship between the amplitude of a potential deflection and its time rate of change at varying distances in the region of the membrane surface. Since we were unable to find prior theoretical treatment of the relationships between the two, we computed the relationships for a uniformly propagating transmembrane action potential in bundles of different sizes using Equation 5 (see theoretical section of Methods). The details of the simulation model of the cylinders of different sizes have been presented in a recent paper [6]. In brief, the simulation results showed that for equivalent values to be achieved by two bundles of markedly different size, the reduction in distance from the membrane surface became more pronounced in going from the original potential waveform to the first derivative to the second derivative. Thus, a large potential deflection with a relatively small amplitude of the first and second derivatives indicates that the observation site is relatively far from a large bundle and, conversely, a small potential deflection with a relatively large amplitude of the first and second derivatives indicates proximity to a small bundle.

Combined experimental-theoretical analysis

The computer simulations [6] suggested that experimentally it should be possible to distinguish variations in the size of a source (bundle size) from variations in the distance of the source from a measurement site by analysis of the amplitude, velocity, and acceleration of each deflection of a polyphasic waveform in non-uniform anisotropic preparations. Figure 8A shows an experimentally measured polyphasic waveform (top) along with the unsmoothed curves of the first (middle) and second (bottom) time derivatives measured in a preparation from a 62-year-old male. The absolute values of the derivative peaks associated with the smallest potential deflections during interval 2 became progressively larger than the other derivatives (arising from larger potential deflections) in going to the first derivative and then to the second derivative. In the middle panel (Figure 8A), the negative peak of the first derivative of deflection 3 and the negative peaks during interval 2 have a similar amplitude. However, the negative peaks of the derivative during interval 2 represented a marked relative increase compared to the very low amplitude of the original potential deflections and, conversely, the negative peak of the derivative of 3 represented considerable relative decrease compared to the

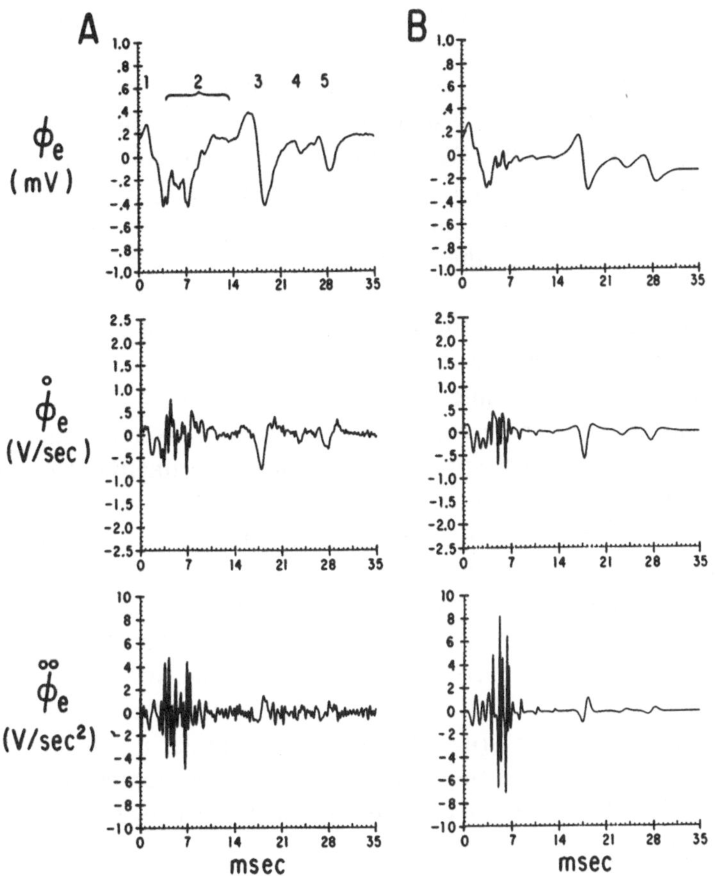

Figure 8. Measured (A) and computed (B) highly complex polyphasic waveform (top) with associated first time derivative (middle) and second time derivative (bottom). At the top of Panel A the numbers identify each deflection that was accounted for experimentally as being due to an identifiable separate atrial bundle. Panel B shows the simulated fit of the experimental data. The experimental waveforms were measured in a preparation from a 62-year-old subject. See text for description. (Reproduced from Circ Res 58: 356–371 (1986), by permission of the American Heart Association, Inc.)

large amplitude of its original potential deflection. The continued progression of the relative changes was especially pronounced in going from the first to the second derivative; the largest second derivative peaks occurred with the smallest original potential deflections, which were produced by sources closest to the observation site. In this case, the microelectrode tip was located in a region of transverse propagation that occurred in a muscle bundle generating the waveforms during interval 2. Based on photographs of the geometry of the preparation under study and the local excitation times at each site that produced each of the 5 deflections identified in the complex waveform (Figure 8A, top), a rigorous test of the theoretical predictions related to the original potential waveform and its derivatives was made by a simulation based on the known location of the bundles of origin (only approximately known for area 2) and the measured times of each deflection, with approximations of different bundle sizes used as an index of source strength. The forward simulation began with a numerical solution for the fast sodium current of a uniformly propagating action potential and ended with superposition of the individual waveforms (Equation 5), which were computed on the basis of ten radial distances for the surface of each cylinder representing each deflection. To make the simulation practical, we simplified as much as possible:

1. We used a value of 25 μm for the radius of all the smallest bundles nearest the measurement site and we represented the largest bundles by two sizes, one with a radius of 150 μm and the other with 250 μm.
2. The local time of depolarization of each bundle was assigned as the time of $-d\Phi_e/dt_{max}$ of each deflection in the original experimental waveform (top of Figure 8A); however, we adjusted the time of $\dot{V}_{max}$ within the error limits (20 μsec) of the experimental sampling rate for the potential deflections during interval 2 to obtain the best visual fit.

The final computed result is shown in Figure 8B for comparison with the experimental curves in Figure 8A. We conclude that the excellent qualitative and quantitative fit of the waveforms strongly supports the concept that in the region close to the membrane currents the amplitude of the extracellular potential deflection is determined primarily by the magnitude of the membrane ionic currents (source size) and the first and second time derivatives (velocity and acceleration) of the deflection are determined primarily by the distance from the current sources.

Discussion

A point established by these results is that the anisotropic electrical properties of human atrial muscle change with advancing age to produce increasingly complex pathways of excitation spread at a microscopic level. The age-related differences in the extracellular waveforms and their derivatives indicate that with advancing age there is progressive electrical uncoupling of the side-to-side connections between groups of parallel oriented atrial fibers, while there was no evidence of electrical uncoupling along the long axis of the fibers. The consequence was an increase in the number of longitudinally oriented insulated boundaries that correlated with the development of extensive collagenous septa that separated small groups of fibers [6]. (The size of each group was approximately that of the small cylinders used in the simulation of Figure 8.) Electrophysiologically this resulted in a pronounced zigzag course of propagation in the transverse direction. This provides a simple but most effective structural mechanism in the presence of normal action potentials for further reducing the effective conduction velocity in the transverse direction to the range of very slow conduction that is routine in the AV node and in very depressed fibers [26].

The results also emphasize the importance of detailed analysis of extracellular potentials because they provide precise measurements at a very small size scale that allow mapping of the spread of excitation in multiple directions. For example, in uniform anisotropic preparations from children, we found no evidence during excitation spread in the transverse direction that propagation proceded along the axis of individual cells. These experimental results, thereby, failed to justify the model of Geselowitz and Miller [24] that microscopically each cell will be excited by colliding waves moving in opposite directions along the long cell axis when propagation is in the transverse direction. As shown in Figure 3, phase-plane plots also failed to provide evidence that collisions occur during transverse propagation in bundles with uniform anisotropic properties. Experimental results at a microscopic level further failed to confirm the theoretical predictions of the Diaz-Rudy-Plonsey model [27] of the effects of the intercalated disks as a possible cause of the direction-dependent shape differences in V_m, the basis for the initial hypothesis of anisotropic discontinuous propagation [3]. We found no evidence during propagation along the long axis of the cells that the intercalated disks cause local delays or that they cause irregularities in the extracellular waveforms as predicted by that model. The delays in excitation spread and the irregularities of the extracellular waveform we found were related to transverse propagation and the absence of side-to-side electrical coupling between small groups of fibers.

Although the results do not fit those of existing theoretical models of anisotropic discontinuous propagation, they are encouraging for investigating excitation spread at a microscopic size scale and for predicting anisotropic drug effects. For example, we found that theoretically there is a unique relationship between Φ_e and its first and second time derivatives as a function of the size of the active bundle. That there is a unique relationship likely accounts for the excellent qualitative and quantitative theoretical fit of the experimental complex polyphasic waveform and its first and second derivatives shown in Figure 8. This implies, in turn, that the relationship between a given experimental extracellular deflection and its first and second derivatives should be useful as an inverse method to estimate the size of underlying active bundles [6].

A major clinical implication of the results is that the progressive change from uniform to nonuniform anisotropic properties makes it possible with increasing age for reentry to occur in progressively smaller regions. Our preliminary studies on this indicate that in nonuniform anisotropic preparations of older subjects (but not from uniform anisotropic preparations from the young group) 'micro-reentry' can occur within an area of 1–2 mm^2 within a single muscle bundle [28]. This size scale for reentry is much smaller than the 25–30 mm^2 area shown previously by West and Landa [29] and Allessie et al. [30] to be the minimum size needed to accomodate reentry in rabbit atrial muscle. This structural mechanism (nonuniform anisotropy) should provide a microscopic basis for understanding numerous mechanisms that involve complex interactions of structure and cellular electrophysiological properties. These include the long-known greater incidence of atrial tachyarrhythmias in older people than in children and the association of increased fibrosis and atrial arrhythmias [31].

Acknowledgment

This work was supported by U.S. Public Health Service Grants HL11307, HL32973, and HL07063.

References

1. Mines GR (1914): On circulating excitations in heart muscles and their possible relation to tachycardia and fibrillation. Trans Roy Soc Canada 8: 43–53.
2. Schmitt FO, Erlanger J (1928): Directional differences in the conduction of the impulse through heart muscle and their possible relation to extrasystolic and fibrillary contractions. Am J Physiol 87: 326–347.
3. Spach M, Miller WT III, Geselowitz DB, Barr RC, Kootsey JM, Johnson EA (1981): The discontinuous nature of propagation in normal canine cardiac muscle. Evidence for recurrent discontinuities of intracellular resistance that affect the membrane currents. Circ Res 48: 39–54.
4. Spach MS, Miller WT III, Dolber PC, Kootsey JM, Sommer JR, Mosher CE Jr (1982): The functional role of structural complexities in the propagation of depolarization in the atrium of the dog. Cardiac conduction disturbances due to discontinuities of effective axial resistivity. Circ Res 50: 175–191.
5. Masuda MO, Paes de Carvalho (1975): Sinoatrial transmission and atrial invasion during normal rhythm in the rabbit heart. Circ Res 37: 414–421.
6. Spach MS, Dolber PC (1986): Relating extracellular potentials and their derivatives to anisotropic propagation at a microscopic level in human cardiac muscle. Evidence for electrical uncoupling of side-to-side fiber connections with increasing age. Circ Res 58: 356–371.
7. Ralston A (1965): First course in numerical analysis. McGraw-Hill Book Co., New York, pp. 76–85.
8. Lorente de Nó R (1947): Analysis of the distribution of the action currents of nerves in volume conductors. Stud Rockefeller Inst Med Res 132: 384–497.
9. Rosenfalck P (1969): Intra- and extracellular potential fields of active nerve and muscle fibers: a physico-mathematical analysis of different models. Akademisk Forlag, Copenhagen.
10. Hodgkin AL, Huxley AF (1952): A quantitative description of the membrane current and its application to conduction and excitation in nerve. J Physiol (Lond) 117: 500–544.
11. Ebihara L, Johnson EA (1980): Fast sodium current in cardiac muscle. A quantitative description. Biophys J 32: 779–790.
12. Fozzard HA, January CT, Makielski JC (1985): New studies of the excitatory sodium currents in heart muscle. Circ Res 56: 475–485.
13. Läuger P (1985): Ionic channels with conformational substrates. Biophys J 47: 581–591.
14. McAllister RE, Noble D, Tsien RW (1975): Reconstruction of the electrical activity of cardiac Purkinje fibres. J Physiol (Lond) 251: 1–59.
15. Beeler GW, Reuter H (1977): Reconstruction of the action potential of ventricular myocardial fibres. J Physiol (Lond) 268: 177–210.

16. Brown AM, Lee KS, Powell T (1981): Sodium current in single rat heart muscle cells. J Physiol (Lond) 318: 479–500.
17. Fozzard HA, Friedlander I, January CT, Makielski JC, Sheets MF (1984): Second-order kinetics of Na^+ channel inactivation in internally dialysed canine cardiac Purkinje cells (Abstract). J Physiol (Lond) 353: 72P.
18. Meves H (1978): Inactivation of the sodium permeability in squid giant nerve fibres. Prog Biophys Molec Biol 33: 207–230.
19. Ebihara L, Shigeto N, Lieberman M, Johnson EA (1983): A note on the reactivation of the fast sodium current in spherical clusters of embryonic chick heart cells. Biophys J 42: 191–193.
20. Spach MS, Barr RC, Johnson EA, Kootsey JM (1973): Cardiac extracellular potentials. Analysis of complex wave forms about the Purkinje networks in dogs. Circ Res 33: 465–473.
21. Geselowitz DB, Barr RC, Spach MS, Miller WT III (1982): The impact of adjacent isotropic fluids on electrograms from anisotropic cardiac muscle. A modeling study. Circ Res 51: 602–613.
22. Jenerick H (1963): Phase-plane trajectories of the muscle spike potential. Biophys J 3: 363–377.
23. Jenerick H (1964): An analysis of the striated muscle fiber action current. Biophys J 4: 77–91.
24. Geselowitz DB, Miller WT III (1982): Active electrical properties of cardiac muscle. Bioelectromagnetics 3: 127–132.
25. Spach MS, Kootsey JM (1985): Relating the sodium current and conductance to the shape of transmembrane and extracellular potentials by simulation: Effects of propagation boundaries. IEEE Trans Biomed Eng BME-32: 743–755.
26. Cranefield PF (1975): The conduction of the cardiac impulse. The slow response and cardiac arrhythmias. Futura, Mt. Kisco, NY, p. 304.
27. Diaz PJ, Rudy Y, Plonsey R (1983): Intercalated discs as a cause for discontinuous propagation in cardiac muscle: a theoretical simulation. Ann Biomed Eng 11: 17–189.
28. Spach MS, Dolber PC (1984): Discontinuous propagation and nonuniform anisotropy: A basis for micro-reentry in human cardiac muscle (Abstract). Circulation 70: II–345.
29. West TC, Landa JF (1962): Minimal mass required for induction of a sustained arrhythmia in isolated atrial segments. Am J Physiol 202: 232–236.
30. Allessie MA, Bonke FIM, Schopman FJG (1977): Circus movement in rabbit atrial muscle as a mechanism for tachycardia. III. The 'leading circle' concept: A new model of circus movement in cardiac tissue without the involvement of an anatomical obstacle. Circ Res 41: 9–18.
31. Bailey GWH, Braniff BA, Hancock EW, Cohn KE (1968): Relation of left atrial pathology to atrial fibrillation in mitral valvular disease. Ann Int Med 69: 13–20.

Discussion

Wit: In addition to the source size and the distance in determining the magnitude of the extracellular potential, have you given any consideration to the effect of the substances that might fill the intercellular spaces on the extracellular potential? For example, in your model of the aging atrial myocardium, as well as in the healed infarcted tissue that we study, the extracellular space becomes filled with a connective tissue matrix. Does that have any effect on the size of the extracellular potentials?
Spach: I didn't show any of that. The morphological analysis was done by Dr Paul Dolber. The major thing to come out of it was that with increasing age, the distribution of the collagen changes with increasing age and especially in the preparations from subjects over 50 years old. The frequency and distribution of collagen septa fit quite nicely with the distances between insulated boundaries calculated from the polyphasic deflections of the waveforms. It is interesting that the size of the bundles of cells in the nonuniform anisotropic tissues varied between 25 and 125 μm (separated by collagen). Thus, the collagen marks areas where there can be no side-to-side electrical couplings (i.e., nexuses) between groups of cells. As far as the resistivity of collagen is concerned, it should be relatively low because structurally collagen is porous; that is, there are many openings in the septa comprised of collagenous fibers. So, the collagen is not what is making the insulated boundaries but rather it marks the area where there is an absence of intercellular connections in a side-to-side direction for intracellular current flow. Longitudinally, we have found no evidence of any conduction delays. It is the delays in conduction between lateral sites that relates to the distribution of collagen. Furthermore, with the development in atrial muscle of nonuniform anisotropic properties, it is not the increase in collagen, but the redistribution of collagen as longitudinally-oriented septa that correlated with the development of polyphasic extracellular waveforms during transverse propagation.
Lab: Have you found any changes in action potential duration?
Spach: That is a difficult question since we have not found evidence to make us believe that there are atrial specialized tracts or specialized fibers in animal or human atrial tissues. What we found in all the preparations, from two years to 62 years, was that the action potentials had the same repolarization shape at the same stimulus rate. At slow rates, there was no 'plateau' shape. Rather, a 'hump' shape occurred. At high rates, the shape changed to that with a 'plateau'. Our findings were consistent with prior analyses of Carmeliet with respect to the effect of changes in the concentration of potassium in extracellular space. The question may refer to the occurrence of repolarization shape changes when the upstroke shape changes, due to direction differences in propagation. We find the repolarization shape to stay the same, except for a slight difference during the initial 15 msec after the peak of the upstroke. (Just after the peak of the upstroke, there

is more rapid early repolarization with the greater amplitude of the upstroke during transverse propagation.) However, I should emphasize that we have not performed a detailed analysis to determine if there are small changes during phase-three repolarization for different directions of propagation in anisotropic bundles.

2. The role of the interstitial space in electrical models of cardiac sources

R. PLONSEY and R.C. BARR

Abstract

For multicellular cardiac tissue bounded by extracellular fluid, it is expected that extracellular potentials at the periphery will be very small and can be neglected in its contribution to an evaluation of sources. This paper examines the behavior of the interstitial potential as a function of depth in an idealized semi-infinite tissue model. The results demonstrate that even at depths of 100 μm the interstitial potentials are no longer negligible. And for depths greater than around 1 mm the linear core-conductor approximation seems well justified.

Introduction

For a single excitable fiber, lying in an unbounded volume conductor, and carrying a propagating action potential, the transmembrane current emerging into the extracellular space behaves as a source function. If the fiber is very thin, its own presence in the extracellular space can be ignored and the field established by a transmembrane current element is the *infinite medium* point-source field. Thus, if i_m is the transmembrane current per unit length the potential field $d\Phi$ is given by

$$d\Phi = \frac{i_m dz}{4\pi\sigma_e r}, \tag{1}$$

where z is the axial coordinate and r is the distance from the source point (ϱ, z) (expressed in axially symmetric cylindrical coordinates) to the field point (ϱ', z') and σ_e is the conductivity of the (extracellular) medium. Integration results in

$$\Phi = \int \frac{i_m(z)dz}{4\pi\sigma_e r}, \tag{2}$$

where

$$r = \sqrt{(\varrho - \varrho')^2 + (z - z')^2}; \tag{3}$$

a result that is frequently quoted in the literature [1].

If, rather than a single fiber there are several parallel fibers, then (2) can be applied to each and the total potential found by superposition. But for an increasing number of closely spaced fibers, a source element, identified by $i_m dz$, can no longer be thought to lie in an unbounded medium since the presence of many fibers cannot be ignored.

A rigorous consideration of one or many fibers shows that, provided axial symmetry for each fiber can be assumed, an axial source density for a fiber of cross-section A_i can be expressed as [1]

$$j(z) = A_i \partial^2(\sigma_i \Phi_i - \sigma_e \Phi_e)/\partial z^2. \tag{4}$$

This is an equivalent source that lies in a uniform unbounded medium (it is often referred to as a line-source model). Consequently, the field from a source element (for single or multiple fibers) is simply

$$d(\Phi) = [A_i(\sigma_i \partial^2\Phi_i/\partial z^2 - \sigma_e \partial^2\Phi_e/\partial z^2)dz]/4\pi\sigma_e r. \tag{5}$$

If Φ_e can be ignored then, since $i_m = \sigma_i A_i \partial^2\Phi_i/\partial z^2$, (5) and (1) become identical. This suggests that equation (1) can be applied provided $\Phi_e \ll \Phi_i$. In fact, for a single fiber, one can demonstrate [1] that $\Phi_e \ll \Phi_i$ and hence that (1) should be satisfactory, and since we already know this to be true, the criterion seems validated. But for increasing numbers of closely-packed fibers, neither the inequality or (1) will continue to be true.

If we imagine a bundle consisting of a very large number of parallel fibers then, except near the periphery, the interstitial current is essentially axial and the potential field is governed by the linear-core-conductor equations. That is [2]

$$\Phi_e = -\frac{r_e}{r_e + r_i} V_m \tag{6}$$

and

$$\Phi_i = \frac{r_i}{r_e + r_i} V_m, \tag{7}$$

where r_e, r_i are interstitial, intracellular resistances per unit length. For this condition (5) can be expressed as

$$d\Phi = [Gf_e \partial^2 V_m/\partial z^2 dz]/4\pi\sigma_e r, \tag{8a}$$

where

$$G = \sigma_i A_i \sigma_e A_e/(\sigma_i A_i + \sigma_e A_e). \tag{8b}$$

A_e is the value of interstitial cross-sectional area associated with each fiber, while f_e is the reciprocal of the fractional interstitial cross-sectional area (i.e. if the total intracellular and interstitial cross-sectional area is A, then $f_e = A/A_e$). In (8b) G is an effective parallel impedance of the intracellular and interstitial paths.

For fibers near the periphery of such a multifibered preparation presumably (1) applies, while for sufficiently deep fibers (8) applies. This paper examines an idealized semi-infinite preparation, for which a rigorous solution is possible, in order to develop some guidance regarding the behavior of the interstitial potentials as a function of depth into the tissue. Such information is indispensable in the evaluation of source strength within, say, cardiac muscle, which consists of multiple layers of excitable fibers.

Bidomain semi-infinite model

We consider a uniform semi-infinite region of cardiac tissue consisting of z oriented fibers that extend from $y = 0$ to $y = \infty$. The region $-\infty<y<0$ consists of extracellular fluid, assumed uniform and isotropic. A uniform plane wave is taken to be propagating in the x direction; its isochrones are planes orthogonal to x.

Note that propagation is chosen to be transverse to the fiber axis, a condition that mirrors much of actual conduction through whole heart tissue [3]. Transverse propagation is supported by cardiac tissue because of the high degree of intercellular communication (continuity) arising from the presence of gap junctions. One can, consequently, consider the preparation as if equivalent uniform fibers lie in the direction of propagation (i.e. x) [4]. This is illustrated in Fig. 1.

A further simplification is possible by ignoring the detailed structure of the cardiac fibers and considering the preparation to be a continuum. One can view the interconnected intracellular space as a uniform domain. Similarly, the interstitial space, which is actually a complex invaginated structure, can be viewed as a uniform continuum (domain). Each domain is separated at all points by the membrane. This view of cardiac tissue is a macroscopic one that deals with space averaged quantities; it has been described and called the *bidomain model* of cardiac muscle [5]. It is perhaps best described by the following expression for intracellular (subscript i) and interstitial (subscript e) current densities, bearing in mind the assumed uniformity in the z direction. We have

$$\bar{J}_i = -[g_{ix}\partial\Phi_i/\partial x\bar{a}_x + g_{iy}\partial\Phi_i/\partial y\bar{a}_y] \tag{9}$$

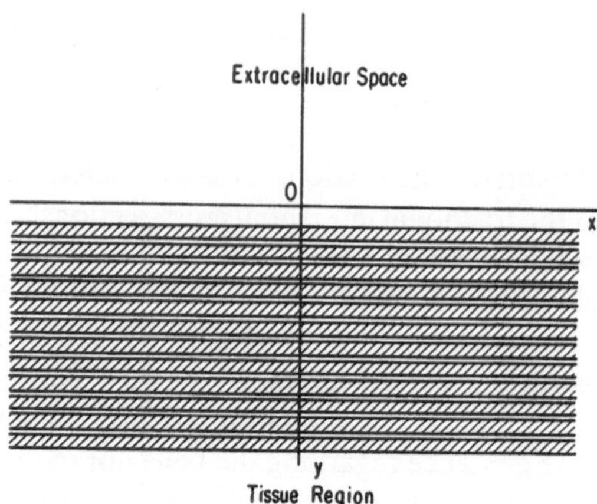

Figure 1. The semi-infinite region y>0 is occupied by cardiac tissue with an equivalent fiber orientation in the x direction. The region y<0 is occupied by extracellular fluid. Uniformity exists in the z direction. A uniform plane wave is assumed propagating in the +x direction.

and

$$\bar{J}_e = -[g_{ex}\partial\Phi_e/\partial x\bar{a}_x + g_{ey}\partial\Phi_e/\partial y\bar{a}_y], \tag{10}$$

where the conductivities are defined on the total tissue space [6]. Note that these parameters reflect the accepted anisotropic structure of both intracellular and interstitial space, As a consequence of the continuity of current, transmembrane current leaving one space enters the other. Consequently,

$$\nabla \cdot \bar{J}_i = -\nabla \cdot \bar{J}_e. \tag{11}$$

Solution for the interstitial potential field

Experimental study of the intracellular action potential of cardiac tissue shows little change in action potential morphology with changing load [6]. Consequently, we assume that the (temporal) transmembrane action potential to be identical for all sites in the tissue preparation (whether near the surface or deep to the surface). Consequently, we have

$$V_m(x,y,t) = V_m(x - \theta t) \tag{12}$$

everywhere, where θ is the velocity of the plane wave propagation (assumed uniform in the x direction).

Following Roth and Wikswo [7], let the scalar function ψ be defined as

$$\psi = \Phi_i + \frac{g_{ex}}{g_{ix}}\Phi_e = V_m + \frac{g_{ix} + g_{ex}}{g_{ix}}\Phi_e, \tag{13}$$

where we have used $V_m = \Phi_i - \Phi_e$. We now introduce a linear transformation from x, y to X, Y defined by

$$X = x \tag{14}$$

and

$$Y = \sqrt{(g_{ix} + g_{ex})/(g_{iy} + g_{ey})}\; y. \tag{15}$$

If (9) and (10) are substituted into (11) one obtains

$$g_{ix}\partial^2\Phi_i/\partial x^2 + g_{iy}\partial^2\Phi_i/\partial y^2 + g_{ex}\partial^2\Phi_e/\partial x^2 + g_{ey}\partial^2\Phi_e/\partial y^2 = 0 \tag{16}$$

and if (13) is introduced into (16), then we have

$$g_{ix}\partial^2\psi/\partial x^2 - g_{ex}\partial^2\Phi_e/\partial x^2 + g_{iy}\partial^2\psi/\partial y^2 - \frac{g_{iy}g_{ex}}{g_{ix}}\frac{\partial^2\Phi_e}{\partial y^2} +$$

$$g_{ex}\partial^2\Phi_e/\partial x^2 + g_{ey}\partial^2\Phi_e/\partial y^2 = 0. \tag{17}$$

We now perform the transformation defined by (14) and (15) on the terms involving ψ in (17). The result is

$$g_{ix}\frac{\partial^2\psi}{\partial X^2} + g_{iy}\left(\frac{g_{ix} + g_{ex}}{g_{iy} + g_{ey}}\right)\frac{\partial^2\psi}{\partial Y^2} + \left(g_{ey} - \frac{g_{iy}g_{ex}}{g_{ix}}\right)\frac{\partial^2\Phi_e}{\partial y^2} = 0. \tag{18}$$

Now, substitute for Φ_e in (18) the value obtained in (13). Furthermore, in view of (12), set $\partial V_m/\partial y = 0$. The final result is

$$\frac{\partial^2\psi}{\partial X^2} + \frac{\partial^2\psi}{\partial Y^2} = 0,\ Y>0. \tag{19}$$

Letting $\nabla^2 \equiv \partial^2/\partial X^2 + \partial^2/\partial Y^2$ and using (13) and (19) leads to the desired relationship

$$\nabla^2\psi = 0 = \nabla^2 V_m + \left(\frac{g_{ix} + g_{ex}}{g_{ix}}\right)\nabla^2\Phi_e. \tag{20}$$

Equation (20) shows that the desired interstitial potential field satisfies Poisson's equation in the two-dimensional X, Y space. This partial differential equation has an integral-form solution, namely [8]

$$\Phi_e = -\left(\frac{g_{ix}}{g_{ix} + g_{ex}}\right)\frac{1}{2\pi}\int \nabla^2 V_m \, ln\,(R)\, dX'dY', \tag{21}$$

where

$$R = \sqrt{(X - X')^2 + (Y - Y')^2} \tag{22}$$

is the distance from a source point (X', Y') to a field point (X, Y).

Equation (21) describes the interstitial field arising from ($\nabla^2 V_m$) viewed as a primary source in a medium of infinite extent. It is necessary to add to this solution a contribution reflecting the secondary sources at y = 0 (the interface between tissue and extracellular bath) which arise from the boundary conditions. At this interface the normal component of current density is continuous and this requires that

$$g_{ey}\partial\Phi_e/\partial y = g_{ey}\sqrt{\frac{g_{ix} + g_{ex}}{g_{iy} + g_{ey}}}\ \partial\Phi_e/\partial Y = \sigma_o\partial\Phi_o/\partial y, \tag{23}$$

where the subscript o represents the extracellular medium. From equation (23) we can identify $g_{ey}\sqrt{(g_{ix} + g_{ex})/(g_{iy} + g_{ey})}$ as the equivalent tissue conductivity. Furthermore, this boundary condition will be automatically satisfied if image sources are defined which lie at the mirror image of the primary sources and have a magnitude factor, F, given by [9]

$$F = \frac{g_{ey}\sqrt{(g_{ix} + g_{ex})/(g_{iy} + g_{ey})} - \sigma_o}{g_{ey}\sqrt{(g_{ix} + g_{ex})/(g_{iy} + g_{ey})} + \sigma_o}. \tag{24}$$

So, finally, for field points in the tissue region (Y>0) we have

$$\Phi_e(X, Y) = -\frac{1}{2\pi}\left(\frac{g_{ix}}{g_{ix} + g_{ex}}\right)\left[\int_0^{\infty}\int_{x'} \frac{\partial^2 V_m}{\partial x'^2}\, ln\,(R)dx'dY' + F\int_{-\infty}^{0}\int_{x'} \frac{\partial^2 V_m}{\partial x'^2}\, ln\,(R)dx'dY'\right]. \tag{25}$$

Numerical model and evaluation

In order to examine the behavior of Φ_e in (25), we define an analytic expression for a cardiac action potential (phase 0) as

$$V_m(x) = 100e^{-8(x/\theta)^4}\text{mV};\ x \geqslant 0, \tag{26}$$

where a uniform plateau is assumed for $x \leqslant 0$. In (26) V_m is in mV, x is in mm, and θ in m/sec. The parameters were chosen to achieve a rise-time of around 1 msec, which is usually observed. The source function is found from

$$\partial^2 V_m/\partial x^2 = 3200(x^2/\theta^4)[32(x/\theta)^4 - 3]e^{-8(x/\theta)^4};\quad x \geqslant 0. \tag{27}$$

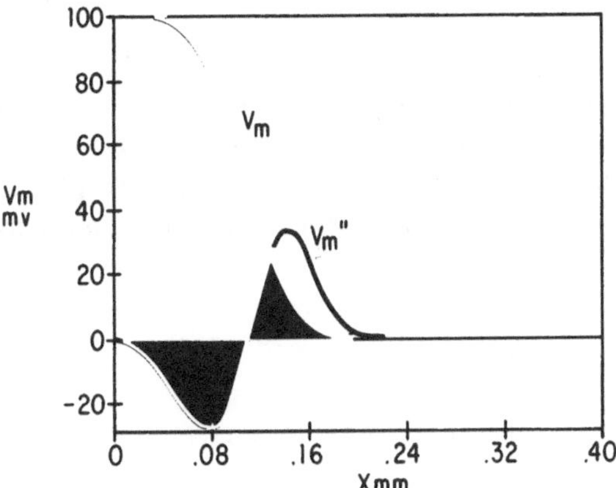

Figure 2. Plot of analytical expressions for $V_m(x)$ and $\partial^2 V_m(x)/\partial x^2$ used in the simulation (see equations (26) and (27)). The ordinate values are in millivolts for V_m and relative values for $\partial^2 V_m/\partial x^2$.

A plot of V_m (26) and $\partial^2 V_m/\partial x^2$ (27) is given in Fig. 2, for $\theta = 20$ cm/sec, a cross-fiber value frequently reported [10] and which we adopt here in our simulation.

Conductivity parameters were derived from the experimental data of Clerc [4] but with the assumption that cells occupy 80% of the tissue volume, a value currently expected (rather than the 70% assumed by Clerc). In bidomain format [6] these are

$$g_{ix} = 2.21 \times 10^{-4}\,\text{S/mm},\quad g_{iy} = 2.21 \times 10^{-4}\,\text{S/mm},\quad g_{iz} = 1.94 \times 10^{-4}\,\text{S/mm},$$
$$g_{ex} = 1.57 \times 10^{-4}\,\text{S/mm}, g_{ey} = 1.57 \times 10^{-4}\,\text{S/mm}, g_{ez} = 4.17 \times 10^{-4}\,\text{S/mm}. \quad (28)$$

These values along with those in (26) when substituted into (6) and (7) lead to an interstitial core-conductor potential of $100 \times (0.221/(0.221 + 1.57)) = 12.3$ mV associated with the rising phase of V_m. The extracellular fluid was assumed to have a conductivity, σ_o, of 2×10^{-3} S/mm, as a result of which $F = -0.745$ is obtained from (24).

The evaluation of Φ_e can now be made by numerical integration of (25), and this was actually done. However, a more satisfactory approach is first to integrate over x′ by parts. Following this it becomes possible to integrate with respect to Y′. The result is to reduce the required numerical integration to one dimension and to eliminate the infinite integrals. This final result is

$$\Phi_e(x, Y) = \frac{1}{2\pi}\left(\frac{g_{ix}}{g_{ix} + g_{ex}}\right)\left[\int_{x'} (1 - F)\frac{\partial V_m}{\partial x'}\tan^{-1}\left(\frac{Y}{x - x'}\right) dx' - \pi(1 + F)\,(V_m(x) - \bar{V}_m)\right]. \quad (29)$$

It is necessary to subtract out the constant component of $V_m(x)$ in the second term of (29) because any constant is necessarily eliminated from the first term.

Discussion of results

Based on the data given in the previous section, the interstitial potential was evaluated for y = 0, 0.1, 0.2, 0.5, 1, 5 mm by numerical integration of (29) (and with essentially identical results from (25)). These are plotted in Fig. 3. The values obtained for y = 5 mm approach the linear core-conductor value expected at large y, namely

$$\Phi_e(x, y_{large}) = -100 \frac{g_{ix}}{g_{ix} + g_{ex}} e^{-8(x/\theta)4}$$
$$= -(12.3\, e^{-8(x/\theta)4} - 6.2)\, mV \tag{30}$$

(where the added constant gives $\Phi_e(x)$ the property of zero average value, a necessary characteristic of fields determined from sources which are described by derivatives $\partial^2 V_m/\partial x^2$ or $\partial V_m/\partial x$ that eliminate constant components).

The value of Φ_e at y = 0 corresponds to that expected from half the sum of the core-conductor field from the primary and the secondary (image) source. this quantity is

$$\Phi_e(x, 0) = -\frac{1}{2}(1 + F)(12.3\, e^{-8(x/\theta)4} - 6.2)\, mV \tag{31}$$

and since F = −0.745, it comes out

$$\Phi_e(x, 0) = -(1.56\, e^{-8(x/\theta)4} - 0.78)\, mV. \tag{32}$$

One notes that, indeed, the results shown in Fig. 3 are consistent with (30) and (32). Both (30) and (32) can also be obtained from an evaluation of (29).

Figure 3 reflects a general result that was expected: At y = 0, Φ_e is small, and fibers at the surface can be treated as if they were isolated, lying in an unbounded medium. Conversely, for large y, the linear-core-conductor relations of (6) and (7) apply and peak-to-peak values Φ_e of 12 mV are expected and obtained. In fact, values roughly in this range are actually seen with conventional unipolar interstitial (plunge electrode) recordings [11].

Figure 3 suggests a criteria for y to be 'large', namely that y>1 mm. However, even for y as small as 10–20 μm in depth, we note that Φ_e lies close to its asymptotic linear-core-conductor value in the phase 0 region.

The question of how to treat a thin layer of cardiac tissue is not directly answered by Fig. 3, but is at least suggested. For tissue, say 400 μm in thickness (with extracellular fluid on each side) one might expect the interstitial potentials shown in Fig. 3 for $0<y<0.2$. In particular, it would not be correct to assume $\Phi_e \approx 0$. The assumption of linear-core-conductor conditions everywhere would be a better assumption, though even here deviations clearly exist. In any event,

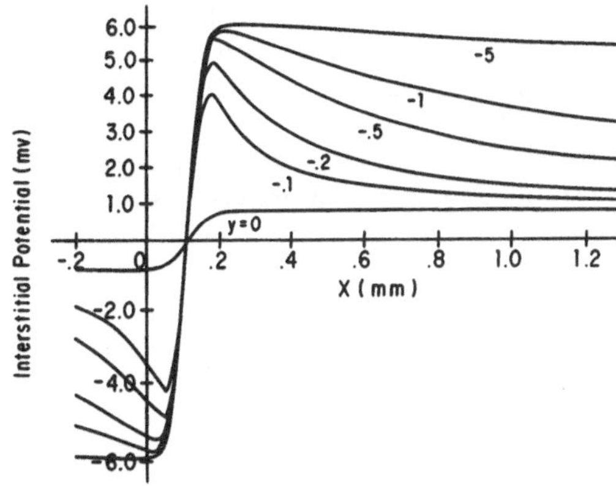

Figure 3. Plot of interstitial potential in a semi-infinite bidomain model of uniform cardiac tissue as described in Fig. 1, for various depths of y = 0, 0.1, 0.2, 0.5, 1, 5 mm. The x coordinate is in mm and corresponds to the $V_m(x)$ shown in Fig. 2. The potential values shown are in mV.

the conclusion that the interstitial space must be explicitly considered seems inescapable. A more detailed extension of this presentation is given elsewhere (12).

Acknowledgment

This study was supported by grants HL 11307 and HL31286 from the National Institutes of Health.

References

1. Plonsey R (1974): The active fiber in a volume conductor. IEEE Trans on Biomed Engr BME-21: 371–381.
2. Hodgkin AL, Rushton WAH (1946): The electrical constants of a crustacean nerve fiber. Proc Roy Soc B 133: 444–479.
3. Durrer D et al. (1970): Total excitation of the isolated human heart. Circulation 41: 899–912.
4. Clerc L (1976): Directional difference of impulse spread in trabecular muscle from mammalian heart. J Physiol 255: 355–336.
5. Tung L (1978): A bidomain model for describing ischemic myocardium d-c potentials, Ph. D. dissertation. Mass Inst of Tech, Cambridge, MA.
6. Plonsey R, Barr RC (1984): Current flow patterns in two-dimensional anisotropic bisyncytia with normal and extreme conductivities. Biophysical J 45: 557–571.
7. Roth BJ, Wikswo JP Jr (1985): A bidomain model for the extracellular potential and magnetic field of cardiac tissue. IEEE Trans on Biomed Engr BME-33: 467–469.
8. Morse PM, Feshbach H (1953): Methods of theoretical physics. Mc Graw-Hill Book Co., New York, NY.

9. Plonsey R (1969): Bioelectric phenomena. McGraw-Hill Book Co., New York, NY.
10. Spach MS, Miller WT III, Miller-Jones E, Warren RB, Barr RC (1979): Extracellular potentials related to intracellular action potentials during impulse conduction in anisotropic canine cardiac muscle. Circ Res 45: 188–204.
11. Spach MS, Barr RC (1975): Ventricular intramural and epicardial potential distributions during ventricular activation and repolarization in the intact dog. Circ Res 37: 243–257.
12. Plonsey R. Barr RC (1987): Interstitial potentials and their change with depth into cardiac tissue. Biophysical J 51: 723–731.

Discussion

Clark: I am wondering what the effect of intercalated disc resistance would be along a cable model of this cylindrical structure? It would seem that your model is a rather macroscopic one, wherein you assume low disc resistance and effectively replace the cellular meshwork by a single 'equivalent cell'.
Plonsey: This is a very simple model. It is known as the bidomain model. It is in fact a macroscopic model, because we have not only simplified the behavior in the axial direction, which is where the intercalated disc would essentially be thought to lie, but have simplified things in the lateral direction (assuming structural and field uniformity) and we are therefore looking at a homogenate, i.e. a macroscopically uniform continuum tissue model. So effects that would be introduced by the intercalated disc are considered only through the contribution to the averaged conductivity; the discrete effect will not be revealed in this model. This model is already more complicated than usually assumed and the discrete effect of the intercalated disc is a still further complication.

3. Parasympathetic control of the SA node cell in rabbit heart – a model

C.R. MURPHEY and J.W. CLARK JR

Abstract

A mathematical model of the sinoatrial (SA) node cell based on the modeling studies of Di Francesco and Noble [1] for the Purkinje fiber, and Noble and Noble [2] for the rabbit SA node, is developed along with models of the utilization of the autonomic neurotransmitters acetylcholine and norepinephrine by elements of the cell membrane. Studies of the phase-sensitivity for the SA node cell model to vagal burst stimulation are conducted, with and without a constant background level of norepinephrine. The results reported are of a preliminary nature, but they mimic published data regarding the free-running behavior of the primary cells of the SA node as well as, their response to phasic vagal burst stimuli.

Introduction

Mathematical models of the Hodgkin-Huxley type [3] were first applied to cardiac muscle by Noble [4] in a study of the cardiac Purkinje fiber. This model was later revised by McAllister, Noble and Tsien [5], and most recently by Di Francesco and Noble [1], based on an accumulated wealth of improved voltage clamp data. The reader unfamiliar with this work is directed to the aforementioned references as well as a book by Noble [6]. In addition, a review of the ionic basis of electrical activity in cardiac tissue based on voltage clamp data is provided by Coraboeuf [1].

The McAllister, Noble, Tsien (MNT) model of the Purkinje fiber has been applied to the characterization of a variety of other cardiac tissues including ventricular cells [8] and sinoatrial node cells [9, 10]. The Purkinje fiber, having the most complex cardiac action potential waveform, may also be viewed as having a full complement of membrane ionic currents. Since the MNT model provided a reasonable characterization of the electrical behavior of the Purkinje fiber waveform based on information available at the time [5], it seemed logical to attempt to model the behavior of other cardiac cells by appropriately deleting or inactivating selected membrane channels, according to known electrophysiological characteristics of a particular type of cell. A major difficulty in this approach in the past has been the paucity of reasonably accurate voltage-clamp data from other tissues (nodal, atrial, etc.) on which to base changes in the many parameters associated with the MNT model. However, rather significant progress has been made in the area of cardiac electrophysiology in the past decade, particularly in the area of membrane biophysics. The accuracy of voltage clamp methods has improved steadily, as have experimental dissection methods and techniques, first with small strips of tissue and more recently with enzymatic dispersion methods that allow one to isolate and study the electrical behavior of virtually any type of cardiac cell (e.g. ventricular [1] atrial [12, 13]; SA and AV node [14]; Purkinje fiber [15]). Recent experimental findings have also required that the classical MNT model be revised in several respects, incorporating for the first time mathematical models of the ATP-dependent Na^{+}-$K+$ pump, a Na^{+}-Ca^{++} exchange mechanism and intra- and extracellular concentration changes for Na^{+}, Ca^{++} and K^{+}. These modifications have been incorporated in the work of Di Francesco and Noble [1] on Purkinje fibers, and this new model has been extended to a characterization of the sinoatrial (SA) node cell by Noble and Noble [2].

The objectives of this paper will be to modify the aforementioned Di Francesco-Noble (DN) model appropriately for the study of the SA node cell membrane response to phasic parasympathetic (vagal) stimulation, with and without a background level of norepinephrine in the bathing medium of the cell. The results of these simulation studies are consistent with experimental data in the literature, and suggest that the model may prove useful in explaining the electrogenetic basis of dynamic vagal-sinus node interactions.

Modeling aspects

The basic node cell model

The electrical equivalent circuit for the membrane of a lumped SA node cell consisting of a membrane capacitance C_m (nF) in parallel with several voltage and time dependent membrane conductances as well as pump, ion-exchange and background currents is shown in Fig. 1. The parameters associated with the cell geometry are contained in Table 5. Under space clamp conditions, the differential equation describing the membrane potential (V) s:

$$\frac{dV}{dt} = -\frac{I_f + I_K + I_{K1} + I_b + I_{NaK} + I_{NaCa} + I_{Na} + I_{si} + I_{stim} + I_{ACh}}{C_m}, \tag{1}$$

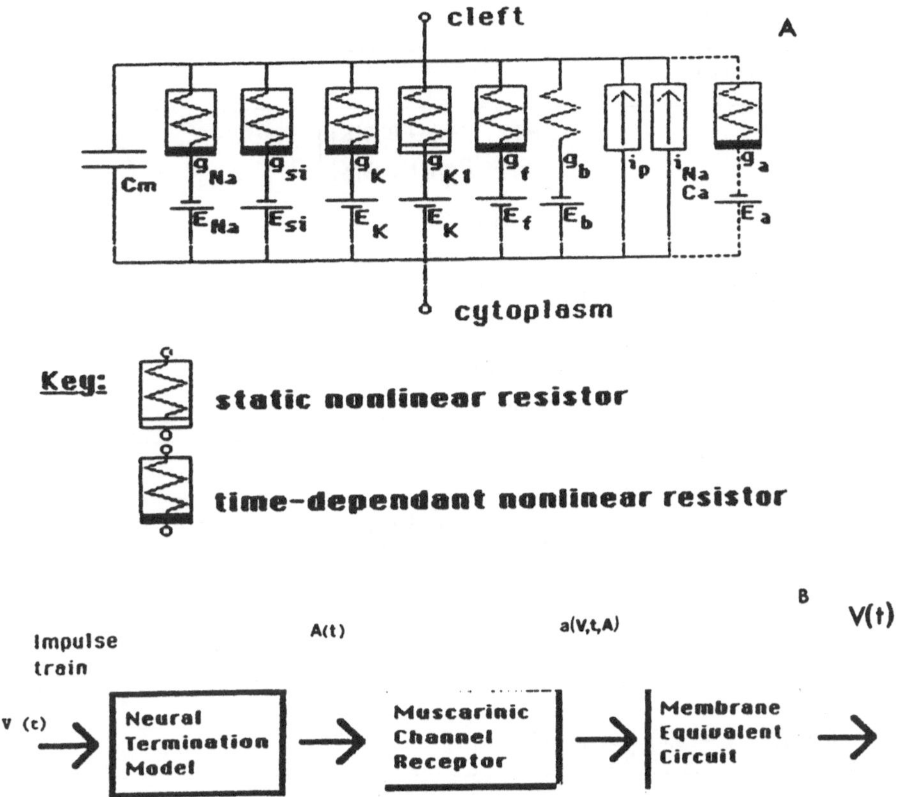

Figure 1. A: equivalent network model of the idealized SA node cell membrane including a separate ACh-sensitive muscarinic channel I_a. B: Block diagram of the overall model including models for ACh release and diffusion from vagal nerve terminations, the ACh receptor complex at the outer membrane surface and muscarinic membrane channel dynamics. Here v(t) represents the vagal neural input to the SA node cell in terms of discrete action potentials, A(t) is the ACh concentration at the ACh-receptor site on the membrane surface, a(A, V, t) is the gating variable associated with the muscarinic channel (dotted lines in A, and V is the transmembrane potential.

where I_{Na}, I_{si} and I_k are the sodium, calcium and potassium currents, respectively; I_{K1} is the instantaneous inward-rectifying background potassium current, I_b is the sum of the *Na* and *Ca* background currents, I_{NaK} is the ATP-dependent Na^+-K^+ pump current; and I_{NaCa} is the *Na-Ca* exchanger current. The specific equations for these currents and the constants associated with them are given in Tables 1–5, where the inward currents are given in Table 1, the delayed outward potassium current I_K and the background currents are given in Table 2, the pump and ion exchange currents in Table 3, the concentrations for Na^+, K^+ and Ca^{++} in the left and intracellular media are given in Table 1, the delayed ouward potassium current I_K and the background currents are given in Table 4, and miscellaneous model parameters are listed in Table 5. One will note from Tables 1 and 2 that the

Table 1. Inward currents

I_{Na}: sodium inward current

$$I_{Na} = m^3 h\, g_{Na}(V - E_{mh}) \qquad E_{mh} = \frac{RT}{F} \ln\left[\frac{[Na]_o + 0.12[K]_c}{[Na]_i + 0.12[K]_i}\right]$$

$$\dot{m} = \alpha_m (1 - m) - \beta_m m \qquad \dot{h} = \alpha_h (1 - h) - \beta_h h$$

$$\alpha_m = \frac{200.0\,(V + 41.0)}{1 - e^{-0.1(V+41.0)}} \qquad \beta_m = 8000.0e^{-0.056(V+66.0)}$$

$$\alpha_h = 20.0e^{-0.125(V+75.0)} \qquad \beta_h = \frac{2000.0}{320.0e^{-0.1(V+75.0)}}$$

I_{si}: slow inward current

$$I_{si} = (dff_2 + d')\,(I_{si,Ca} + I_{si,K}) \qquad \eta_{si} = 1 + \frac{\delta_{si}\,[NE]_o^{n_{si}}}{[NE]_o^{n_{si}} + K_{NE,si}^{n_{si}}}$$

$$I_{si,Ca} = \frac{4.0\,\eta_{si} P_{si}\,(V - 50.0)\,\frac{F^2}{RT}\,\left([Ca]_i\, e^{\frac{100.0F}{RT}} - [Ca]_o\, e^{-2(V-50.0)\frac{F}{RT}}\right)}{1 - e^{-(V-50.0)\frac{2F}{RT}}}$$

$$I_{si,K} = \frac{0.01\,\eta_{si} P_{si}\,(V - 50.0)\,\frac{F^2}{RT}\,\left([K]_i e^{\frac{50.0F}{RT}} - [K]_o\, e^{-(V-50.0)\frac{F}{RT}}\right)}{1 - e^{-(V-50.0)\frac{F}{RT}}}$$

$$\dot{d} = \alpha_d (1 - d) - \beta_d d \qquad \dot{f} = \alpha_f (1 - f) - \beta_f f$$

$$\alpha_d = \frac{30.0\,(V + 24.0)}{1 - e^{-0.25(V+24.0)}} \qquad \alpha_f = \frac{6.25\,(V + 34.0)}{e^{0.25(V+34.0)-1}}$$

$$\beta_d = \frac{12.0\,(V + 24.0)}{e^{0.1(V+24.0)} - 1} \qquad \beta_f = \frac{50.0}{1 + e^{-0.25(V+34.0)}}$$

$$\alpha_{d|V=-24.0} = 120.0 \qquad \alpha_{f|V=-34.0} = 25.0$$

$$\beta_{d|V=-24.0} = 120.0 \qquad d' = \frac{d'_{max}}{1 + e^{-0.15(V+15.0)}}$$

$$\dot{f}_2 = \frac{\bar{f}_2 - f_2}{\tau_{f_2}} \qquad \bar{f}_2 = \frac{K_{m.f_2}}{[Ca]_i + K_{m.f_2}}$$

$$\tau_{f_2} = \frac{K_{m.f2}}{\alpha_{f_2}([Ca]_i + K_{mf_2})}$$

Hodgkin-Huxley type gating variables m, h, d, f and n are solutions of first order differential equations of the form:

$$\dot{z}(V, t) = \alpha_z(1 - z) - \beta_z z, \qquad (2)$$

where z = m, h, d, f, n, y, a and the rate functions α_z and β_z are functions of transmembrane potential V. The nomenclature follows the classical H-H formulation for cardiac muscle employed in the MNT model, and more recently the

Table 2. Outward and background currents

I_K: delayed rectifier current

$$I_K = x\bar{I}_K \qquad \dot{x} = \alpha_x\,(1 - x) - \beta_x x$$

$$\bar{I}_K = I_{k,max}\frac{[K]_i - [K]_c e^{-0.04(V-35.0)}}{140.0}\left[1 + \frac{\delta_k\,[NE]_o^{nk}}{[NE]_o^{nk} + K_{NE,K}^{nk}}\right]$$

$$\alpha_x = \frac{0.5\,(V + 22.0)}{1.0 - e^{-0.2(V+22.0)}} \qquad \beta_x = \frac{0.178\,(V + 22.0)}{e^{0.067(V+22.0)} - 1.0}$$

I_f: hyperpolarizing-activated current

$$I_f = y\bar{I}_f \qquad \dot{y} = \alpha_y\,(1 - y)\,\beta_y y$$

$$\bar{I}_f = \frac{[K]_c}{[K]_c + K_{mf}}\,g_{f,k}\,(V - E_f)\left[1 + \frac{\delta_f\,[NE]_o^{nf}}{[NE]_o^{nf} + K^{nf}}\right]$$

NE,f

$$\alpha_y = 0.05\,e^{-0.067(V+E_y)} \qquad \beta_y = \frac{1.0\,(V + E_y)}{1 - e^{-0.2\,(V+E_y)}}$$

$$E_y = 52.0\left[1 + \frac{\delta_y\,[NE]_o^{ny}}{[NE]_o^{ny} + K_{NE,y}^{nf}}\right] \qquad \beta_{y|V=-E_y} = 2.5$$

I_{K1}: time independent background potassium current

$$I_{K1} = \frac{[K]_c}{[K]_c + K_{m,K1}}\;\frac{g_{K1}\,(V - E_K)}{1 + e^{(V - E_K + 10.0)\frac{2F}{RT}}}$$

$I_{b,Na}$: background sodium current $\qquad$ $I_{b,Ca}$: background calcium current

$$I_{b,Na} = g_{b,Na}\,(V - E_{Na}) \qquad I_{b,Ca} = g_{b,Ca}\,(V - E_{Ca})$$

$$I_b = I_{b,Na} + I_{B,Ca}$$

Di Francesco-Noble (DN) model. Differences between the kinetic behavior of the current components are thus reflected in the individual rate functions $\alpha_z(V)$ and $\beta_z(V)$ which are specified in Tables 1 and 2.

Parasympathetic stimulation

A major objective of this report is the study of the effect of parasympathetic stimulation on the shape and time course of the action potential of the SA node cell. It is generally accepted that the hyperpolarizing effect of acetylcholine (ACh) release on cardiac tissues is due to an increase in potassium conductance, however the specific mechanism remains controversial. One group of studies supports the view that ACh opens ACh-specific channels separate from the normal potassium channels [16, 17]; while other studies suggest that it directly affect the kinetics of the normal potassium channel [18, 19]. In our model we have chosen the first alternative, namely, a separate channel hypothesis and ACh is assumed to have no direct influence on any other channel; this chemically-sensitive channel is also voltage-dependent, and is commonly referred to as the 'muscarinic channel'. A block diagram model of the parasympathetic neural terminations, the muscarinic ACh-sensitive membrane receptor complex and the muscarinic membrane channel dynamics are shown in Fig. 1(b). Here v(t) represents the vagal neural input to the SA node cell in the form of discrete action potentials, A(t) is the ACh concentration at the receptor site on the outer membrane surface, a(A, V, t) is a gating variable for the muscarinic membrane channel and V(t) is the transmembrane potential. The muscarinic channel is also shown in Fig. 1(a) (in dotted lines) as an additional channel shunting the membrane capacitance. The equations describing the parasympathetic stimulation system are given in Table 4 and are based on previous work [9, 10]. Thus, this neural stimulation model allows one to apply discrete patterned vagal stimuli to

Table 3. Pump and exchanger currents

I_{NaK}: sodium-potassium pump current

$$I_{NaK} = \bar{I}_{NaK} \frac{[K]_c}{[K]_c + K_{m,K}} \frac{[Na]_i}{[Na]_i + K_{m,Na}} \left[1 + \frac{\delta_{NaK} [NE]_o^{nNaK}}{[NE]_o^{nNaK} + K_{NE,p}^{nNaK}}\right]$$

I_{NaCa}: sodium-calcium exchanger

$$I_{NaCa} = \frac{k_{NaCa} \left(e^{\gamma \frac{VF}{2RT}} [Na]_i^n [Ca]_o - e^{(\gamma - 1)\frac{VF}{2RT}} [Na]_o^n [Ca]_i\right)}{1 + d_{NaCa} \left([Na]_o^n [Ca]_i + [Na]_i^n [Ca]_o\right)}$$

the SA node cell model to discern the effect of these stimuli on the waveshape and time course of the action potential of the SA node cell.

Sympathetic stimulation

Since it is generally agreed that the dynamics of the sympathetic control of the SA node cell response are much slower than the dynamics of the parasympathetic response, it is assumed that sympathetic stimulation by itself will not have the

Table 4. Compartmental equations for ionic species

$$[\dot{Na}]_i = \frac{-(I_{Na} + I_{b.Na} + I_{f.Na} + I_{si.Na} + 3I_{NaK} + 3\,I_{NaCa})}{V_iF}$$

$$[\dot{Ca}]_i = \frac{-(I_{si.Ca} + I_{b.Ca} - 2I_{NaCa} + I_{up} - I_{rel})}{2V_iF}$$

Calcium binding equations

$$I_{rel} = \alpha_{rel}\,[Ca]_{rel}\,\frac{[Ca]_i^r}{[Ca]_i^r + K_{m.Ca}^r} \qquad I_{up} = \alpha_{up}\,[Ca]_i\,(\overline{[Ca]}_{up} - [Ca]_{up})$$

$$I_{tr} = \alpha_{tr}\,p\,([Ca]_{up} - [Ca]_{rel}) \qquad \dot{p} = \alpha_p\,(1-p) - \beta_p p$$

$$\alpha_p = \frac{0.625\,(V + 64.0)}{e^{0.25(V+64.0)} - 1} \qquad \beta_p = \frac{5.0}{1 + e^{-0.25(V+64.0)}}$$

$$\alpha_{p|V=-64.0} = 2.5 \qquad \alpha_{up} = \frac{2FV_i}{\tau_{up}\,\overline{[Ca]}_{up}}$$

$$\alpha_{tr} = \frac{2FV_{rel}}{\tau_{rep}} \qquad \alpha_{rel} = \frac{2FV_{rel}}{\tau_{rel}}$$

$$[\dot{Ca}]_{up} = \frac{I_{up} - I_{tr}}{2V_{up}F} \qquad [\dot{Ca}]_{rel} = \frac{I_{tr} - I_{rel}}{2V_{rel}F}$$

$$[\dot{Ca}]_i = \frac{-(I_{si.Ca} + I_{b.Ca} - 2I_{NaCa} + I_{up} - I_{rel})}{2V_iF}$$

Potassium binding equations

$$[\dot{K}]_c = P_{diff}\,([K]_b - [K]_c) + \frac{I_{m.K}}{V_iF} \qquad [\dot{K}]_i = \frac{-I_{m.K}}{V_iF}$$

$$I_{m.K} = I_{K1} + I_K + I_{f.K} + I_{si.K} + I_{b.K} + 2I_{NaK}$$

phasic influence on the waveshape and time course of the SA node cell action potential. Therefore, in the present report we will consider only the case of tonic sympathetic stimulation that essentially provides a constant background level of norepinephrine (NE). The model equations affected by a change in norepinephrine concentration in the bathing medium [NE] are given in Tables 1 and 2. The specific currents affected by NE are the slow inward current I_{si}, the delayed rectifier current I_k, and the background current I_f which is activated upon hyperpolarization. Unlike ACh, norepinephrine is assumed to affect the behavior of three existing membrane channels. The binding reaction for NE to a receptor site is assumed to be modeled by an independent first-order process described by Michaelis-Menten kinetics. The gating variables of the slow inward and delayed rectifier (I_k) channels are assumed to be unaffected by [NE] based on the findings of Kass and Wiegers [20] on Purkinje fibers, namely that the dynamics of these channel currents appear to be independent of [NE] and only the gain function for the channel is affected. The dynamics of the background current i_f are affected by [NE] according to Noma et al. [21] and Brown et al. [22] and consequently, the rate constants α_y and β_y in Table 2 appear as functions of [NE].

Computational aspects

The modeling equations were implemented in the C programming language on a Vax 11-750 using 15 digit precision for all variables, the numerical integration scheme employed was a hybrid form consisting of Rush-Larsen approximations for the gating variables ([23] and a fifth-order Runge-Kutta-Merson method [24]). The stepsize in time was adjusted by taking into account both the error

Table 5. Parameters

$V_T = 0.80\ a^2 l$	$V_c = 0.05\ V_T$	$V_i = 0.95\ V_T$	$V_{up} = 0.05\ V_T$
$V_{rel} = 0.02\ V_T$	$V_{Ca} = 0.1\ V_i$	$g_{Na} = 7.0\ \mu S$	$P_{si} = 8.0\ sec^{-1}$
$\alpha_{f2} = 10.0\ sec^{-1}$	$K_{m.f_2} = 0.001\ mM$	$I_{k.max} = 30.0\ nA$	$g_{K1} = 20.0\ \mu S$
$\tau_{up} = 0.007\ sec$	$\tau_{rep} = 0.1\ sec$	$\tau_{rel} = 0.075\ sec$	$\overline{[Ca]}_{up} = 5.0\ mM$
$K_{NaCa} = 0.015$	$d_{NaCa} = 0.001$	$P_{diff} = 10.0\ sec$	$C_m = 0.0056\ nF$
$[K]_b = 2.4\ mM$	$g_a = 0.75\ \mu S$	$g_{b.Na} = 0.03\ \mu S$	$g_{f.K} = 30.0\ \mu S$
$g_{f.Na} = 30.0\ \mu S$	$d'_{max} = 0.04$	$g_{b.Ca} = 0.02\ \mu S$	$[K]_c = 2.4\ mM$
$\bar{I}_{NaK} = 75.0\ nA$	$K_{m.Na} = 40.0\ mM$	$K_{m.K} = 1.0\ mM$	$\gamma = 0.5$
$K_{mf} = 45.0\ mM$	$K_{m.Ca} = 0.001\ mM$	$[Na]_o = 140.0\ mM$	$[Ca]_o = 2.0\ mM$
$M_{Ach} = 1.74\ 10^{-16}\ mM$	$k_{Ach} = 12.32\ sec^{-1}$	$k_H = 1.62\ sec^{-1}$	$\alpha_a = 17.0\ sec^{-1}$
$D = 9.15\ 10^{-9}\ cm^2/sec$	$x_{Ach} = 0.0001\ cm$	$k_{d.Ach} = 1.7\ 10^{-3}\ mM$	$\lambda = 0.0133\ mV^{-1}$
$\delta_{si} = 0.37$	$n_{si} = 1.2$	$K_{NE.si} = 1.26\ 10^{-7}\ M$	$\delta_K = 0.12$
$n_K = 1.15$	$K_{NE.K} = 1.33\ 10^{-7}\ M$	$\delta_f = 0.24$	$n_f = 1.15$
$K_{NEf} = 1.33\ 10^{-7}\ M$	$I_{K.max} = 30.0\ nA$	$a = 0.2\ mm$	$l = 0.1\ mm$

estimate provided by the Runge-Kutta-Merson method and the allowable rate of change of transmembrane voltage with each step.

Results

Figure 2 illustrates the free-running behavior of the SA node cell model. The general waveshape of the transmembrane potential agrees very well with published data for the rabbit SA node cell. The channel currents contributing to the total membrane current I_m are also shown. Clearly, the fast component of the slow inward current I_{si} is responsible for the leading edge of the action potential, the slight plateau region is contributed by the influence of the *Na-Ca* exchanger current and the presence of incomplete inactivation of the slow inward current. Incomplete voltage-dependent inactivation is taken into account in the model via the function $d'(V)$ appearing in the equation for I_{si}; the terminology adopted comes from the MNT model. This appears to be a very necessary feature of the model for producing plateau behavior in pacemaking cells. The adoption of the function $d'(V)$ is a temporary measure on our part as we await quantitative descriptions of the inactivation variable f for this tissue as it exhibits incomplete voltage-dependent inactivation at higher membrane voltages. Moreover, that voltage-dependent activation is a general feature of slow-inward *Ca* channels and is now being called into question by findings that inactivation of calcium channels is mediated by calcium in several noncardiac preparations [25]. Investigations on frog atrium [26] and calf Purkinje fibers [27, 28] partially confirm that this also occurs in the heart, on slow inward channels. Inactivation in these channels is therefore most likely both voltage and calcium dependent and future models should attempt to incorporate these experimental findings. In Fig. 2 the repolarization of membrane potential is accomplished by the increase in the delayed potassium current I_K, and the slow decrease in the 'tail' of this current is the main factor is governing the rate of depolarization of membrane potential V during phase 4 depolarization.

The true course of membrane hyperpolarization produced by vagal stimulation cannot be determined in the normal free-running cell. To study this effect experimentally one might add appropriate amounts of tetrodotoxin (TTX) and verapamil to the bathing solution of an isolated nodal preparation, in order to block the fast and slow inward currents. In the model the parameters $\bar{g}_{Na}$ and P_{si} (Table 1) may be set equal to zero, thus simulating the effect of blocking these channels with drugs. Implementing this approach, the effect of single-burst vagal stimulation of the quiescent SA node cell membrane is shown in Fig. 3. In panel A, the transmembrane potential response to a single vagal stimulus is shown. One will note that the membrane response begins only after a latency L of approximately 90 msec and its magnitude grades in a nonlinear fashion with the number of pulses delivered per burst (i.e. 1, 3, 5, 9 ppb). Fig. 3B shows the time course of

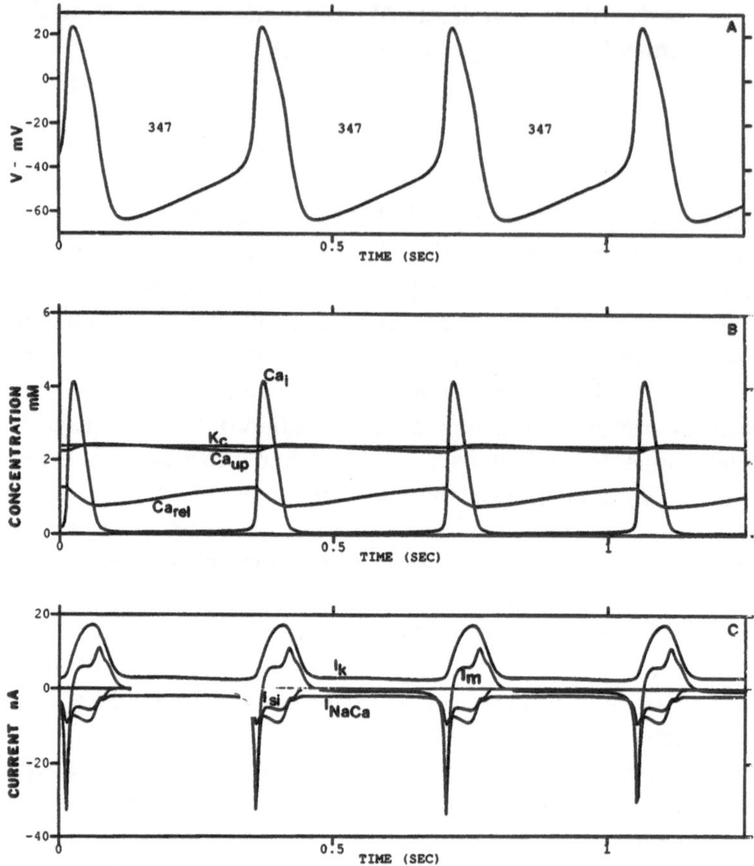

Figure 2. Free running behavior of the SA nodal cell model. The numbers seen in the figure refer to the cycle length (347 msec). Panel A, transmembrane potential; Panel B shows the time course of concentration changes in the internal calcium concentration, Ca_i (μM). Calcium in the uptake and release compartments Ca_{up} (mM) and Ca_{rel} (mM) and the potassium ion concentration Kc (mM). Panel C shows a number of currents: I_m is the total transmembrane current in nA, I_{si} is the slow inward current, I_{NaCa} is the sodium-calcium exchanger current in nA, and I_K is the inward rectified delayed potassium current.

the current through the muscarinic, ACh-sensitive channel in response to single-burst vagal stimulation at 1, 3, 5 and 9 pulses per burst (ppb), while panel C shows the time course of the ACh concentration at the outer surface of the cell membrane.

Figure 4 demonstrates the phase-sensitivity of the innervated SA node cell, in that the length of the test cycle in which the vagal stimulus is applied varies, depending on the portion of the cycle in which the stimulus is delivered. This figure illustrates the model response to a vagal burst (5 ppb) applied with various delays (−70, 0, 100, 200 msec) after the last spontaneous discharge, i.e. the

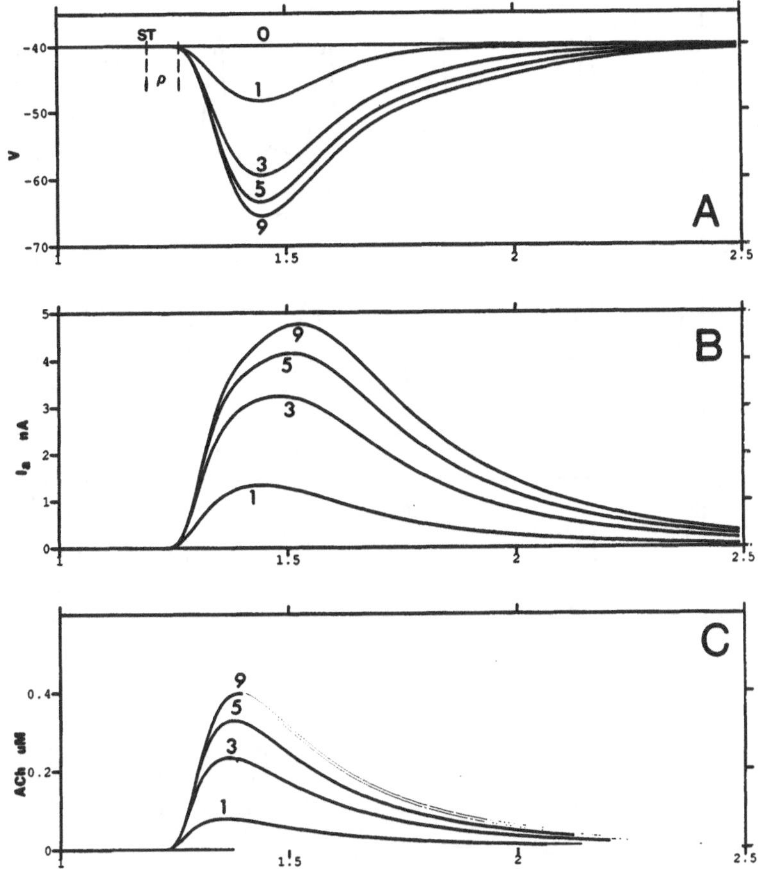

Figure 3. Temporal response of the model to a single vagal burst when the inward channels I_{Na} and I_{si} have been blocked. A: The hyperpolarizing change in membrane potential in response to the stimulus delivered at t = 0; note the latency, L, in the response (~90 msec). The majority of this latency is due to the diffusion of ACh across the gap between the neural release site and the outer membrane surface of the cell. B: the time course of the muscarinic channel current. C: the time course of the concentration of acetylcholine at the cell surface. The response at more than three pulses per burst shows marked saturation.

control heart period. Figure 5 examines the effects of vagal stimulation more closely by showing the temporal relationships between the transmembrane potential (V), the total membrane current (I_m), and the muscarinic channel current (I_a), as a single vagal burst (5 pbb) is delivered with a phase delay $\Phi = 0$ msec. Approximately four cycles of a control waveform are shown in panels A and B for reference, along with the superimposed test waveforms resulting from the single vagal burst stimulation. The point marked ST in fig. 5A refers to the time of stimulus delivery. One will note the delay prior to the rise in muscarinic channel current I_a (panel B) and the fact that this current diminishes substantially in

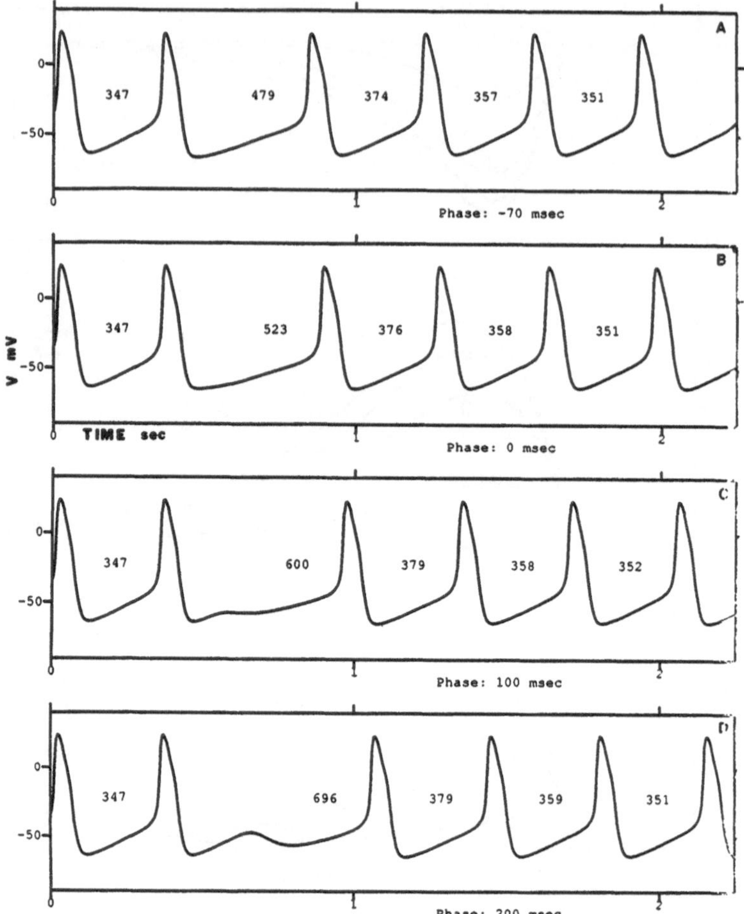

Figure 4. Phase sensitivity of the innervated SA node cell model as single-burst vagal stimuli (5 ppb) are applied with various stimulus delays: A, −70; B, O; C, 100; D, 200 msec. A zero delay corresponds to stimulus delivered at the onset of the test cycle P. Note there is a latency of approximately 90 msec in response to the applied vagal stimulus. This latency is a major contributor to the functional no-effect period ϱ associated with the test cycle.

succeeding heartbeats. The model-generated curves of Fig. 3(b) are in general agreement with the experimental results of Jalife and Moe [29] for the isolated sinus node of the young cat.

The conventional methods used to display information regarding the phase sensitivity of pacemaking cells are the pacemaker response curves (Fig. 6(A)) and the vagal inhibition curve (Fig. 6(B)). The pacemaker response curve (PRC) is concerned with the relative change in length of the test cycle (the cycle in which the stimulus is delivered) as a function of stimulus phase measured with respect to the onset of the test cycle. On the other hand, the vagal effect curve of Brown and

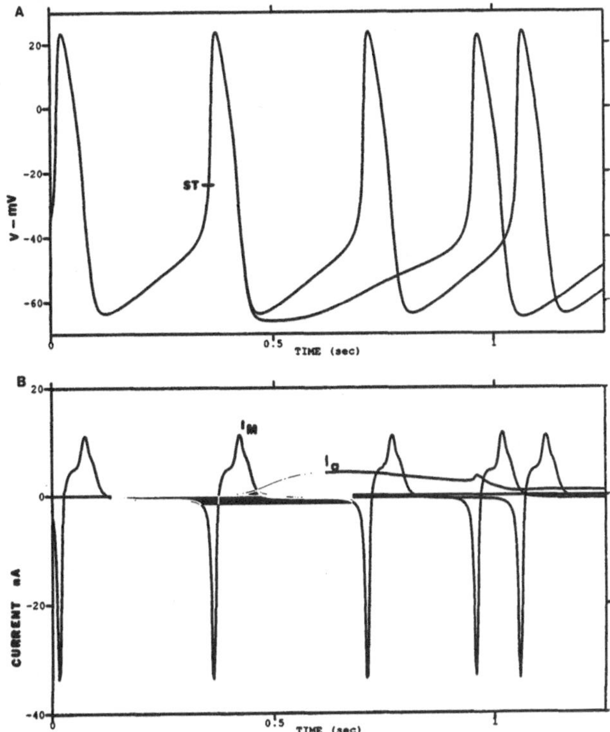

Figure 5. temporal relationships between transmembrane potential V, total membrane current I_m and muscarinic channel current Ia as a single vagal burst (5 ppb) is delivered at the point marked ST in the top record. Control records of V and I_m are superimposed in panels A and B for reference.

Eccles [30] is concerned with the relative change in cycle length (period) over several beats.

In the pacemaker response curve of Fig. 6(A) the ordinate is the relative change in the cycle length from control $\triangle P$ given by

$$\triangle P = \frac{P_1 - P_0}{P_0} \tag{3}$$

where P_0 is the control cycle length or period. The abscissa is the normalized stimulus delay which may be varied over the range $-\varrho/P_0 \leqslant \varphi \leqslant (P_0 - \varrho)/P_0$ where ϱ is the 'no effect' period, wherein a stimulus delivered late in the cycle has no effect on the current test cycle, but does have an effect on succeeding cycles. The PRC is concerned however only with one cycle, the test cycle of length P_1 in which the stimulus is delivered. As the stimulus latency is increased from zero, the resulting periods increase untill a maximum is reached (see Fig. 6(A)); beyond this delay where the maximum slowing of the cycle occurs, a rapid decrease in the response occurs and the stimulus is in the no-effect zone discussed above.

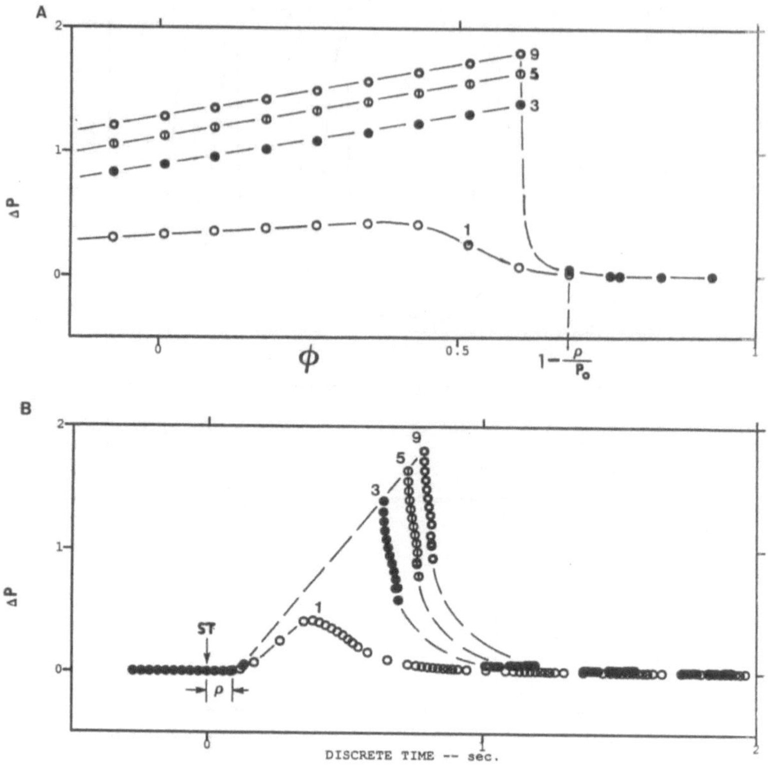

Figure 6. A: family of model-generated phase response curves (PRC's) constructed by sweeping across the test cycle. The response of the model is given in terms of the normalized change in the period of the test cycle (ΔP) relative to the control period (P_0). Here ϱ is the no effect period. The majority of this time interval is taken by L, the latency in the response of the membrane to vagal burst stimulation (see Fig. 3). B: family of model-generated vagal effect curves for 1, 3, 5 and 9 ppb. The ordinate is the normalized change in heart period and the abscissa is the discrete time calculated according to equation (3). Data for four heart periods are shown. For more details see [10, 30].

Similarly, test stimuli delivered prior to the beginning of the test cycle P, (i.e. $-\varrho/P_0<\varphi<0$), have no effect on the control heart period P_0, but do have an effect on P. A phase φ equal to zero means that the stimulus is delivered at the beginning of the test cycle.

Figure 7 shows the influence of the addition of norepinephrine to the bathing medium of the cell. The bath concentration is 10 μM and steady state conditions are assumed. It is apparent from panel A that as a result of the addition of NE to the bath, cycle length has diminished from the control value of 347 msec to a period of 263 msec. In comparing Figures 2 and 7 (panel C) one will note that the currents I_{si} and I_K have also increased as a result of their dependency on [NE]. These currents however do not change as much as the current I_f which is the main factor influencing membrane current flow during phase 4 depolarization in the

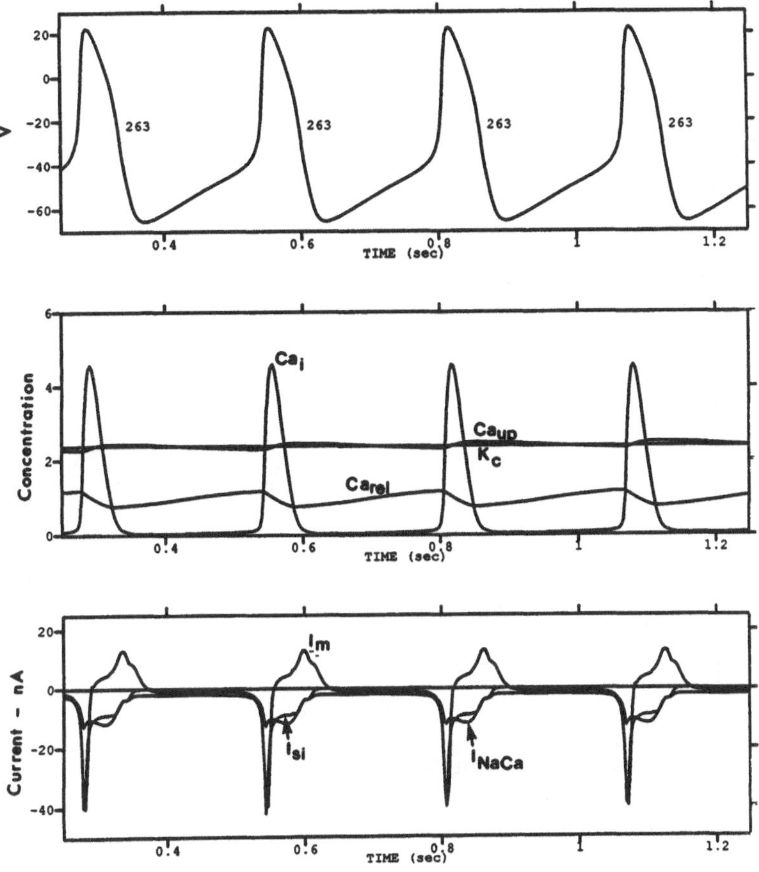

Figure 7. Steady-state model behavior in the presence of 10 μM norepinephrine.

presence of significant concentrations of NE. Under control conditions (no autonomic influence) the main factor affecting phase 4 depolarization is the slow decrease in potassium channel conductance i.e. the slow tail of the I_K waveform). The steady-state dose-response curve curve for the norpinephrine concentration [NE] and the cycle length of the resulting train of nodal action potentials is shown in Fig. 8. As concentration increases from a threshold level of 0.01 μM to a saturation dose of approximately 10.0 μM, cycle length changes from 347 msec to 263 msec, a change of approximately 24% from the control level. One will also observe from Fig. 9 that background levels of [NE] strongly affect the phase sensitivity of the cell membrane to vagal burst stimuli, and the form of the changes seen in the PRC's of Fig. 9(A) are in general agreement with the experimental findings of Stuesse et al. [31].

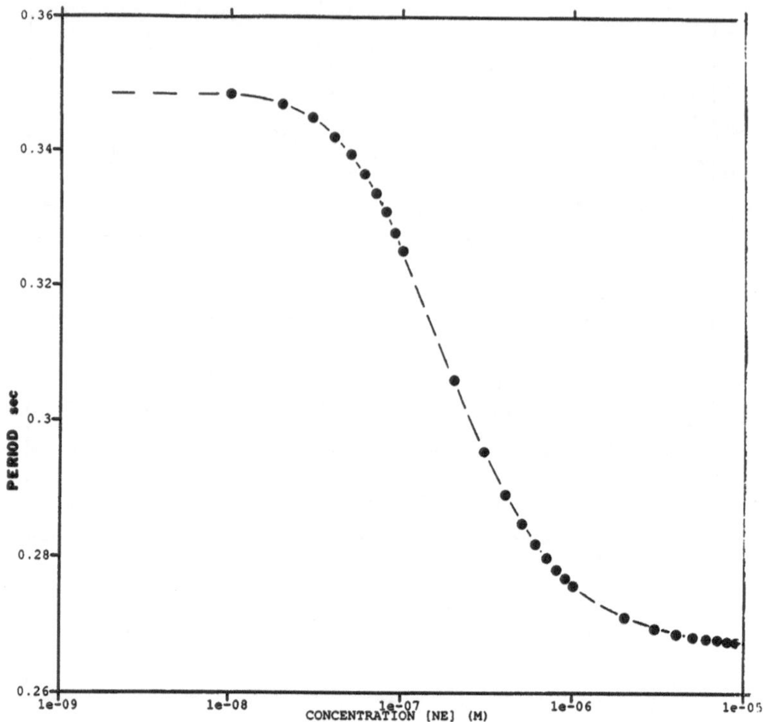

Figure 8. Dose-response curve for norepinephrine concentration and steady-state cycle length of the SA node cell action potential.

Discussion

A preliminary, first approximation model for the response of the rabbit SA node cell to phasic vagal burst-like stimuli, with and without background levels of norepinephrine is presented. The basic cell model is heavily based on the new Di Francesco-Noble (DN) model for Purkinje fibers [1] and the adaptation of that model to the SA node cell by Noble and Noble [2]. The DN model introduces fluid compartments (including a cleft space), Ca^{++}-binding storage and release, as well as a *Na-K* membrane pump and a *NaCa* exchanger mechanism, as important elements in the description of the electrical behavior of cardiac cells. Previous models on this subject [9, 10, 32, 33] have not described the SA node in such detail. The benefit that accrues by using the DN model is a much more comprehensive description of factors affecting the state variables of the model, during the course of an action potential as well as over longer periods of time.

In autonomic stimulation of the SA node cell, periods of time involving several heart beats are of interest. The vagal stimulation model employed, namely that used in previous work [10], is capable of producing both phase response and vagal

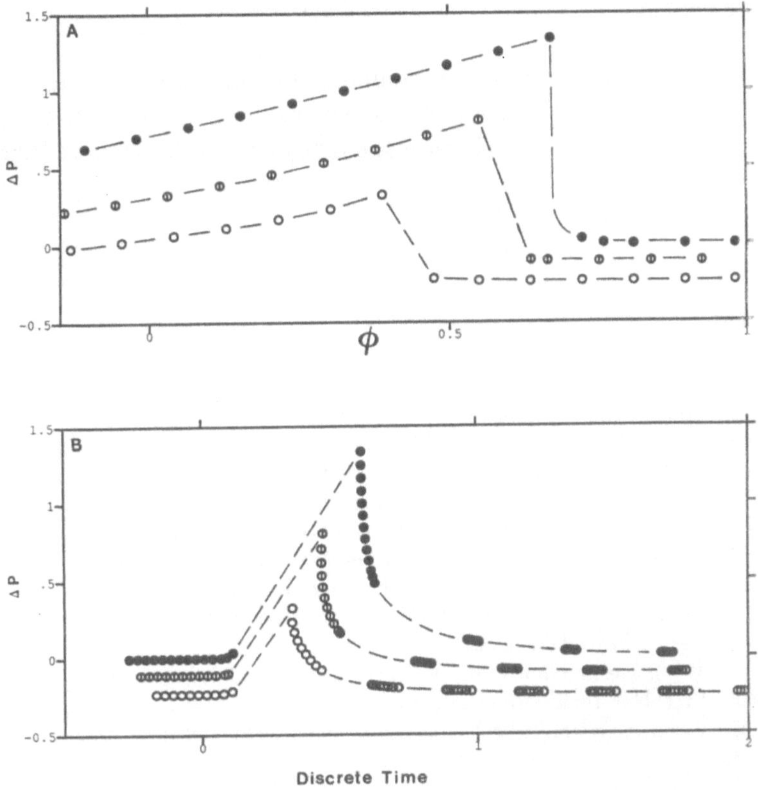

Figure 9. Pacemaker response curves (A) and vagal effect curves (B) in response to single burst vagal stimulation at 5 ppb, under three background conditions regarding norepinephrine concentration [NE] = 0 (filled circles), 0.174 (crossed circles), and 10 μM (open circles).

effect curves that describe the experimental findings of many investigators quite well (see Fig. 6(A) and (B)). Our efforts to mathematically model the effect of norepinephrine on the waveshape and cycle length of the SA node cell is based on the experimental findings of Brown and Di Francesco [22] and Noma et al. [16]. The extension of the modified model to the case where the effect of the background levels of NE on the phase sensitivity of the cell to vagal burst stimuli (Fig. 9) seems to have bourne good fruit, since the model-generated pacemaker response curves generally agree with the experimental findings of Stuesse et al. [31].

The results reported here are admittedly preliminary. However, a modeling approach of this type may eventually be of use not only in describing the electrical behavior of pacemaking cells in the heart, but also as a conceptual tool for the study of more complex subjects such as the effect of parasympathetic-sympathetic interactions on nodal tissue, and subsequently their effect on heart rate.

Acknowledgments

The authors would like to thank Randall Rasmusson and Dr Wayne Giles of the Department of Medical Physiology, University of Calgary, Calgary, Alberta, Canada for their continued assistance and many helpful discussions. The authors are also indebted to Dr Dennis Noble for his assistance. This work was supported in part by NSF Grant ECS8405435.

References

1. Di Francesco D, Noble D (1985): A model of cardiac electrical activity incorporating ionic pumps and concentration changes. Phil Trans Roy Soc B 307: 353–398.
2. Noble D, Noble S (1984): A model of S.A. node electrical activity using a modification of the Di Francesco-Noble (1984) equations. Proc Roy Soc B 222: 295–304.
3. Hodgkin AL, Huxley AF (1952): A quantitative description of membrane current and its application to conduction and excitation. J Physiol (London) 117: 500–554.
4. Noble D (1962): A modification of the Hodgkin-Huxley equations applicable to Purkinje fiber action and pacemaker potentials. J Physiol (London) 160: 317–352.
5. McAllister RE, Noble D, Tsien RW (1975): Reconstruction of the electrical activity of cardiac Purkinje fibers. J Physiol (London) 251: 1–59.
6. Noble D (1979): The initiation of the heartbeat (2nd ed.). Clarendon, Oxford.
7. Coraboeuf E (1982): Ionic basis of electrical activity in cardiac tissue. In: Levy MN, Vassalle M (eds) Excitation and neural control of the heart. American Physiological Society, Bethesda, Md, pp. 1–35.
8. Beeler WG, Reuter H (1977): Reconstruction of the action potential of ventricular myocardial fibers. J Physiol (London) 268: 177–210.
9. Bristow DG, Clark JW (1982): A mathematical model of the primary pacemaking cell in the SA node of the heart. Amer J Physiol 243: H207–H218.
10. Bristow DG, Clark JW (1983): A mathematical model of the vagally driven primary pacemaker. Amer J Physiol 244: H150–H161.
11. Lee KS, Week TA, Kao RI, Eaikee NA, Brown AM (1979): Sodium current in single heart muscle cells. Nature (London) 278: 269–271.
12. Hume JR, Giles W (1981): Active and passive electrical properties of single bullfrog atrial cells. J Gen Physiol 78: 19–42.
13. Hume JR, Giles W (1983): Ionic currents in single isolated bullfrog atrial cells. J Gen Physiol 81: 153–194.
14. Taniguchi J, Shinichiro K, Noma A, Irisawa H (1981): Spontaneously active cells isolated from the sino-atrial and atrio-ventricular nodes in the rabbit heart. Jpn J Physiol 31: 547–558.
15. Sheets MF, January CT, Fozzard HA (1983): Isolation and characterization of single canine cardiac Purkinje cells. J Physiol (London) 53: 544–548.
16. Noma A, Kotake H, Irisawa H (1980): Slow inward current and its role mediating the chronotropic effect of epinephrine in the rabbit sinoatrial node. Pflügers Archiv 388: 1–9.
17. Osterrieder W, Noma A, Trautwein W (1980): On the kinetics of the potassium channel activated by acetylcholine in the SA node of the rabbit heart. Pflügers Archiv 386: 101–109.
18. Garnier D, Nargeot J, Ojeda C, Rougier O (1978): The action of acetylcholine on background and conductance in frog atrial trabeculae. J Physiol (London) 174: 381–396.
19. Mubagwa K, Carmeliet E (1983): Effects of acetylcholine on electrophysiological properties of rabbit Purkinje fibers. Circ Res 53: 740–751.

20. Kass RS, Wiegers SE (1982): The ionic basis of concentration-related effects of noradrenaline on the action potential of calf Purkinje fibers. J Physiol (London) 322: 541–558.
21. Noma A, Trautwein W (1978): Relaxation of the ACh-induced potassium current of the rabbit sinoatrial node. Pflügers Archiv 377: 193–200.
22. Brown H, Di Francesco D (1980): Voltage-clamp investigations of membrane currents underlying pace-maker activity in the rabbit sino-atrial node. J Physiol (London) 308: 331–351.
23. Rush S, Larsen H (1978): A practical algorithm for solving dynamic membrane equations. IEEE Trans on BME 25: 389–393.
24. Lance GN (1960): Numerical methods for high speed computers. Iliffe and Sons, London.
25. Ashcroft FM, Stanfield PR (1980): Calcium dependence on the inactivation of calcium currents in skeletal muscle fibers of the insect. Science 213: 224–226.
26. Fischmeister R, Mentrard D, Vassort G (1981): Slow inward current ionactivation in frog heart atrium. J Physiol (London) 320: 27P–28P.
27. Marban E, Tsien RW (1981): Is the slow inward current of heart muscle inactivated by calcium? Biophysiol J 33: 143 (Abstract).
28. Tsien RW, Marban E (1982): Digitalis and slow inward current in heart muscle: evidence for regulatory effects of intracellular calcium on calcium channels. In: Hagihara Y, Ebashis (eds) Advances in pharmacology and theraputics II, Vol. 3 Cardio-renal and cell pharmacology. Pergamon Press, Oxford, pp. 217–215.
29. Jalife J, Moe GK (1980): Phase effects of vagal stimulation on pacemaker activity of the isolated sinus node of the young cat. M Res 45: 595–608.
30. Brown GL, Eccles JC (1934): The action of a single vagal volley on the rhythm of the heart beat. J Physiol (London) 82: 211–240.
31. Stuesse SL, Wallick DW, Zeiske H, Levy MN (1981): Changes in vagal phasic chronotropic responses with sympathetic stimulation in the dog. Amer. J Physiol 241: H850–H856.
32. Yanigahara K, Noma A, Irisawa H (1980): Reconstruction of sinoatrial node pacemaker potential based on the voltage clamp experiments. Jpn J Physiol 30: 841–857.
33. Michaels DC, Matayas EP, Jalife J (1984): A mathematical model of the vagal control of sinoatrial pacemaker activity. Circ Res 55: 89–101.

4. Effects of the discrete cellular structure on electrical propagation in cardiac tissue

Y. RUDY and W. QUAN

Abstract

The effects of the discrete cellular structure on propagation of electrical excitation in cardiac muscle were studied in a 1-dimensional fiber model containing a periodic intercalated disc (ID) structure. Globally, the macroscopic velocity of propagation follows the behavior associated with propagation in a continuous tissue (except for high values of disc resistance). In addition, the computed spatial extracellular potential is a smooth bi-phasic waveform and does not reflect the underlying discrete cellular structure of the tissue. Other results of the simulations demonstrate the discontinuous nature of propagation. $\dot{V}_{max}$ displays a bi-phasic behavior as a function of increasing ID resistance. An initial 'paradoxical' increase in $\dot{V}_{max}$ (with a simultaneous decrease in conduction velocity) is followed by a decrease which leads to decremental propagation and conduction block. The time constant of the foot of the action potential (τ_{foot}) increases monotonically with increasing ID resistance. An increase in the leakage current to extracellular space brings about a significant decrease in the action potential duration and a loss of the plateau. This major effect is accompanied by a relatively smaller decrease in conduction velocity. Collision of two activation wavefronts results in a significant (100%) increase in $\dot{V}_{max}$ and a very small (0.6%) decrease in τ_{foot}.

Introduction

The anatomical structure of the myocardium as an assembly of discrete cells separated by a periodic intercalated disc structure was established in 1954. However, until recently the propagation of electrical excitation in cardiac muscle has been characterized as though it occurred in a syncytium. The effects of the structural discontinuities introduced by the discs were not considered important, and activation was analyzed on the basis of continuous models utilized successfully for nerves (classical continuous cable theory). Recent experimental results [1, 2] showed electrical properties of cardiac muscle that could not be explained on the basis of classical continuous cable theory. For example, $\dot{V}_{max}$ (maximum rate of change of the temporal action potential) was observed to *increase* as propagation velocity *decreased* due to a wider angle of propagation relative to the fiber axis. This result is in contrast to the direct relationship between $\dot{V}_{max}$ and velocity predicted by continuous models and often used in the interpretation of results obtained in cardiac tissue. In addition, the importance of the anisotropic structure of cardiac muscle in determining conduction velocity and source configuration [3–5], as well as its possible role in causing conduction abnormalities [1] was recently established. The anisotropy is caused largely by the higher density of discs traversed by a wavefront propagating perpendicular to as compared to parallel to the fiber axis. The anisotropy reflects, therefore, the discrete nature of the myocardium. It is clear that the effects described above and the underlying mechanisms involved can only be examined using a model which includes microscopic discontinuities (intercalated discs) at the cellular level. In this paper a model of this nature is utilized to study the effects of the periodic disc structure on propagation in cardiac muscle.

Methods

The model (Figure 1) consists of a one dimensional fiber that includes 40–100 individual cells (each 100 μm long, and 16 μm in diameter). Neighboring cells are connected by an intercalated disc structure modelled as a T-resistance network (two axial resistances representing the intercytoplasmic channels (connexons), and a radial leakage resistance to the extracellular space). Each individual cell was discretized into 3 Beeler and Reuter [6] membrane patches. This division of the cell was tested for convergence. It permits the study of spatial variations within a single cell, and allows to separately study effects of the myoplasm and of the intercalated disc resistance. By combining the Beeler and Reuter membrane model with the core conductor model [7] and the periodic intercalated disc structure, we were able to develop equations for the propagating action potential V_m (x,t) at every membrane patch. The method of Cooley and Dodge [8] and the simplifying algorith of Rush and Larsen [9] were used to compute V_m (x,t) numerically.

Results

Effects of variations in the intercalated disc resistance

Under normal physiological conditions the contributions from the myocardial cell

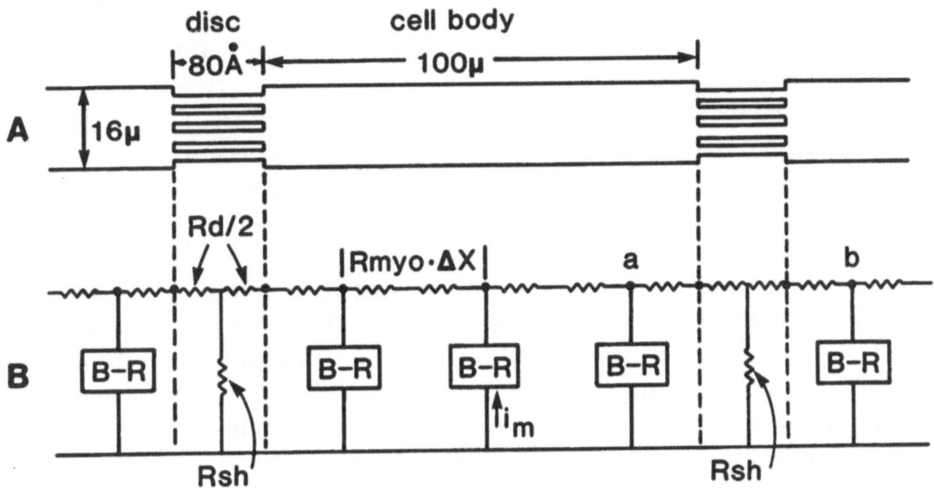

Figure 1. A: discrete cable model of cylindrical cardiac cells, each 100 μm in length and 16 μm in diameter, interconnected by an intercalated disc structure which contains intercellular bridges (connexons). B: core conductor network with 3 Beeler and Reuter (B-R) membrane patches per cell, and a T-network representing the intercalated disc between cells. R_d = disc resistance, R_{myo} = myoplasm resistance, and R_{sh} = leakage resistance to extracellular space.

myoplasm and from the intercalated disc to the total effective axial resistance are roughly equal. However, while the myoplasm occupies a length of 100 μm per cell in the direction of propagation, the gap junction between cells is only 80 Å in dimension, introducing a recurrent periodic discontinuity in the axial resistance. Moreover, the junctional resistance can be modulated and obtain very high values in abnormal cases such as ischemia and infarction leading to very slow conduction and, in the extreme case, to complete decoupling of neighboring cells and a resulting conduction block. It is clear, therefore, that the discrete recurrent junctional resistances must play an important role in the activation process in cardiac tissue. This section deals with the effects on propagation caused by changes in junctional resistance. In the stimulations below the myoplasm resistance was kept constant at the typical value of 200 ohm · cm, while the disc resistance was varied over a wide range of values (see Figures below).

Macroscopic velocity and microscopic velocity

Two different velocities were defined: microscopic velocity θ_{micro} representing the velocity of propagation inside a single cell, and macroscopic velocity θ_{macro} (or average velocity θ) representing the average velocity of propagation over many cells. The effects of variations in the effective axial resistivity (brought about by changing the disc resistance for a constant myoplasm resistance of 200 ohm · cm) on θ_{micro} and θ_{macro} are shown in Figure 2 (curves 1 and 2, respectively). The continuous case (no discs were included in the model) is shown for comparison in curve 3, and follows the inverse square root relationship between conduction velocity and axial resistance as expected. As the disc resistivity was varied from 0.1 ohm · cm^2 to 360 ohm · cm^2 θ_{micro} and θ_{macro} exhibit opposite changes. The microscopic velocity increases with increasing disc resistance reflecting the fact that the current is more confined to the single cell and therefore more current is available to depolarize the cellular membrane. The macroscopic (average) velocity, on the other hand, decreases with increasing disc resistance as a result of an increased time delay at the disc. In the range of effective axial resistivity from 210 ohm · cm to 1000 ohm · cm the macroscopic velocity follows closely the inverse square root relationship of continuous cable theory. However, beyond this range changes in the disc resistance result in a greater decrease in velocity than predicted by the inverse square root relationship. It will be shown below (section on decremental propagation) that in the range of 380 ohm · cm^2 to 400 ohm · cm^2 of disc resistance decremental conduction is obtained in the discontinuous model, and beyond this range complete block occurs. Note (Figure 2) the discontinuous 'saltatory' nature of propagation with high velocity of propagation inside a cell, and slower propagation over many cells. For the typical value of 2 ohm · cm^2 disc resistance the microscopic velocity is twice macroscopic velocity. This ratio increases and the saltatory nature of propagation becomes more pronounced with increasing disc resistance (Figure 2).

$\dot{V}_{max}$ and velocity

The maximum rate of rise of the action potential $\dot{V}_{max}$ and the average macroscopic velocity θ_{macro} are shown in Figure 3 (curves 1 and 2 respectively) as a function of the effective axial resistance (again varied by increasing the disc resistance while keeping the myoplasm resistance constant at 200 ohm · cm). The continuous case is shown for comparison in Figure 4. $\dot{V}_{max}$ displays a bi-phasic behavior. In the range of disc resistance from 0.1 ohm · cm^2 to 70 ohm · cm^2 $\dot{V}_{max}$ *increases* and conduction velocity *decreases*. This 'paradoxical' behavior is opposit to the direct relationship between $\dot{V}_{max}$ and conduction velocity that is predicted by continuous cable theory when the membrane sodium conductance is varied. Note that for small values of disc resistance velocity is high and $\dot{V}_{max}$ levels off, approaching the value associated with propagation in a continuous cable (see Figure 4). For high values of disc resistance a second phase is exhibited and $\dot{V}_{max}$ decreases with increasing disc resistance. This part of the curve reflects the transition to decremental conduction and eventually to a complete conduction block. For a certain value of disc resistance (70 ohm · cm^2) $\dot{V}_{max}$ attains a maximum. For this high resistance value the cell is separated to a large degree from its downstream neighbor and $\dot{V}_{max}$ approaches the value that could be obtained

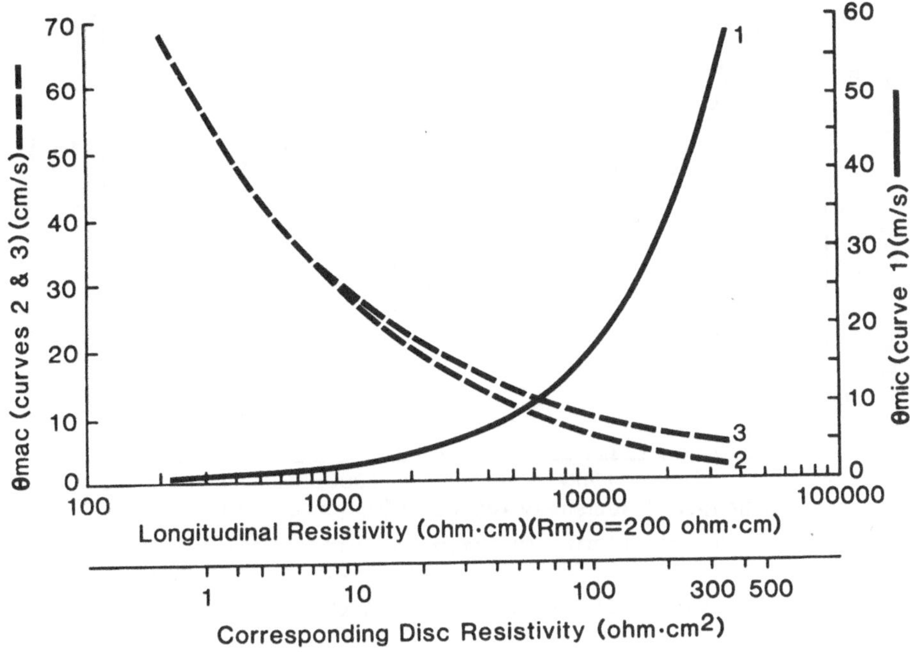

Figure 2. The effects of variations in axial (longitudinal) resistivity on microscopic velocity (θ_{mic} curve 1) and on average macroscopic velocity (θ_{mac} curve 2). The continuous case (no discs included in the model) is shown for comparison (curve 3) and follows the inverse square root relationship of continuous cable theory. The effective longitudinal resistivity is varied by varying the disc resistivity while the myoplasm resistivity is kept constant at 200 ohm · cm. Both effective longitudinal resistivity and the corresponding disc resistivity are indicated.

under space-clamp condition. Note that in the continuous case (Figure 4) the velocity drops according to the inverse square root relationship and $\dot{V}_{max}$ remains constant, independent of variations in axial resistance.

The foot of the action potential (τ_{foot})

Figure 5 shows the behavior of τ_{foot} (curve 1) as a function of axial resistance (again varied by increasing the disc resistance). The macroscopic velocity is also shown (curve 2). For comparison, the continuous case is shown in Figure 6. Note that τ_{foot} increases monotonically with increasing disc resistance in the actual discontinuous case, accompanied by a decrease in velocity. As expected, no change in τ_{foot} is observed in the continuous case (Figure 6). The sensitivity of the τ_{foot} measurement to its distance from the stimulus site is simulated in Figure 7. For a stimulus of $900\,\mu A/cm^2$ τ_{foot} measured at a distance of 2 mm from the stimulus site is about 10% smaller than that at 4 mm away. This long range effect

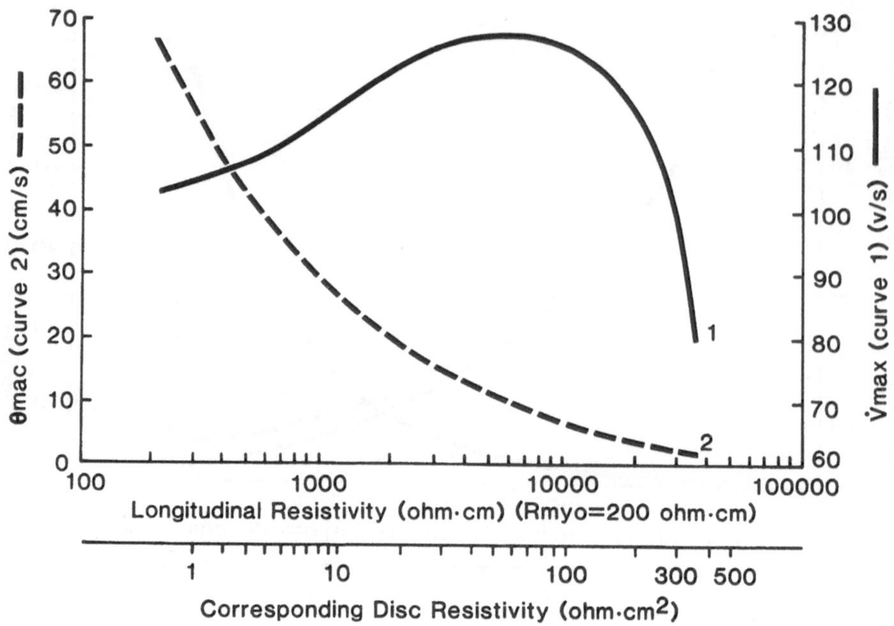

Figure 3. Effects of variations in disc resistivity on the macroscopic velocity of propagation (curve 2) and on the maximum rate of rise of the action potential $\dot{V}_{max}$ (curve 1).

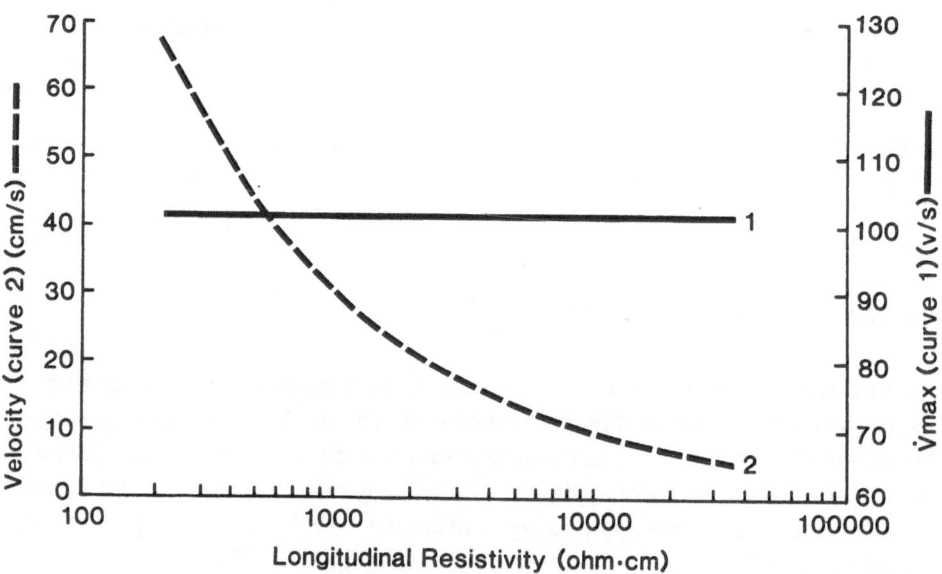

Figure 4. $\dot{V}_{max}$ (curve 1) and conduction velocity (curve 2) as a function of axial resistivity for a continuous cable (no discs are included in the model).

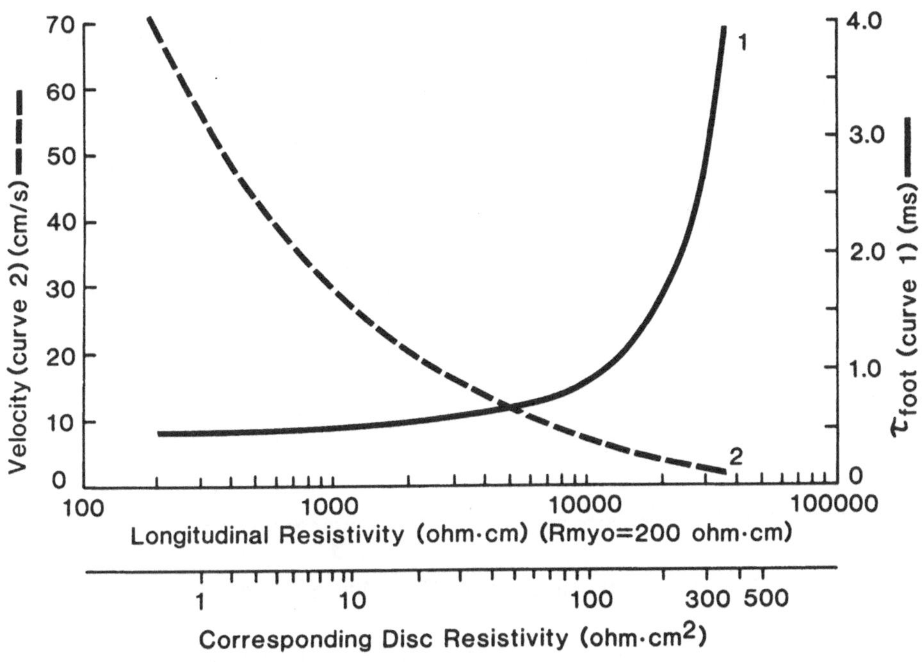

Figure 5. Effects of variations in disc resistivity on the macroscopic velocity (curve 2) and on the time constant of the foot of the action potential τ_{foot} (curve 1).

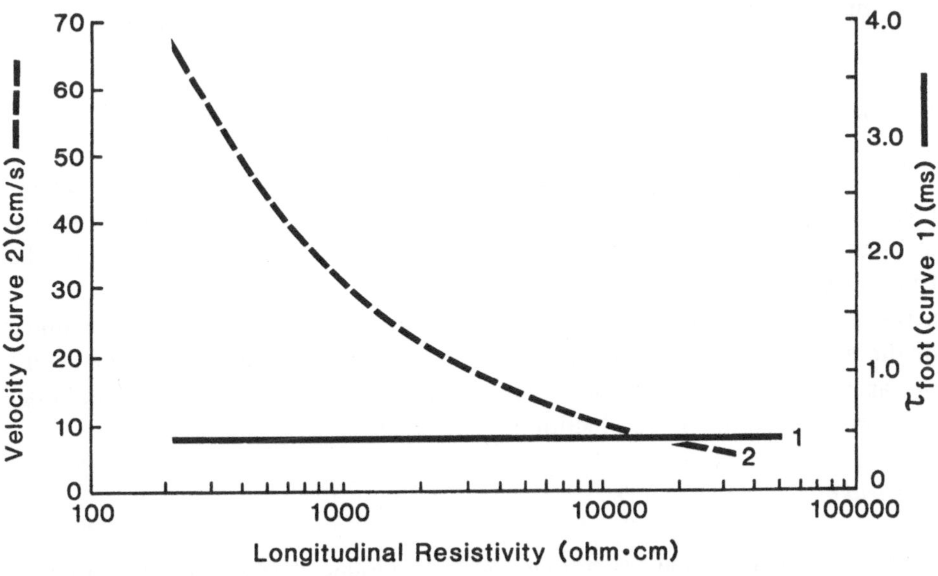

Figure 6. τ_{foot} (curve 1) and conduction velocity (curve 2) as a function of axial resistivity for a continuous cable.

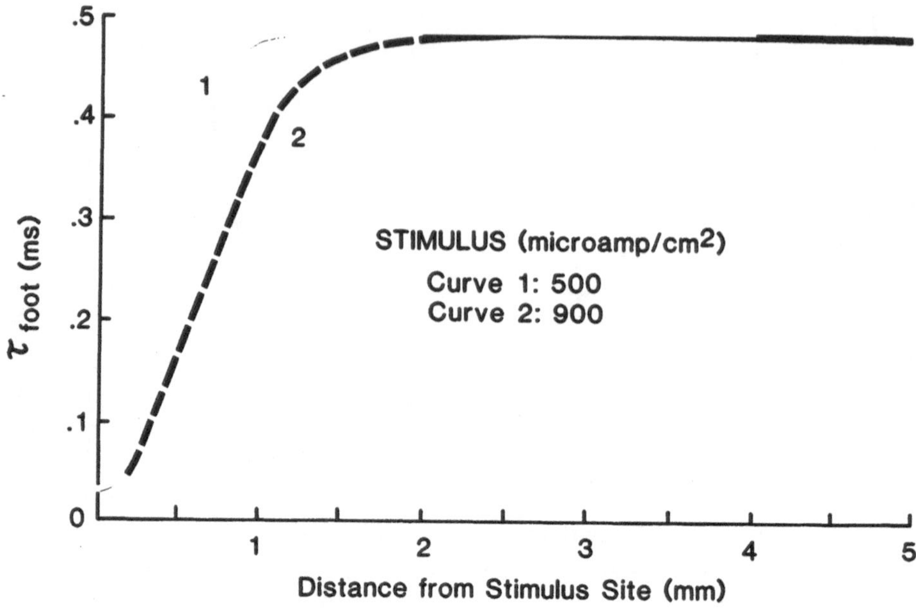

Figure 7. The effect of the stimulus on τ_{foot} as a function of distance from the stimulus site. Stimuli of two different strengths are considered: 500 $\mu A/cm^2$ and 900 $\mu A/cm^2$ (curves 1 and 2 respectively).

of the stimulus has to be considered in measurements of τ_{foot} from a cardiac tissue of complex geometry.

Decremental propagation

For the range of very high disc resistivity (380 ohm · cm^2 to 400 ohm · cm^2) decremental propagation is obtained in our model simulations. This situation is shown in Figure 8. The velocity of propagation decreases progressively with distance from the stimulus site (the velocity could be as low as 1.5 cm/sec). In addition, the action potential duration and amplitude decrease. Note the spike like appearance of the action potential which is consistant with the experimental observations of Sasyniuk and Mendez [10]. For values of disc resistance greater than 400 ohm · cm^2 complete conduction block occurs.

The leakage resistance (R_{sh})

An increase in the leakage current to the extracellular space may occur in areas of damaged myocardium due to a decrease in the leakage resistance at the disc. The effects of such changes on the propagated action potential are simulated below. The major effect is on the action potential duration as shown in Figure 9. Curves 1

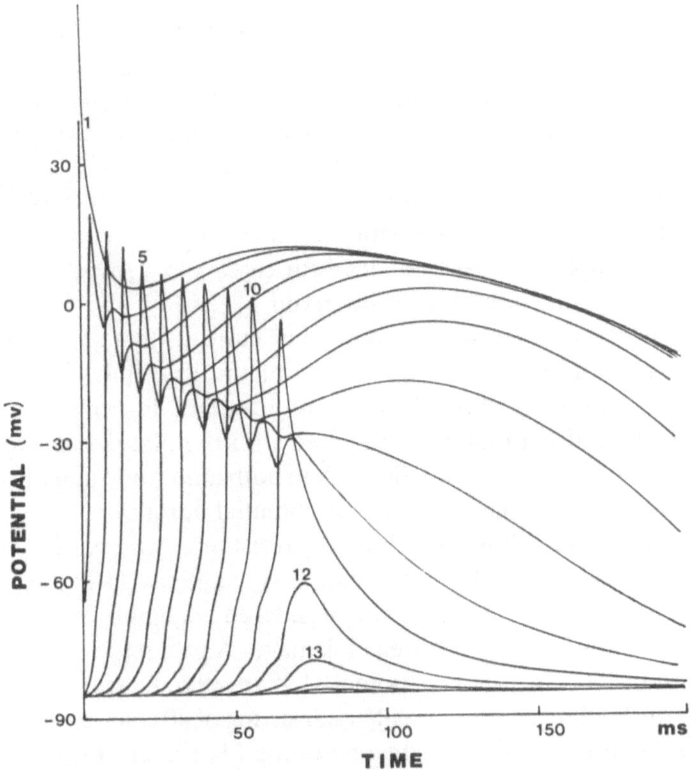

Figure 8. Decremental propagation caused by a very high resistivity (R_d = 380 ohm · cm²). The numbers in the body of the figure indicate the cell number relative to the stimulus site.

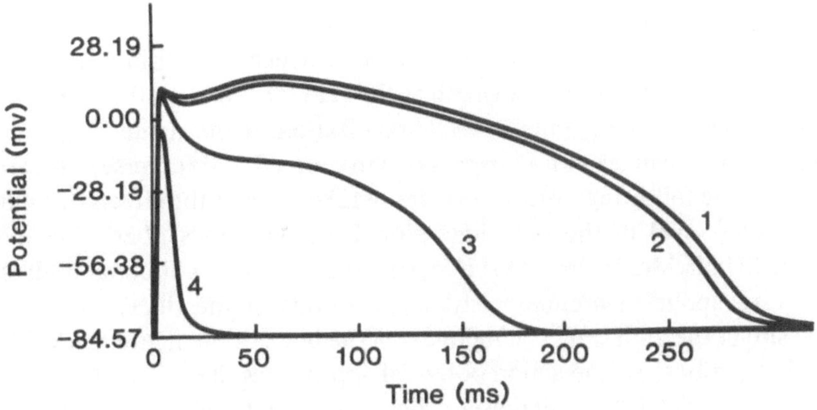

Figure 9. Effects of variations in leakage resistance (R_{sh}) on the propagating action potential. Curves 1 to 4 correspond to progressively decreasing values of R_{sh} (see text).

to 4 correspond to progressively decreasing values of the leakage resistance ($R_{sh} = 10^8, 10^7, 10^6$ and 10^5 kΩ, respectively). As a result of the increase in leakage current, the duration of the action potential decreases progressively until the plateau is completely lost (curve 4). Note the small changes when R_{sh} is decreased from 10^8 to 10^7 kΩ. In contrast, for R_{sh} smaller than 10^7 kΩ the action potential duration decreases quickly and this change is accompanied by a decrease in the amplitude of the plateau. A progressively increasing effect on the velocity of propagation is also observed with the values of 55.47 cm/sec; 55.40 cm/sec; 54.80 cm/sec; and 48.12 cm/sec obtained for cases 1 to 4 respectively. For lower values of R_{shunt} conduction block is observed.

The effects of variations in R_{sh} on the ionic currents that constitute the Beeler and Reuter membrane model are shown in Figure 10. While the sodium current (I_{Na}) decreases by only about 10% in the range of R_{sh} considered, the slow currents (I_s, I_{x1} and I_{k1}) that are associated with the plateau and repolarization phases are strongly affected and diminish in both amplitude and duration, bringing about the large change in the action potential duration.

In the simulations above the leakage resistance was varied at every disc location in the fiber. A different situation is examined in Figure 11. Here the leakage current at all disc locations is considered negligible except at the end of the fiber, simulating a localized area of damage. A progressive decrease in action potential duration and plateau potential is observed as the action potential aproaches the 'leaking' end. For a fiber consisting of 40 cells, and for $R_{sh} = 10^5$ kΩ the action potential duration at the end of the fiber is shorter by about 20 msec than the duration at the 5th cell away from the stimulus site (the duration is measured at −60 mV).

Collision

Due to the complex geometry of the myocardial structure collisions of propagation wavefronts are likely to occur both at the cellular level and the global tissue level. In particular, the geometry and organization of the tissue suggests that multiple collisions can occur for propagation in a direction transverse to the fibers orientation. The following simulation (Figure 12) examines the effects of collision at the cellular level in the one dimensional discontinuous fiber. The model consists of 40 individual cells with symmetrical boundary conditions at both ends. Stimuli were applied simultaneously at both ends of the fiber, leading to a collision site at the 20th cell. The numbers in the body of the figure mark the cell number in the fiber. As the action potential approaches the collision site several changes are observed. $\dot{V}_{max}$ increases progressively and is almost doubled at the collision site. In addition, $\dot{V}_{max}$ is obtained at progressively higher values of potential (marked by the line connecting the cells from 10 to 20 in the figure), and the amplitude (relative to the zero potential) increases as well. In contrast to the

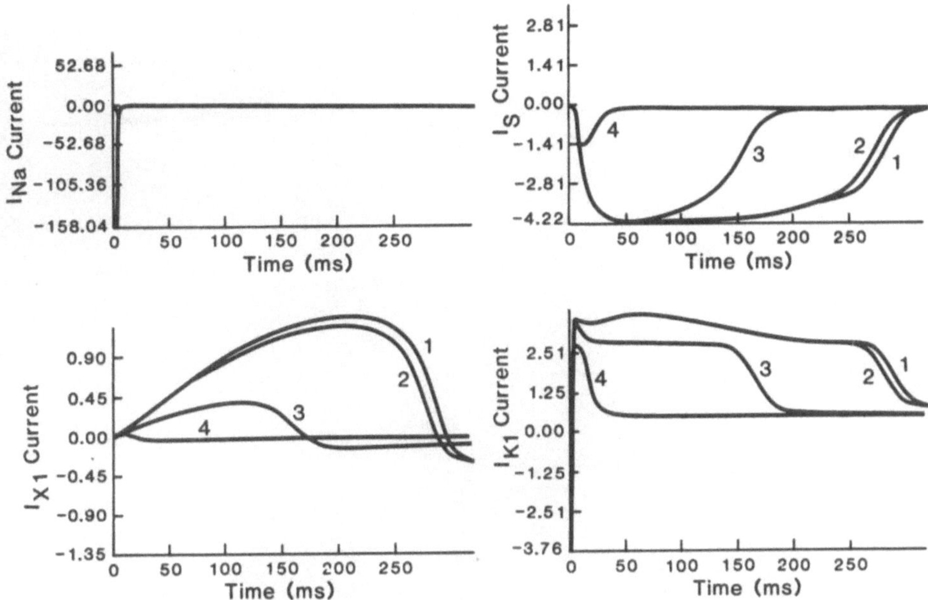

Figure 10. Effects of variations in R_{sh} on the ionic currents that constitute the Beeler and Reuter model of the ventricular action potential. Curves 1 to 4 correspond to progressively decreasing values of R_{sh} as in Figure 9 above.

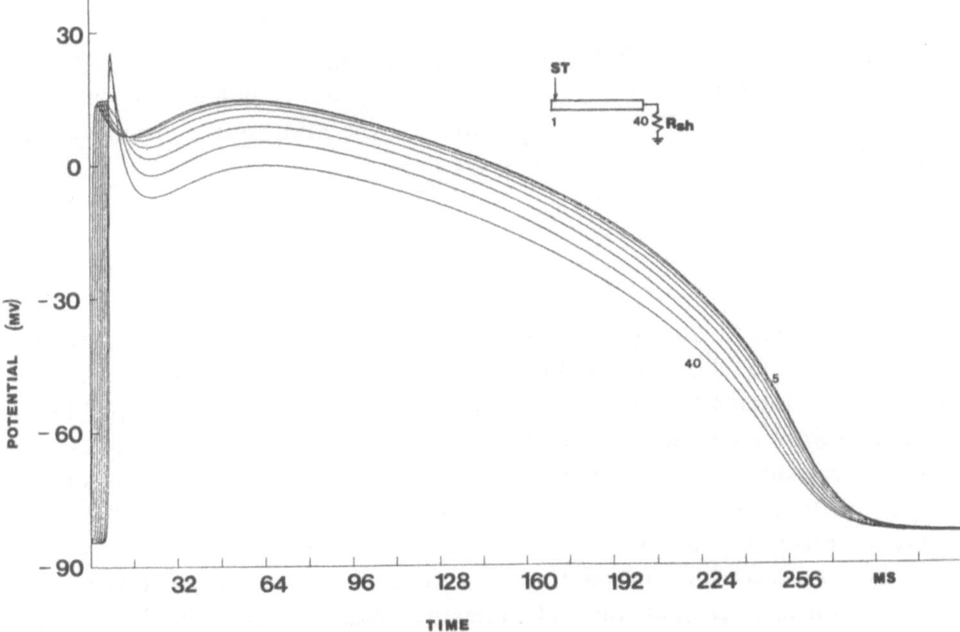

Figure 11. The effect of a 'leaking end' on the propagating action potential. The model contains 40 cells and is stimulated at cell number 1. A leakage resistance ($R_{sh} = 10^5$ kΩ) is present at the 40th cell (see inset). The numbers in the body of the figure indicate the cell number relative to the stimulus site.

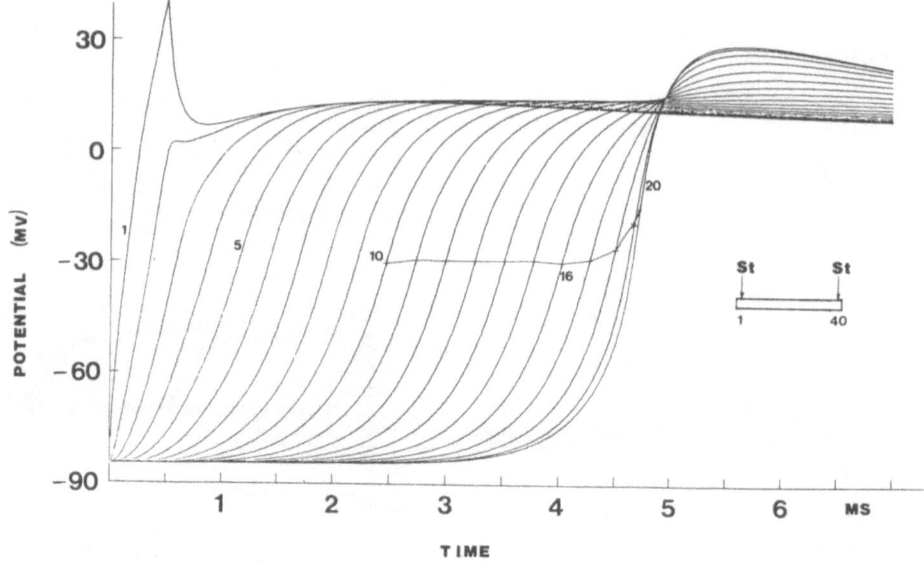

Figure 12. The effects of collision on the propagating action potential. The fiber is stimulated simultaneously at both ends (see inset). The numbers in the body of the figure indicate the cell number in the fiber. The line connecting cells 10 through 20 marks the potential at which $\dot{V}_{max}$ is obtained. The collision site is at cell number 20.

large increase in the value of $\dot{V}_{max}$, τ_{foot} shows a very small decrease of only 0.6%. The variations of these four variables ($\dot{V}_{max}$, the membrane potential V_m at $\dot{V}_{max}$, τ_{foot}, and the maximum potential amplitude V_{max}) as a function of distance from the collision site are summerized in Figure 13.

Extracellular potential

The rising phase of a spatial propagating action potential obtained from the discontinuous model is shown in Figure 14. Note the sharp discontinuities introduced at each intercalated disc location (arrows). In contrast, the action potential computed from a continuous model (no discs included) is smooth an does not exhibit sharp changes in slope (inset to Figure 14). The equivalent dipolar source density along the fiber is proportional to the slope of the action potential. The source density is therefore very large at the disc. However, only a small fraction of the cell cross section is occupied by the connexons at the gap junction and is available for axial current flow. The effective cross section at the disc is only 0.01%–0.03% of the total cross section based on morphological studies [11]. Taking this factor into account, the contribution to the extracellular field from sources at the disc becomes negligible [12], and the computed spatial extracellular

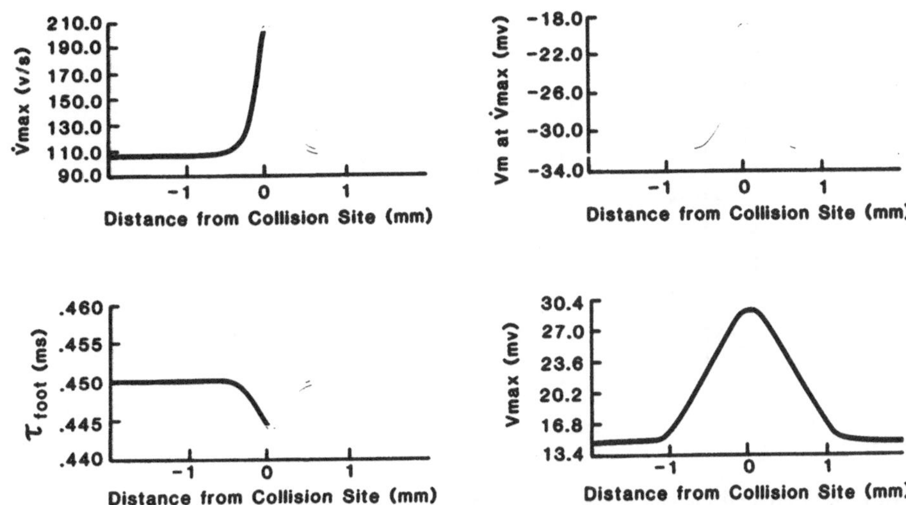

Figure 13. A summary of the effects of collision (as a function of distance from the collision site) on $\dot{V}_{max}$, V_m (membrane potential) at which $\dot{V}_{max}$ is obtained, τ_{foot}, and V_{max} (maximum potential amplitude).

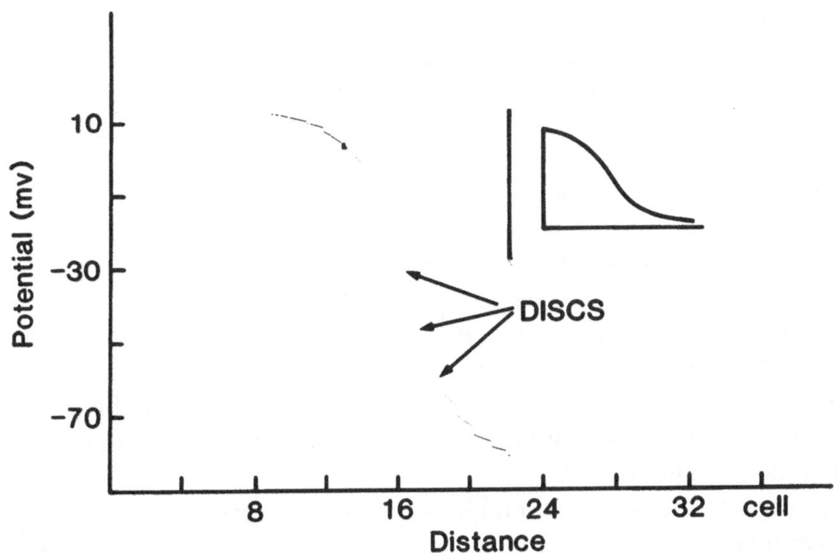

Figure 14. Spatial action potential wavefront obtained from the discontinuous model. Note major discontinuities in leading edge at disc locations (arrows). A smooth action potential is shown for comparison (inset).

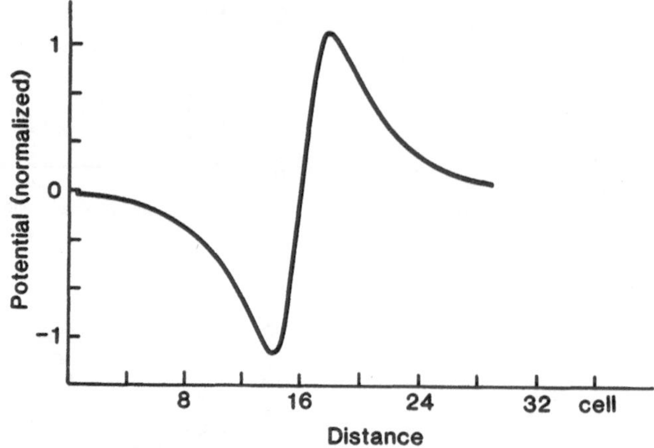

Figure 15. Computed spatial extracellular potential at the surface of the discontinuous fiber.

potential at the surface of the fiber (Figure 15) is a smooth biphasic waveform that does not reflect the underlying discontinuous structure.

Discussion

The simulations described above demonstrate the importance of the structural discontinuities introduced by the intercalated discs in determining the characteristics of propagation in cardiac muscle. The propagation is discontinuous in nature with high velocity inside a cell, and slower average (macroscopic) velocity over many cells. This discontinuous behavior becomes progressively more pronounced with increasing disc resistance. It should be emphasized, however, that over the normal physiological range of disc resistivity the discrete structure of the myocardium is not manifest in the behavior of the macroscopic velocity of propagation which follows closely the inverse square root relationship of continuous cable theory. Only for high values of disc resistance ($>20\,\mathrm{ohm \cdot cm^2}$) a deviation from this relationship is observed, and for very high disc resistance ($>380\,\mathrm{ohm \cdot cm^2}$) decremental propagation and conduction block are obtained. In addition, the extracellular potential even at the surface of the fiber does not reflect the underlying discontinuities and resembles the smooth bi-phasic waveform of the continuous case.

In contrast to the above, several important characteristics of the propagating action potential are strongly influenced by the underlying discrete nature of the fiber. For a certain range of disc resistivity a 'paradoxical' increase in $\dot{V}_{max}$ with decreased velocity caused by higher disc resistance is observed. The behavior in this range can be explained on the basis of higher degree of confinement of the axial current flow. Since the relative contribution of the discs to the effective resistivity is higher in the direction transverse to the fibers, slow conduction with high $\dot{V}_{max}$ should occur in this direction. This behavior was observed experimentally by Spach et al. [1]. It should be noted that for high values of disc resistivity ($>70\,\text{ohm}\cdot\text{cm}^2$) $\dot{V}_{max}$ starts to decrease and a gradual transition to decremental propagation and eventually conduction block is observed. This complex non-monotonic behavior of $\dot{V}_{max}$ implies that the common practice of using $\dot{V}_{max}$ as an index of conduction velocity (based on the direct relationship between the two that is obtained from classical continuous cable theory) may not always be valid for cardiac muscle.

Another important parameter is the foot of the action potential (τ_{foot}). In our simulations τ_{foot} increases with increasing disc resistance. This result is in disagreement with the experimentally observed decrease in τ_{foot} for propagation transverse to the fibers in the 2-dimensional tissue preparation of Spach et al. [1]. The complex geometry of cell connections and branching in two dimensions suggests that many collisions may occur in this preparation, especially in the case of transverse propagation. This motivated us to examine the effects of collisions in our 1-dimensional discrete model. As a result of the collision $\dot{V}_{max}$ is almost doubled. This result is consistent with the 80% increase in $\dot{V}_{max}$ observed by Spach et al. A slight decrease in τ_{foot} is observed at the collision site in the simulation. While the direction of the change is in agreement with the experiment, quantitatively the simulated effect is negligible compared to the 30% change that is observed experimentally. The question whether multiple collisions in the two dimensional geometry can bring about the observed change awaits further investigation.

The simulations related to the effects of increased leakage current at the disc examine a situation that is not documented experimentally. However, it is possible that under abnormal conditions structural changes in the disc may occur that bring about a decrease in the leakage resistance (R_{sh}). The major effect of an increase in the leakage current is to significantly shorten the duration of the propagating action potential. Such localized changes in regions of the myocardium can bring about non-uniformities in refractory periods and precipitate conditions of vulnerability to arrhythmias (reentry).

Acknowledgment

This study was supported by the National Institute of Health Grant HL 33343.

References

1. Spach MS, Miller WT III, Geselowitz DB, Barr RC, Kootsey JM, Johnson EA (1981): The discontinuous nature of propagation in normal canine cardiac muscle. Evidence for recurrent

discontinuities of intracellular resistance that affect the membrane currents. Circ Res 48: 39–54.

2. Spach MS, Kootsey JM, Sloan JD (1982): Active modulation of electrical coupling between cardiac cells of the dog. A mechanism for transient and steady state variations in conduction velocity. Circ Res 51: 347–362.
3. Plonsey R, Rudy Y (1980): Electrocardiogram sources in a two-dimensional anisotropic activation model. Med Biol Engr Comput 18: 87–95.
4. Plonsey R, Barr RC (1984): Current flow patterns in two-dimensional anisotropic bisyncytia with normal and extreme conductivities. Biophys J 45: 557–571.
5. Barr RC, Plonsey R (1984): Propagation of excitation in idealized anisotropic two-dimensional tissue. Biophys J 45: 1191–1202.
6. Beeler GW, Reuter H (1977): Reconstruction of the action potential of ventricular myocardial fibers. J Physiol (London) 286: 177–210.
7. Hodgkin AL, Rushton WHA (1946): The electrical constants of a crustacean nerve fiber. Proc R Soc London, Ser B 133: 444–508.
8. Cooley JW, Dodge FA (1966): Digital computer solutions for excitation and propagation in the nerve impulse. Biophys J 6: 583–599.
9. Rush S, Larsen H (1978): A particular algorithm for solving dynamic membrane equations. IEEE Trans BME 25: 389–392.
10. Sasyniuk BI, Mendez C (1971): A mechanism for re-entry in canine ventricular tissue. Circ Res 28: 3–15.
11. Haas HG, Meyer R, Einwächter HM, Stuckem W (1983): Intercellular coupling in frog heart muscle: Electrophysiological and morphological aspects. Pflügers Archiv 399: 321–335.
12. Plonsey R, Barr RC (1985): Effect of junctional resistance on source-strength in a linear cable. Ann Biomed Eng 13: 95–100.

5. Electrical field model for electric interactions between myocardial cells

N. SPERELAKIS

Abstract

An electric field model for the electrical transfer of excitation between contiguous excitable cells was proposed in which there is no requirement for low-resistance connections between the cells. The major requirement is that the pre- and post-junctional membranes be ordinary excitable membranes. The electric field that develops in the narrow junctional cleft between contiguous cells during the rising phase of the action potential in the pre-junctional membrane acts to depolarize the post-junctional membrane to threshold. The electric field model has been further developed by incorporating the effect of K^+ accumulation in the clefts. The combined effects of the electric field and K^+ accumulation were examined in a chain of six cells. Propagation occurred down the chain at velocities of about 25 cm/sec, at surface to junctional membrane capacitance ratios ranging from 62.5 : 1 to 80 : 1. When the surface to junctional membrane capacitance ratio of 80 : 1 was kept constant but the total capacitance was increased 2×, 3×, and 4× the corresponding velocities were: 25.5 (1×), 15.6 (2×), 9.6 (3×), and 2.9 cm/sec (4×). When K^+ accumulation was not incorporated, propagation occurred only when the capacitance ratio was 80 : 1 and at a slower velocity. Hence, allowing K^+ to accumulate in the junctional clefts facilitates transmission of excitation from one cell to the next and enhances propagation velocity. These results are in agreement with our previous theoretical analysis that showed that K^+ accumulation in the junctional clefts could be an important facilitory mechanism for transmission of excitation, and with the fact that propagation velocity increases markedly to an optimal value when $[K]_o$ is elevated to about 8 mM. The electric field model is also consistent with the findings of Spach et al. [1] that propagation in cardiac muscle is saltatory or discontinuous in nature, and with those of Diaz et al. [2] who concluded that propagation jumps from intercalated disk to intercalated disk, with most of the propagation time being consumed at the cell junctions. Although it is not known whether the electric field model actually applies biologically, given the morphological arrangement of the cells with very closely spaced junctional membranes, it is difficult to rule it out. Hence, the electric field model provides a possible alternative mechanism for electrical interactions among contiguous excitable cells that either are not normally connected by low-resistance tunnels or have lost such connections under pathological conditions.

Introduction

The vertebrate myocardium is an assembly of short individual cells, separated at their ends by the intercalated disks (IDs). The fluid in the ID gap is continuous with the bulk interstitial fluid, and the gap thickness averages about 200 Å [3]. Regions in which the two membranes come into closer proximity (about 20 Å), the gap junctions, are found abundantly in mammalian hearts, but such specialized contacts are rare and much smaller in area in lower vertebrates (see for references [4, 5]). A step on the rising phase of the action potential, resembling a post-junctional potential, becomes prominent under conditions of impeded propagation [6]. Increase in gap width occurs in conditions that depress propagation [4], and the cell-to-cell transmission process is labile [7, 8]. Contiguous cells become functionally disconnected at the IDs following focal injury [9] and under other experimental conditions [4].

There are two major schools of thought with respect to the mechanism whereby excitation spreads from one cell to the next. One school, summarized by Weidmann [10], believes that the cells are connected by low-resistance pathways at the gap junctions (by means of small-diameter tunnels), such that local-circuit current accompanying the action potential can readily spread from one cell to the next. The second school of thought, summarized by Sperelakis [8, 11], believes that the cells do not require low-resistance connections. If so, then there must be some type of unique mechanism involved. For example, K^+ ion accumulation in the junctional cleft during the rising phase of the action potential might help to rapidly depolarize the post-junctional membrane to its threshold [13]. An analysis of the resistance and potential profiles within the cleft at the intercalated disk was made [14]. Sperelakis and Mann [15, 16] presented a new model which would allow electrical transmission to occur between contiguous excitable cells, without the requirement of low-resistance connections, provided that the pre- and post-junctional membranes were ordinary excitable membranes. In this electric field model, the electrical potential developed in the narrow junctional gap between cells, during excitation of the prejunctional membrane, serves to depolarize the postjunctional membrane to threshold by means of a 'patch clamp' effect. The present article is an expansion and updating of my article published three years ago [11].

Some evidence against low-resistance coupling

This section will provide a brief review and summary of some of the key evidence that suggests that adult myocardial cells are not normally connected by low-resistance pathways. In the case of reverted (partially dedifferentiated) myocardial cells in reaggregate culture, about half of double-microelectrode impalements showed moderate to strong degrees of electrotonic coupling, i.e., the ratio of $\Delta V_2/\Delta V_1$ was high, whereas very weak or no electronic coupling was observed in the highly differentiated reaggregates [17].

Morphological evidence

In electron microscopy of cardiac muscle, in certain conditions such as muscular dystrophy or hypertonicity, pathologically-appearing cells are often observed surrounded by normal-appearing cells [3, 18]. The cell membranes along the cell surface and intercalated disks are the sharp boundaries between the normal-appearing and abnormal-appearing cells. The morphological changes may include: super-contracted myofibrils, swollen SR, and swollen and disrupted mitochondria. The fact that the individual cell is the smallest unit to exhibit pathology or die is more consistent with lack of low-resistance connections to neighboring cells.

In cat hearts rapidly fixed during induced ventricular fibrillation, sharp discontinuities in sarcomere length were observed across the intercalated disks [19]. That is, one cell might be in a contracted state (e.g., average sarcomere length of 1.8 μm), whereas a contiguous cell across an intercalated disk was in a relaxed state (e.g., sarcomere length of 2.1 μm). It is difficult to conceive how this could occur if low-resistance connections existed between cells, since then the two cells should have been at nearly the same membrane potential, and hence have about the same state of contraction.

As stated previously, gap junctions are either absent or present at very low incidence, and tiny in size, in cardiac muscle of lower vertebrates (e.g., amphibians and reptiles) ([20]; see for additional references [4]). If this is correct, and since transmission from myocardial cell to myocardial cell does occur in these hearts, if is difficult to assume that the gap junction is the morphological basis for transmission from cell to cell.

In sheep Purkinje fibers exposed to two electron-opaque tracers (ruthenium red and lanthanum nitrate), Baldwin [21] found that cells near a cut end, but allowed to heal, took up the tracers whereas the other cells did not. In tissue prefixed in glutaraldehyde dye coupling occurred even though glutaraldehyde fixation should have converted all communicating junctions to the blocked or uncoupled state. No differences could be detected morphologically between gap junctions in injured (and presumably uncoupled) and un-injured areas. These findings seem to place some doubt on the role of gap junctions in the transmission of excitation.

Presence of junctional potentials

Junctional potentials are not expected in cables, e.g., if the cells were freely interconnected by low-resistance pathways. In reality, steps on the rising phase of the cardiac action potential are frequently observed [6, 22–24]. The steps (or prepotentials) become much more prominent under conditions of impeded propagation. The junctional potential represents the excitatory interaction between contiguous cells, and triggers the action potential in the post-junctional cell. In the context of the electric field hypothesis discussed below, the junctional potential may reflect the potential change across the post-junctional membrane (passive plus active).

Excitatory junctional potentials (EJPs) are illustrated in Fig. 1 for cultured heart cell monolayers. They can be observed as steps on the rising phase of the action potentials. The EJPs can also be revealed by hyperpolarizing the membrane sufficiently to inhibit development of action potentials (Fig. 1A–B). When such an experiment is done, there is an abrupt disappearance of the spikes, leaving only the driving EJPs (Fig. 1B). The sudden disappearance of spikes also argues against low-resistance connections between cells, because if such connections existed, then the amplitude of the action potential should have decreased progressively as anodal block spread further and further away into neighboring cells with increasing steps of hyperpolarizing current. This was never observed [24]. Therefore, it seems unlikely that the cells were connected by low-resistance pathways, even though transmission of excitation occurred from cell to cell.

Sometimes EJPs without spikes occurred naturally, indicative of a partial block of transmission (Fig. 1D–F). In such cases, local excitatory potentials are sometimes superimposed on the EJPs, and they can be suppressed by hyperpolarization (Fig. 1E). Depolarizing pulses circumvent the partial block (Fig. 1D). Contractions of the impaled cell did not occur when only EJPs were recorded, although the neighboring cells contracted; however, contractions did occur when spikes were generated.

Hypertonicity partial block

Intracellular microelectrode recordings simultaneous with surface ECG recordings were made on isolated frog hearts before and during perfusion with hypertonic solutions [25]. In isotonic solution the intracellular action potentials were always in synchrony with the surface ECG potentials. However, in hypertonic solution an impaled cell sometimes fired action potentials at a fraction of the

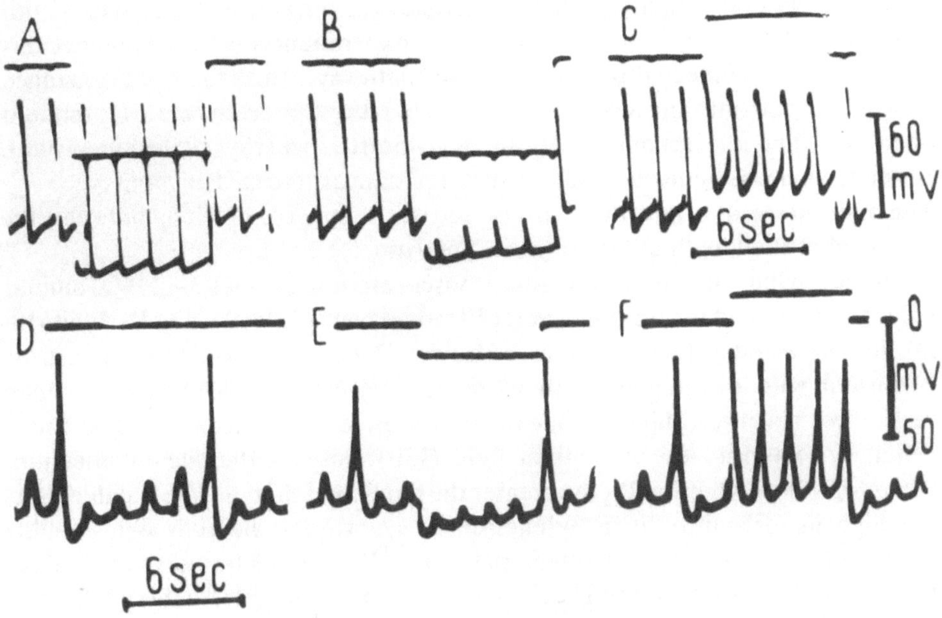

Figure 1. Presence of driving junctional potentials in monolayer cultures of embryonic chick ventricular cells, showing the spread of excitation to the impaled cell from a neighboring cell. Upper trace indicates relative intensity of current pulse; upward deflection, depolarizing current and downward deflection, hyperpolarizing current. A–C: sequential photos from one impalement. Hyperpolarizing pulses of 4.8 nA (A) and 7.6 nA (B); the larger pulse suddenly abolishes firing and reveals the driving junctional potentials. Depolarizing pulse of 3.6 nA applied in C. D–F: sequential photos from an impalement illustrating the variable magnitudes of the junctional potential. D: no current applied; amplitude of prepotential increases during diastolic depolarization between spikes. E: hyperpolarizing pulse of 2.0 nA diminishes the local excitatory response and produces complete transmission block. Anodal-break excitation occurs at end of pulse. F: depolarizing pulse of 1.8 nA causes each junctional potential to trigger a spike, thus circumventing the naturally-occurring partial block. Taken from Sperelakis [8].

ECG frequency. During the time that the impaled cell failed to fire an action potential there was only a very small (1–2 mV) potential change in this cell; this indicates that the large electric field generated by the heart, as evidenced by the ECG, was only slightly reflected in the quiescent impaled cell. This suggested that the impaled cell was electrically isolated from its neighbors, even though it had a large resting potential and was capable of firing large action potentials, thus showing that it was functionally connected to the surrounding cells.

High input resistance

The resistance between two closely-spaced microelectrodes was measured in frog ventricular muscle when one microelectrode was intracellular and when both were intracellular [26]. The rationale for this experiment was that if the myocardial cells were connected by low-resistance pathways, then the total resistance measured when only one electrode was impaled (the input resistance, R_{in}) should decrease when the second electrode was inserted nearby (<0.5 mm away). Instead, what was found was that the total resistance increased to about twice R_{in}. This indicates either that there are no low-resistance connections between the cells or that the length constant (λ) is $\ll 500\,\mu m$.

The R_{in} values obtained for cardiac muscle are high, about 3–12 MΩ; similar values are obtained for cultured heart cell monolayers [8, 24, 26, 27]. De Mello [9, 28] has reported values of about 3 MΩ for Purkinje fibers. The high R_{in} is consistent with the junctional membranes (intercalated disks) being of high resistance, because a high R_{in} means that most of the current injected intracellularly exits into the interstitial fluid (ISF) close to the site of injection. Therefore, the higher the R_{in} the greater the likelihood that the intercalated disks are high in resistance. In a 3-dimensional syncytium, the cells being highly interconnected with low-resistance pathways, R_{in} should be very low (or R_m would have to be extremely high). In a true cable $R_{in} = \frac{1}{2} r_m^{0.5} r_i^{0.5}$; therefore, for a fiber of given diameter and r_m, R_{in} is a fuction of r_i. Since the resistance of the intercalated disks (r_{md}) is in series with, and indistinguishable from, r_i, a high R_{in} would reflect a high r_{md}. An additional approach was also used to infer that the intercalated disk membranes are high in resistance [11].

Electrotonic spread of current

The most direct method of determining whether current can spread easily from one cell to another is to measure the electrotonic spread of injected current. This was done in frog and cat ventricular muscles (trabeculae) using double microelectrodes cemented together at a fixed interelectrode distance [29–31]. Electrode 1 was placed in a bridge circuit so that voltage (ΔV_1) could be recorded while polarizing current was injected; electrode 2 was used only for voltage recording (ΔV_2). At interelectrode distances of 60 μm or greater (longitudinal orientation), currents of up to 16 nA never produced a change in E_m at electrode 2 (i.e., $\Delta V_2 = 0$), even though ΔV_1 was large. That is, the degree of electrotonic interaction ($\Delta V_2/\Delta V_1$) was always nearly zero. At shorter distances, two types of behavior were observed depending on the impalement: either $\Delta V_2/\Delta V_1$ was large (e.g., 0.3–1.0) or the ratio was nearly zero. For example, Fig. 2 illustrates two impalements at an interelectrode distance of 7 μm, one of which showed a large electrotonic interaction (Panel A), and one which exhibited almost zero interaction (Panel B). The shorter the interelectrode distance the greater was the incidence of observed interactions. When the electrodes were placed perpendicular to the fiber axis, significant electrotonic interactions were never observed at

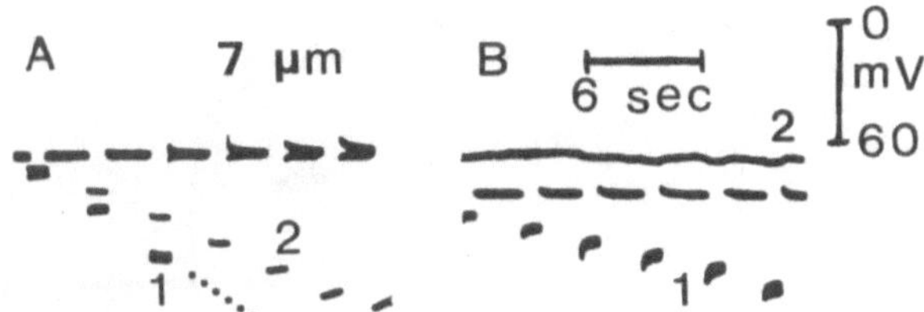

Figure 2. Typical experiments measuring spread of electrotonic current between two closely-spaced intracellular microelectrodes in intact myocardium at rest. The experiments illustrated were on frog ventricular trabeculum at an interelectrode distance of 7 μm. Electrode 1 was in a bridge circuit and was used to apply current and record potential (ΔV_1) simultaneously; electrode 2 was used to record voltage (ΔV_2), a short distance away. In some impalements (A), the degree of electrotonic interaction during the application of hyperpolarizing pulses (ratio of ΔE_m recorded by each electrode, namely $\Delta V_2/\Delta V_1$) was high, being nearly 100% in some cases. In other impalements (B), the degree of interaction was low, approaching 0%. Several step increments of current were applied in A and B. The bridge became unbalanced during the last four steps in A. Figure modified from Tarr and Sperelakis [29].

distances greater than 10 μm. Thus, it was concluded that electrotonic interactions between the two electrodes occurred only when the two microelectrodes had impaled the same cell.

Several criteria independently confirmed when the two electrodes had impaled the same cell. One such criterion was the recording of simultaneous and congruous subthreshold oscillations. Another criterion was the decline of resting potenial due to injury subsequent to the double impalement. The latter is illustrated in Fig. 3, in which impalements were made in frog ventricular muscle at an interelectrode distance of 11 μm. As shown in Panel A, the interaction at rest and during the plateau was zero in this case in which both cells had high resting potentials. In another penetration (Panel B), the cell impaled had a low resting potential due to the double impalement, and the interaction was substantial.

A fortuitous result is illustrated in Panels C and D of Fig. 3. These are sequential records from one impalement showing that while the two electrodes were in the same cell the interaction was large (Panel C), but when one electrode spontaneously left that cell and impaled a neighboring cell (due to the contraction) the degree of interaction went to zero (Panel D). These data suggest that there are no low-resistance connections between contiguous myocardial cells.

Resistivity measurements

Longitudinal resistivity (ϱ_l) measurements were made in bundles of cardiac muscle (trabeculae and papillary muscles) before and during equilibration in 8-fold higher resistance solution [7, 32]. It was found that ϱ_l increased 6.3-fold (Table 1), indicating that most of the applied current passed through the extra-

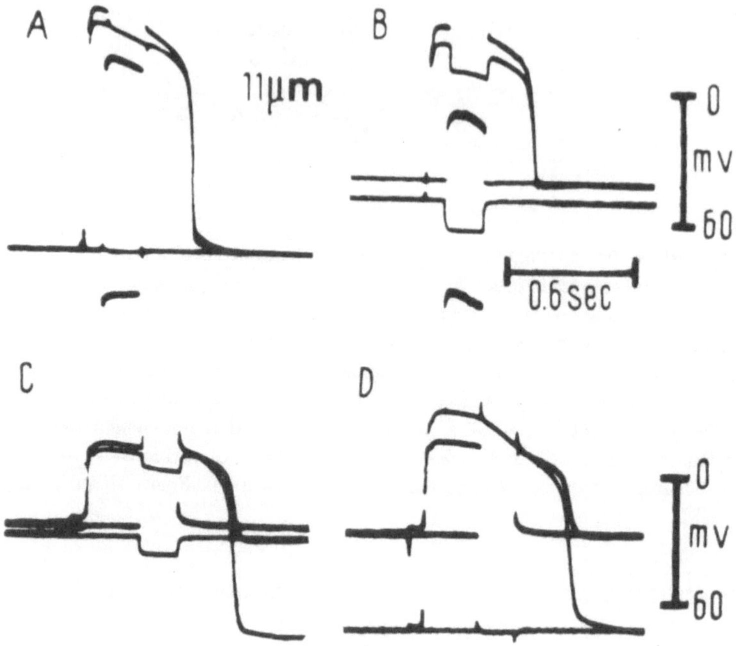

Figure 3. Three experiments (A, B, and C–D) measuring the spread of electrotonic current between two closely-spaced intracellular microelectrodes in intact frog ventricular trabeculae at rest and during the action potential plateau. The interelectrode distance was 11 μm. Two successive sweeps of the oscilloscope superimposed in each photograph. A: interaction at rest and during the plateau was nearly 0%. B: in another impalement in which the cell was injured by the two electrodes, the resting potential was low and the degree of interaction was high. C–D: in another impalement in which the cell was injured, the resting potential was low, and the degree of interaction was high (electrode 1 deflection not shown because of bridge imbalance). The contraction accompanying the action potential caused one of the electrodes to become dislodged from that cell and penetrate into a neighboring cell which had a normal resting potential; the degree of interaction then became nearly zero. Figure modified from Tarr and Sperelakis [29].

cellular space. That is, if ϱ_l had increased 8-fold, then *all* of the current would have passed through the interstitial fluid (ISF) space, even though the cross-sectional area of the cell space is much larger than that of the ISF space. In contrast, in skeletal muscle, which is composed of long cellular cables, ϱ_l increased only 1.6-fold (Table 1), indicating that most of the applied current passed through the intracellular space. Therefore, these findings suggest that the myocardial cells are not connected by low-resistance pathways.

Impedance measurements

The longitudinal tissue impedances (Z) of parallel-fibered cat papillary muscles and ventricular trabeculae were measured at different sinusoidal frequencies [7]. In normal Ringer solution, it was found that the impedance decreased as frequency was increased, so that the ratio of impedances at 10,000 Hz to 10 Hz ($Z_{10\,KHz}/Z_{10\,Hz}$) was 0.75. This suggests that there are transversely oriented membranes in cardiac muscle (presumably the intercalated disks) that have a high capacitance (C_{md}) and a high resistance (R_{md}). After equilibration in isosmotic sucrose solution to increase the resistance of the interstitial fluid (ISF) the $Z_{10\,KHz}/Z_{10\,Hz}$ ratio decreased even further to 0.48. That is, in sucrose, a greater fraction of

Table 1. Summary of measurements on the longitudinal and transverse resistivities of cardiac muscle fiber bundles compared to skeletal muscle, and calculations based on these measurements.

A. In normal Ringer solution (isotonic control)		
ϱ_l (Ω-cm)	296 ± 19 (25)	200 ± 12 (26)
ϱ_t (Ω-cm)	3351 ± 240 (29)	4285 ± 236 (23)
ϱ_t/ϱ_l	11.4	21.4
B. In tenfold diluted Ringer (+ sucrose to isotonicity)		
ϱ_l (Ω-cm)	1865 ± 99 (7)	321 ± 34 (11)
ϱ_t (Ω-cm)	3672 ± 171 (26)	5506 ± 434 (11)
ϱ_t/ϱ_l	2.0	17.1
C. Ratio of B to A:		
ϱ_l/ϱ_l	6.28	1.60
ϱ_t/ϱ_t	1.10	1.27
ϱ_{isf} (Ω-cm)	311 (33,700)	468 (17,100)
ϱ_{cell} (Ω-cm)	6140 (3,730)	349 (5,710)
$\varrho_{cell}/\varrho_{isf}$ (measured)	19.8 (0.11)	0.75 (0.33)
(calculated assuming junctions are zero resistance)		
Vol_{isf} (% extracellular space)	16.1 (1.3)	17.8 (4.1)
ϱ_j (Ω-cm-junc)	5970	53
R_{mj} (Ω-cm²)	45	–
R_{mj} (Ω-cm²) (corrected for convolutions)	288	–
C_{mj} (μF/cm²)	6.8	–

* Since in sartorius, $\varrho_{cell} \simeq \varrho_{isf}$, then if in sucrose $\varrho_{isf} \to \infty$, the maximum ϱ_l^{su}/ϱ_l would be 2.0. ϱ_l^{su} is the longitudinal resistivity in ion-free isosmotic sucrose solution.

ϱ_{isf} calculated assuming that the resistivity of the extracellular pathway goes up 8.5 times in isosmotic solution in which all ion concentrations have been diluted 10-fold.

ϱ_j calculated assuming a myoplasmic resistivity (R_i) of 140 Ω-cm (at 37° C) for cat cardiac muscle and 240 Ω-cm (at 22° C) for frog sartorius; these values become 167 and 296 Ω-cm, respectively, when corrected for the ISF space (R_i/Vol_{isf}).

R_{mj} (uncorrected calculated assuming 67 junctions/cm (cell length of 150 μm) and no convolutions of disk. The corrected R_{mj} calculated on the assumption of a 6.4-fold increase in surface area due to convolutions obtained from the tortuosity ratio of 2.5 for cat cardiac muscle measured by Sperelakis and Rubio. The R_{mj} value is for only one membrane of the junction.

Values given in parentheses are the calculated values for the transverse direction.

Table modified from Sperelakis and Macdonald [32].

the applied current must pass through the cell-to-cell pathway, and so the tissue impedance should be more sensitive to the frequency. In contrast to these results on cardiac muscle, the longitudinal tissue impedance of frog skeletal muscle (sartorius) was independent of frequency, consistent with the absence of transverse cell membranes, i.e., the fibers are long cables.

From the above resistivity and impedance data, calculations gave the following values for cardiac muscle: $R_{md} = 288\,\Omega \times cm^2$; $C_{md} = 6.8\,\mu F/cm^2$; $Vol_{ISF} = 16\%$ (Table 1). The resistance of the cell pathway was about 20× greater than that for the ISF pathway, whereas in skeletal muscle, this ratio was only 0.75 (Table 1) [8, 32].

Transverse resistivity

In parallel-fibered muscle bundles, the electrical resistance or resistance to diffusion should be several times greater in the radial compared to the axial directions relative to fiber orientation. Therefore, the extracellular fluid of a muscle bundle itself acts as a cable, and one must distinguish between length constants of the tissue and of the cells (or fibers). To examine this point, a physical model to represent the extracellular fluid of a bundle of parallel cardiac muscle fibers was constructed by using glass rods and Tyrode solution [8]. With the packing of rods used, the electrical resistivity of the 'tissue' in the transverse direction was seven times that in the longitudinal direction. In actual cardiac muscle, this ratio can be much larger because of the smaller ECF space and the more flattened profile of cell cross-sections. The ratio can theoretically approach infinity with special packing.

An electrical analog circuit representing diffusion in the extracellular fluid of a bundle of cardiac muscle fibers was also constructed [8]. Bullet-shaped potential profiles (at 1/e) were obtained from the electric analog for any longitudinal section passing through the core of the 'bundle' of 0.5 mm radius for different resistance ratios. If the length constant (λ) is arbitrarily taken as the point where the potential falls to 1/e (37%), this analog gives an average tissue λ for a bundle of 500 μm radius of about 0.53 mm (λ' at the core of over 0.9 mm) if the ratio of diffusion coefficients in the longitudinal/radial directions is taken as 8. Weidmann [33] actually found that λ_{Br} for Br^- diffusion in 0.4 mm radius cardiac bundles, Br^- being used as an extracellular marker, was approximately 0.5 mm.

Theoretical calculations were also made for diffusion in parallel-fibered muscle bundles using the diffusion equations [8]. Calculations were made for bundles having radii of 0.4 mm and 1.0 mm. The curves were sums of exponentials, but approached a single exponential at the larger ratios. There was reasonably close agreement between the theoretical calculations and the electrical analog measurements. Therefore, the long apparent 'length constants' measured by any extracellular means can be due entirely to ion movements through the extracellular fluid and need not have any direct bearing on the resistance of the intercalated disks.

The transverse resistivity of cardiac muscle bundles was 11.4-fold greater than the longitudinal resistivity, thus indicating that the tissue bundle acts as a cable (Table 1) [32]. Because of this electrical anisotropy, this could account, at least in part, for the fact that measurements of length constant made with extracellular application of current give relatively long values of about 0.8–1.6 mm (e.g., see [10]). That is, it is possible that measurements of λ, made by extracellular application of current, do not allow conclusions as to the cell-to-cell coupling resistance (see [8]). With intracellular application of current, very short equivalent λ values are obtained [8, 29, 34].

Cable analysis in cardiac bundles

It was demonstrated using physical analogs (glass rod model) and electrical analogs that muscle bundles composed of parallel fibers act as a cable [8]. Such muscle bundles behave as a cable because the resistivity of the tissue in the transverse (or any radial) direction is much higher (10–20×) than that in the longitudinal direction [32]. In other words, the diffusion coefficient for a small ion, such as Na^+ or Cl^- through the interstitial fluid (ISF) space, would be much lower in the transverse direction because of the tortuosity factor. A theoretical and mathematical analysis of this problem of diffusion in a bundle was also made [35]. Thus, the ISF space of the bundle acts as a cable because, from within the core of the bundle, the transverse resistance is 10–20× greater than the longitudinal resistance. This fits the definition of a cable, which is two relatively low-resistance conductors separated by a relatively high transverse resistance. The second longitudinal conductor is the fluid bathing the outer surface of the bundle. Therefore, the cable properties of the muscle cells themselves must be distinguished from those of parallel-fibered muscle bundles.

The cable behavior of muscle bundles can explain why measurements of the length (space) constant (λ) by extracellular methods give values much longer (e.g., 0.8–1.6 mm) than those obtained by intracellular injection of current (e.g., 70–200 μm, which is about the length of one cell). (For a summary of these values, the tissue used, and the references, see Table 5 in the article by Sperelakis [8].) Therefore, depending on whether the current was applied intracellularly or extracellularly, opposite conclusions would be reached with respect to the resistivity of the cell-to-cell junctions (e.g., the intercalated disks in the case of cardiac muscle) and whether contiguous cells were connected by low-resistance pathways. (When a very large current is injected intracellularly (e.g., >1 μA), it behaves as an extracellularly-applied current and produces a measurable membrane potential change in adjacent cells, which gives a long apparent length constant value that is artifactual.) It has been concluded in a number of publications, based on the findings of a long λ from extracellular application of current or ^{42}K [8, 33], that the cells are connected by low-resistance pathways, since λ was several times greater than one cell length. Arguments were developed and proposed in the article by Sperelakis [8] that the cell-to-cell resistance cannot be determined from experiments in which current is applied extracellularly.

To further analyze this problem, a bundle of closely-packed parallel fibers embedded in an interstitial fluid (ISF) space, and bathed in a large volume conductor, was modeled by an electrical circuit analog. To simplify the model, only one fiber tract imbedded deep within the bundle core, consisting of 20 cells linked end to end in a chain configuration, was represented and linked to the equivalent circuit for the ISF space at each cell in the chain. The electrical circuit representing the configuration of passive cell elements plus the surrounding extracellular space is shown in Figure 4. Since all voltage measurements were made under steady-state conditions, the capacitive elements in the cell membrane could be ignored. These studies were carried out by Sperelakis and Picone [36].

The results showed that for cells not connected with low-resistance pathways, a relatively long λ can be obtained if current is applied extracellularly. That is, the length constant of the external bundle cable (λ_b) determines the apparent λ value measured intracellularly (λ_f) in such a situation. Therefore, λ values measured by extracellular application of current should not be used to determine whether contiguous cells are connected by low-resistance pathways.

λ_f and λ_b had values of about 3.2 cl under standard conditions, which included a ratio of resistivities of the bundle ($r_{ot}/2r_{ol}$ ratio) of 10 : 1 (Figs 5, 6). When the $r_{ot}/2r_{ol}$ ratio was increased to 20 : 1, λ_f and λ_b increased to 4.5 cl. If the cell length is about 200 μm, then a λ_f of 4.5 cl is equivalent to 0.90 mm, which is in the vicinity of the experimentally measured values.

The length constant of the inner fiber cable is strongly influenced by the outer bundle cable. In fact, there is a 1 : 1 dependence of λ_f on λ_b (see Fig. 7). The outer bundle cable facilitates the electrotonic spread of current along the fiber, allowing more current flow down the fiber's length than would otherwise occur, giving an apparent λ_f of about 3.2 cell lengths (cl) under standard conditions. Indeed, in the absence of this outer bundle cable, the apparent length constant of the fiber falls greatly (λ_f <1 cl). Thus, λ_b has a large influence on λ_f. In contrast, the inner fiber cable has a negligible influence on the outer bundle cable; its presence or absence does not substantially alter the bundle length constant.

Lowering r_{md} had very little effect on λ_b, with or without r_{jc} connected. Lowering r_{md}, with or without r_{jc} connected, had little effect on λ_f, until r_{md} was lowered to 1/800th or less of its standard value. In contrast, when the outer bundle cable was disconnected, lowering r_{md} had a large effect on λ_f, as expected from the cable equation. Since the present analysis applies regardless of the actual mechanism of cell-to-cell interaction, i.e. whether the resistance between cells is low or high, one cannot conclude about the nature of cell-to-cell coupling from measurements of length constant in a muscle bundle using extracellularly applied current.

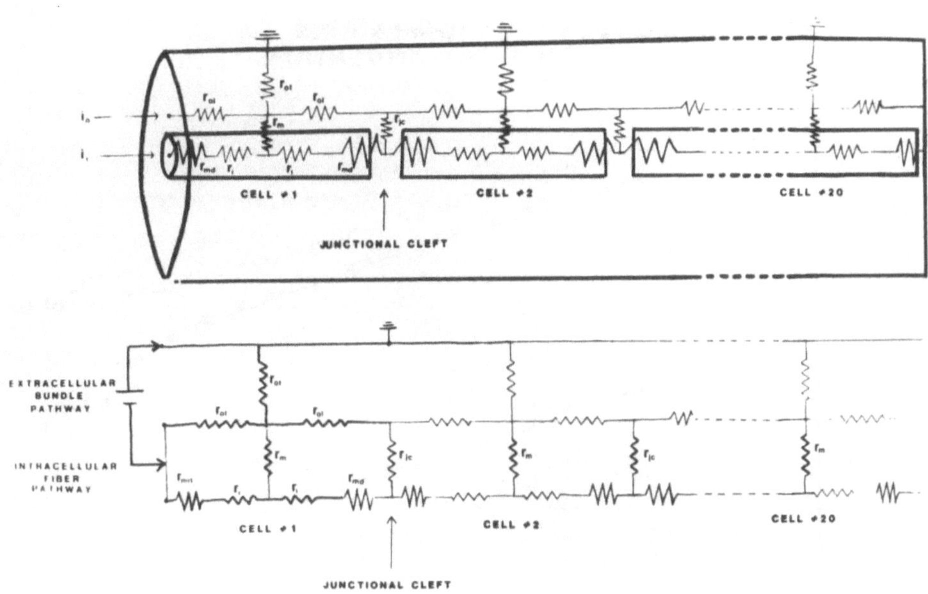

Figure 4. Circuit used for the electrical analog model for cable analysis of bundles of cardiac muscle or smooth muscle. A fiber pathway, composed of a chain of 20 cells in series connected end to end, is depicted deep within the core of a muscle bundle composed of many fibers orderly packed in parallel to one another in part A. The circuit details are shown more clearly, with the cells and bundle superimposed, in part B. The surface of the muscle bundle is bathed in a large volume of Ringer solution which serves as a large volume conductor and is at ground potential. In the standard model, the end (junctional) membranes have a high resistivity equal to that of the surface cell membrane, i.e., the contiguous cells are not connected by low-resistance tunnels; r_{md} is the resistance of these membranes, prorated for surface area. As depicted, r_{jc} is the radial resistance of the junctional cleft. r_m is the transmembrane resistance of each cell surface membrane; r_i is the equivalent internal longitudinal resistance (myoplasmic) of half of the cell length; r_{ol} is the equivalent external (outside) longitudinal resistance of the interstitial fluid (ISF) between fiber tracts; r_{ot} is the equivalent (outside) transverse resistance of the ISF space. Because of tortuosity in the transverse direction through the bundle, the ratio of resistivities ($r_{ot}/2r_{ol}$) is about 10. The values used for all circuit parameters are listed in Table 1. Current was injected into one end of the bundle by applying a battery between ground and the intracellular fiber pathway (i_i) and extracellular bundle pathway (i_o), as depicted. Taken from Sperelakis and Picone [36].

If the current is injected intracellularly only into cell 1 of the 20-cell chain, then an enormous discontinuity in potential along the inner fiber cable occurs, which is confined primarily to cell 1 but slightly to cell 2 as well (Fig. 8). However, beginning with cell 3 and beyond, the voltage profiles and λ_b and λ_f values are unchanged from those depicted in Figures 5 and 6. Therefore, currents injected intracellularly behave as if they were applied extracellulary with respect to cells distant from the point of current injection. The results were similar when current was injected intracellularly into cell 11, except that the discontinuity was symmetrical, as expected, on both sides of the current injection point. This distortion

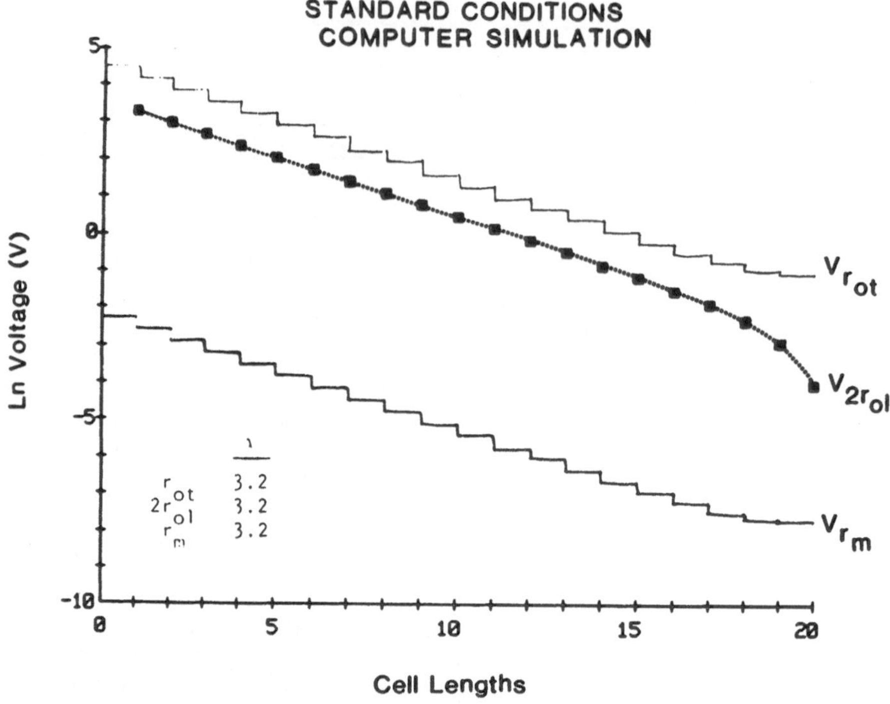

Figure 5. Computer simulation of fall-off of steady-state voltage with distance (cell lengths) under standard conditions. At lower left, values for the length constant (λ) are shown, as measured from the spatial decay of voltage across the extracellular transverse resistances (r_{ot}),the paired extracellular longitudinal resistances ($2r_{ol}$), and the membrane resistance (r_m), respectively. As can be seen, there is some disturbance of the exponential decay of potential at the termination of the bundle. Two curves in the figure were drawn to reflect the discontinuities in potential along the outer bundle cable and inner fiber cable, due to the use of lumped single resistors to represent the resistive parameters for each cell and its surrounding fluid. Taken from Sperelakis and Picone [36].

quickly dissipates as the current flows away from the point of injection. The large voltage discontinuity in the injected cell and somewhat in its immediate neighbor is caused by the high-resistance junctions in the model (under standard conditions), i.e., the lack of low-resistance connections between cells. The slightly larger voltage drop in the neighboring cell is the result of an increased amount of current flowing directly between the injected cell and its neighbor across the cell junction.

Hence, length constant measurements, made using bundles of muscle fibers, are not sufficient to make any conclusions regarding the degree of cell-to-cell coupling in the fibers. As was shown above, this is because the relatively long length constant of the bundle (e.g., 0.8–1.6 mm, depending on bundle diameter and cell packing [8]) is the primary determinant of the voltage decay measured intracellularly along the fiber. In cases where low-resistance connections between

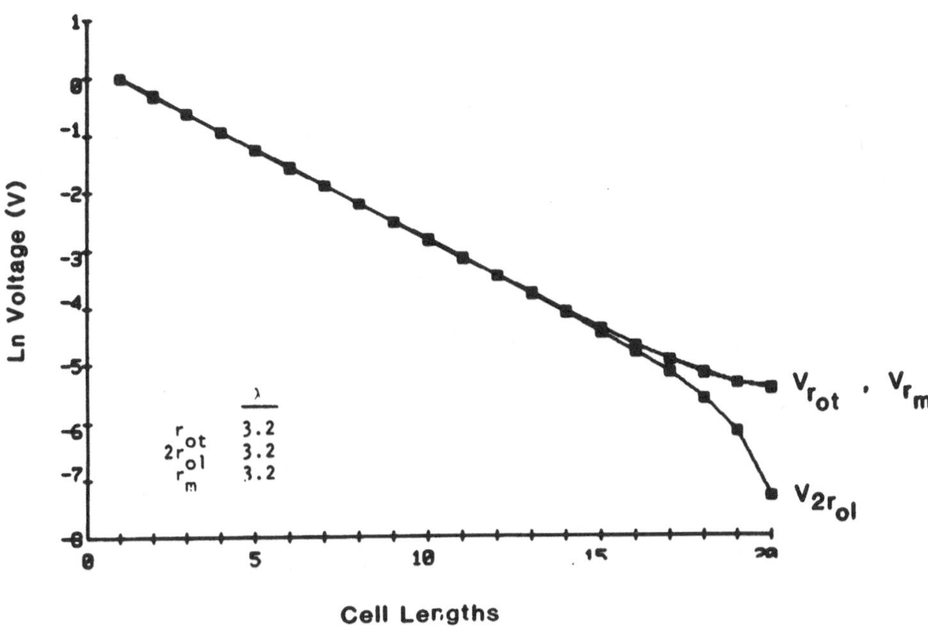

Figure 6. Fall-off of steady-state voltage with distance (cell lengths) under standard conditions plotted in a normalized fashion with respect to the voltage across cell 1. At lower left, values for the length constant (λ) are shown, as measured from the spatial decay of voltage across the extracellular transverse resistances (r_{ot}), the paired extracellular longitudinal resistances ($2r_{ol}$), and the membrane resistances (r_m). Taken from Sperelakis and Picone [36].

contiguous cells are assumed not to exist, a long apparent length constant would still be obtained. That is, a long length constant does not reflect low-resistance connections between cells in a fiber, but rather reflects the long length constant of the bundle.

Thus, measurements of cell-to-cell coupling, based on the use of an Abe-Tomita bath chamber [37], should be re-evaluated. This overriding influence of the bundle length constant probably accounts for results obtained by a number of laboratories, in which they found that conditions which varied the number of gap junctions had little or no apparent effect on the length constant as measured in an Abe-Tomita chamber [37–39]. For example, Daniel et al. [38] noted that the length constants for the circular and longitudinal layers of the large intestine are nearly identical despite the large difference in the number of gap junctions in these tissues.

In summary, the long length constant values obtained for bundles of parallel-packed fibers by extracellular application of polarizing current (e.g., 0.8–1.6 mm)

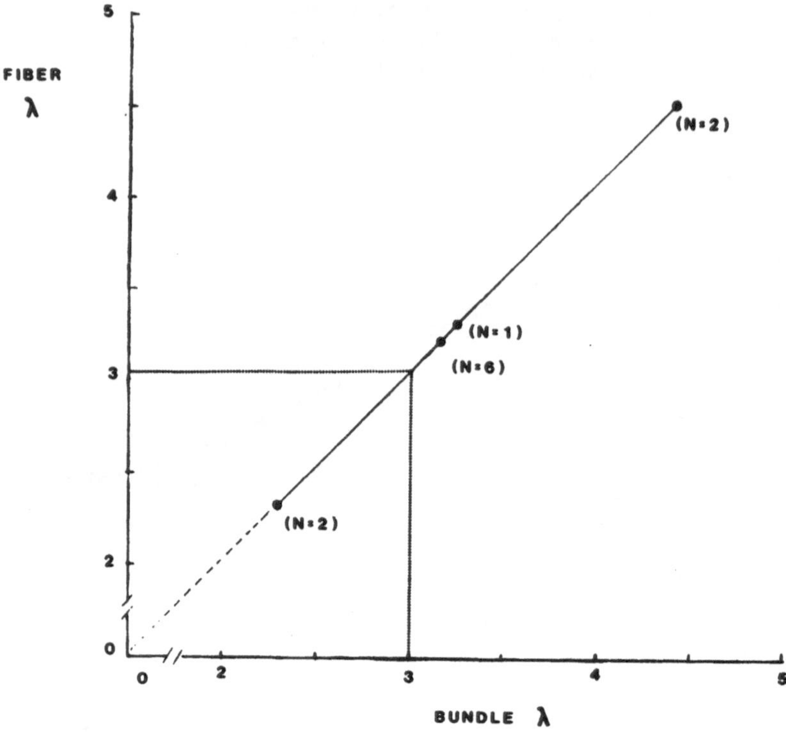

Figure 7. Graphic plot of the data from the computer simulations showing the dependence of the length constant of the cell pathway (fiber λ) on the length constant of the interstitial fluid pathway (bundle λ). The straight line drawn through the data points has a slope of 1.0 and extrapolates through the origin, and indicates that the bundle λ completely determines the measured fiber λ. The values for λ are given in arbitrary units of cell length. The numbers given in parenthesis near each data point indicate the number of data points averaged, all of which were identical values. Bundle λ was changed by varying the r_{ot}/r_{ol} ratio. Taken from Sperelakis and Picone [36].

are primarily due to the long length constant of the extracellular space, not of the fiber. Thus, these values do not necessarily reflect low-resistance junctions between the short cardiac muscle or smooth muscle cells. Such measurements of length constant, therefore, should not be used as a measure of cell-to-cell resistance. Thus, traditional measurements of cell-to-cell coupling should be questioned, and probably accounts for results obtained by several investigators in which they found that conditions which varied the number of gap junctions had little or no apparent effect on the cell-to-cell resistance.

High-resistance coupling

From the above, it appears that there is some doubt about the validity of the low-

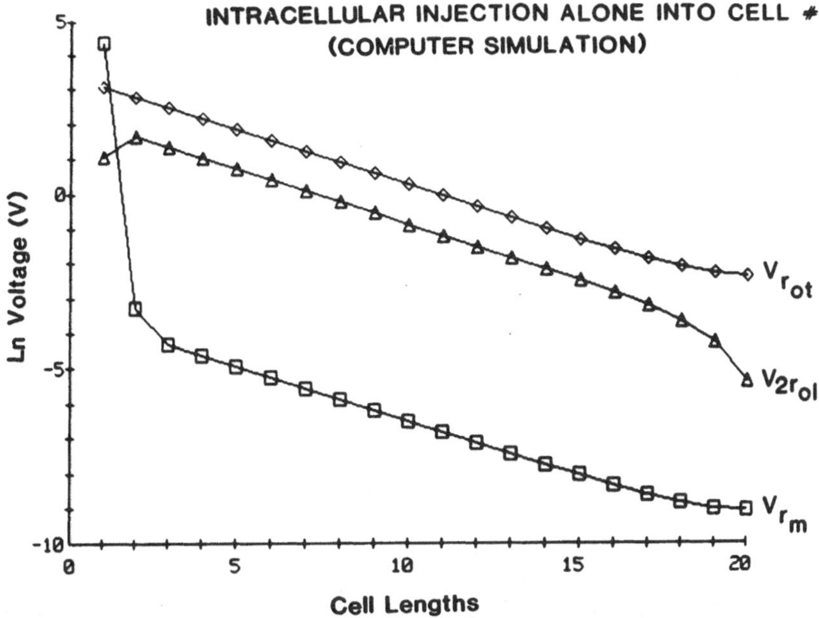

Figure 8. Potential profile observed when current was applied to the inner fiber cable only, by injecting intracellularly into Cell 1. The fall-off in potential along the inner fiber cable (V_{r_m}) is indicated by the square symbols, and the fall-off along the outer bundle cable is indicated by the diamonds ($V_{r_{ot}}$) and triangles ($V_{2r_{ol}}$). There was an enormous discontinuity in potential along the inner fiber cable between the first few cells. Currents injected intracellularly behave as if injected extracellularly with respect to distant cells. Taken from Sperelakis and Picone [36].

resistance coupling hypothesis for adult cardiac muscle. The purpose of this section is to present several alternative possibilities based on high-resistance coupling between the cells.

K^+ accumulation model

A normal cell constituent such as K^+ ion could serve as a chemical messenger. During depolarization, the electrochemical driving force for net outward K^+ current increases instantaneously. Therefore, efflux of K^+ across all surfaces of the cell will suddenly increase during the rising phase of the action potential, if K^+ conductance (g_K) remains constant. The K^+ effluxing across the surface sarcolemma will tend to diffuse rapidly into and mix with the bulk ISF. However, the K^+ effluxing into the narrow intercalated disk (ID) cleft will accumulate and tend to depolarize the post-junctional membrane. A theoretical analysis [12] indicated that the K^+ concentration in the ID cleft would increase from a baseline level of 4 mM to about 10 mM within 1 msec (for a g_K of 0.01 S/cm^2 and gap width of 100 Å)

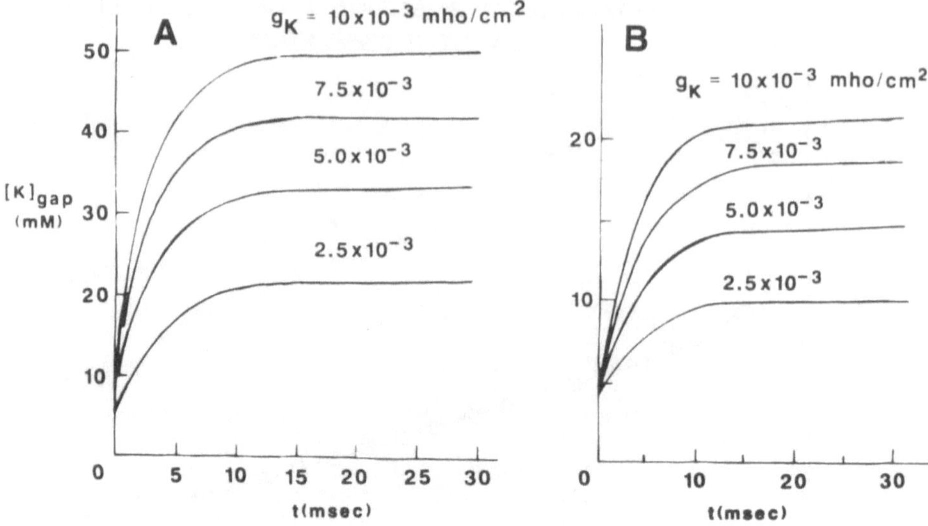

Figure 9. Potassium accumulation in the intercalated disk cleft during excitation of the pre-junctional cell based on theoretical calculations. K^+ concentration in the center of the junctional gap ($[K]_{jc}$) is given as a function of time in msec. It was assumed that the initial $[K]_{jc}$ value was 4 mM, and the resting potential was −90 mV. The curves were calculated for the four different K^+ conductance (g_K) values indicated. A: gap width of 50 Å. B: gap width of 200 Å. Figure modified from Macdonald et al. [12].

(Fig. 9). Such a K^+ accumulation is sufficient to decrease E_K across the post-junctional membrane by about 20 mV, which is close to the critical depolarization required to reach threshold. The K^+ accumulation was even greater if the effective junctional gap width was decreased. Thus, K^+ accumulation may be at least a contributory factor in the transmission process.

Page and McCallister [40] proposed that transient ion accumulations occurring in the ID cleft might be electrophysiologically important. By use of K^+-sensitive micro-electrodes, Kline and Morad [41] demonstrated that a K^+ accumulation of 1–2 mM occurs in the ISF of frog ventricular strips during each action potential. They suggested that much greater K^+ accumulations would occur in narrow clefts such as at the cell junctions.

Consistent with the view that K^+ accumulation in the ID cleft may be important in the transfer of the signal are the observations that propagation velocity

a. increases (to a maximum) when $[K]_o$ is elevated about two-fold, and
b. decreases to about 50% when cardiac muscle bundles are equilibrated in two-fold hypertonic solution to increase the cleft volume [13].

It was demonstrated that extracellular K^+ accumulation mediates a specific neuronal interaction between giant interneurons of the cockroach (Periplaneta) that are not electrotonically coupled by low-resistance connections [42]. A single action potential was capable of generating a large depolarization in an adjacent neuron. Intracellular injection of TEA^+ increased the duration of the action potential of the injected cell while reducing the postsynaptic depolarization, thus indicating that K^+ accumulation was the mechanism of the postsynaptic potential.

Electric field model

In the electric field model, the electrical field that develops in the narrow cleft between two contiguous cells during the course of an action potential in one cell is the mechanism for the transfer of excitation. The circuit used for the model is depicted in Fig. 10. When the prejunctional membrane fires, the cleft between the cells becomes negative with respect to ground (the interstitial fluid surrounding the cells), and this negative cleft potential acts to depolarize the post-junctional membrane (by an equal amount) to its threshold. This, in turn, brings the surface membrane of the post-junctional cell to threshold. The inner surface of the post-junctional membrane remains at nearly constant potential with respect to ground. Thus, virtually no local-circuit current flows through the post-junctional cell, and intercellular transmission occurs electrically without low-resistance connnections between cells.

A number of mechanisms can be invoked to allow the pre-junctional membrane to fire a fraction of a millisecond before the immediately adjacent surface membrane, including: a slightly lower threshold (increased $\bar{g}_{Na}$), slightly lower capacitance (time constant), slightly faster kinetics of activation of the fast Na^+ conductance of the junctional membranes, or K^+ accumulation in the junctional cleft.

In a further development of the model, the modified Hodgkin-Huxley equations [43, 44] were incorporated to make the model conform more closely with known membrane behavior, and the effect of varying the dynamics of the gates of the cation channels on transmission capabilities of the model was determined [45, 46].

Subsequently, we expanded the model to a chain of six cells, and we altered its mathematical formulation to allow greater flexibility in varying the individual cell membrane parameters. It was demonstrated that the electric field model allows propagation at a constant velocity down the entire chain of cells (Fig. 11). In addition, we examined the effect of increasing the extracellular resistances and the radial cleft resistance on propagation, including doing a 'sucrose-gap' type of simulation. With the parameters used, propagation occurred at a velocity of about 0.17 m/sec. Raising the extracellular resistances, ROL and ROR, along the entire 6-cell chain up to 4-fold slowed propagation only slightly; however, when the radial cleft resistance, RJC, was varied concomitantly (as should occur in the biological situation) then there was a marked slowing of propagation velocity, e.g., to 3.3 cm/s (24% of control) in 4.0× resistance. Variation of RJC alone had a similar effect (Fig. 12). The optimal RJC value for peak velocity was 10 MΩ. Higher values of RJC depressed the velocity, although the effect was relatively

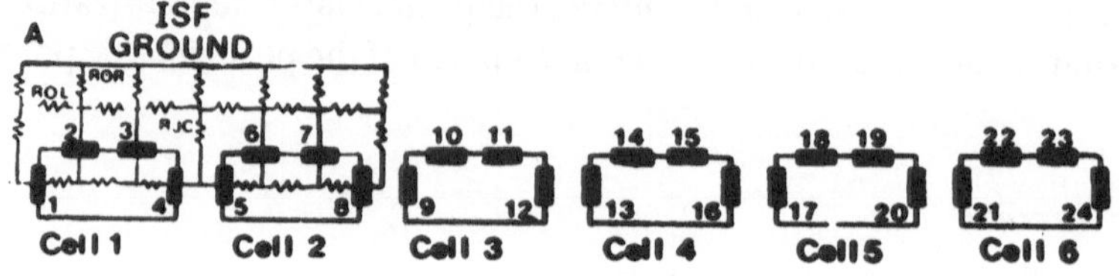

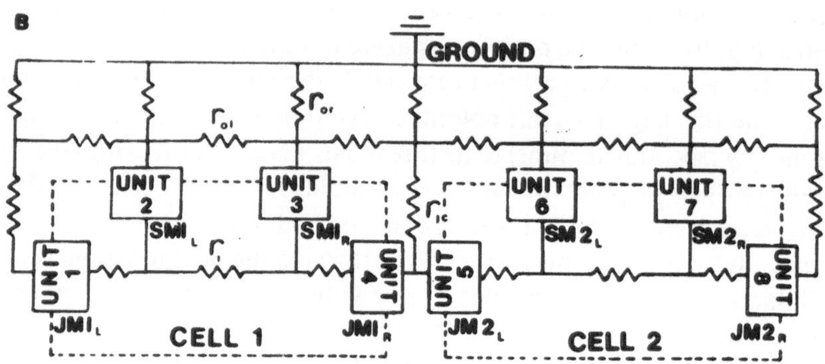

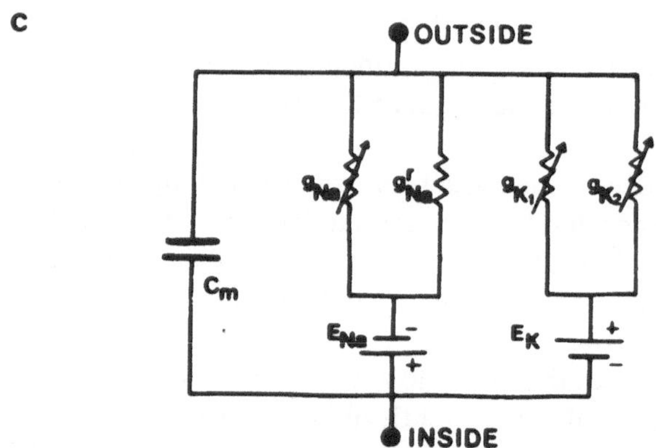

Figure 10. Schematic diagram of the chain of six myocardial cells modelled for computer simulation of the electric field interactions between cells in the narrow junctional clefts. A: the chain of 6 cells, numbered sequentially. Each cell was composed of four Hodgkin-Huxley (H-H) units, one for each junctional membrane and two for the surface membrane (one for the left half of the cell, and the other for the right half of the cell). The H-H units are numbered serially from 1 to 24 in the 6 cells. B: enlarged diagram of the first two cells in the chain, showing the four H-H units for each cell, the external resistance (r_{ol} and r_{or}) and internal resistance (r_i), and the radial junctional cleft resistance (r_{jc}). Ground is the bulk interstitial fluid bathing the bundle. C: the equivalent circuit for each H-H unit is depicted. C_m = membrane capacitance; E_{Na}, E_K = the equilibrium potentials for Na^+ and K^+; g^r_{Na} = resting Na^+ conductance; g_{Na} = voltage-dependent Na^+ conductance; g_{KI} = inward-going K^+ conductance; g_K = outward-going delayed rectifier K^+ conductance. Figure taken from Sperelakis et al. [58].

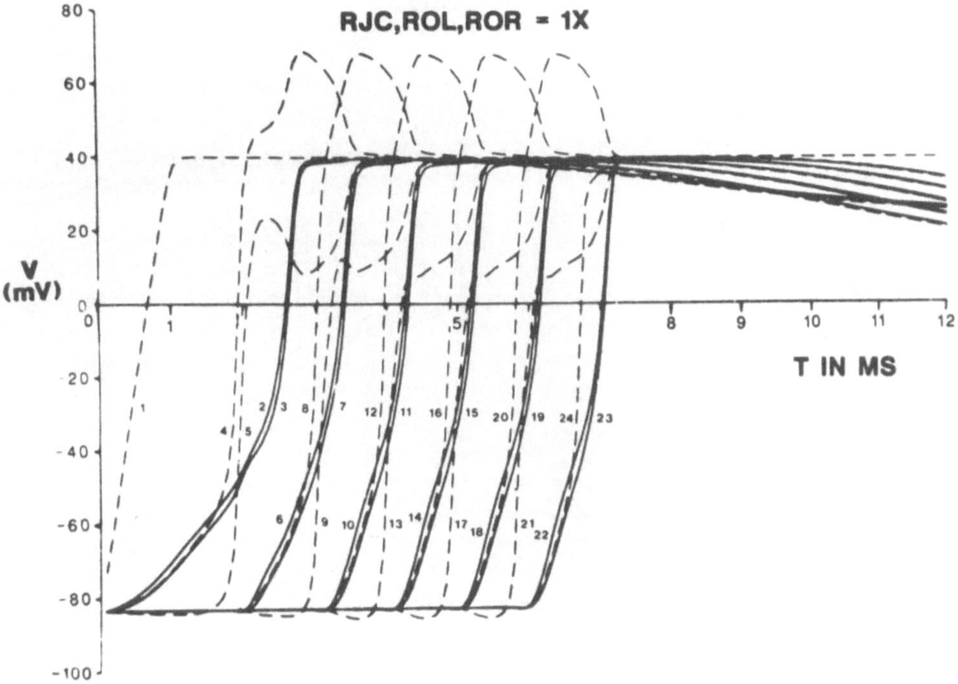

Figure 11. Successful propagation of action potentials at constant velocity along a chain of six cells under standard conditions of the model. All external resistances [ROL (r_{ol}), ROR (r_{or}), RJC (r_{jc})] are equal to 1x. The ordinate gives the membrane potential (in mV) and the abscissa gives the time (in msec). Unit 1 is driven by an applied ramp depolarization. The traces are numbered 1 to 24 to indicate the respective H-H units. Propagation velocity was 17.1 cm/sec. Figure taken from Sperelakis et al. [58].

small at 2-fold RJC (20 MΩ) (Fig. 13). Lowering RJC to about 0.6× (6 MΩ) slowed the propagation velocity slightly, but further lowering of RJC to 5 MΩ and lower caused failure of propagation (Fig. 13). Lowering of ROL and ROR up to 8-fold had essentially no effect on velocity of propagation (Fig. 13).

In a sucrose-gap type of simulation, raising the resistance of the extracellular fluid bathing the middle two cells, up to 3 times the normal value, slowed down propagation velocity in the sucrose-gap region (Fig. 14). Raising this resistance to 4 times blocked propagation through this region. $+\dot{V}_{max}$ of both the surface membrane and junctional membrane decreased as a function of the external resistance. Part of the slowing of propagation velocity and $+\dot{V}_{max}$ of the action potentials and block in the sucrose gap region may be attributed to the lowering of the Na^+ equilibrium potential (E_{Na}) that results from lowering of $[Na]_o$ (in order to raise r_o). This lowers the electrochemical driving force ($E_m - E_{Na}$) for inward fast Na^+ current during the rising phase of the action potential, and hence lowers $+\dot{V}_{max}$ and peak overshoot potential of the action potentials (APs). (r_o was

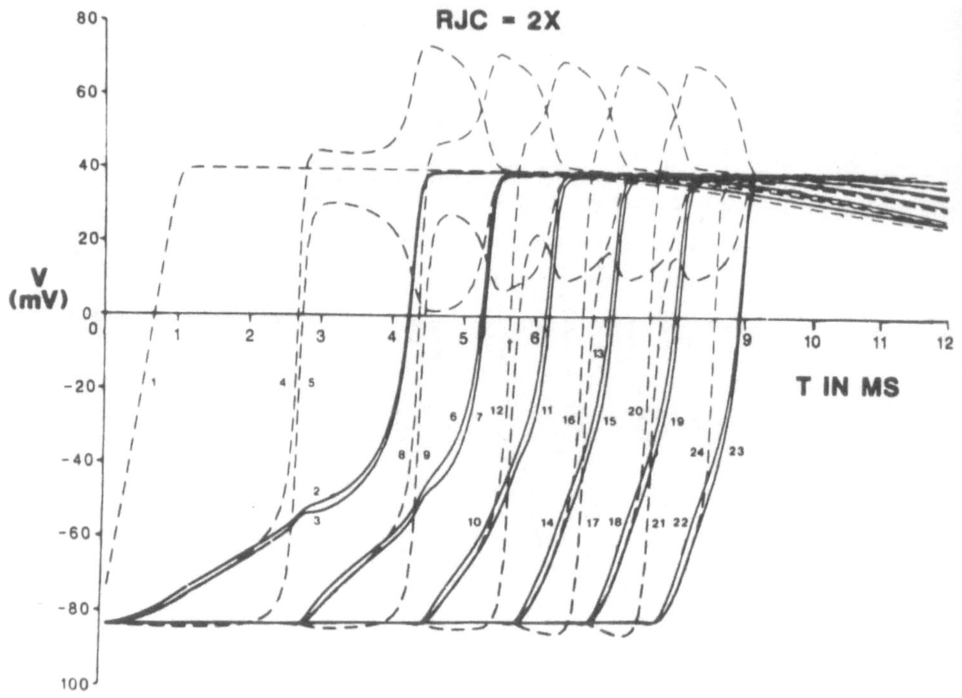

Figure 12. Propagation of action potentials under conditions in which the radial junctional cleft resistance (RJC) alone was increased by 2-fold along the entire chain of 6 cells. This had a significant effect to slow down propagation velocity ($\bar{\theta}$). $\bar{\theta}$ was 16.1 cm/sec, as compared to 17.1 cm/sec under the standard conditions (RJC = 1x) illustrated in Fig. 11. Figure taken from Sperelakis et al. [58].

increased by lowering $[Na]_o$ and $[Cl]_o$ only; $[K]_o$, and hence E_K, was not changed.) The other reason for the lowering of propagation velocity in the sucrose-gap region is the fact that RJC of the junction in the center of the gap (between cells 3 and 4) was increased proportionally to ROL and ROR, and hence this acts to slow propagation, as described above for the experiment in which the external resistances were varied uniformly along the entire chain of 6 cells.

Thus, the electric field model allows propagation of excitation at constant velocity down a chain of cells not connected by low-resistance tunnels, and propagation velocity is dependent on the extracellular resistance, and particularly on RJC. Hence, this model can account for many of the facts observed biologically.

Combined K^+ accumulation and electric field models

We have recently combined the K^+ accumulation model with the electric field model. By incorporating the likely possibility of rapid K^+ accumulation in the

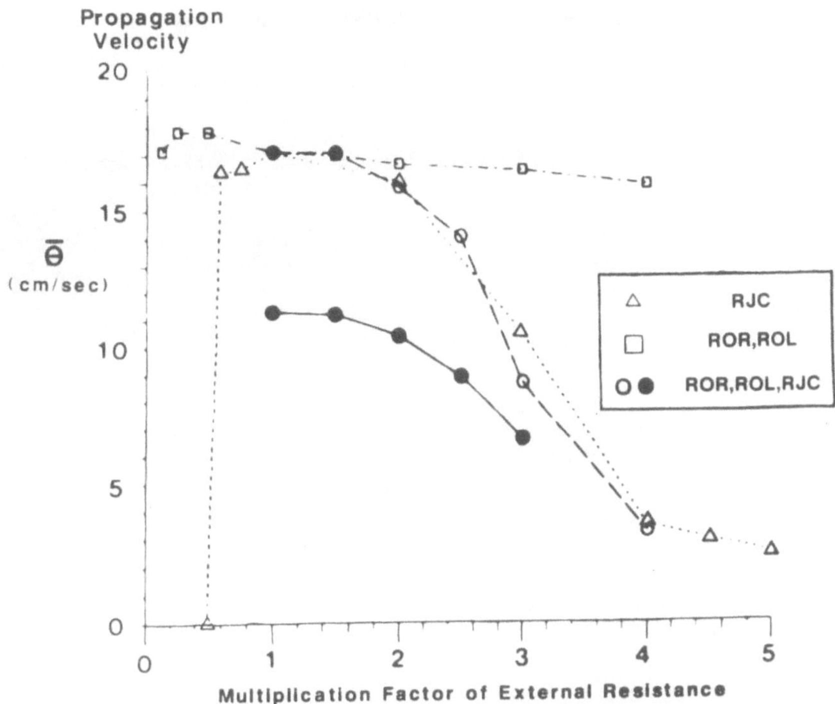

Figure 13. Graphic summary of data for average propagation velocity ($\bar{\theta}$) as a function of the external resistances along the entire chain of 6 cells. The value of 1.0 on the abscissa represents the standard resistance parameters used in the model. When ROL, ROR, and RJC were increased simultaneously to 1.5×, 2.0×, 2.5×, 3.0×, and 4.0× times the standard values, $\bar{\theta}$ was greatly decreased (circle symbols in figure). When only ROL and ROR were increased, there was only a slight decrease in $\bar{\theta}$ (square symbols). Decrease in ROL and ROR to $^1/_2$×, $^1/_4$×, and $^1/_8$× times also had little effect on $\bar{\theta}$. When RJC alone was increased (triangle symbols), the decrease in $\bar{\theta}$ was about as great as when all three external resistances were varied. Lowering RJC to 0.7× and 0.6× had little effect, but lowering to 0.5× produced an abrupt failure of propagation. Thus, there was only a relatively small effect of RJC between 6 MΩ (0.6×) and 20 MΩ (2×). When $\bar{g}_{Na}$ of the junctional membranes was set to equal to that for the surface membranes (400 mS/cm^2), $\bar{\theta}$ was slowed (filled circles). Figure taken from Sperelakis et al. [58].

junctional cleft into the electric field model, we expected that this will facilitate the transmission process. In turn, this should allow all electrical properties of the junctional membranes to be identical to those of the surface membrane and yet achieve successful transmission. The safety factor for transmission should also be enhanced.

The six cell chain simulation was modified to allow for K^+ ion accumulation in the ID clefts. K^+ ions were allowed to diffuse out of the pre- and post-junctional membranes into the junctional cleft. Computer simulations were made with and without K^+ accumulation to determine the effect of K^+ ion accumulation in the

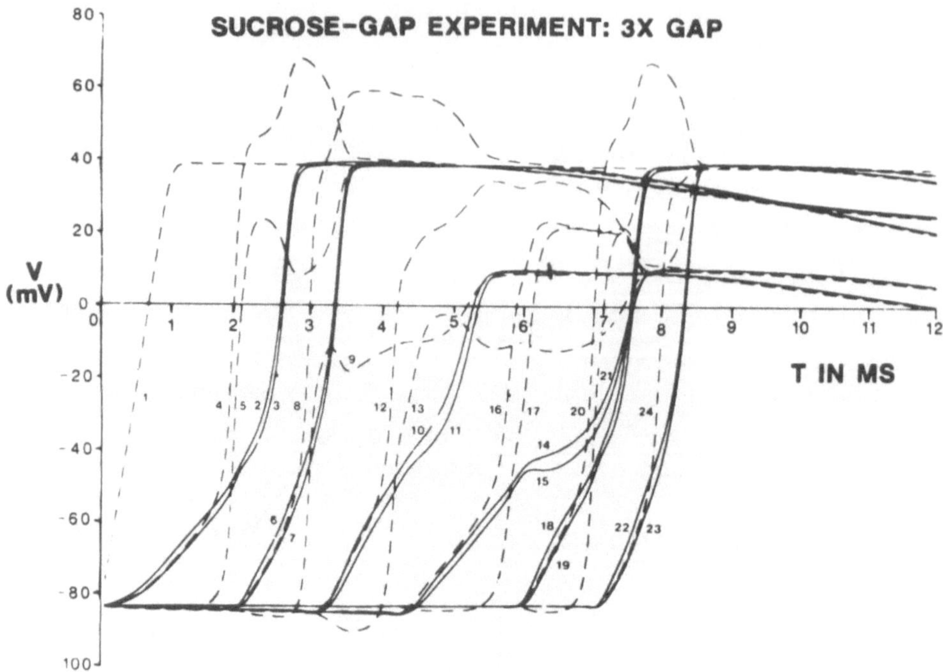

Figure 14. Sucrose-gap-type of experiment in which the external resistances (ROL, ROR, RJC) were increased by 3-fold along only the middle two cells (Cells 3 and 4) of the 6-cell chain. The external resistances were raised by the equivalent of replacing two-thirds of the NaCl in the solution bathing the sucrose-gap region with an equi-osmolar amount of sucrose. Since the Na^+ equilibrium potential (E_{Na}) was decreased in the sucrose-gap region (assumes that $[Na]_i$ remained constant), this accounts for the smaller overshoot of the action potentials in Cells 3 and 4. Note that propagation velocity (θ) and $+\dot{V}_{max}$ were decreased in the two cells in the sucrose gap. θ in the sucrose gap was 6.7 cm/sec, compared to 19.8 cm/sec for the cells outside of the sucrose gap. Increasing the gap resistances to 4× caused failure of propagation in the sucrose gap region (not depicted). Figure modified from Sperelakis et al. [58].

intercalated disk clefts on propagation by the electric field mechanism. Different surface to junctional membrane capacitance ratios were used to determine the effect of this parameter on the velocity of propagation and to make propagation erratic in the absence of K^+ accumulation, so that the effect of K^+ accumulation could be assessed.

The differential equations modeling the system were of the form:

$$\frac{dE}{dt} = \bar{C}^{-1}(I - \bar{G}E), \tag{1}$$

where $\bar{C}^{-1}$ is the inverse of the capacitance matrix, $\bar{G}$ is the conductance matrix, E is the vector of voltages across the units. The derivation of the conductance matrix was given previously [16, 45].

To study the effect of K^+ accumulation, five more differential equations were used to describe the state of the system, one for each of the gaps found between the six cells [47]. The five new differential equations were of the form:

$$\frac{d[K]_{jc}}{dt} = \frac{1}{vF}(I_{Kpre} + I_{Kpost} - I_{Kpump}). \tag{2}$$

Derivation of this equation is as follows. If $[K]_{jc}$ is the concentration of K^+ in the junctional cleft and v is the volume of the cleft, then v $[K]_i$ is the total amount of K^+ in the cleft (Q). The K^+ will move into the cleft through both the pre- and post-junctional membranes (first from prejunctional membrane). If the area of a membrane facing a cleft is A, then:

$$\frac{dQ}{dt} = A(J_K^{in} - J_K^{out}), \tag{3}$$

where J_K^{in} and J_K^{out} are the amount (in moles) of K^+ per unit time per unit area moving into the cleft and out of the cleft. If the cells are very close together compared to the cleft membrane areas, then $J_K^{out} = 0$. That is, there is no significant diffusion of K^+ out of the mouth of the cleft in the short time being considered (<1 msec). The final equation obtained is:

$$\frac{dQ}{dt} = \frac{1}{F}(I_K^{pre} + I_K^{post} - I_K^{pump}). \tag{4}$$

It is assumed that the K^+ pumped is equal to the leak of K^+ down its resting electrochemical gradient into the junctional cleft:

$$I_K^{pump} = 2\,[g_{K(r)}]\,[E_r - E_K], \tag{5}$$

where the subscript r refers to the value at rest. The factor of 2 reflects the two junctional membranes.

Computer plots of the K^+ accumulation in the five junctional clefts ($[K]_{jc}$) were made. There is a K^+ efflux into the junctional cleft from the prejunctional cell during the rising phase of its action potential down an electrochemical gradient for K^+ $[(E_m - E_K)]$. There was a very large (>72 mM) and rapid (<1.0 msec) rise in $[K]_{jc}$ in each cleft in succession that correlated with propagation down the cell chain. This large increase in $[K]_{jc}$ would act to depolarize the postjunctional membrane, and so facilitate transmission of excitation by the electric field model.

Simulations were made to determine whether K^+ accumulation in the cleft has a profound effect on propagation down the entire chain of 6 cells. The results of some of these experiments are illustrated in Figures 15–17. In these figures, the upper panels (Part A) represent the situation without allowing for K^+ accumulation in the junctional cleft, and the lower panels (Part B) represent the situation

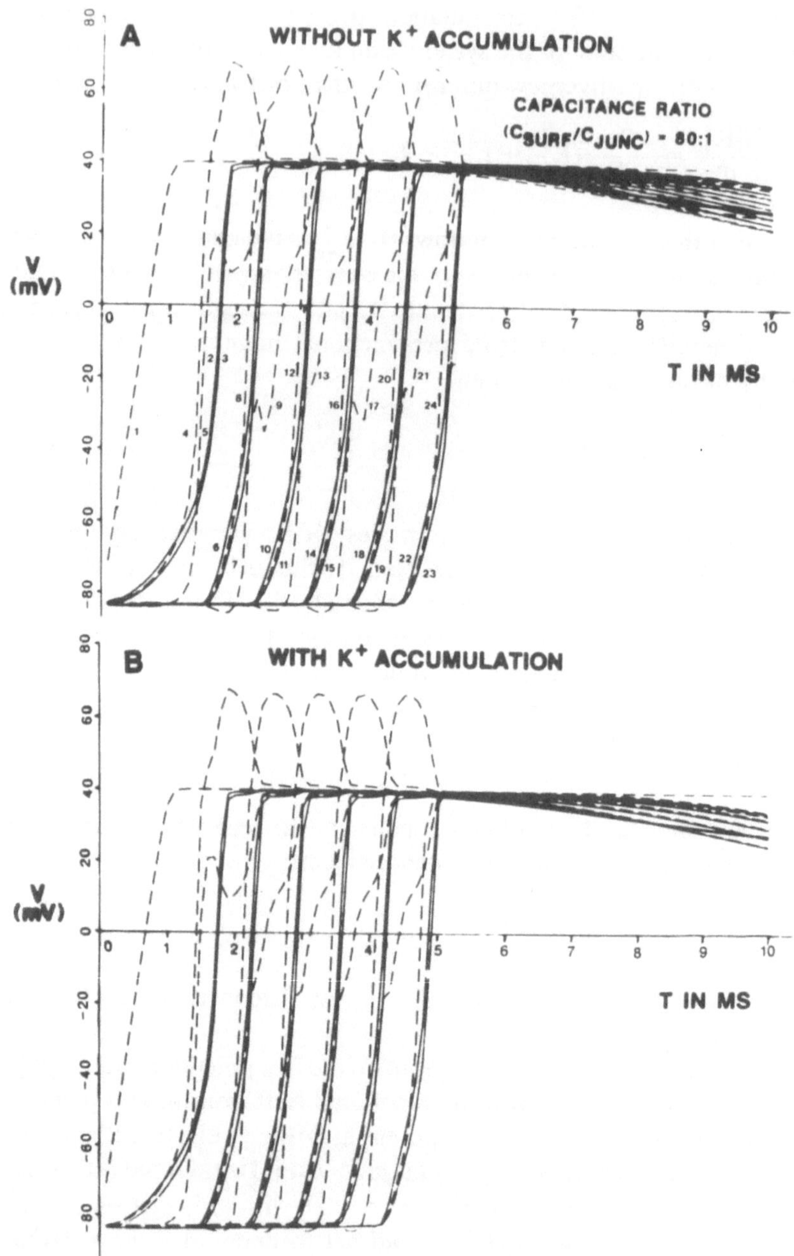

Figure 15. Effect of allowing K^+ accumulation on propagation velocity. Capacitance ratio (surface membrane to junctional membrane) of 80:1 (200 pf/2.5 pf). A: successful propagation of action potentials at constant velocity along the chain of six cells. Propagation velocity was 23.7 cm/sec. K^+ accumulation was not incorporated in this simulation. B: effect on propagation when K^+ accumulation in the cleft was incorporated. Note that the propagation velocity was slightly faster in this case: 25.5 cm/sec. Taken from Sperelakis et al. [47].

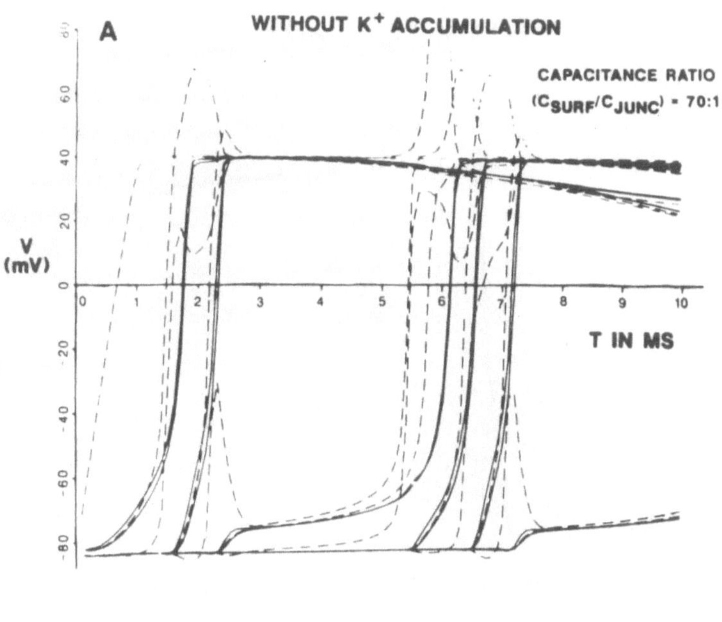

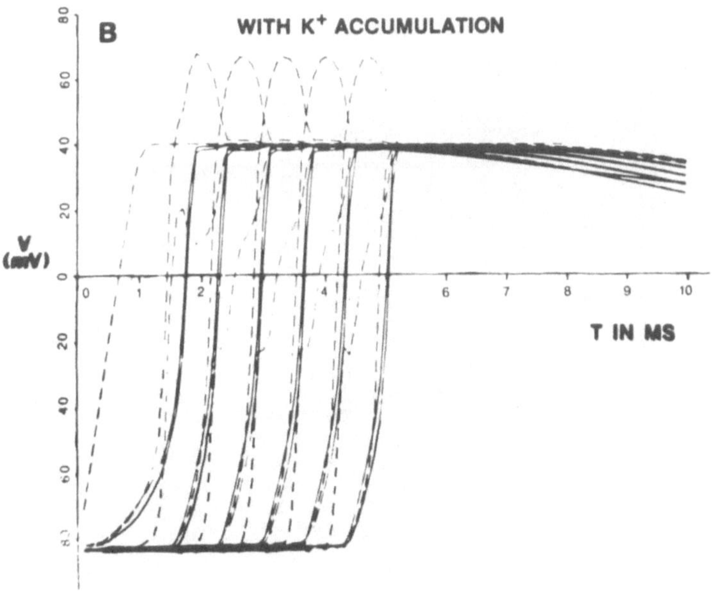

Figure 16. Effect of allowing K^+ accumulation when parameters were set so that propagation was erratic. Capacitance ratio of 70 : 1. A: erratic propagation of the action potential along the chain of cells without K^+ accumulation. B: uniform and fast propagation along the chain with K^+ accumulation. Propagation velocity was 24.6 cm/sec. Taken from Sperelakis et al. [47].

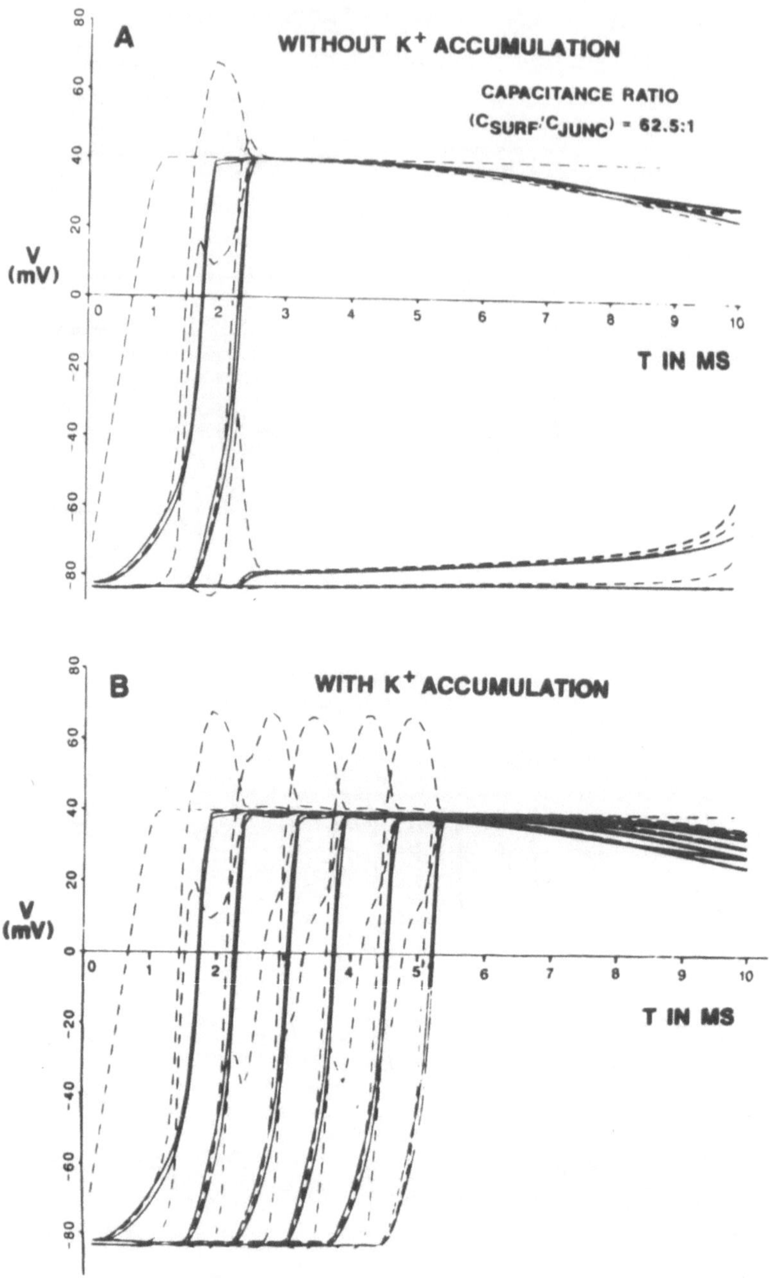

Figure 17. Effect of allowing K^+ accumulation when parameters were set so that firing was erratic. Capacitance ratio of 62.5:1. A: erratic and failure of propagation without K^+ accumulation. B: uniform and fast propagation of the action potential down the cell chain with K^+ accumulation. The propagation velocity was 23.7 cm/sec. Taken from Sperelakis et al. [47].

with incorporation of K^+ accumulation. The capacitance ratio of surface membrane to junctional membrane (C_{surf}/C_{junc}) was held constant in any such comparison. The capacitance ratios were 80 : 1 (Fig. 15), 70 : 1 (Fig. 16), and 62.5 : 1 (Fig. 17). In Figure 15, it can be seen that incorporation of K^+ accumulation speeded up the velocity of propagation. In Figures 16–17, it can be seen that allowing for K^+ accumulation changed erratic and partially blocked propagation into a regular fast propagation. The results of these experiments are summarized in Table 2. Thus, K^+ accumulation in the junctional clefts facilitates and speeds propagation by the electric field mechanism.

The effects of varying the capacitance ratio, C_{surf}/C_{junc}, on propagation was also determined. The ratio was lowered by raising the value of C_{junc} (Table 2). The effect of varying C_{surf}/C_{junc} can be discerned for the situation without K^+ accumulation by comparing the upper panels in Figures 15–17. The C_{surf}/C_{junc} ratios illustrated are: 80 : 1 (Fig. 15A), 70 : 1 (Fig. 16A), and 62.5 : 1 (Fig. 17A). At a ratio of 80 : 1 (Fig. 15A), propagation was smooth and fast. At lower ratios, propagation became slowed and progressively more erratic (Fig. 16A) and eventually blocked (Fig. 17A). The effects of varying the ratio of C_{surf}/C_{junc} can be discerned for the situation with K^+ accumulation by comparing the lower panels in Figures 15–17. These results are summarized in Table 2. Thus, these experiments demonstrate that smoothness and speed of propagation is strongly dependent on the ratio of capacitances of the surface membrane to junctional membrane. The higher this ratio, that is, the lower the value of the junctional membrane capacitance (C_{junc}), the smoother and faster the propagation.

Figure 18 summarizes the results of varying the total cell capacitance while maintaining an 80 to 1 ratio of surface membrane capacitance (C_{surf}) to junctional membrane capacitance (C_{junc}). There was a marked slowing of propagation

Table 2. Summary of all simulations assessing incorporation of K^+ accumulation.

Capacitance (pf)			Incorporation of K^+ accumulation	Propagation velocity (cm/sec)	$\dot{V}_{max}$ (V/sec)
Junctional	Surface	Ratio of Surf./Junc.			
2.5	200	80 : 1	No	23.7	472
2.5	200	80 : 1	Yes	25.5	
2.86	200	70 : 1	No	Erratic	475
2.86	200	70 : 1	Yes	24.6	
3.08	200	65 : 1	No	Erratic	476
3.08	200	65 : 1	Yes	23.7	
3.2	200	62.5 : 1	No	Blocked	455
3.2	200	62.5 : 1	Yes	23.7	
3.33	200	60 : 1	No	Blocked	452
3.33	200	60 : 1	Yes	Erratic	

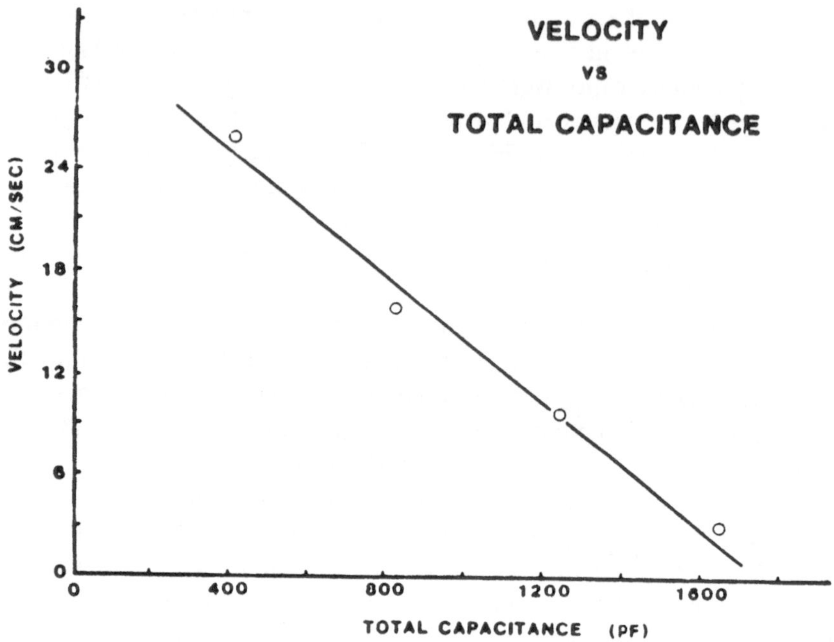

Figure 18. Plot of propagation velocity (ordinate) versus total capacitance (abscissa). The total cell capacitance is the sum of the four parallel capacitances: two surface membranes (C_{surf}) and two junctional membranes (C_{junc}). The standard (1x) values for C_{surf} and C_{junc} were 200 pf and 2.5 pf, respectively, giving a C_{total} of 405 pf. C_{total} was doubled (810 pf), tripled (1215 pf), and quadrupled (1620 pf) in the simulations. As can be seen, there was a linear decrease in velocity with increase in cell capacitance. Taken from Sperelakis et al. [47].

velocity when the total capacitance was increased. Doubling the absolute capacitance values caused a drop in propagation velocity from 25.5 to 15.6 cm/sec (Fig. 19). Tripling the capacitances descreased the propagation velocity to 9.6 cm/sec. Quadrupling the capacitance values slowed propagation velocity down to 2.9 cm/sec. Thus, propagation velocity is critically dependent on the absolute values of the membrane capacitances, as well as on the ratio of C_{surf}/C_{junc}.

The results demonstrate that propagation of action potentials with the electric field model is facilitated by the K^+ accumulation in the junctional gap between the pre- and post-junctional cells. The results also indicate that increasing the total capacitance of both the surface and junctional membranes slows down the rate of propagation. The present results are in agreement with and extend our previous theoretical analysis that showed that K^+ accumulation, by itself, might be an important facilatory mechanism for transmission of excitation between myocardial cells [12]. The fact that propagation velocity increases markedly to an optimal value as the K^+ concentration in the bathing solution ($[K]_o$)is elevated [13] is consistent with K^+ accumulation playing a role in the transfer of excitation from cell to cell. The combined electric field/K^+ accumulation model provides a

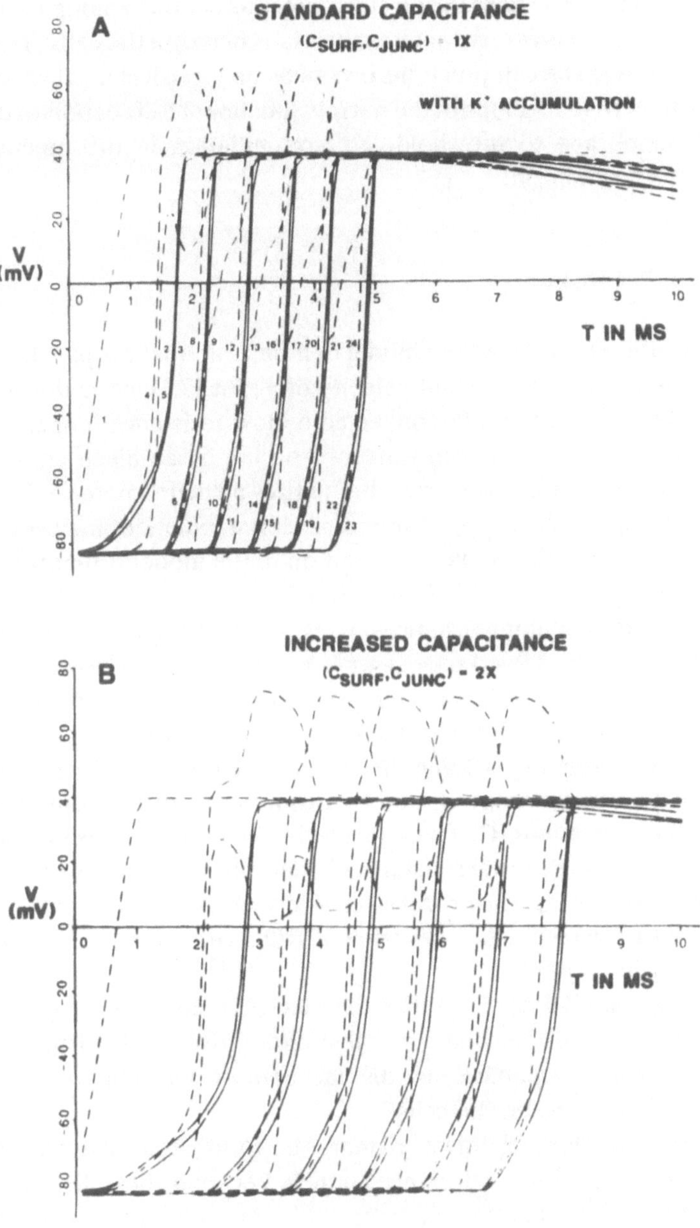

Figure 19. Effect of increasing the capacitance of the surface membrane by a factor 2. With K^+ accumulation. A: fast propagation down the cell chain under standard conditions: capacitance ratio of surface membrane (C_{surf}) to junctional membrane (C_{junc}) of 80 : 1 (200 pf/2.5 pf). Propagation velocity was 25.5 cm/sec. B: slowed propagation when the capacitance of both the surface membranes and junctional membranes were increased 2-fold (C_{surf})/C_{junc} still 80 : 1). Propagation velocity was slowed to 15.6 cm/sec. Taken from Sperelakis et al. [47].

possible alternative mechanism for electrical interactions among excitable cells that does not require low-resistance connections between the cells. Transmission of excitation across the cell junctions occurs by an electrical mechanism, namely the electric field that develops in the narrow junctional cleft depolarizes the post-junctional membrane to threshold. K^+ accumulation in the junctional clefts facilitates this mechanism.

Discussion and summary

The results with our electric field model demonstrate that propagation of action potentials can occur at a constant velocity of about 17.1 cm/sec down a chain of excitable cells that are not interconnected by low-resistance tunnels. Transmission of excitation across the cell junctions occurs by an electrical mechanism, namely when the pre-junctional membrane fires an action potential, the electric field that develops in the narrow junctional cleft depolarizes the post-junctional membrane to threshold. The key assumption in the model is that the junctional membranes are ordinary excitable membranes.

Raising the extracellular resistances, ROL and ROR, along the entire chain of 6 cells by up to 4-fold slowed propagation velocity slightly. However, when the radial cleft resistance, RJC, was increased either alone or concomitantly with ROL and ROR, then there was a marked slowing of propagation velocity. In a real biological experiment, raising the ROL and ROR (e.g., by partial replacement of NaCl in the bathing solution by isosmotic sucrose) should also cause a proportional increase in RJC. These results indicate that RJC is the most important parameter of the external resistances in determining velocity of propagation. In addition, it is clear that the model is relatively insensitive to the actual values of ROL and ROR selected, since lowering of ROL and ROR by up to 8-fold also had relatively little effect.

Although we don't know whether the electric field model applies to actual biological cells, it does provide a possible alternative mechanism for electrical interactions among excitable cells; this mechanism does not require low-resistance connections between the cells.

The other possible mechanism, namely the local-circuit current hypothesis, requires that there be low-resistance tunnels between the cells. A theoretical analysis of the potential in the junctional cleft between myocardial cells, assuming that the junctional membranes were non-excitable and low in resistance, was done by Heppner and Plonsey [48] and by Woodbury and Crill [49]. For such a modified cable situation, they found that the maximum resistivity of the junctional membranes that would allow successful transmission (for a cleft thickness of 80 Å) was about $3\,\Omega \times cm^2$, i.e., about 1/100–1/1000 times that of the surface membrane. The value of $3\,\Omega \times cm^2$ is in good agreement with values calculated for a similar arrangement by Weidmann [33] and Sperelakis [8] (for other references, see [4]).

The electric field hypothesis can account for a number of experimental facts concerning propagation in cardiac muscle, namely that

a. propagation velocity is about 0.3 m/sec;
b. propagation is bi-directional;
c. the transmission process is labile and often can exhibit partial or complete block;
d. increasing the separation of the junctional membranes under pathological or experimental conditions, thus decreasing RJC, impedes and blocks transmission;
e. there is a prepotential step on the rising phase of the action potential;
f. synaptic-like vesicles are not observed at the intercalated disks.

In addition, and more importantly, the electric field hypothesis is consistent with the lack of measurement of low resistance between myocardial cells in adult heart tissue by a number of different approaches (for a summary of these, see [4, 8] and foregoing sections).

The electric field model is also consistent with recent observations of Spach et al. [1] who found that the rate of rise of the cardiac action potential was greater with transverse propagation, although propagation in the transverse direction was much slower than in the longitudinal direction, i.e., propagation velocity could be separated from rate of rise. They also reported that propagation in cardiac muscle is saltatory or discontinuous in nature. These findings are consistent with the predictions given by Sperelakis and colleagues (e.g., see [8]), namely that myocardial cells behave as truncated cables with little or no low-resistance coupling between the cells.

Diaz, Rudy and Plonsey [2] also concluded, from a theoretical analysis of a model based on resistive coupling between cells, that 'continuous cable theory does not adequately describe propagation in cardiac musle' and that excitation jumps from intercalated disk to intercalated disk, i.e., saltatory propagation occurs. They found that propagation inside a single cell was ten times faster than the average velocity over many cells, i.e., most propagation time is consumed at the cell junctions. This is also consistent with the predictions given by Sperelakis and colleagues for truncated cables (see [8]). In the model of Diaz et al. [2], propagation velocity was greatly slowed at r_{jc} values below 170 MΩ, and failed at r_{jc} values below 17 MΩ. These r_{jc} values are considerably higher than those required in our electric field model (>5 MΩ).

The electrotonic length (L, dimensionless) was measured in pig ventricular muscle using the Rall analysis [50]. It was found that L. varied between 0.81 and 2.26 in 8 cells analyzed, with a mean value of about 1.4. Input resistance ranged between 8.8 and 39 MΩ, and τ_m from 1.2 to 3.7 msec. From the low value of L, the authors concluded that the myocardial cell does not terminate in a dendritic-like arborization, i.e., there must not be low-resistance connections with neighboring cells to produce a 3-dimensional syncytium.

A study highly quoted in support of low-resistance coupling in cardiac muscle is that of Barr et al. [51] showing that a sucrose-gap of about 100–200 μm blocked propagation in frog atrial strands unless a low shunt resistance was placed across the sucrose-gap region. However, it seems this experiment shows only that in a biological system current must flow in order to produce a potential change. Regardless of interpretation, the fact that the sucrose-gap region had to be short in order for the experiment to work, indicates that the length constant (λ) cannot be long, as claimed by some investigators.

Another study highly quoted in support of low-resistance coupling is that of Weidmann [33], who showed that the steady-state distribution of ^{42}K along ventricular muscle bundles (across a membrane separating a loading compartment) was exponential with a length constant of about 1.55 mm, whereas that for ^{82}Br was only 0.55 mm. However, it seems difficult to conclude what the resistivity of the intercalated disk is from this experiment because of the anistropic muscle bundle acting as a cable (problem discussed above) and because longitudinal diffusion can occur through capillaries, etc.

A number of other studies have been done using dye diffusion as a presumed indicator of low-resistance coupling (for references, see [4]). However, it is interesting that no evidence of electrotonic coupling was found among pyramidal cells of the guinea pig hippocampus, although the fluorescent dye Lucifer Yellow injected into one soma spread to neighboring cells (dye coupling) [52]. Therefore, dye studies must be interpreted with caution.

Although the parameters of the electric field model were selected specifically for cardiac muscle, the principles of this model have general applicability to interactions between other types of closely-apposed excitable cells. The only requirements are that their cell membranes be in close apposition over a small fraction of the total surface area, and that the junctional membranes be ordinary excitable membranes. The model might also apply to intracellular interactions between the cell membrane and sarcoplasmic reticulum (SR) membrane. Electrical field interactions between neurons in vertebrate brain, both excitatory and inhibitory, have been described by Korn and Faber [53], but these are ephaptic in nature, depending on current flow through the second neuron and on the resistance of the extracellular space. Dudek and co-workers [54–56] have shown that electrical fields contribute to the generation of synchronous epileptiform bursting in adjacent hippocampal neurons in which chemical transmision was blocked. Propagation in smooth muscle tissues also may be dependent on electric field effects. For example, Daniel and co-workers [57] noted that propagation occurs in the absence of ultrastructurally defined gap junctions in several types of smooth muscles, such as the taenia coli. Since numerous close appositions, but not low-resistance tunnels, are present in these tissues, it is possible that electrical field effects are important for propagation in this tissue.

Acknowledgments

The work of the author and his colleagues summarized and reviewed in this article was supported in part by N.I.H. grant HL-31942. The author wishes to acknowledge the collaborations with his colleagues, particularly Dr James E. Mann, Jr.

References

1. Spach MS, Miller WT III, Geselowitz DB, Barr RC, Kootsey JM, Johnson EA (1981): The discontinuous nature of propagation in normal canine cardiac muscle. Evidence for recurrent discontinuity of intracellular resistance that affects the membrane currents. Circ Res 48: 39–54.
2. Diaz PJ, Rudy Y, Plonsey R (1981): A cardiac propagation model with intercalated discs. (Abst) 34th ACEMB meeting, Houston (September 21–23), pp. 217.
3. Sperelakis N, Rubio R (1971): Ultrastructural changes produced by hypertonicity in cat cardiac muscle. J Mol Cell Cardiol 3: 139–156.
4. Sperelakis N (1979): Propagation mechanisms in heart. Ann Rev Physiol 41: 441–457.
5. Forbes MS, Sperelakis N (1985): Intercalated discs of mammalian heart: A review of structure and function. Tissue and Cell 17: 605–648.
6. Hoshiko T, Sperelakis N (1961): Prepotentials and unidirectional propagation in myocardium. Am J Physiol 201: 873–880.
7. Sperelakis N, Hoshiko T (1961): Electrical impedance of cardiac muscle. Circ Res 9: 1280–1283.
8. Sperelakis N (1969): Lack of electrical coupling between contiguous myocardial cells in vertebrate hearts. In: McCann FV (ed.) Comparative physioloy of the heart: Current trends, Experientia Suppl. 15. Birkhauser Verlag, Basel, pp. 135–165.
9. De Mello WC (1972): The healing-over process in cardiac and other muscle fibers. In: De Mello WC (ed.) Electrical phenomena in heart. Academic Press, New York, pp. 323–351.
10. Weidmann S (1969): Electrical coupling between myocardial cells. Prog Brain Res 31: 275–281.
11. Sperelakis N (1983): The possibility of propagation between myocardial cells not connected by low-resistance pathways. In: Myocardial Injury (ed. J.J. Spitzer), Plenum Press, pp. 1–23.
12. Macdonald RL, Hsu D, Mann JE, Sperelakis N (1975):An analysis of the problem of K^+ accumulation in the intercalated disk clefts of cardiac muscle. J Theor Biol 51: 455–473.
13. Sperelakis N, Mayer G, Macdonald R (1970): Velocity of propagation in vertebrate cardiac muscles as functions of tonicity and $[K^+]_o$. Am J Physiol 219: 952–963.
14. Mann JE Jr, Foley E, Sperelakis N (1977): Resistance and potential profiles in the cleft between two myocardial cells: electrical analog and computer simulations. J Theor Biol 68: 1–15.
15. Sperelakis N, Mann JE Jr (1977): Evaluation of electric field changes in the cleft between excitable cells. J Theor Biol 64: 71–96.
16. Mann JE, Sperelakis N (1979): Further development of a model for electrical transmission between myocardial cells not connected by low-resistance pathways. J Electrocardiol 12: 23–33.
17. McLean MJ, Sperelakis N (1980): Difference in degree of electrotonic interactions between highly differentiated and reverted cultured heart cell reaggregates. J Memb Biol 57: 37–50.
18. Forbes MS, Sperelakis N (1972): Ultrastructure of cardiac muscle from dystrophic mice. Am J Anat 134: 271–290.
19. Sperelakis N, Rubio R, Redick J (1970): Sharp discontinuity in sarcomere lengths across intercalated disk of fibrillating cat hearts. J Ultrastruct Res 30: 503–532.
20. Forbes MS, Sperelakis N (1971): Ultrastructure of lizard ventricular muscle. J Ultrastruct Res 34: 439–451.
21. Baldwin KM (1981): Cell-to-cell tracer movement in cardiac muscle: Ruthenium red vs lanthanum. Cell Tiss Res 221: 279–294.

22. Hoshiko T, Sperelakis N (1962): Components of the cardiac action potential. Am J Physiol 203: 258–260.
23. Sperelakis N, Shumaker K (1968): Phase-plane analysis of cardiac action potentials. J Electrocardiology 1: 31–42.
24. Sperelakis N, Lehmkuhl D (1964): Effect of current on transmembrane potentials in cultured chick heart cells. Gen Physiol 47: 895–927.
25. Sperelakis N, Hoshiko T, Keller RF Jr, Berne RM (1960): Intracellular and external recordings from frog ventricular fibers during hypertonic perfusion. Am J Physiol 198: 135–140.
26. Sperelakis N, Hoshiko T, Berne RM (1960): Non-syncytial nature of cardiac muscle: membrane resistance of single cells. Am J Physiol 198: 531–536.
27. Van der Kloot WG, Dane BD (1964): Conduction of the action potential in the frog ventricle. Science 146: 74–75.
28. DeMello WC (1975): Effect of intracellular injection of calcium and strontium on cell communication in heart. J Physiol 250: 231–245.
29. Tarr M, Sperelakis N (1964): Weak electronic interaction between contiguous cardiac cells. Am J Physiol 207: 691–700.
30. Sperelakis N, Tarr M (1965): Weak electronic interaction between neighboring visceral smooth muscle cells. Am J Physiol 66: 119–134.
31. Tarr M, Sperelakis N (1967): Decreased intercellular resistance during spontaneous depolarization in myocardium. Am J Physiol 212: 1503–1511.
32. Sperelakis N, Macdonald RL (1974): Ratio of transverse to longitudinal resistivities of isolated cardiac muscle fiber bundles. J Electrocardiol 7: 301–314.
33. Weidmann S (1966): The diffusion of radiopotassium across intercalated disks of mammalian cardiac muscle. J Physiol 187: 323–342.
34. Tanaka I, Sasaki Y (1966): On the electrotonic spread in cardiac muscle. J Gen Physiol 49: 1089–1110.
35. Macdonald RL, Mann JE Jr, Sperelakis N (1974): Derivation of general equations describing tracer diffusion in any two-compartment tissue, with application to diffusion in cylindrical muscle bundles. J Theor Biol 45: 107–131.
36. Sperelakis N, Picone J (1986): Cable analysis in cardiac muscle and smooth muscle bundles. I.T.B.M. 7: 433–457.
37. Abe Y, Tomita T (1968): Cable properties of smooth muscle. J Physiol (London) 196: 87–100.
38. Daniel EE, Daniel VP, Duchon G, Garfield RE, Nichols M, Malholtra SK, Oki M (1976): Is the nexus necessary for cell-to-cell coupling of smooth muscle? J Membr Biol 28: 207–239.
39. Sims SM, Daniel EE, Garfield RE (1982): Improved electrical coupling in uterine smooth muscle is associated with increased numbers of gap junctions at parturition. J Gen Physiol 80: 353–375.
40. Page E, McCallister LP (1973): Studies on the intercalated disk of rat left ventricular myocardial cells. J Ultrastruct Res 43: 388–411.
41. Kline R, Morad M (1976): Potassium efflux and accumulation in heart muscle. Biophys J 16: 367–372.
42. Yarom Y, Spiro ME (1982): Extracellular potassium ions mediate specific neuronal interaction. Science 216: 80–82.
43. Noble D (1962): A modification of the Hodgkin-Huxley equations applicable to Purkinje fiber action and pacemaker potentials. J Physiol 160: 317–352.
44. Beeler GW, Reuter H (1977): Reconstruction of the action potential of ventricular myocardial fibers. J Physiol 268: 177–210.
45. Ruffner JA, Sperelakis N, Mann JE Jr (1980): Application of the Hodgkin-Huxley equations to an electric field model for interaction between excitable cells. J Theor Biol 87: 129–152.
46. Mann JE, Sperelakis N, Ruffner JA (1981): Alterations in sodium channel gate kinetics of the Hodgkin-Huxley equations on an electric field model for interaction between excitable cells. IEEE Trans. Biomed. Eng. 28: 655–661.

47. Sperelakis N, LoBrocco B, Mann JE, Marschall R (1985): Potassium accumulation in intercellular junctions combined with electric field interactions for propagation in cardiac muscle. Innov et Tech en Biol et Med 6(1): 24–43.
48. Heppner DB, Plonsey R (1970): Simulation of electrical interaction of cardiac cells. Biophys J 10: 1057–1075.
49. Woodbury JW, Crill WE (1970): The potential in the gap between two abutting cardiac muscle cells. Biophys J 10: 1076–1083.
50. Beder SD, Skinner JE (1981): Cardiac cellular electrophysiology in awake conscious pigs: membrane cable properties. Circulation 64: IV-116, Abstract 428.
51. Barr L, Dewey MM, Berger W (1965): Propagation of action potentials and the structure of the nexus in cardiac muscle. J Gen Physiol 48: 797–823.
52. Knowles WD, Funch PG, Schwartzkroin PA (1982): Electrotonic and dye coupling in hippocampal CA 1 pyramidal cells *in vitro*. Neursci 7(7): 1713–1722.
53. Korn H, Faber DS (1980): Electrical field effect interactions in the vertebrate brain. Trends in Neuroscience 3(1): 6–9.
54. Snow RW, Dudek FE (1984): Electrical fields directly contribute to action potential synchronization during convulsant-induced epileptiform bursts. Brain Res 323: 114–118.
55. Taylor CP, Dudek FE (1984): Synchronization without active chemical synapses during hippocampal afterdischarges. J Neurophysiol 52: 143–155.
56. Traub RD, Dudek FE, Taylor CP, Knowles WD (1985): Simulation of hippocampal afterdischarges synchronized by electrical interactions. Neurosci 14: 1033–1038.
57. Daniel EE, Daniel VP, Duchon G, Garfield RE, Nichols M, Malholtra SK, Oki M (1976): Is the nexus necessary for cell-to-cell coupling of smooth muscle? J Membr Biol 28: 207–239.
58. Sperelakis N, Marschall R, Mann JE (1983): Propagation down a chain of excitable cells by electric field interactions in the junctional clefts: effect of variation in extracellular resistances, including a 'sucrose-gap' simulation. IEEE Trans Biomed Eng 30: 658–664.

6. The role of distributed conduction velocities in simulated epicardial activation maps

D. ADAM

Abstract

The effects of the spatial arrangement of myocardial fibers and of the inferred 3-dimensional distribution of conduction velocities on epicardial activation patterns are described. A simplified geometry is considered, that of an ellipsoidally shaped left ventricle (LV), attached to a sectioned ellipsoidal right ventricle. The modeled myocardial volume is sectioned into different layers and areas, each filled with different 'cells', thus allowing to describe the distribution of velocities and orientation similar to physiological and anatomical data. The propagation velocity along the myocardial fiber is assumed to be 3 times the transverse velocity. Once simulation starts, a stimulated 'cell' activates all its neighbors, thus generating patterns of activation within and on the surfaces of the myocardium. The simulated activation maps from the myocardial surfaces are found to be sensitive to the underlying distribution of conduction velocities, specifically when abnormal velocities are introduced at certain 'infarcted' areas. The existence of ectopic foci is readily identified by the distortion of the normal patterns. The maps, however, are much less sensitive to minute changes in the location of the foci of activation within the normal conduction system. While the simulated epicardial and endocardial maps are affected by the spatial distribution of the conduction velocities, the surface maps are specifically sensitive in displaying the existence of abnormally propagating myocardial activity.

Introduction

This study examines the relationship between simulated activation maps, as calculated on the surfaces of an idealized heart, and (some of) the processes which influence the generation of these maps. The activation maps do not include all the information contained within the potential maps. They may serve however, as data for calculating the electrical sources within the myocardium (the inverse problem), as they were found to produce a good description of the underlying processes [1]. The importance of the epicardial and endocardial maps is becoming more evident as their clinical use is more common [2], and commercial systems for epicardial recordings are available. Data has been accumulating concerning the success of surgical interventions guided by recordings and analysis made by such systems [3]. As most of the information required for estimating the myocardial sources is contained in the epicardial surfaces [1], the measurements must be made on the epicardium and may therefore be carried out only during open chest surgery procedures.

Measurements of surface activation maps, or for that matter also of potential maps, are hampered by technical problems and limitations. The number of electrodes and data acquisition channels is limited and therefore the spatial resolution is usually low. The electrodes affect the normal activity of the myocardium and quite often also damage it. These difficulties have limited the use of this technique and the experimental data available in the literature. It is therefore quite impossible to locate experimental data concerning the sensitivity of the epicardial maps to the various parameters which govern their production. While tissue properties like directional conduction velocities [4], conductivities [5] and even membrane characteristics [6, 7] are well documented, the complexity and inaccuracy of intact heart measurement do not allow us this data. The complexity is increased when pathologies are studied, when spatial distribution of properties is altered and the initiation of activity is shifted. There has been, therefore, the need for models of the electrical processes within the heart, the analysis of their sensitivities, the description of the spread of their excitation and the potentials they generate. Such models should perform well both under normal conditions as well as conduction pathologies, like Bundle Branch Block, regional obstruction of Purkinje fibers and myocardial infarction. The models and their generated surface maps have to perform just as well under conditions of ectopic activity and prematurity.

A model which generates the surface maps with high spatial resolution may produce the necessary data needed for the different studies of the forward problem (e.g. producing the body surface potential maps) or the inverse problem (e.g. calculating the myocardial surfaces maps or even the myocardial sources). The ultimate goal of electrocardiography is to estimate the myocardial electrical sources from body surface potential maps; as this estimation problem is ill-posed, several suggestions have been made for calculating the epicardial activation maps [8] or the activation maps together with the action potential amplitudes [9] by accepting some restrictions. These volume conduction models and their respective limitations may also be studied and evaluated by the use of the present model of the myocardial activation process.

When trying to compare measured myocardial surfaces' physiological data with data generated by models, the choice is limited to finite-elements models, which may include true geometry, inhomogeneity of the tissue or non -isotropy of the myocardial fibers [10, 11]. Presently, 3-dimensional models are usually limited to simple, idealized geometry [12]. The analytical models, which in many cases include physiologically important properties (like membrane conductances) as part of the model parameters [13, 14], are usually limited in scope to one-dimensional or two-dimensional models. They seldom include the distribution of parameters found in the biological sytem.

Different models of the myocardial activation processes have been described in the literature; a few of these produce also the myocardial and the surface potential maps [15] or activation maps [16,17,18]. In order to take into account some of the important properties that govern the myocardial activation processes (e.g. anisotropy, distribution of properties) the present model has been constructed. Although the basic principals are similar to the model reported elsewhere [11], the model was modified significantly (see Methods). In its present form the model uses 3-dimensional finite-elements to describe the activation processes in the left and right ventricles while generating excitation time maps (i.e. equiactivation times or isochrones) on the myocardial surfaces during the QRS period. The model is used here to describe the effects of the spatial arrangement of myocardial fibers and of the inferred 3-dimensional distribution of conduction velocities on epicardial activation patterns. The model is also used to determine the sensitivity of the epicardial maps to conduction pathologies, like Bundle Branch Block, regional obstruction of Purkinje fibers and myocardial infarction. Last, the model and its generated surface maps are tested under conditions of ectopic activity and prematurity.

Methods

The activation process of the left ventricle (L.V.) and right ventricle (R.V.) is simulated here by utilizing a finite-elements model. The basic concepts of the model have been described elsewhere [11], but for convenience a short description is given below, emphasizing the modifications made. The model incorporates 3-dimensional geometry of the myocardial volume, with the L.V. as an idealized ellipsoid and the R.V. as a sectioned, narrower ellipsoid. The model is constrained by a few assumptions, which are detailed and justified below.

Model assumptions

1. The myocardial geometry is described by non-contracting ellipsoids, as the simulations include the activation processes during the QRS, before mechanical contraction is initiated (see Fig. 1). The myocardial volume is sectioned to about 1.2 mm 'cells', by a grid of $98 \times 78 \times 98$.
2. The L.V. 'cells' are grouped into 4 confocal layers, while each of the layers is

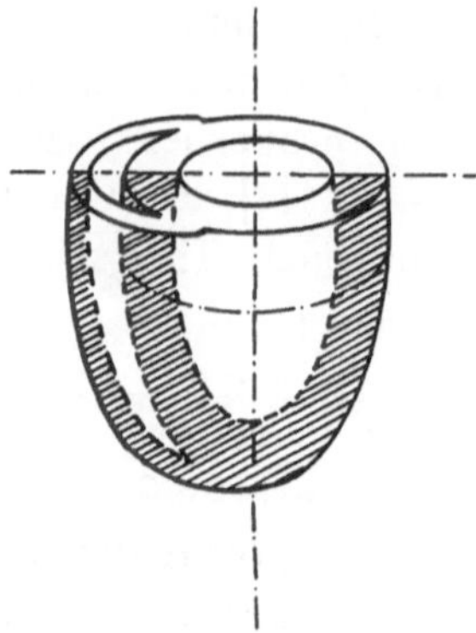

Figure 1. The geometry of the model is depicted here: the left ventricle as idealized ellipsoid; the right ventricle as a narrower, sectioned ellipsoid.

divided into 14 subgroups. The R.V. contains 2 layers, each of 7 subgroups. In each subgroup all 'cells' have similar properties, selected out of a Gaussian distribution.

3. The parameters by which a subgroup is defined are: direction of high velocity – the direction of the myocardial fibers at that location, which imposes propagation velocity three times higher than in all other directions; propagation velocity (a relative value – multiplication of the simulation basic time step); absolute refractory period (R.P.) – mean and standard deviation of the mean (S.D.); activation time (mean and S.D.), the time period during which the 'cell' activates its neighbors that are not during their own R.P.
4. The direction of high velocity is chosen out of 14 possible directions, in a way that closely resembles the fibers orientation within the myocardium. The fiber orientation is spiral with different tilt at the various layers [19]. In a passive 'fiber' (or group of 'cells'), forward and backward propagation is allowed.
5. The inner-most layer, the 'endocardium', is characterized by a higher conduction velocity (between 2–4 times the velocity of myocardial fibers [20]), with direction of higher velocity pointing mostly from apex to base [21]. The interaction between the 'Purkinje' network and the 'myocardium' may be in both directions, as the myocardial cells may re-activate the Purkinje cells [22]. The model does not contain the more central parts of the conduction system, i.e. the A.V. node, the HIS bundles or left and right bundle branches.
6. The propagation from one 'cell' to the next does not depend on membrane properties, but on the geometrical relationships and on whether the neighboring 'cells' are active or passive. The implications of this assumption are that the membrane properties do not appear explicitly as parameters of the simulation, but only indirectly through their effect on (mean) conduction velocity and (mean) refractory period over a length of a few 'cells'. On the other hand, the computational complexity is reduced by orders of magnitude.

Model formulation and simulation

The assumptions mentioned above define the rules used for producing the activation process in the present model. The flexibility in defining different geometries, and sections within these geometries, allows the selections of parameters which describe different tissue properties at each section. Thus before each simulation the conduction velocities, for the high speed direction and for all other directions, are selected by setting the mean and S.D. of the mean for each section. In order to initiate the activation process, stimulation points must be defined. For the normal case, these points are defined on the endocardium, within the layer which represents the Purkinje conduction network. Once this is done, after the next simulation time step and then after all following steps, the 'cells' which are active effect their neighbors according to the rules stated above. In this manner the activity spreads to all 'cells' which are not refractory. As the activation sequence is studied here only during the QRS period, the repolarization processes are not included, but secondary activation wavefronts may appear either when premature beats are studied or when regional refractory periods are very short and reactivation occurs.

The simulations used here have been completed within reasonable time by extensively using the Virtual Memory features of the computer employed (VAX-780/VMS). Typically a simulation study might require 20 minutes CPU, although some might run for little more than an hour. The results were plotted by a modified PLOT-10 and SAS-Graph plotting libraries.

Results

Different tissue characteristics and stimulation conditions have been selected to demonstrate the effects of conduction velocities on the epicardial activation maps. The simulations have usually started with all 'cells' inactive, and four 'cells' being stimulated. The four points, which are the stimulation points for most of the studies reported here, are located on the central frontal cross-section plane; two are located in the lower 1/5 of the L.V. endocardium (Purkinje 'cells') on the free wall and septum, respectively, while the other two are similarly located in the R.V. Once simulation is initiated, all parameters remain constant. Since the present report emphasizes the activation process (during the QRS), the simulations have been terminated after a certain time period (90 simulation time steps) long enough to activate all the myocardium. The pattern of propagation of the activation process within the myocardium may be extracted from the simulation results by focusing on the time of activation of each 'cell' in the model. As the results describe the processes in three dimensions, any visual presentation of results requires either 2-dimensional cross-sectional data or (spread out) surface data, with the third axis denoting the time of activation.

The simulation of the myocardial activation process during normal performance requires selection of parameters similar to those found under normal physiological conditions. The selection has been of long refractory periods (50 times the simulation step), small S.D. of the mean for the distribution of the refractory periods within the population, short activation times, Purkinje network of 'cells' on the endocardial layer with fiber orientation from apex to base and typical distribution of conduction velocities, as described and justified elsewhere [23, 19]. Typical results of simulations with parameters within the normal range are presented in Fig. 2. In this figure and the following ones, (a) and (b) display the time of activation of the different 'cells' on the anterior epicardial layer of the ventricles and on a central frontal cross-section plane of the two chambers, respectively: the higher the point, the later it was activated (with arbitrary scales); (c) displays the epicardial activation map (i.e. equiactivation times or isochrones) of the two ventricles, calculated from (a). In Fig. 2(b) the slope at the endocardial layers indicates the rapid propagation from the points of stimulation to base, while across the myocardial wall the slope is steep, i.e. propagation is slow. While in the cross-section of the free wall the activity propagates smoothly, in the septum the two wavefronts collide. These differences can hardly be seen in the epicardial maps. The last area to be activated is the epicardial layer near the base on the anterior side.

When the conduction system is completely abolished in both ventricles, different resulting activity maps are generated, as seen in Fig. 3. One feature is quite evident, the early activation above the septum, due to the initial stimulation on both sides of the wall while the conduction system is not present. Although such a condition is rare clinically, it serves as an example of the sensitivity of the maps. A more common pathological condition is that of Right Bundle Branch Block, here modeled by no conduction system in the right cavity (myocardial fibers only). Fig. 4 presents the results. The propagation of activity on the epicardial layers above the R.V. looks very similar to that of the previous figure, while the activity over the L.V. looks more like the normal case. The pattern is clear and meaningful.

Various clinical conditions may be tested by an early second stimulation (Premature Ventricular Contraction), usually associated with automaticity of cells injured by an ischemic episode, or conduction abnormality. To simulate such a condition, a second, early stimulation has been applied to the R.V. of the model. The stimulation points are, as usual, in the Purkinje fibers network on the endocardial free wall and septum. The activation sequence at the central cross-section is depicted in Fig. 5(b), representing a particular moment in which the first (regular) beat has activated the whole myocardium, while the second early R.V. P.V.C. has activated most of the R.V. and only part of the L.V. (in this figure the initiation of a third stimulation is seen). The activation maps at the epicardial layers are clearly demonstrating the underlying processes. It is interesting to note that as long as the premature activation does not penetrate the

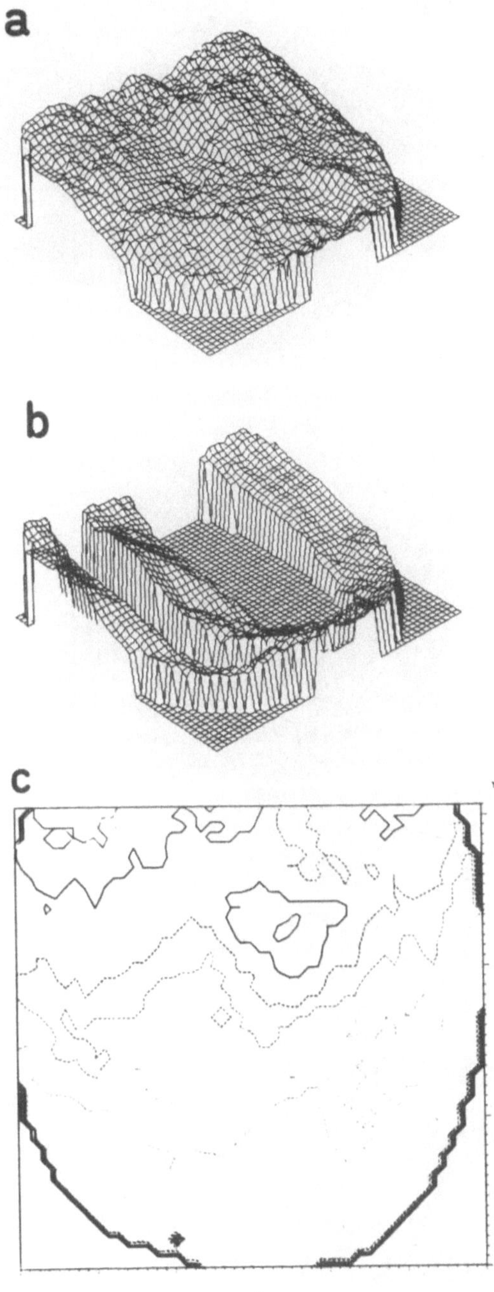

Figure 2. Time of activation of different 'cells', (a) in the anterior epicardial layer of the ventricles and (b) in a central frontal cross-section plane of the two chambers: the higher the point, the later the 'cells' were activated (arbitrary scale); (c) epicardial activation map (i.e. equiactivation times or isochrones) of the two ventricles, calculated from (a). Simulation results under normal conditions.

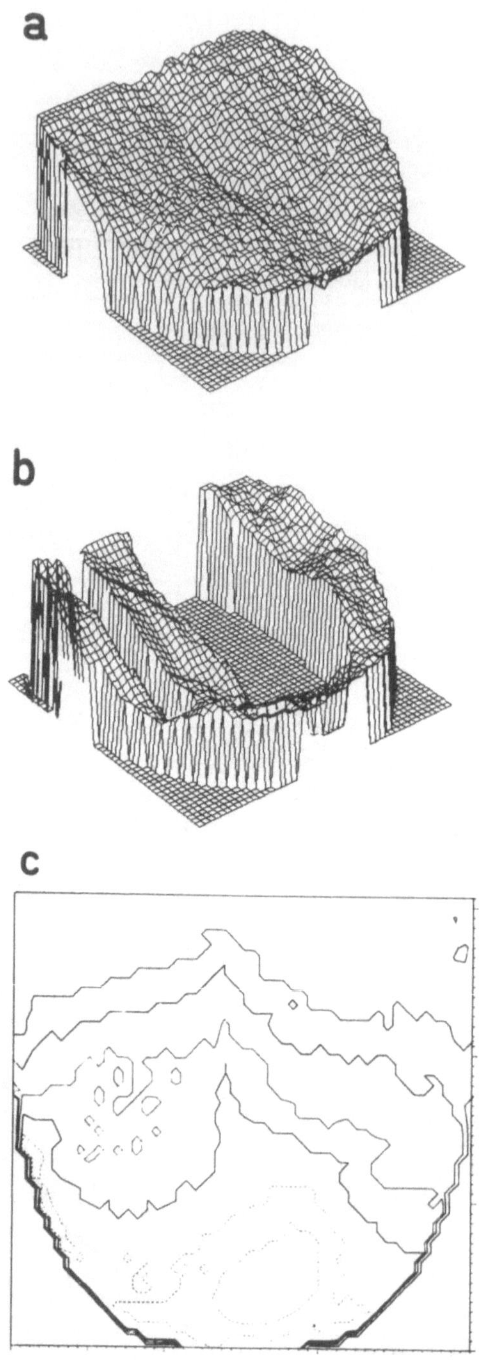

Figure 3. Same as Fig. 2 but under different conditions: the conduction system is completely abolished in both ventricles, resulting in different activity maps. The early activation above the septum is quite evident in these maps.

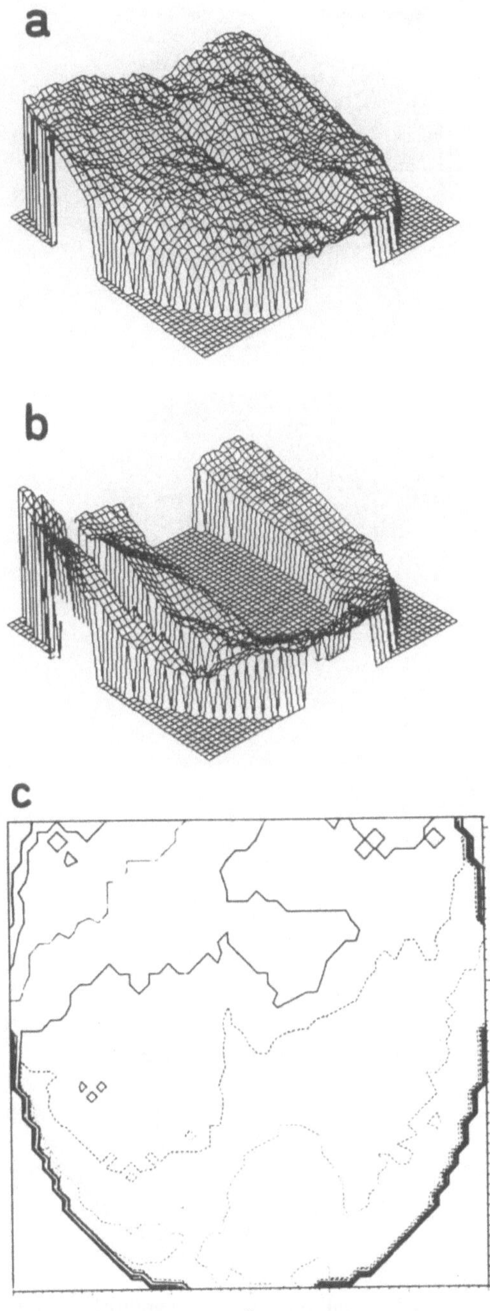

Figure 4. Same as Fig. 2 but under different conditions: the conduction system in the R.V. is blocked or abolished, simulating a common pathological condition of Right Bundle Branch Block. The propagation of activity on the epicardial layers above the R.V. looks very similar to that of the previous figure, while the activity over the L.V. looks more like the normal case.

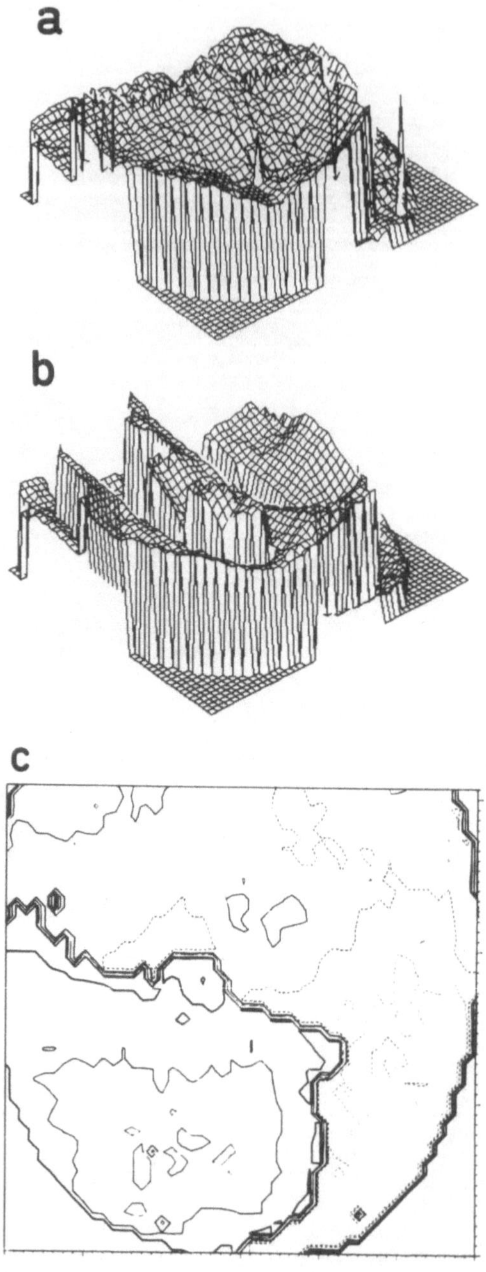

Figure 5. Same a Fig. 2 but under different conditions: simulation of an early, abnormal beat (P.V.C.). A second, early stimulation has been applied to the R.V. of the model. The stimulation points are as usual in the Purkinje fibers network on the endocardial free wall and septum. A particular moment is represented in which the first (regular) beat has activated the whole myocardium while the second early R.V. P.V.C. has activated most of the R.V. and only part of the L.V. (in (b) an initiation of a third stimulation is also seen).

Purkinje network, the propagation is slow.

A different, common, clinical condition is that of chronic myocardial infarction, which usually manifests itself by an area of necrotic tissue with very low conduction velocities surrounded by areas of high excitability. This condition implies short R.P. and leads very often to re-entry, leading usually to ventricular tachycardia and fibrillation. Fig. 6 depicts such a condition. The infarction is penetrating the width of the left lateral side of the L.V. damaging also the conduction system at that area (seen as the highest plateaus in this figure, symbolizing areas which have been activated very late in the previous beat). Because of the anisotropy of the tissue, the activation propagates somewhat quicker around one side of the infarction than the other, leading to a wavefront which starts circulating that area (Fig. 6(d, e, f)). This condition, together with short R.P., leads to 'fibrillation', when 'cells' are reactivating each other in a random way (Fig. 6(g, h, i)). The epicardial maps (Fig. 6(c, f, i)), representing in this figure lateral views of the L.V. free wall, demonstrate clearly the underlying activity. It is worth while noting that the R.V. free wall is the last area to be affected by the circling wavefront as well as by the deterioration into 'fibrillation'.

Discussion

The emphasis of this study is on the spatial distribution of epicardial activation times and their relationship to the myocardial processes which generate them. The simulated surface activation maps are found to be sensitive to the underlying distribution of conduction velocities. Although this result is expected from other (more idealized) models, and from experimental measurements [1, 24, 25], it is interesting to note that they were produced by a 3-dimensional geometry of complex intra-structure, including layers with different fiber orientation. As both ventricles have, in the model, similar conduction system and are stimulated simultaneously, the last epicardial areas to be activated are on the anterior and posterior L.V. free walls near the base. The limitation on the number of stimulation sites in the model may explain the differences between the present results and those of detailed experiments [24, 25]. The maps, however, are much less sensitive to minute changes in location of points of initiation of activity in the normal conduction system. This is held true as long as the stimulation point is limited to the central cross-section. Once the stimulation points are allowed to occupy any point on the endocardium, the patterns of activity vary significantly. These conditions were excluded from the present study.

Once pathologies are introduced, the simulation results reveal many properties and advantages of the model. The resultant maps are specifically altered when abnormal velocities are introduced at certain 'infarcted' areas. When the area is defined by just minor reduction of conduction velocities at the epicardial layers, there are minute changes in the maps. Once the velocities change significantly

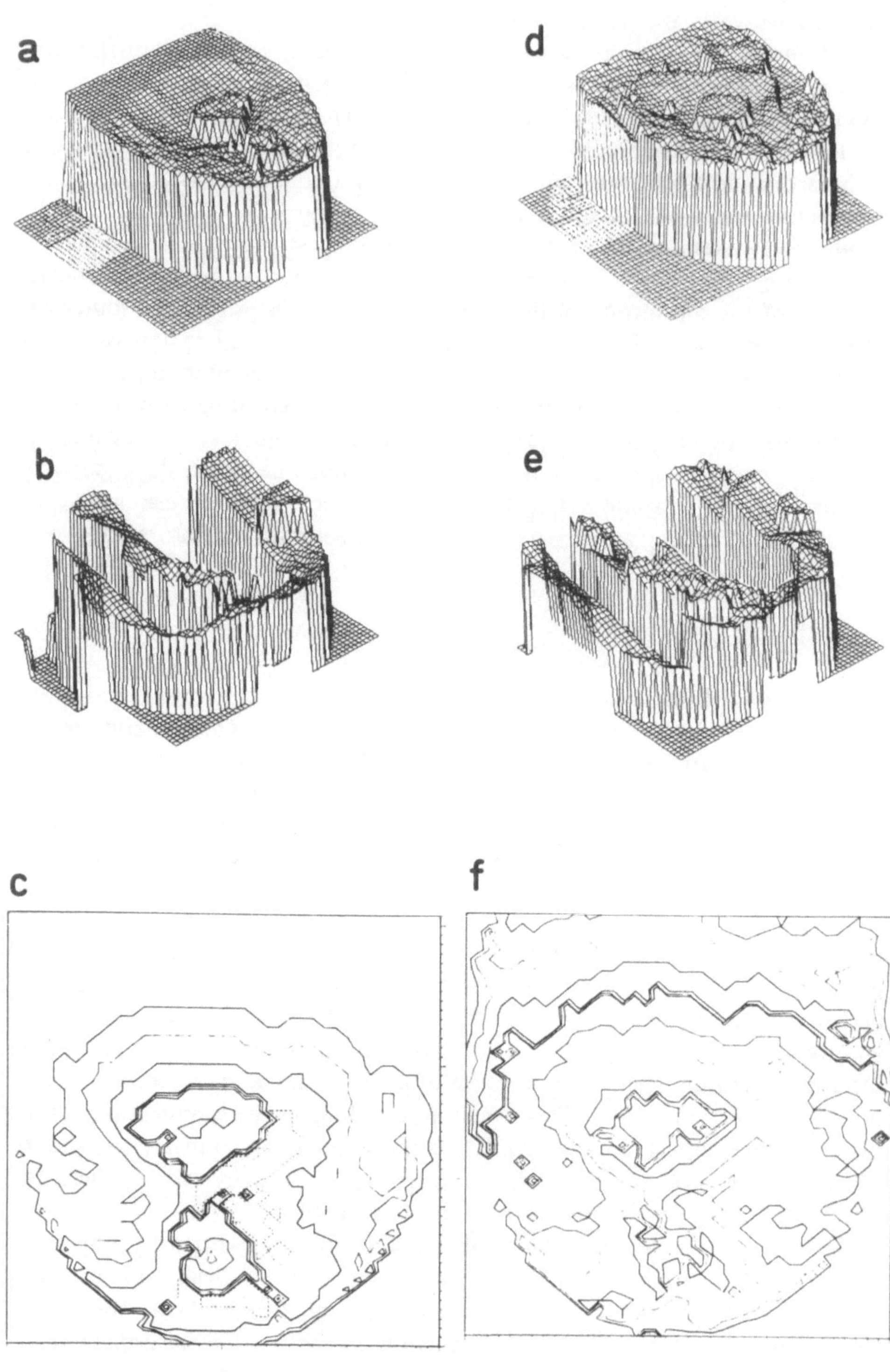
a
d
b
e
c
f
y
y

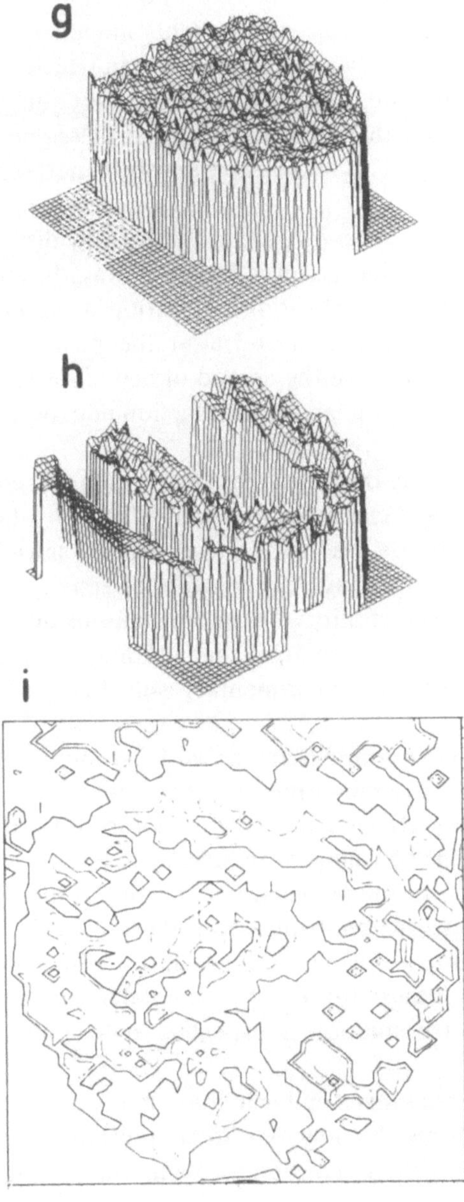

Figure 6. A sequence of results and maps is presented, of an infarcted and excitable (short R.P.) myocardium. (a, d, g): depicts the time of activation of different 'cells' in the anterior epicardial layer of the ventricles: the higher the point, the later the 'cells' were activated (arbitrary scales); (b, e, h): similarly, in a central frontal cross-section plane of the two chambers; (c, f, i): epicardial activation maps (i.e equiactivation times or isochrones) of the two ventricles, calculated from (a), (d) and (g), respectively. In (a, b, c), early after the stimulation, the activity wavefront propagates regularly in the myocardium, except the infarcted area. In (d, e, f), due to anisotropy, the wavefront starts a 're-entry'. In (g, h, i), due to fragmentation and short R.P., 'fibrillation' occures, in which neighboring 'cells' re-activate each other.

and the 'infarction' penetrates through the whole width of the myocardial wall, the changes are global. Because of the nonhomogeneity of the tissue at the different layers and areas, a condition may arise in which the activation process advances more rapidly around one side of the 'infarction' than the other, thus leading to re-entry. As conduction velocities are pre-assigned, and do not depend on the local membrane potentials, re-entry may be generated only around a very-slow conducting tissue.

The existence of ectopic foci is readily identified by distortions of the normal patterns. The success of the model is in generating different propagation velocities and patterns for the activation wavefront in the myocardium before it penetrates the conduction system and after the penetration. As the P.V.C. originates in the R.V., most of the spread of activity is slow; once the activity reaches the L.V. endocardium and its conduction network, the activation wavefront spreads rapidly.

Several conclusions may be drawn from the results presented here. While the simulated epicardial and endocardial maps are affected by the spatial distribution of the conduction velocities, the maps are specifically sensitive in displaying the existence of abnormally propagating myocardial activity. These consequences mean that although the variability with time and among different subjects may be high, pathologies produce a more significant alteration of the maps. This result is, to some extent, supported by experimental results [25], but quantitative evaluation is impossible.

A more general conclusion may be drawn from the results presented above. The generated maps vary smoothly over the ventricular surface only during normal activity, while when pathological conditions are introduced the maps include large variations of values over short spatial distances. The high spatial frequencies found in the maps generated by the model under 'pathological' conditions would make it impossible to produce a meaningful solution of the inverse solution. As measured data under such conditions produce similar results [1], this conclusion holds also for the experimental measurements. Therefore the accuracy of the inverse solution is expected to be good only under normal conditions.

As epicardial potential maps and activation maps are becoming a more clinically useful tool, while also helping to validate solutions of the forward or inverse problems, the study of their sensitivities to the underlying processes becomes more important. The present simulation results and the surface maps they generate are useful as base for quantitative evaluation of models of myocardial activation processes [16, 17, 18], and of solutions of the forward problem [12]. The present model and its maps may serve as an important link in validating solutions of the inverse problem [12], either in its present form or with the addition of body surface potentials.

Acknowledgment

This study was supported in part by the Michael Kennedy-Leigh Fund, London, and by the Technion VPR-Micay Archie Biomedical Research Fund. It was sponsored by the MEP Group, Woman's Division, ATS, New York.

References

1. Barr RC, Spach MS (1978): Inverse calculation of QRS-T epicardial potentials from body surface potential distributions for normal and ectopic beats in the intact dog. Circ Res 42: 661–675.
2. Hinsen R, Silny J, Rau G, v. Essen R, Merx W, Effert S (1982): Exercise electrocardiography and monitoring of myocardial infarction with a clinical mapping system. In: Models and measurements of the cardiac electric field. Plenum press, New York, pp. 191–203.
3. Vondenbusch B, Silny J, v. Essen R, Ludwig B, Rau G, Effert S (1985): ECG-mapping during coronary dilatation: improvement of diagnosis and therapy control. Computers in Cardiology, IEEE press.
4. Sano T, Takayama N, Shimamoto T (1959): Directional differences of conduction velocity in the cardiac ventricular syncytium studied by microelectrodes. Circ Res 7: 262–267.
5. Clerc L (1976): Directional differences of impulse spread in trabecular muscle for mammalian heart. J Physiol (London) 255: 335–346.
6. Spach MS, Miller WT, Dolber PC, Kootsey JM, Sommer JR, Mosher CE (1982): The functional role of structural complexities in the propagation of depolarization in the atrium of the dog. Circ Res 50: 175–191.
7. Spear JF, Michelson EL, Moore EN (1983): Reduced space constant in slow conducting regions of chronically infarcted canine myocardium. Circ Res 53: 176–185.
8. Cuppen JJM, van Oosterom A (1984): Model studies with the inversely calculated isochrones of ventricular depolarization. IEEE Trans Biomed Eng, V. BME-31: 652–659.
9. Geselowitz DB (1985): Use of time integrals of the ECG to solve the inverse problem. IEEE Trans Biomed Eng, V. BME-32: 73–75.
10. Ritsema van Eck HJ (1972): Digital computer simulation of cardiac excitation and repolarization in man. M.Sc. thesis, Dalhousy U., Halifax, Nova Scotia, Canada.
11. Adam D, Barta E (1986): The effects of anisotropy on myocardial function. Submitted to Annals of Bioengineering.
12. Rudy Y, Plonsey R (1979): The eccentric spheres model as the basis for a study of the role of geometry and inhomogeneities in electrocardiography. IEEE Trans Biomed Eng, V. BME-26, 392–399.
13. Plonsey R,, Barr RC (1984): Current flow patterns in two-dimensional anisotropic bisyncytia with normal and extreme conductivities. Biophys J 45: 557–571.
14. Geselowitz DB, Miller WT (1983): A bidomain model for anisotropic cardiac muscle. Ann Biomed Eng, 11: 191–206.
15. Van Oosterom A, van Dam RT (1976): Potential distribution in the left ventricular wall during depolarization. Electrocardiology Adv Cardiol 16: 27–31.
16. Solomon JC, Selvester RH (1973): Simulation of measured activation sequence in the human heart. Am Heart J 85: 518–523.
17. Steinhaus BM, Spitzer KW (1983): Simulation of activation sequence effects in heart tissue. IEEE Frontiers of Eng. and Comp. in Health Care, pp. 199–204.
18. Okajima M, Fujino T, Kobayashi T, Yamada K (1968): Computer simulation of propagation process in excitation of the ventricles. Circ Res 23: 203–211.

19. Streeter DD, Spotnitz HM, Patel DJ, Ross J, Sonnenblick EH (1969): Fiber orientation in the canine left ventricle during diastole and systole. Circ Res 24: 339–347.
20. Joyner RW, Veenstra R, Rawling D, Chorro A (1984): Propagation through electrically coupled cells. Biophys J 45: 1017–1025.
21. Otsuka N, Hara T (1965): Gross demonstration of the mammalian atrioventricular bundle by a periodic acid procedure. Schiff Stain Technol 40: 305–311.
22. Veenstra RO, Joyner RW, Rawling DA (1984): Purkinje and ventricular activation sequence of canine papillary muscle. Circ Res 54: 500–515.
23. Adam D, Barta E (1987): The effects of anisotropy on myocardial activation. In: Sideman S, Beyar R (eds.) Simulation and control of the cardiac system. CRC Pub, Fl.
24. Arisi G, Macchi E, Baruffi S, Spaggiari S, Taccardi B (1983):Potential fields on the ventricular surface of the exposed dog heart during normal excitation. Circ Res 52: 706–715.
25. Spach MS, Barr RC (1975): Analysis of ventricular activation and repolarization from intramural and ectopic potential distributions for ectopic beats in the intact dog. Circ Res 37: 830–843.

Discussion

Clark: Could you say a word or two about the endocardial activation sequence that you use to drive the model. What approximations did you use with regard to the excitation of wall elements? Did you assume a sequential fashion? You assumed a propagation velocity, but you had to drive the model with an endocardial activation sequence to begin with. How are they interrelated? What data was it based upon and what are the algorithms for the spread through the wall?
Adam: The endocardial layer was covered with, what might be called, Purkinje fiber network which means it's spread of activation was about three times as fast as in the myocardial layers (2.5 : 1). The main orientation of the Purkinje fibers was mostly from the apex to the base of the ventricle, but not necessarily only in that direction. The chances are that the excitation would go much quicker from the apex to the base, as verified by several reports from the Joyner group, Otsuka and Hara, Kubbertus and others. The propagation process from one cell to its neighbors is according to the Higgins principle. It means that once a cell is active, it will activate its neighoring cells in the next timestep and it will do that in a 3 : 1 ratio in the preferred direction. This process is fixed in time and therefore its speed is fixed. On the other hand, the overall propagation velocity is not fixed and is determined according to tissue characteristics and condition. In all the normal cases, the initiation of activity was achieved by simultaneously stimulating only four points, two at the left ventricle and two at the right ventricle, on the Purkinje conduction system. From there the activation spreads out quicker through the Purkinje conduction system and slower through the myocardial fibers.
Rudy: Do you make any attempt to represent the conduction system with realistic geometry? Is there any penetration of the Purkinje network into the myocardial wall as part of the model so as to allow bidirectional conduction.
Adam: The conduction system distal to the Purkinje fibers network is represented in the model in as true a fashion as possible. These fibers are oriented from apex to base, with a speed of propagation 2.5 times that in the myocardial fibers. The activation also propagates in other directions, but slower. The layer, with the Purkinje fibers is the inner-most layer, covering the endocardium. The endocardium is shaped in the present simulation as an ellipsoid, and so is the layer of the conduction system. The interaction between the Purkinje (conduction) layer and the endocardium is achieved by propagation of activity between the two kinds of cells, but at low conduction velocities. There is also the possibility of activation from the myocardium back to the conduction system, so it is a bi-directional conduction. The penetration of the Purkinje fibers into the subendocardial layers is achieved by higher-than-usual transverse (radial) conduction velocities in these layers. The functional role of these fibers is, therefore, simulated.

7. Effects of anisotropy on functional reentrant circuits: preliminary results of computer simulation studies

W.J.E.P. LAMMERS, A.L. WIT and M.A. ALLESSIE

Abstract

The effects of uniform anisotropy of conduction was studied on functional reentry in a computer model. The model simulated conduction of the cardiac impulse in a 30 × 30 matrix of cells, connected to each other by a specified resistance that determined the time lag between excitation of one cell and another (conduction velocity). Each cell also had a predetermined time course for recovery of excitability (refractory period). Functional reentry was initiated in an isotropic matrix (equal conduction latencies in all directions) by exciting a cell adjacent to a transient line of conduction block. Functional reentrant circuits had properties of 'leading circle' reentry. The wave length of the circulating excitation (refractory period × conduction velocity) was only slightly shorter that the path length of the circuit, did not vary greatly as the impulse conducted around the circuit and only a very small excitable gap was present. During established reentry, the sheet was made anisotropic (conduction in the horizontal direction was 5 times more rapid than in the vertical direction). This caused the reentrant circuit to assume an oval shape. Furthermore, the wave length of the circulating excitation changed markedly in different regions of the circuit, expanding during rapid horizontal conduction and contracting during slow vertical conduction. As a result of the slow vertical conduction and the resultant short wave length, a large excitable gap appeared. The results predict, therefore, that functional reentrant circuits in anisotropic tissue will have an excitable gap.

Introduction

Conduction of the cardiac impulse is strongly influenced by the structural interrelationships of the myocardial fiber bundles. A fundamental characteristic is that impulse propagation is more rapid along the long axis of myocardial fibers than perpendicular to the long axis [1]. This anisotropic property has been further subdivided by Spach et al. [2, 3]. According to their definitions *uniform anisotropy* occurs in cardiac muscle in which the fibers are all arranged parallel to each other. *Nonuniform anisotropy* occurs when non conductile barriers such as those formed by connective tissue influence conduction or when myocardial fibers are not arranged in parallel.

The anisotropic properties of cardiac muscle may play an important role in the genesis of reentrant arrhythmias. Spach et al. [2] proposed that it may cause the conduction block of premature impulses that may initiate reentry because of a low safety factor for conduction in the longitudinal direction. Conduction perpendicular to fiber orientation can also be slow enough even in normal tissue to cause reentry [2]. Slowed conduction caused by anisotropy in the epicardial border zone of canine infarcts may be an important factor leading to *functional* reentry in this region [4–8]. Not only might anisotropy cause reentry but also reentrant circuits in anisotropic tissue might have different properties than circuits in tissue that is not strongly anisotropic. For example, the reentrant circuits in the epicardial border of infarcts often have excitable gaps e.g. during reentrant tachycardias electrically stimulated impulses can invade the reentrant circuit and reset or terminate the arrhythmia (unpublished observations). This experimental result is contrary to a predicted property of functional circuits – it has been shown that in atrial reentry caused by the leading circle mechanism, an excitable gap does not exist because the head of the wave front usually travels in the relatively refractory tail [8]. We propose that excitable gaps in the functional circuits of infarcts might be a consequence of the anisotropy-induced slow conduction which might not be prominent in the atrial free wall. However, it is not possible in experimental studies to change the anisotropic properties of the tissue and determine the effects on reentrant circuits – an intervention that would directly show the influences of anisotropy on reentry. We have, therefore, used a computer model of excitation in a sheet of excitable elements to study the effects of anisotropy on reentry.

The electrical excitation model

The model permits the investigation of the propagation of excitation waves in a 2 dimensional matrix. The model consists of a sheet of 900 cells arranged in a regular matrix of 30 × 30 (Fig. 1A). Every cell is connected to eight neighbors (Fig. 1B), except at the boundaries of the matrix. The following parameters are assigned to each cell.

1. A parameter designating the cell as *'active' or 'inactive':* cells that are 'active' can be excited and those that are 'inactive' cannot. This makes it possible to construct reentrant circuits with various geometrical configurations, such as circuits around a hole in the matrix. Cells can be designated as being inactive for a finite period of time and thereafter, may become active. In this way,

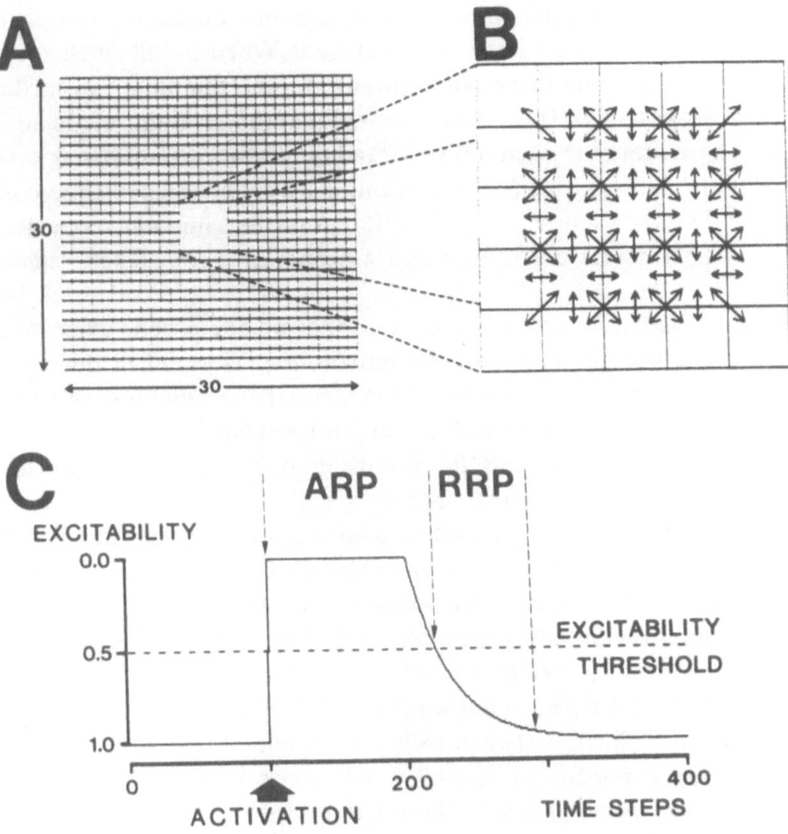

Figure 1. The 30 × 30 matrix of cells used in the simulation studies is shown in A. The center of this matrix is magnified in B to show the connections between cells (arrows). These connections are in vertical and horizontal directions as well as in the oblique directions at each corner. In C the time course of excitability in one cell is depicted. The vertical axis is the state of excitability with 1.0 being fully excitable and 0.0 being completely inexcitable. On the horizontal axis is time expressed as arbitrary units that occur during the simulation (time steps). At the moment of activation, excitability drops to zero and remains at that level for a pre-assigned time period. This is followed by a gradual increase in excitability with a time course given by a simple exponential function. The cell is absolutely refractory from the moment of activation until the exponential recovery phase has reached the excitability threshold (ARP). Thereafter the cell is in its relatively refractory period until the 95% excitability level is reached.

temporary regions of block can be induced.

2. Conduction latencies (expressed in arbitrary time units, called time steps) to the eight neighboring cells: this is the amount of time required for one cell to excite the next when the cells are fully excitable. An additional time latency is added to this basic latency when cells have not completely recovered excitability from a previous activation (see below). These local conduction properties may be different in different directions.

3. A time period and a time constant: together they determine the course of excitability after the cell has been activated. When a cell fires, either by activation from a neighboring cell or by an external 'stimulus', the excitability of the cell drops to zero (Fig. 1C) and remains at this level during the assigned period. Thereafter, the excitability is gradually restored, following a simple exponential function with a rate determined by the assigned time constant (Fig. 1C). These parameters can be different or the same in every cell.

Two general parameters are used which are operative for all the cells in the matrix:

1. Duration of activation: this is the time allowed for a cell, when fired, to activate a neighboring cell. In the simulations performed in this study the duration of activation was set at 1 time step. If the neighboring cell is not receptive within this time period, it will not be excited.
2. Threshold of excitability: this threshold determines the minimum level of excitability required for activation (Fig. 1C).

The threshold of excitability, together with the time course of excitability, determines the absolute and relative refractory time periods in each cell (Fig. 1C). The absolute refractory period (ARP) starts at the moment a cell is activated and ends when the exponentially increasing excitability reaches the threshold of excitability. During this period the cell is inexcitable. The relative refractory period starts after the ARP and ends when excitability has reached a level of 0.95.

The conduction velocity between cells is determined by the basic latency as assigned to every connection (see no 2) and the excitability of the cell at the moment it is activated according to the relationship:

$$\text{Conduction time} = \frac{\text{Basic latency}}{\text{Excitability level}}.$$

In the fully excitable state (excitability = 1.0, see Fig. 1C) the conduction time is equal to the basic latency. If the cell is partially excitable, the conduction time is increased depending on the initial excitability level according to the above equation.

Two major events occur at each time step during an actual simulation.

1. The excitability level is updated in every cell.
2. If a cell has fired in the previous time step, the possibility of conduction to its neighbors is tested. If one of these neighboring cells is fully or partially excitable, the conduction time between the two cells is calculated. The conduction time is added to the activation time of the firing cell to obtain the predicted activation time of the receiving cell. Usually this new activation time exceeds the current simulation time. The cell is, therefore, not yet allowed to fire; instead this *predicted* activation time is stored until the simulation time reaches the predicted time, at which moment the cell will fire. During the time that the excited cells waits to fire, the same cell may be approached by other

impulses coming from a different direction which may lead to an update of the predicted fire time. The cell is allowed to fire when the running simulation time reaches the earliest predicted activation time.

The simulation program was written in Fortran IV. It was run on a PDP 11/04 computer using a Tektronix 4010 terminal as operator console and a Ramtek 9050 graphic processor for color display of the sequence of propagation and the state of excitability in the 900 cells.

Results

Properties of the conductive matrix – the sheet of 'excitable' cells

For the simulations that we describe in this report, we utilized several sheets of excitable cells with different intrinsic properties. One sheet was isotropic; this means that the latency time in all directions was equal and therefore conduction velocity in all directions was the same. The pattern of activation in this isotropic sheet after the center cell was excited (center stimulation) is shown in Fig. 2A. Activation occurs in concentric circles away from the center. We also used anisotropic sheets (uniform anisotropy) in which conduction in the vertical axis was made slower than conduction in the horizontal axis by increasing the latency time in the vertical axis relative to the horizontal. The latency time changes monotonically between the two axes. The activation pattern after excitation of the center element in an anisotropic sheet with a 3 : 1 latency ratio is shown in Fig. 2B. The isochrones are elliptical with the long axis of the ellipse in the horizontal direction because of the more rapid activation (shorter latency time).

Simulation of functional reentry in an isotropic matrix

Reentrant excitation was initiated in an isotropic sheet by activating (stimulating) a cell in the sheet adjacent to a long line of block which was caused by making a line of cells temporarily inexcitable (Fig. 3). In the figure, the location of the inexcitable cells are shown by the black line and the site of stimulation is indicated by the 'S'. Activation proceeded away from this site toward the end of the line of block which was programmed to disappear by the time activation had travelled along its entire length. The activation wave then moved back towards its site of origin (right to left) on the opposite side of the original line of block. As it travelled back toward the stimulation site, the activation wave was prevented from exciting cells it had already activated because these remained inexcitable for 132 time units (absolute refractory period – see Fig. 1). By the time the excitation wave arrived opposite to the stimulus site (toward the left margin of the sheet) the cells that were initially activated had recovered excitability. Activation then

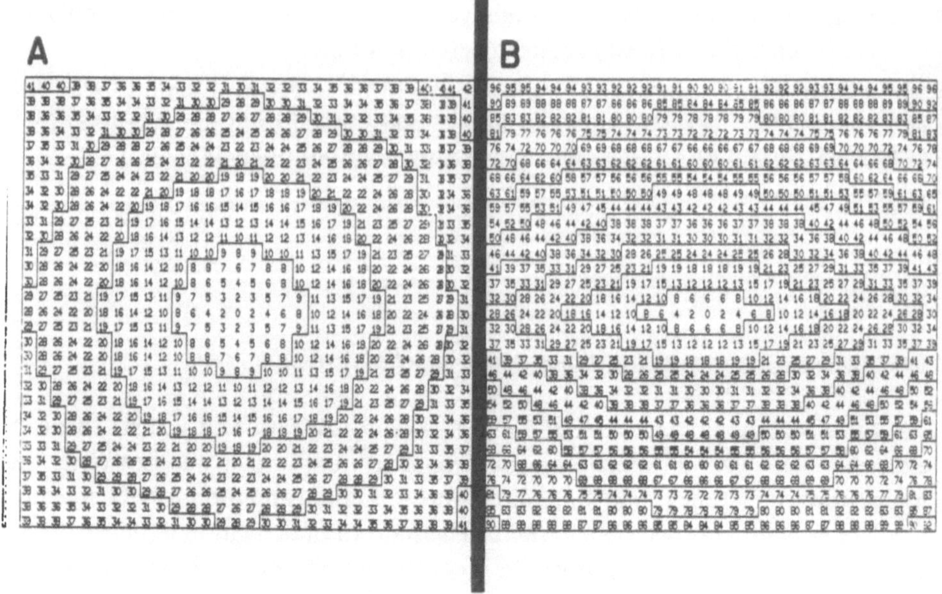

Figure 2. Activation patterns after excitation of the center cell in two different sheets. In A the sheet is isotropic, the latency value (see Fig. 1) is equal in all directions. There is uniform spread of activation away from the central stimulus. In B, the sheet is anisotropic. Latency in the vertical direction was made 3 times longer then in the horizontal direction; activation in this direction is, therefore, slower than in the horizontal direction. In this figure, the activation times of each of the cells is plotted as excitation moves away from the stimulus site. The same number of activation times make up the excitation maps shown in the following figures. However, only the isochrones are shown for the sake of clarity.

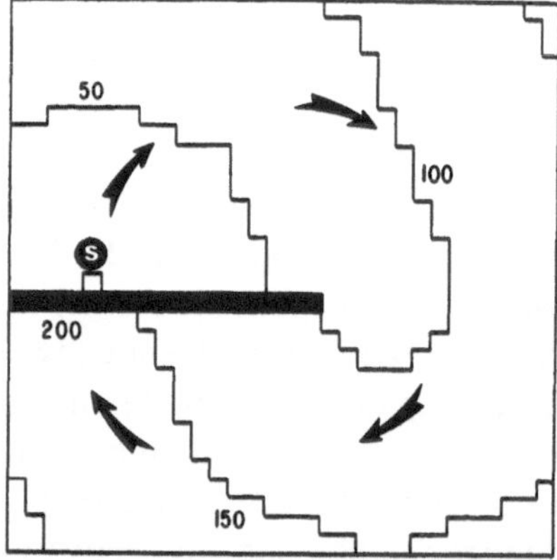

Figure 3. Initiation of functional reentry in an isotropic sheet. At the beginning of the stimulation, a line of elements perpendicular to the left border was made inexcitable. This line is shown in black. An element adjacent to the line (S) was excited. Activation occurred in the sequence indicated by the arrows and the isochrones. Before activation reached the 100 isochrone the line of block was removed.

occurred across the line and once more in the left to right direction. Continuous reentry was thereby established.

Figure 4A shows the pattern of activation of the isotropic sheet during the stable reentry. Activation occurs in a spiral pattern with wavefronts propagating in all directions away from the center. We will concentrate on the events occurring at the origin of the spiral where the smallest diameter reentrant circuit is located. This has been called the leading circle [8, 9] and we will use this terminology despite the fact that this smallest circuit is not really circular. This circuit of excitable elements is indicated by the black bars in Figure 4A. It is also shown, enlarged, in Figure 4B where the time of activation of each cell comprising the circuit is indicated for one complete revolution. The arrows show the sequence with which one cell is exciting the next. For this cycle excitation begins in the top row of cells (cell labelled 5) and continues in a clock wise direction to the cell indicated by the 134. The complete revolution time around the circuit is 137 time units. Activation is occurring around a long, narrow line between the two horizontal rows of cells. This is a line of block because activation from one row cannot cross over to excite cells in the other row except at the ends. The block is functional –cells on one side of the line are refractory while activation is occurring on the other side of the line, preventing activation from crossing or short circuiting the line.

As the wave of excitation proceeds around the functional circuit, it leaves in its wake a 'tail' of functionally refractory cells, e.g. cells that have recently been excited and have not yet recovered excitability (to the excitability threshold). Thus a part of the circuit is always inexcitable and this part moves around the circuit following the excitation wave. How much of the circuit is inexcitable is determined by the *wave length* of the propagating excitation wave which is defined as the distance traveled by the excitation wave during the time the tissue restores its excitability sufficiently to propagate another impulse. The wave length is equal to the functional refractory period × the conduction velocity [10]. In order for reentry to continue, the wave length cannot be longer than the path length. That is, there must always be some excitable tissue in front of the activation wave or else activation would die out. In the experimental studies on leading circle reentry in rabbit atria it was shown that the size of the reentrant circuit was determined by the conduction velocity and refractory period of the impulse and that the size was not much longer than the wave length [8, 9].

We found this same characteristic in our simulation of functional reentry in an isotropic sheet. The size of the circuit was just large enough to accommodate the wave length of the simulated excitation wave, with a small part of the circuit in front of the activation wave always existing in the excitable state. Therefore, propagation around the circuit could continue. Figure 5 shows the state of excitability of cells in the leading circle at different representative times during propagation around the circuit. All inexcitable cells are indicated in black. Excitable cells in the circuit are designated by the unfilled boxes that have the

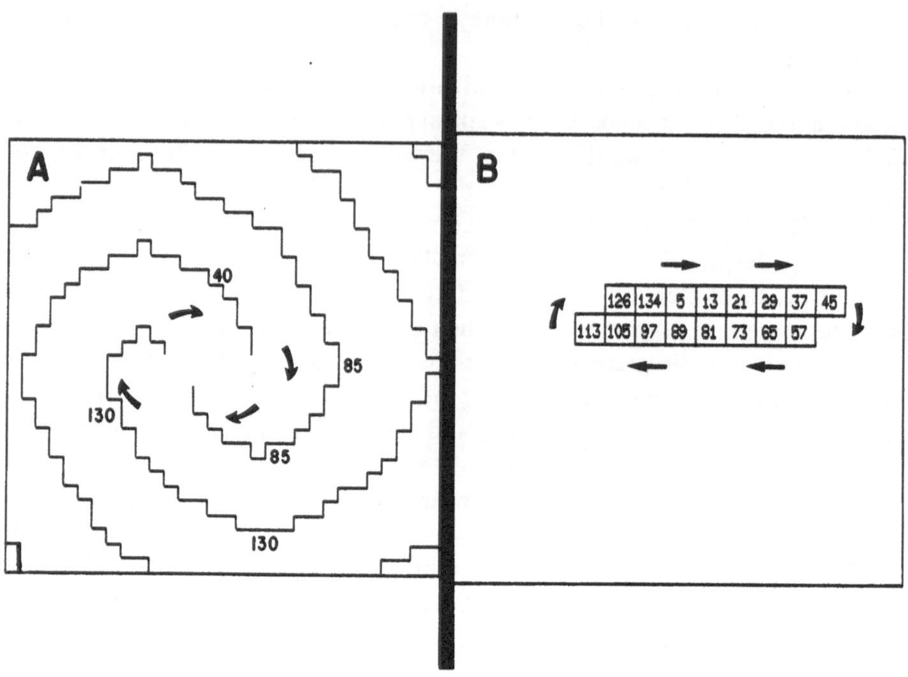

Figure 4. A: pattern of reentry (initiation shown in Fig. 3) in the isotropic sheet. The leading circle of excitable elements are indicated in black and the relative times of activation of these elements are shown in the enlarged version of the leading circle in B.

state of excitability printed in them. This state of excitability is determined by the exponential time course for recovery shown in Fig. 1. Since the excitability threshold in this simulation was 0.5, cells were only excitable when this threshold was exceeded. In Figure 5, the decimal has been omitted in indicating the state of excitability. The total range of excitability is from 6 (just excitable) to 10 (fully excitable). There is at least one cell with an excitability greater than 5 just in front of the head of the wave front at each time shown. For example, in Fig. 5A, the wavefront is moving from right to left along the bottom row of cells. At the time shown, the head of the excitation wave is preceded by two cells designated as having an excitability of 6, meaning the cells are relatively refractory and can be excited. Excitability of other cells outside the leading circle that are relatively refractory are also plotted and inscribe the same spiral of activation around that center region that was described in Fig. 4. At the time period shown in Fig. 5B, the excitation wave has just arrived at the last cell at the left of this row. There is one cell with an excitability of 6 in front of the wavefront at this time. In Fig. 5C and 5D activation is occurring from left to right along the top column of cells and at each time depicted there are two partially [6] excitable cells in front of the activation wave.

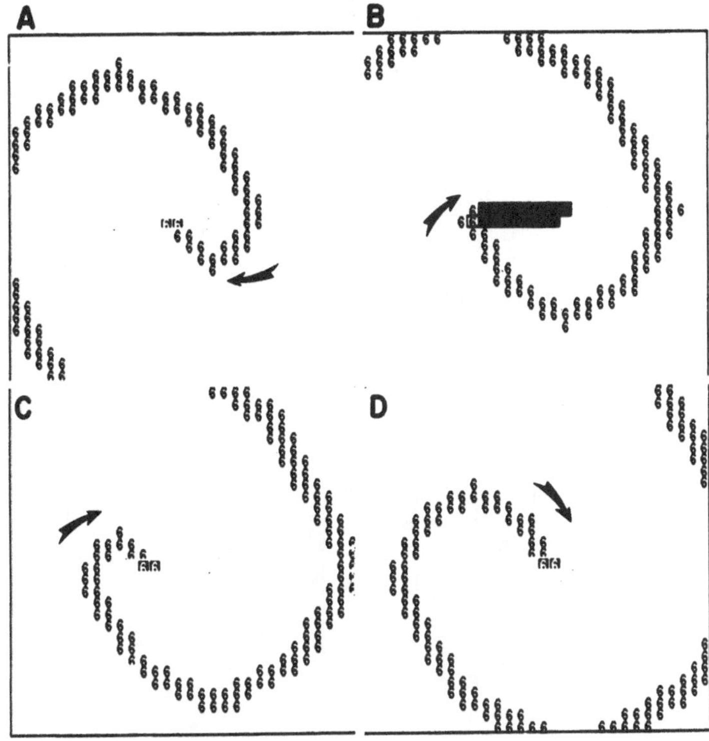

Figure 5. The excitable gap in the leading circle and in the rest of the isotropic sheet during functional reentry. In each panel, the leading circle of excitable elements is indicated by the black bars (see Fig. 4 for explanation of this format). The white boxes with the numbers indicate the elements comprising the excitable gap and their relative excitability for different locations of the wave front in the circuit. The arrows indicate the direction of activation. In each panel, the activation wave is just moving into the partially excitable elements.

At this time we will introduce the term 'excitable gap'. This term is used to describe the part of the circuit which remains excitable during reentry [11]. The gap may be either completely or partially excitable. The part of the circuit which is excitable is determined by the relationship between the wave length of the impulse and the path length of the circuit. The larger the path length with respect to the wave length, the greater is the part of the circuit that remains excitable. As shown in Fig. 5, during the simulation of functional reentry, no cells in the circuit are completely excitable and thus there is no completely excitable gap. However, there are partially excitable cells in front of the activation wave and these constitute a *partially excitable gap*. Figure 6 shows the extent of this partially excitable gap in this simulation as activation moves around the reentrant circuit. The cells that constitute the leading circle are numbered from 1–16 as shown in the top of the diagram. The arrow points out the direction of activation of these

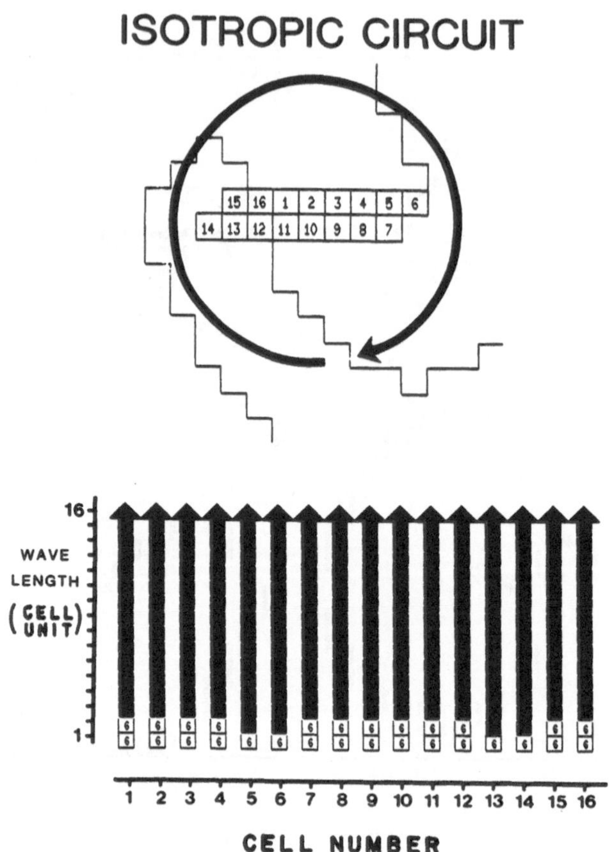

Figure 6. The wave length of refractory cells and the partially excitable gap during functional reentry in an isotropic circuit. At the top, the cells comprising the leading circuit are numbered from 1 to 16 (see Fig. 5). At the bottom, the wave length is indicated by the length of the black arrow (the number of each cell is on the horizontal axis). The unfilled boxes comprise the gap of partially excitable cells.

elements. These cells are also indicated by number on the horizontal axis of the graph below. This graph shows the duration of the wave length as excitation proceeds from one cell to the next. On the vertical axis of this graph is the wave length expressed as the number of cells it encompasses. The wave length along the circuit is indicated by the length of the vertical black arrows. The size of the excitable gap is shown by the unfilled boxes that contain the state of excitability. As activation is progressing between the first 4 cells (cell number 1–4 on the horizontal axis), the wave length extends over 14 of the 16 cells in the circuit (length of the black arrow on the vertical axis). The other 2 cells are excitable with an excitability level of 6. The wave length increases to 15 cells when activation of elements 5 and 6 occurs, and the excitable gap decreases to one cell. Then the wave length decreases again to 14 cells when cells 7–12 are activated and once more increases when cells 13 and 14 are activated. The gap increases and decreases concomitantly.

This simulation clearly shows that during circus movement in a sheet of isotropic tissue there is only a small excitable gap all around the circuit. The excitable gap only shows minimal variations in width caused by slight variations in conduction velocity.

Effects of anisotropy on functional reentry

After functional reentry was established in the isotropic sheet, the sheet was made anisotropic while reentry continued. The change in the sheet caused a change in the characteristics of the reentrant circuit. The effects of an anisotropic sheet with a 5:1 conduction ratio (slow conduction in the vertical direction) is shown in Fig. 7. Activation now occurs in an oval pattern around the center leading circle (Fig. 7A), rather than the circular pattern shown in Fig. 4A. The oval is a consequence of the disparity in conduction velocities between the horizontal and vertical directions; the long axis of the oval is in the direction of most rapid conduction. Figure 7B shows the activation times for one cycle for the cells that comprise the leading circle. The size of the central leading circuit has decreased by one cell and conduction time around the circuit has increased to 179 time units.

The state of excitability of cells comprising the leading circle at several representative times is indicated in Fig. 8. The format of the figure is the same as Fig. 5. In Fig. 8A, activation is turning around the left corner and is preceded by one partially excitable cell (excitability level is 6). In Fig. 8B, as activation is moving from left to right in the horizontal direction it is now preceded by 6 partially excitable cells, 3 of which have an excitability of 8. As the activation wave approaches the right corner of the leading circle and turns around it, the number of partially excitable elements preceding it decreases (Fig. 8C, D). Figure 9 (format is the same as Fig. 6) shows the extent of the partially excitable gap and the wave length at each cell in the leading circuit. Both are changing throughout the reentrant circuit, with the minimum wave length and maximum partially excitable gap occurring when cells 7 and 14 are activated (excitable gap consists of 6–7 cells, 3 with an excitability of 6 and 4 with an excitability of 8). The maximum wave length and minimum partially excitable gap occurs at cells 5 and 6 and 12 and 13 (excitable gap is one cell with an excitability of 6). It is therefore apparent that anisotropy has increased the excitable gap.

The changes in the wave length and the partially excitable gap during reentry in the anisotropic matrix are a consequence of the marked changes in conduction velocity in the leading circuit. Moving in the horizontal direction there are 6 time units between activation of adjacent elements. The conduction velocity slows markedly when activation occurs in the vertical direction. At the left there are 44

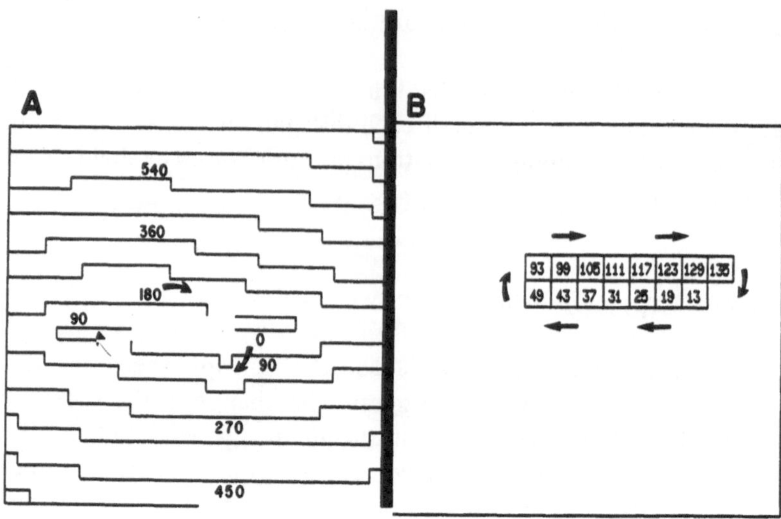

Figure 7. Pattern of reentry (initiation shown in Fig. 3) in an anisotropic sheet with a 5 : 1 activation ratio. The leading circle of excitable elements are indicated in black and the relative times of activation of these elements are shown in the enlarged version of the leading circle in B.

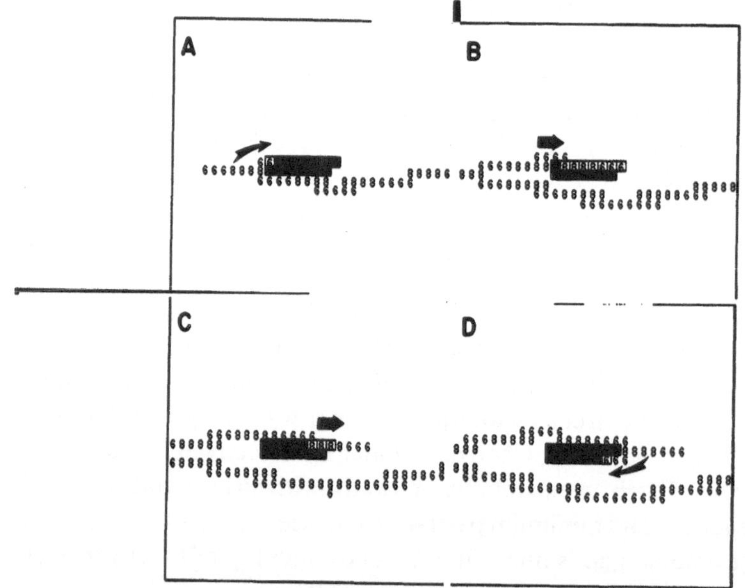

Figure 8. The excitable gap in the leading circle and in the rest of the anisotropic sheet during functional reentry. In each panel, the leading circle of excitable elements is indicated by the black bars. The white boxes with the numbers indicate the elements comprising the excitable gap and their relative excitability for different locations of the wave front in the circuit. The arrows indicated the direction of activation. In each panel, the activation wave is just moving into the partially excitable elements.

ANISOTROPIC CIRCUIT

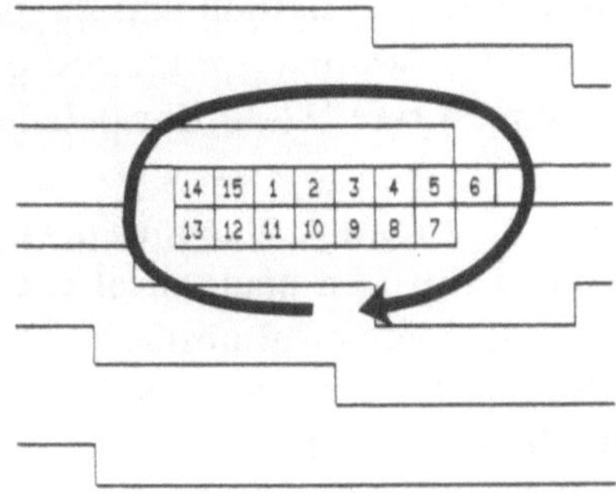

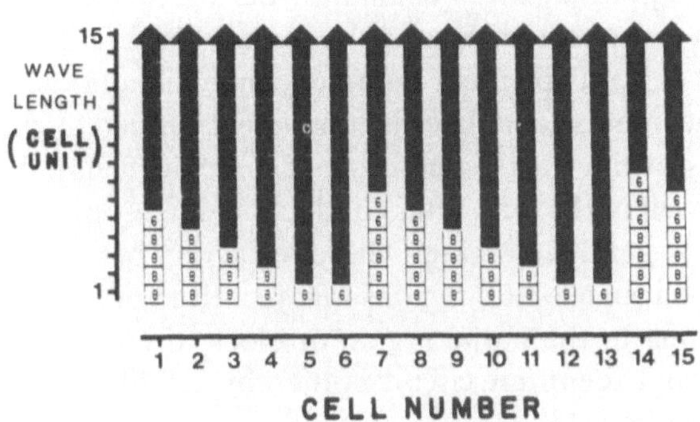

Figure 9. The wave length of refractory and the partially excitable gap during functional reentry in an anisotropic sheet (5 : 1 latency ratio). The format is the same as Fig. 6.

time units between elements 13 and 14 and at the right there are 57 time units between elements 6 and 7. The very slow activation is a consequence of the anisotropy. As a result the wave length shortens drastically and the partially excitable gap increases at these times. These changes then outlast the return of rapid conduction velocity; wave length gradually increases and partially excitable gap decreases during rapid excitation in the horizontal direction.

Discussion

The cardiac impulse normally arises in the sinus node and spreads throughout the heart over well defined routes. The conducting impulse leaves in its wake refractory tissue that cannot be reexcited for 200–500 msec. As a result, when the last remnants of heart muscle are excited, the impulse finding itself completely surrounded by refractory fibers, dies out. Under certain conditions, however, an impulse that has excited the heart once does not die out but finds a pathway of excitable fibers over which it may return to reexcite part or all of the heart. This phenomenon is called reentrant excitation and the pathway through which the impulse propagates while it is 'waiting' for the rest of the heart to regain excitability is the reentrant circuit (see [12–14] for detailed reviews on mechanisms causing reentry).

In general, there are two basic kinds of reentrant circuits, an anatomical circuit and a functional circuit [8, 13]. An anatomical circuit is comprised of a well defined pathway around an anatomical obstacle. This type of reentrant circuit was first studied by Mines [11] in rings of excitable tissue, the center of the ring formed by the obstacle. In the in situ heart, anatomical circuits may be formed by the bundle branches of the specialized ventricular conducting system [16], by the atria, AV conducting system, ventricles and bypass tracts in patients with WPW syndrome [17], by the tissue around the orifices of the vena cavae [18] or AV communication [19]. In all these examples, during reentrant tachycardia, the impulse circles in one direction around the central barrier. On the other hand, a functional circuit is not dependent on a nonconductile obstacle, but the circuit through which the impulse circulates is completely defined by the electrophysiological properties of the fibers composing the circuit [8, 13]. Thus reentry can occur in the free wall of the atria after conduction of a properly timed premature impulse blocks transiently in regions where refractory periods may be long, and conducts slowly through other regions where refractory periods are shorter, eventually returning to the initial region of block after it has recovered excitability. A functional reentrant circuit is thereby established and reentry may continue by the leading circle mechanism [20, 21].

The properties of reentry resulting from these two different mechanisms and the arrhythmias they cause, have been shown to be very different [8]. These differences are mostly a result of the relationship between the wave length of the conducting impulse and the length of the path comprising the reentrant circuit. As we have already indicated, the wave length is defined as the distance travelled by the depolarization wave during the time needed for the tissue it has excited to restore excitability sufficiently to propagate another impulse [10]. For reentry to continue, this wave length cannot be longer than the path length or else the conducting impulse would run into the refractory tissue in its wake, block and reentry would stop. However, in a reentrant circuit around an anatomical obstacle the wave length may be significantly less than the path length and therefore part of the reentrant circuit is always fully excitable – a gap of full excitability exists [8]. The presence of such a gap has 3 significant influences on the properties of the circuit. First, the revolution time of the impulse around the circuit is determined primarily by the conduction velocity of the impulse and not significantly influenced by (moderate) changes in the refractory period. Second, the reentrant circuit is predicted to be more stable. Third, it is possible to perturb conduction of the reentrant impulse and even stop reentry by applying appropriately timed stimuli to tissue in or around the reentrant circuit. It is this third property that we wish to emphasize in this discussion. During continuous reentry a new impulse may be elicited by a stimulus applied to tissue near the circuit. This stimulated impulse may enter the reentrant circuit if it finds excitable tissue in the circuit. This may easily occur when there is a large excitable gap. Once in the circuit, the stimulated impulse may begin to conduct in both directions around the circuit. In doing so, it can collide in the retrograde direction with the reentering impulse but continue to conduct in the antegrade direction around the circuit. Reentry may continue although the revolution time may be transiently perturbed (prolonged) if the stimulated impulse conducts more slowly around the circuit in relatively refractory tissue. If the stimulated impulse occurs sufficiently early in the excitable gap, it may collide with the reentering impulse in the retrograde direction, but also block in the antegrade direction. Reentrant excitation is terminated as a result. This is the physiological basis for termination of reentrant tachycardias by stimuli applied to the atria or ventricles by a pacemaker [22].

On the other hand, in a functional reentrant circuit caused by the leading circle mechanism, the length of the circuit is not fixed but is determined by the electrophysiological properties of the tissue [8]. The impulse, therefore, circulates in the smallest possible pathway in which the stimulating efficacy is just enough to excite the tissue ahead which is still in its relative refractory phase – 'in this smallest circuit possible which is designated as the leading circle, the head of the circulating wave front is continuously biting in its own tail of refractoriness' [8]. Because of this tight fit, the length of the circulating pathway equals 'the wave length' of the circulating impulse. Functional circuits of this kind may, therefore, not be stable. Because there is a tight fit between the crest and the tail of the impulse, changes in refractory period can have significant influences on the revolution time around the circuit and there is no excitable gap in the circuit. This implies that a wave front (or stimulus) of greater efficacy than the circulating impulse is required to interfere with the leading circle [8]. This property may protect leading circle reentry from being terminated by stimuli applied to the heart during the arrhythmias which it causes and may explain why some reentrant arrhythmias cannot be terminated by pacemakers [23].

The tendency has been to apply the principles learned from studying leading circle reentry in atrial myocardium to functional reentry occurring in other regions of the heart. However, this may not be a valid assumption. We have studied reentrant excitation in the sheet of muscle which survives on the epicardial surface of canine infarcts. This reentry is also functional – there is usually no anatomical obstacle and the reentrant circuit is determined by the functional properties of the cardiac tissue [5, 24]. However, unlike leading circle reentry in the atria a large excitable gap is sometimes present in the circuit allowing reentrant tachycardias to be terminated by electrical stimuli applied to the ventricles. One major difference between the anatomy and electrophysiology of the muscle in which reentry is occurring in the epicardial border zone of the infarcts and in the atrial free wall is the orientation of the myocardial fibers and the influence of this orientation on conduction. In the epicardial border zone, the muscle fibers are oriented in parallel to one another and conduction parallel to the long axis of the myocardial fibers may be 3–5 times more rapid then conduction perpendicular [4]. This difference in conduction velocity dependent on anisotropic structure has been explained [1–3] by the differences in the degree of cell coupling in the different directions. Because of the differences in conduction velocity caused by anisotropy, the conduction velocity of the impulse around the reentrant circuit is not uniform – it is more rapid in that part of the circuit parallel to fiber orientation while slower in that part of the circuit perpendicular to fiber orientation [5]. It has been proposed by Frame and Hoffman that differences in properties in different parts of the circuit might lead to the appearance of an excitable gap [25]. On the other hand in that part of the atria where leading circle reentry has been studied most thoroughly, there is no clear influence of fiber orientation on conduction velocity since the myocardial fibers are arranged in many different directions.

To determine whether the presence of anisotropy might lead to the appearance of an excitable gap, we did the simulation study described in the results. Our computer model for activation of a sheet of excitable cells is not based on simulating transmembrane currents or longitudinal current flow [26, 27], but simply relies on excitation latencies between cells and the interrelationships between excitation and the time course of recovery of excitability of the cells. These are important factors that govern conduction in reentrant circuits. In our simulation in an isotropic sheet of cells, the functional reentrant circuit closely mimicked some aspects of leading circle reentry studied in atrial myocardium. In particular, the size of the leading circle was governed by the properties of conduction and refractoriness of the cells, and the head of the wave front travelled in the partially refractory tail. As shown in Fig. 5, the excitable gap in the isotropic circuit is small, consisting of only one or two cells and the state of excitability in the gap is never more than 0.6. Thus, excitability is just sufficient to allow continued propagation around the circuit. Another important characteristic of this functional reentry is the relative consistent wave length of the impulse throughout the circuit. Although there are small changes in conduction velocity in several regions of the circuit they do not influence the wave length sufficiently to cause major changes in the excitable gap. It is also expected that in leading circle reentry in atrial myocardium, the wave length is relatively constant throughout the reentrant circuit during tachycardia since, at these rapid rates, refractory periods and conduction velocity may be nearly uniform.

In the anisotropic matrix of cells, leading circle reentry also occurs. However, there are marked changes in conduction velocity when activation changes from the fast direction (parallel to fiber orientation) to the slow direction (perpendicular to fiber orientation). As a result of the slowing, the wave length quickly decreases revealing a large excitable gap not evident in the isotropic matrix. Thus, it is predicted that tachycardias caused by functional reentry and occurring in anisotropic tissue may be more stable than in isotropic tissue and may be terminated by pacemaker stimuli.

Acknowledgment

This work was supported by the Foundation for Medical Research (FUNGO) Grant 13-22-76 in the Netherlands and by Program Project Grant HL 30557 from the National Institutes of Health.

References

1. Clerc L (1976): Directional differences of impulse spread in trabecular muscle from mammalian heart. J Physiol (London) 255: 335–346.
2. Spach MS, Miller WT, Geselowitz DB, Barr RC, Kootsey JM, Johnson EA (1981): The discontinuous nature of propagation in normal canine cardiac muscle: Evidence for recurrent discontinuities of intracellular resistance that affect the membrane currents. Circ Res 48: 39–54.
3. Spach MS, Miller WT, Dolber PC, Kootsey JM, Sommer JR, Mosher CE Jr (1982): The functional role of structural complexities in the propagation of depolarization in the atrium of the dog. Cardiac conduction disturbances due to discontinuities of effective axial resistivity. Circ Res 50: 175–191.
4. Ursell PC, Gardner PI, Albala A, Fenoglio JJ Jr, Wit AL (1985): Structural and electrophysiological changes in the epicardial border zone of canine myocardial infarcts during infarct healing. Circ Res 56: 436–451.
5. Dillon S, Ursell PC, Wit AL (1985): Pseudo-block caused by anisotropic conduction: A new mechanism for sustained reentry. Circulation 72: III–279.
6. El-Sherif N, Hope RR, Scherlag BJ, Lazzara R (1977): Reentrant ventricular arrhythmias in the late myocardial infarction period. 2. Patterns of initiation and termination of reentry. Circulation 55: 702–718.
7. El-Sherif N, Smith A, Evans K (1981): Canine ventricular arrhythmias in the late myocardial infarction period. 8. Epicardial mapping of reentrant circuits. Circ Res 49: 255–265.
8. Allessie MA, Bonke FIM, Schopman FJG (1977): Circus movement in rabbit atrial muscle as a mechanism of tachycardia. III. The 'leading circle' concept: a new model of circus movement in cardiac tissue without the involvement of an anatomic obstacle. Circ Res 41: 9–18.
9. Allessie MA, Bonke FIM, Schopman F (1973): Circus movement in rabbit atrial muscle as a mechanism of tachycardia. Circ Res 33: 54–62.
10. Smeets JLRM, Allessie MA, Lammers WJEP, Bonke FIM, Hollen J (1986): The wave length of the cardiac impulse and reentrant arrhythmias in isolated rabbit atrium. The role of heart rate, autonomic transmitters, temperature and potassium. Circ Res 58: 96–108.
11. Mines GR (1913): On dynamic equilibrium in the heart. J Physiol (London) 46: 349–383.
12. Wit AL, Cranefield PF (1978): Reentrant excitation as a cause of cardiac arrhythmias. Am J Physiol 235: H1–H17.
13. Allessie MA, Bonke FIM (1980): Atrial arrhythmias: Basic concepts. In Mandel WJ (ed.): Cardiac arrhythmias: their mechanisms, diagnosis and management. JB Lippincott Co., Philadelphia, pp. 145–166.
14. Janse MJJ (1986): Reentry rhythms. In: Fozzard HA, Haber E, Jennings RB, Katz AM, Morgan HE (eds). The heart and cardiovascular system. Raven Press, New York, pp. 1203–1238.

15. Lewis T (1925): The Mechanism and graphic registration of the heart beat, 3rd ed. Shaw and Sons, London.
16. Moe GK, Mendez C, Han J (1965): Aberrant AV impulse propagation in the dog heart: a study of functional bundle branch block. Circ Res 16: 261–286.
17. Gallagher JJ, Gilbert M, Sevenson RH, Sealy WC, Kasell J, Wallace AG (1975): Wolff Parkinson-White syndrome: the problem, evaluation and surgical correction. Circulation 51: 767–785.
18. Lewis T (1920): Observations upon flutter and fibrillation. Part IV. Impure flutter; theory of circus movement. Heart 7: 293–331.
19. Frame LH, Page RL, Boyden PA, Hoffman PF (1983): A right atrial incision that stabilizes reentry around the tricuspid ring in dogs. Circulation 68: Suppl III–360.
20. Allessie MA, Lammers WJEP, Bonke FIM, Hollen J (1985): Experimental evaluation of Moe's multiple wavelet hypothesis of atrial fibrillation. In: Zipes DP, Jalife J (eds) Cardiac electrophysiology and arrhythmias. Grune and Stratton, Orlando, pp. 265–275.
21. Allessie MA, Lammers WJEP, Bonke FIM, Hollen J (1984): Intra-atrial reentry as a mechanism for atrial flutter induced by acetylcholine and rapid pacing in the dog. Circulation 70: 123–135.
22. Karagueuzian HS, Fenoglio JJ Jr, Weiss MB, Wit AL (1979): Protracted ventricular tachycardia induced by premature stimulation of the canine heart after coronary artery occlusion and reperfusion. Circ Res 44: 833–848.
23. Waldo AL, Maclean WAH, Karp RB, Kouchoukos NT, James TN (1977): Entrainment and interruption of atrial flutter with atrial pacing: studies in man following open heart surgery. Circulation 56: 737–744.
24. Wit AL, Allessie MA, Bonke FIM, Lammers WJEP, Smeets J, Fenoglio JJ Jr (1982): Electrophysiologic mapping to determine the mechanism of experimental ventricular tachycardia initiated by premature impulses. Am J Cardiol 49: 166–185.
25. Frame LH, Hoffman BF (1984): Mechanisms of tachycardia. In: Surawicz B, Pratrap Reddy C, Prystowsky EN (eds) Tachycardias. Martinus Nijhoff, Dordrecht, pp. 7–36.
26. Beeler GW, Reuter H (1977): Reconstruction of the action potential of ventricular myocardial fibers. J Physiol (London) 268: 177–210.
27. Van Capelle FJ, Durrer D (1980): Computer simulation of arrhythmias in a network of coupled excitable elements. Circ Res 47: 454–466.

8. Interaction of oscillatory currents and steady-state membrane conductance in isolated cardiac myocytes: Experimental description and preliminary modeling of syncytial effects

C. NORDIN and R.S. ARONSON

Abstract

Oscillatory currents associated with conditions that increase myoplasmic Ca^{2+} may be an important cause of ventricular arrhythmias. During diastole, the magnitude of voltage deflections generated by such currents will be a function not only of the currents themselves, but also of the net conductance of the membrane, which is reflected in the steady-state current-voltage relationship. We used the two microelectrode voltage clamp technique in isolated guinea pig ventricular myocytes to study the relationship between the magnitude of oscillatory current and the shape of the steady-state current-voltage relationship. This was done under two experimental conditions that induce self-sustained, non-driven action potentials in unclamped cells:

1. exposure to K^+-free, Na^+-deficient modified Tyrode's solution which induces spontaneous action potentials, and
2. exposure to normal Tyrode's solution containing ouabain (10^{-6} M) which induces triggered action potentials that arise from delayed after-depolarizations.

No current oscillations were recorded at the zero-current intercept in normal Tyrode's solution, and the steady-state current-voltage relationship showed that 1.5 nA of inward current was necessary to deflect the membrane voltage from the resting potential to the threshold for action potentials (−65 mV). After exposure to modified Tyrode's solution, spontaneous oscillatory currents with a magnitude as large as 2.0 nA developed at the zero-current intercept, and the shape of the current-voltage relationship was altered so that only 0.5 nA of inward current was needed to bring the resting potential to threshold. After exposure to ouabain (10^{-6} M), transient inward currents with peak magnitudes of 1–4 nA were recorded upon repolarization from depolarizing voltage clamp steps. Exposure to ouabain did not have a significant effect on the shape of the steady-state current-voltage relationship. Thus the magnitude of oscillatory currents in isolated myocytes is such that changes in the current-voltage relationship may be crucial in determining whether or not such currents will generate voltage deflections large enough to provoke action potentials. A simple model was developed to determine the magnitude of voltage deflections in a cell with oscillatory currents, and in adjacent resting cells. The model predicts that increasing resistance of gap junctions, increasing the membrane resistance, or decreasing the number of gap junctons between cells increases the likelihood that current oscillations will evoke propagated action potentials. The model also predicts that under conditions where the resistance of the gap junctions and surface membrane are increased, one or a small number of cells may initiate triggered action potentials which could propagate to adjacent heart muscle and cause ventricular tachycardia.

Introduction

In recent years, investigators in the field of myocardial electrophysiology have characterized two different forms of oscillatory currents in cardiac tissue: damped, transient current oscillations which follow depolarizing voltage steps, especially after exposure to toxic doses of digitalis [1–6]; and spontaneous current oscillations that develop without the need for depolarizing steps [1–3, 7–9]. Both types of current may depend on elevations of myoplasmic Ca^{2+} [10, 11]. While much attention has been focused on the underlying etiology of these current oscillations, relatively little attention has been paid to the process by which the currents are translated into voltage deflections, which ultimately serve as the stimulus for the opening of the voltage-dependent channels that cause the action potential. The magnitude of the voltage deflections is a function not only of the magnitude of the oscillatory currents, but also of the other conductances of the membrane which are time-independent. During diastole, those time-independent conductances determine the shape of the steady-state current-voltage relationship. Changes in the current-voltage relationship could therefore have a major effect on whether or not oscillatory currents associated with conditions of Ca^{2+} overload will induce recurrent action potentials.

To analyze such changes quantitatively, we have used voltage clamp techniques to study the electrical properties of isolated guinea pig ventricular myocytes under conditions that cause both spontaneous and depolarization-related current oscillations. By using individual cells, we can quantitate the absolute magnitude of the current oscillations. Furthermore, we can precisely measure the steady-state current-voltage relationship of the myocytes. Thus, we can determine values for the two variables which ultimately interact to generate voltage deflections.

With this quantitative data, we can then begin to reconstruct the effects of current oscillations generated by individual myocytes when those myocytes are connected to each other in the myocardial syncytium. Thus, our research has focused on two goals: first, to determine experimentally the precise behavior of oscillatory currents and current-voltage relationships in isolated myocytes from guinea pig ventricles; and second, to use simple mathematical models to obtain some insight, based on experimental quantitation, into the behavior of oscillatory currents in the myocardial syncytium.

Methods

Cells were isolated from guinea pig ventricles by a modification of techniques described elsewhere [12–14]. Guinea pigs (400–600 grams) were anesthetized with ether and then killed by cervical dislocation. The hearts were quickly mounted on a Langendorff apparatus and perfused with a Ca^{2+}-free Tyrode's solution of the following composition (mM): Na^+ 143; K^+ 6.0; Mg^{2+} 1.2; Cl^- 122.8; HCO_3^- 25; PO_4^{2-} 1.2; SO_4^{2-} 1.2; glucose 11.0.

Subsequently crude collagenase (Worthington, Type I) was added (125 μg/ml), and the solution was recirculated for 20 minutes. Following this, the hearts were minced with scissors and placed in a stirring apparatus to promote physical dispersion. During this period (30 minutes), $[Ca^{2+}]$ was increased to 100 μM, the collagenase concentration was increased to 255 μg/ml and hyaluronidase, 130 μg/ml, was added. The cells were harvested by gravity sedimentation. After decanting the collagenase containing solution, the cells were then placed in a HEPES buffered Tyrode's solution of the following composition (mM): Na^+ 143; K^+ 6.0; Ca^{2+} 1.0; Mg^{2+} 1.2; Cl^- 124.8; PO_4^{2-} 1.2; SO_4^{2-} 1.2; HEPES 25; glucose 11.0.

For experiments, isolated myocytes were placed in a perfusion chamber mounted on the stage of a Nikon inverted stage microscope. Solutions were perfused continuously at 37° C via a Hamilton valve system. The entire perfusion system and microscope were mounted in a Faraday cage.

Recordings were obtained with conventional microelectrodes filled with 3 M KCl. Tip resistances ranged from 50–100 MΩ. We studied only cells that were electrically quiescent with resting potentials negative to −80 mV following impalement with one or two microelectrodes. In all experiments, cells were initially perfused with control Tyrode's solution of the following composition (mM): Na^+ 151.3; K^+ 4.0; Ca^{2+} 2.4; Mg^{2+} 0.5; Cl^- 147.3; HCO_3^- 12.0; PO_4^{2-} 1.8; glucose 5.5. The composition of the modified Tyrode's solution was as follows (mM): Na^+ 82.6; Tetraethylammonium (TEA^+) 69.0; Cs^+ 4.0; Ca^{2+} 2.4; Mg^{2+} 0.5; Cl^- 78.8; SO_4^{2-} 34.4; PO_4^{2-} 1.8; glucose 5.5; sucrose 34.4. All solutions containing HCO_3 were gassed with 95% O_2 and 5% CO_2.

Action potential data was analyzed from Polaroid photographs of oscilloscopic records. Voltage and current records were obtained on a strip chart recorder (Gould).

Results

Oscillatory currents in isolated guinea pig myocytes

We have used two experimental approaches to study oscillatory currents in isolated myocytes. First, to study spontaneous membrane current oscillations, we developed a modified Tyrode's solution which would, on theoretical grounds, both induce Ca^{2+} overload (low Na^+ [15], zero K^+ [16]) and reduce steady-state membrane conductance (zero K^+ [16, 17], Cs^+ [18], TEA^+ [19]). We have shown that the solution causes reversible, nondriven action potentials in guinea pig ventricular papillary muscles [20]. Second, to study depolarization-dependent transient oscillatory currents we exposed the myocytes to control Tyrode's solution containing ouabain (10^{-6} M).

Figure 1 shows the effects of modified Tyrode's solution on the electrical activity of an unclamped isolated ventricular myocyte. In control Tyrode's solution (Figure 1A) the cell generated normal action potentials following brief depolarizing current pulses delivered through the recording electrode. The membrane potential was stable between action potentials. Following 40 seconds of exposure to modified Tyrode's solution (Figure 1B), the cell depolarized slightly and developed irregular undulations in membrane potential; these were followed by a burst of nondriven action potentials. The self-sustained action potentials persisted for a short time after the cell was re-exposed to control Tyrode's solution between Figure 1B and 1C. Thereafter the diastolic potential gradually hyperpolarized and the self-sustained action potentials terminated with a large afterdepolarization (Figure 1C). Subsequently, the membrane potential of the cell again remained quiescent between stimulated action potentials in control solution (Figure 1D), confirming complete reversibility of the spontaneous activity.

To investigate the changes in membrane currents underlying self-sustained activity induced by the modified Tyrode's solution, we used two microelectrodes to voltage clamp [21] the isolated cells. This technique avoids the obligatory internal dialysis associated with large bore, low resistance suction electrodes [22], and thus permits us to study the effects of native changes in intracellular constituents on current and voltage behavior in the myocytes. Only cells which were electrically and mechanically quiescent in normal Tyrode's solution and which had normal resting membrane potentials following insertion of both electrodes were used for experiments. The cells were initially voltage clamped to the resting potential (i.e. the zero-current intercept). The membrane potential was then shifted in 10 mV increments from −100 mV to more positive potenials by manually changing the clamp potential every 1–2 seconds. Following this, the command potential was returned to the zero current intercept and the cell was exposed to the modified Tyrode's solution. After the first appearance of spontaneous current oscillations, a second current-voltage relationship was obtained by the same protocol.

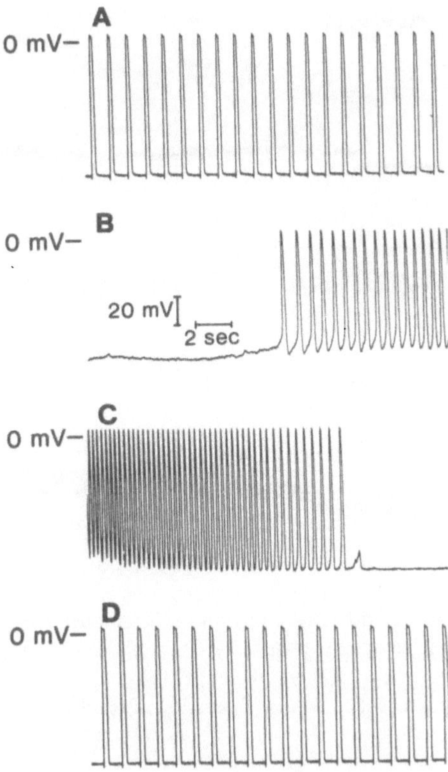

Figure 1. Effect of modified Tyrode's solution on transmembrane voltage of an isolated guinea pig ventricular myocyte. Panels were taken from continuous records obtained in control Tyrode's solution (A), 40 sec after exposure to modified Tyrode's solution (B), 60 sec after reexposure to control Tyrode's solution (C), and 3 min after reexposure to control Tyrode's solution (D). Action potentials in panels A and D were stimulated by 1 msec depolarizing current pulses; stimulation was turned off during exposure to the modified Tyrode's solution.

Figure 2 shows the voltage clamp records obtained in control and modified Tryrode's solution in an isolated guinea pig myocyte. In control solution (Figure 2A), large changes in current were recorded when the membrane potential was clamped to values negative to −70 mV. Very slow irregular oscillations developed at −60 mV. Faster and more regular current oscillations were recorded only when the membrane potential was clamped to −20 mV and more positive. In contrast, in modified Tyrode's solution (Figure 2B), current oscillations developed at all membrane potentials positive to −110 mV; the largest oscillations had a peak-to-peak magnitude of about 1.0 nA. Furthermore, current deflections between incremental clamp potentials were markedly reduced at potentials negative to −70 mV.

Figure 3 shows the steady-state current-voltage relationship obtained from the

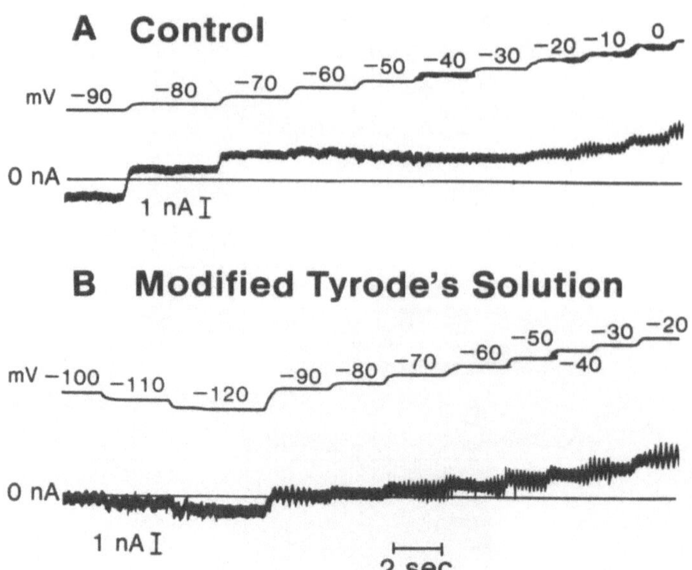

Figure 2. Transmembrane current and voltage records obtained during two microelectrode voltage clamp of the isolated guinea pig myocyte in control Tyrode's solution (A) and 70 sec after exposure to modified Tyrode's solution (B). In each panel, the upper trace is the clamp potential and the lower trace is the transmembrane current. See text for discussion of results.

voltage clamp records of Figure 2. The shape of the current-voltage relationship in control Tyrode's solution is similar to that reported by other investigators for cardiac muscle [23–25]. In contrast, a marked decrease in membrane conductance induced by the modified Tyrode's solution is reflected in the current-voltage relationship by the very shallow slope near and negative to the zero-current intercept.

It is important to note that a precise value can be determined from each current-voltage relationship for the quantity of inward current needed to bring the cell from the resting potential (that is, the zero-current intercept) to the threshold (−65 mV) for activation of the Na^+ channels that generate the upstroke of the normal cardiac action potential. For this cell, the value is 1.5 nA in control Tyrode's solution. Any inward current of less magnitude will fail to elicit an action potential. In modified Tyrode's solution, however, only about 0.5 nA would be needed to bring the membrane potential from the zero current intercept of −90 mV to −65 mV; this is less than half the current required with the current-voltage relationship obtained in the control solution. Thus, this change in the current-voltage relationship will amplify the voltage deflection associated with any oscillatory current and thereby increase the likelihood that current oscillations of any given magnitude will cause action potentials.

As an example of this interaction, we can consider the effect of the current

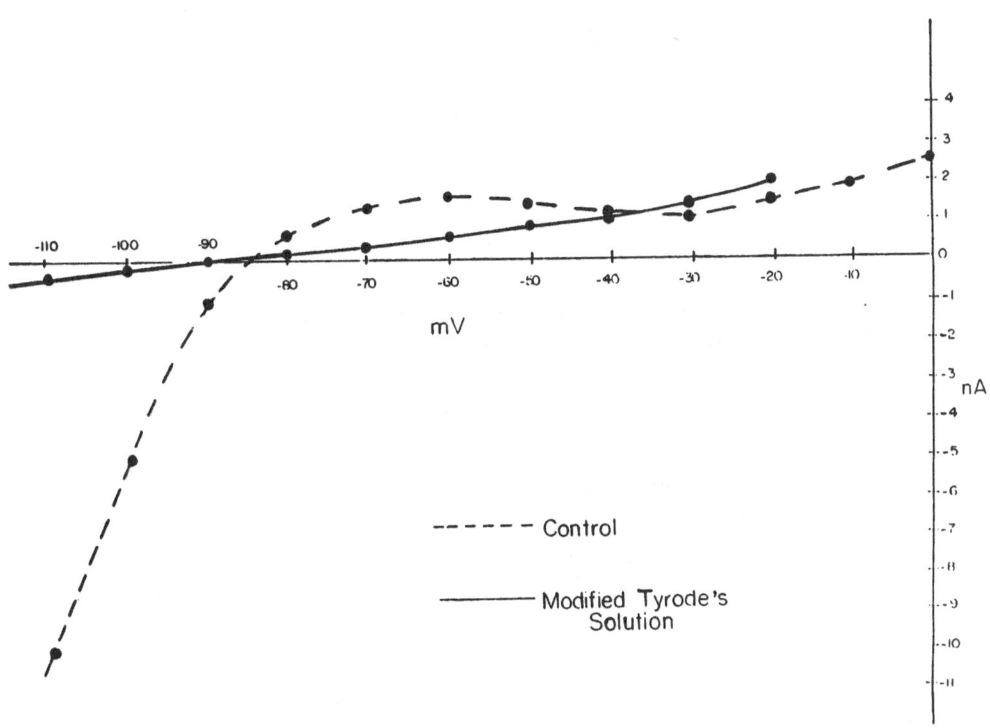

Figure 3. State-current-voltage relationship obtained in normal (dashed line) and modified Tyrode's solution (solid line); the data for the curves were from the records in Figure 2. At membrane potentials where current oscillations developed, the value for the steady-state the current was obtained by visual estimation of the mean value of the current. See text for discussion.

oscillations generated by the cell whose records are shown in Figure 2 and whose current-voltage relationship is plotted in Figure 3. In our analysis of the current-voltage relationship, we plotted the steady-state current value as the mean between the inward and outward peaks of the spontaneous current oscillations. The largest oscillation of this cell at −90 mV in modified Tyrode's solution had a peak-to-peak amplitude of about 1.0 nA. If we assume that inward current flows only during the inward phase of the oscillatory cycle, then the maximum inward current will be about 0.5 nA. Thus, in this cell, spontaneous current oscillations will elicit action potentials only if the current-voltage relationship is altered such that the outward current value at the threshold potential (−65 mV) is 0.5 nA or less. Since this condition is met in modified Tyrode's solution, the current oscillations at −90 mV should be sufficient to elicit action potentials. In contrast, the current-voltage relationship in normal Tyrode's solution is such that an inward current of 0.5 nA will cause a voltage deflection from −85 mV to −80 mV or only 5 mV. Thus, the normal current-voltage relationship stabilizes the cell.

In other experiments, the peak-to-peak magnitude of spontaneous current oscillations in modified Tyrode's solution was as large as 2.0 nA. According to our analysis, these oscillations would generate about 1.0 nA of inward current. We will therefore use 1.0 nA in the model which follows (next section) to represent the magnitude of the inward component of spontaneous current oscillations.

The current-voltage relationship is a nonlinear function of conductances which are voltage dependent. Nevertheless, regardless of the shape of this relationship, the amount of inward current needed to provoke an action potential will be equivalent to the amount of current needed to shift the membrane potential from the value corresponding to the zero-current intercept to the membrane potential that corresponds to the peak level of outward current recorded positive to the zero-current intercept. As in Figure 3, this peak value is generally found at the threshold voltage itself.

This observation allows one to view the changes in the current-voltage relationship induced by the modified Tyrode's solution from the point of view of membrane resistance (r_m). In terms of simple linear modeling of the behavior of oscillatory currents, r_m can be considered as the reciprocal of chord conductance, and can be determined for a given voltage step by evaluating the reciprocal of the slope of the line connecting two points on the current-voltage relationship. In the case of the current-voltage relationship in control solution (Fig. 3), the value of r_m between the membrane potential corresponding to the zero-current intercept (−85 mV) and the membrane potential corresponding to the threshold for the action potential (−65 mV) is 20 mV/1.5 nA or about 13 MΩ. In other cells, the value was betweeen 10 and 20 MΩ, with 15 MΩ being a typical value. In contrast, after exposure to modified Tyrode's solution r_m between the zero-current intercept (−90 mV) and the threshold (−65 mV) is 25 mV/0.5 nA, or 50 MΩ. These values will be used to represent r_m in the model which follows below.

In addition to studying spontaneous action potentials and their underlying sustained oscillatory currents, we also have investigated delayed after-depolarizations and the transient, depolarization-induced oscillatory currents which are believed to cause them [1–6]. For this purpose, we exposed the isolated myocytes to ouabain (10^{-6} M) until delayed after-depolarizations appeared. Figure 4 shows an example of the effects of ouabain (10^{-6} M) on the voltage activity of an unclamped isolated myocyte. In control solution, no fluctuations in diastolic potential were observed after 10 or 20 driven action potentials (Figure 4A). After exposure to ouabain for 4 minutes, a large but sub-threshold delayed after-depolarization was recorded after 20 but not after 10 driven action potentials (Figure 4B). After exposure to ouabain for 7 minutes (Figure 4C), bursts of triggered action potentials developed after 10 and 24 driven action potentials. The bursts of self-sustained action potentials terminated with large after-depolarizations. Following return to control solution, no after-depolarizations were recorded after 10 or 20 driven action potentials (Figure 4D).

We investigated the magnitude of the current that generated the delayed after-depolarizations and triggered action potentials by voltage clamping isolated

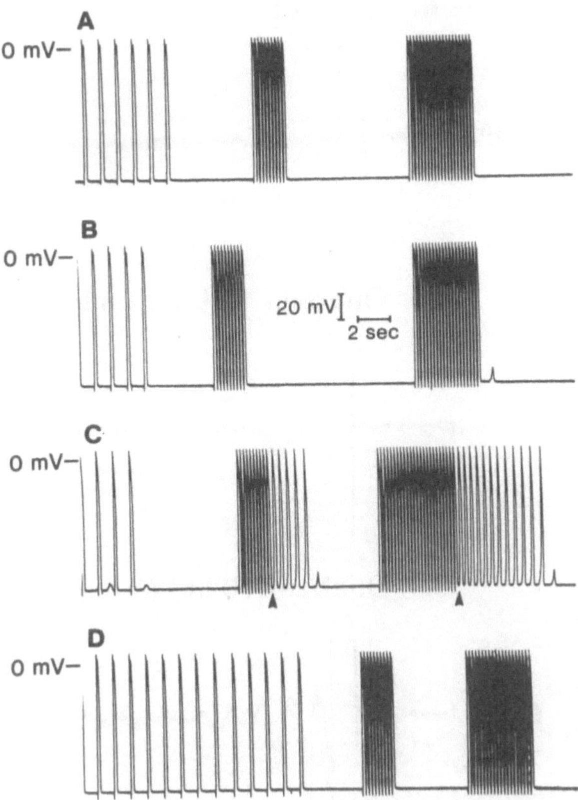

Figure 4. Effects of exposure to ouabain (10^{-6} M) on the transmembrane voltage of an isolated guinea pig myocyte. Each panel was taken from continuous chart recordings in control Tyrode's solution (A), following 4 min of exposure to ouabain (B), following 7 min of exposure to ouabain (C), and 5 min after return to control Tyrode's solution (D). Arrowheads in C indicate the onset of triggered action potentials arising from delayed after depolarizations. All other action potentials were elicited by intracellular depolarizing current pulses lasting 1 msec and applied at intervals of 1,000 msec and 200 msec.

myocytes exposed to ouabain. For these experiments, we used depolarizing voltage clamp steps. Figure 5 shows an example of one such experiment. In this cell, the holding potential was set at the zero-current intercept, −90 mV. The cell was then clamped to 0 mV for 200 msec. In control solution, this protocol failed to elicit any oscillatory currents (Figure 5A). In contrast, after exposure to ouabain for 2 minutes, a single, phasic inward current of about 1 nA developed following the clamp step (Figure 5B). After exposure to ouabain for 8 min, the voltage step was followed by a series of very large current oscillations which decreased in magnitude over several cycles (Figure 5C). Even at this level of intoxication, the zero current intercept remained at −90 mV.

The peak value of inward current observed in this experiment was 4 nA. Thus,

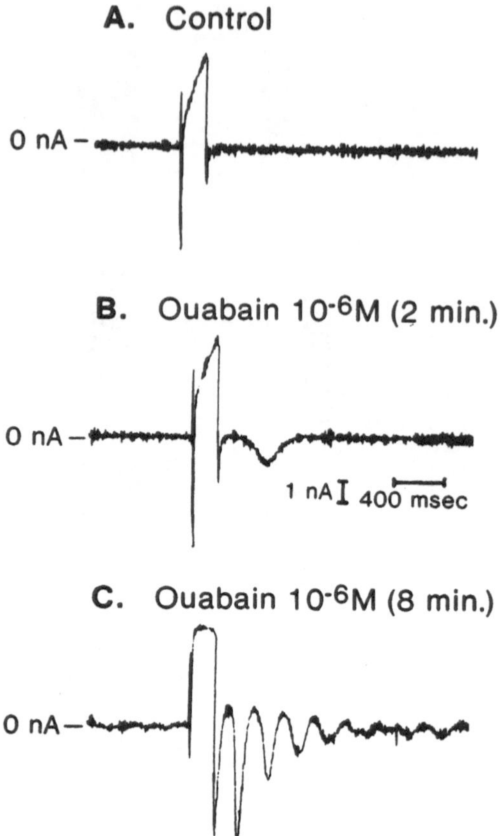

Figure 5. Effects of exposure to ouabain (10^{-6} M) on transmembrane currents during two microelectrode voltage clamp of an isolated guinea pig myocyte. In each panel, the holding potential was −90 mV and the voltage clamp step was to 0 mV for 200 msec; the voltage trace is not shown. See text for discussion of results.

the magnitude of the phasic inward current induced by depolarizing step pulses is larger than the peak-to-peak magnitude of spontaneous current oscillations. Interestingly, in preliminary experiments, ouabain itself seems to cause little or no change in the current-voltage relationship. Neither the zero current intercept nor the total current required to bring the membrane to threshold for action potentials was affected by exposure to ouabain. The normal steady-state current-voltage relationship requires about 1.5 nA of inward current to deflect the membrane potential from the resting potential to the threshold potential (Figure 3); therefore, currents of 1 nA, as in Figure 5B, will only generate subthreshold delayed after depolarizations in unclamped cells. However, the larger currents recorded after longer exposure to ouabain (Figure 5C) are clearly sufficient to bring the membrane potential to threshold, and thus evoke triggered action potentials.

Preliminary mathematical model of the effects of oscillatory currents in a myocardial syncytium

On the basis of this quantitative information we can now begin to address an important and related question: under what conditions can oscillatory currents of the magnitude we have observed in isolated cardiac myocytes generate recurrent non-driven action potentials in the myocardial syncytium? In a syncytium, current generated in any one cell flows not only across the membrane of that cell, but also into the myoplasm of other cells via gap junctions. Such flow of current between cells may be relatively insignificant in conditions associated with global alterations in electrophysiological function and when oscillatory fluctations in current are synchronized, which might be expected in the case of the phasic inward current induced by digitalis glycosides. Yet, even in such conditions, some heterogeneity is probably present in the amount and timing of such current. Clearly, in conditions associated with local damage or focal metabolic perturbations, alterations in current flow between cells may be a crucial determinant of whether or not deflections in membrane voltage can become large enough to induce action potentials.

In considering this problem, it is important to note that other investigators [26, 27] have reported that the resistance to current flow in gap junctions can vary, and in fact may increase under conditions of Ca^{2+} overload. For example, Kameyama [26] showed that the average value of gap junctional resistance (r_j) beween pairs of guinea pig myocytes was $2.1 \pm 1.0\,M\Omega$ in normal external solution with $K^+ =$ 5.4 mM. However he also reported that r_j can reversibly reach values exceeding $15\,M\Omega$ in low Na^+ solution. Thus, conditions associated with increased myoplasmic Ca^{2+} appear not only to induce oscillatory currents, but also to change the resistance to current flow between cells in which the oscillatory currents develop.

An increase of r_j may be extremely important in the processes that underlie the generation of nondriven action potentials. The low value of r_j under normal conditions acts to shunt oscillatory current in any cell away from the surface membrane and to diffuse it between larger groups of cells. Gap junctions of low resistance can thereby reduce transmembrane voltage deflections associated with focal oscillatory currents. Increasing r_j will tend to drive more current across the surface membrane and thereby increase the transmembrane voltage deflection. On the other hand, extremely high values of r_j may prevent action potentials that develop in one cell from propagating to adjacent cells. If values of r_j become very high, each cell in the syncytium will approach the electrical state of the isolated ventricular myocyte, which of course has no gap junctions.

Thus in considering the influence of syncytial relationships on oscillatory voltage activity, one can rephrase the question and ask: is there a reasonable range of values for r_j in myocardial syncytia (such as the peak reversible value of $15\,M\Omega$ observed by Kameyama [26]) that will enable oscillatory currents within individual myocytes to depolarize the membrane potential enough to provoke action potentials which can then excite adjacent resting cells? To approach this problem we have developed a simple model which describes the relationship between oscillatory currents (i_{os}), r_j, r_m, and the number of junctions between cells(n) [28].

The model assumes that two separate processes occur. First, i_{os} generates an action potential (V_{ap}) in a *generator cell* when the voltage deflection caused by i_{os} in this cell (ΔV_{gen}) exceeds the threshold for activation of the Na^+ current that generates the upstroke of the action potential. In a typical cell, this value is about 20 mV. Once generated, V_{ap} then is applied across r_j to an *adjacent resting cell.* V_{ap} will elicit an action potential in the adjacent resting cell if the voltage deflection across its membrane (ΔV_{adj}) also exceeds the threshold voltage. Thus, i_{os} will cause an action potential in the adjacent resting cell only when both ΔV_{gen} and ΔV_{adj} exceed the threshold voltage.

To determine the voltage deflection caused by i_{os} in the generator cell, and by V_{ap} in the adjacent resting cell, one must first evaluate the effective resistance, which we call r_{in}, for each cell. To do this, we calculate r_{in} as a function of three resistance elements: r_m, a given number (n) of r_j, and r'_{in}, an element which is in series with each r_j. A schematic diagram of this configuration is shown in Figure 6. Conceptually, r'_{in} represents a resistance that corresponds to the ensemble effect of all cell-to-cell electrical connections in the syncytium; r_m and r'_{in} connect to the extracellular fluid which we assume to be at ground or zero potential. Therefore r_m and each junctional branch containing $r_j + r'_{in}$ are parallel elements in the circuit. From this model, the value of r_{in} is

$$r_{in} = \frac{1}{\dfrac{1}{r_m} + \sum_{x=1}^{n} \dfrac{1}{r_{jx} + r'_{inx}}}. \tag{1}$$

If all values of r_j and r'_{in} are equal, then

$$r_{in} = \frac{1}{\dfrac{1}{r_m} + \dfrac{n}{r_j + r'_{in}}}. \tag{2}$$

From these equations, it can be seen that precise values of r_{in} depend upon the complex electrical interactions of the total syncytial structure, which will determine the value of the series element r'_{in}. However, for any given values of r_m, r_j, and n, the minimum value for r_{in} is obtained by assuming that r_j forms a short circuit to the extracellular space (ie, $r'_{in} = 0$). The maximum value is obtained by assuming that any contiguous cell has no junctional connections other than to the cell for which r_{in} is being calculated; for this condition, $r'_{in} = r_m$ of the contiguous cell. Thus, the maximum and minimum values of r_{in}, and therefore for the resulting ΔV_{gen} and ΔV_{adj} can be defined regardless of the syncytial architecture.

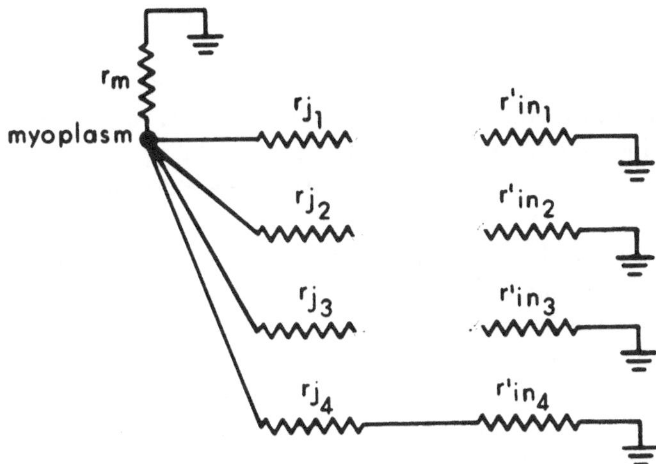

Figure 6. Schematic diagram of the electrical network used to calculate effective cellular resistance (r_{in}) in an individual myocyte connected to four other cells. Resistance is calculated between the myoplasm, represented by the node, and the extracellular space, represented by ground.

To calculate ΔV_{gen}, we apply Ohm's law directly:

$$\Delta V_{gen} = i_{os} \times r_{in}. \tag{3}$$

If ΔV_{gen} is greater than 20 mV, i_{os} will cause an action potential in the generator cell. To determine whether the action potential so generated will propagate, we next calculate ΔV_{adj} when ΔV_{ap} is applied to a circuit comprised of two series resistances: r_j connecting the generator and adjacent resting cell, and r_{in} of the adjacent resting cell. For this circuit,

$$\Delta V_{adj} = \frac{r_{in} \times V_{ap}}{r_j + r_{in}}. \tag{4}$$

The adjacent resting cell will generate an action potential when ΔV_{adj} exceeds 20 mV.

These equations establish several relationships, each of which will be illustrated in the examples which follow (Figures 7–10):

1. The value of ΔV_{gen} always increases with increasing r_j, since a greater proportion of the current from i_{os} flows across the surface membrane which comprises r_m. This relationship holds for any choice of values for the other variables.
2. The value of ΔV_{adj} always decreases as r_j increases, since the voltage drop across the gap junction connecting the generator cell and the adjacent resting cell increases relative to r_{in} as a proportion of V_{ap}.
3. The upper limit for V_{gen} is always determined by the product $r_m \times i_{os}$. ΔV_{gen} approaches this value asymptotically as r_j increases.

4. The upper limit for ΔV_{adj} is equal to V_{ap}, and is approached as r_j approaches zero.
5. The value of ΔV_{gen} is directly proportional to the magnitude of i_{os}.
6. Decreasing the number of gap junctions will always increase r_{in}, and will therefore increase the values for both ΔV_{gen} and ΔV_{adj}.
7. The values for ΔV_{gen} and ΔV_{adj} will both increase if r_m increases.

Thus the model shows that regions of the myocardium are most likely to produce propagated action potentials from oscillatory currents when the number of gap junctions between cells is decreased, when the membrane resistance of cells is increased, and when the resistance of gap junctions between cells is increased as high as possible without exceeding the value necessary to allow propagation of the action potential between cells. Such conditions are probably most likely to occur in diseased regions where electrical connections between cells are disrupted either anatomically by structural alterations or functionally by increased myoplasmic Ca^{2+} which can cause cell-to-cell uncoupling to occur [26].

We can use this simple model to analyze the behavior of myocardial syncytia comprised of cells that have membrane current-voltage relationships and oscillatory currents with the values we have measured in isolated cardiac myocytes. We shall illustrate this behavior with four cases. In each case, we will use the values we determined experimentally in isolated cardiac cells for r_m and i_{os}. We will then examine the way the resulting voltage deflection varies as a function of r_j. V_{ap} is assumed to be 120 mV, a typical value for the amplitude of the action potential in isolated guinea pig myocytes [29].

The four cases we will consider are shown in Figures 7–10. In each case the data are plotted so that ΔV, representing either ΔV_{gen} or ΔV_{adj}, is considered as a function of r_j. The graphs show curves for the maximum and minimum values for ΔV_{gen} and ΔV_{adj} at each value of r_j. The hatched areas therefore represent the possible range of each.

The first two cases, shown in Figures 7 and 8, address the question of whether spontaneous current oscillations of the type we have observed in modified Tyrode's solution might generate propagated non-driven action potentials. We therefore choose the value of i_{os} to be 1 nA, the maximum magnitude of the inward component of current generated by the spontaneous current oscillations in myocytes exposed to this experimental solution. Since normal cell-to-cell connections may be disrupted in damaged areas of the syncytium, we assume that $n = 2$ to simulate a reduction in the number of cell-to-cell connections; that is, the generator and adjacent resting cells are each connected only to one other cell. Finally, we choose values for r_m derived from the normal current-voltage relationship (15 MΩ) and from the altered current-voltage relationship induced by modified Tyrode's solution (50 MΩ). Figure 7 shows the results of the calculations with normal membrane resistance. With these conditions, ΔV_{gen} will not exceed 10 mV at any value of r_j less than 40 MΩ. Thus, the generator cell will fail to elicit an action potential if the resting membrane potential is not significantly depolarized.

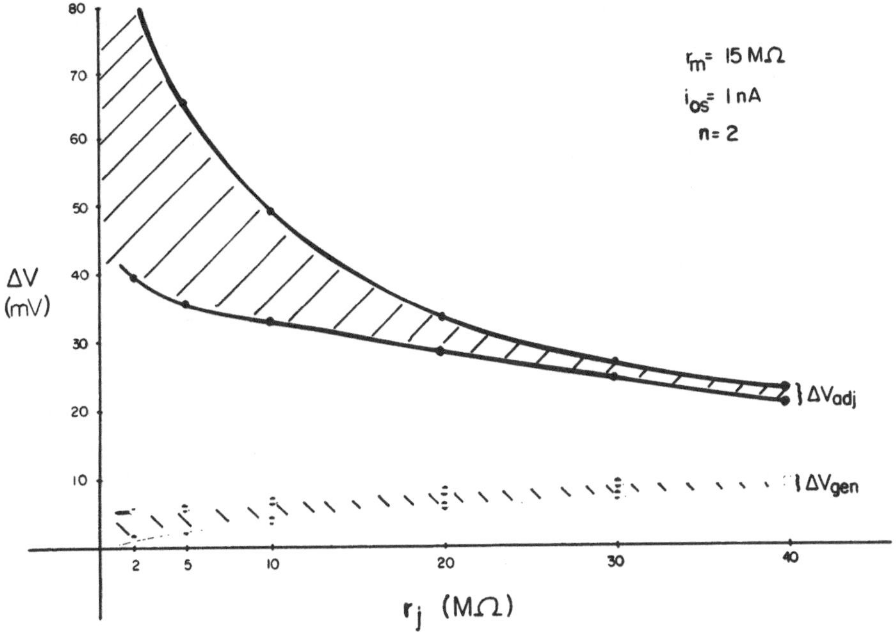

Figure 7. Plots of the voltage deflections (ΔV) as a function of gap junctional resistance (r_j), calculated from equations of the model. The values selected for r_m and i_{os} were measured experimentally. The hatched area between curves indicates the range between minimum and maximum values for ΔV_{gen} and ΔV_{adj}, which are represented as ΔV on the ordinate. For ΔV_{adj} the magnitude of the action potential was assumed to be 120 mV and n was selected as 2 to simulate a certain degree of anatomic disruption between cells.

Figure 8 illustrates curves calculated with the same values for i_{os} and n used in Figure 7 but with an abnormally high r_m of 50 MΩ. In this set of conditions, the range for ΔV_{gen} exceeds 20 mV at $r_j = 20$ MΩ. Thus, ΔV_{gen} can achieve relatively high values in the range of r_j observed in the experiments by Kameyama with low Na^+ solution [26]. The results of Figure 8 also demonstrate that at normal values of r_j (e.g., about 2 MΩ), the deflections in the generator cell would be less than 20 mV, even with increased r_m. In both Figure 7 and Figure 8, the range of values for ΔV_{adj} exceeds 20 mV for all values of r_j less than 40 MΩ. If an action potential is elicited in the generator cell under these conditions, then it will propagate.

Thus, the model predicts that even in regions where the myocardial syncytium is highly disrupted, spontaneous current oscillations of the magnitude we have measured will not cause propagated action potentials unless both r_m and r_j are significantly increased.

On the other hand, phasic inward currents like those seen in Figure 5 are considerably larger than spontaneous oscillatory currents, and therefore have a better chance of eliciting action potentials. Figures 9 and 10 analyze the behavior of syncytia in which one or a small group of cells are generating such phasic

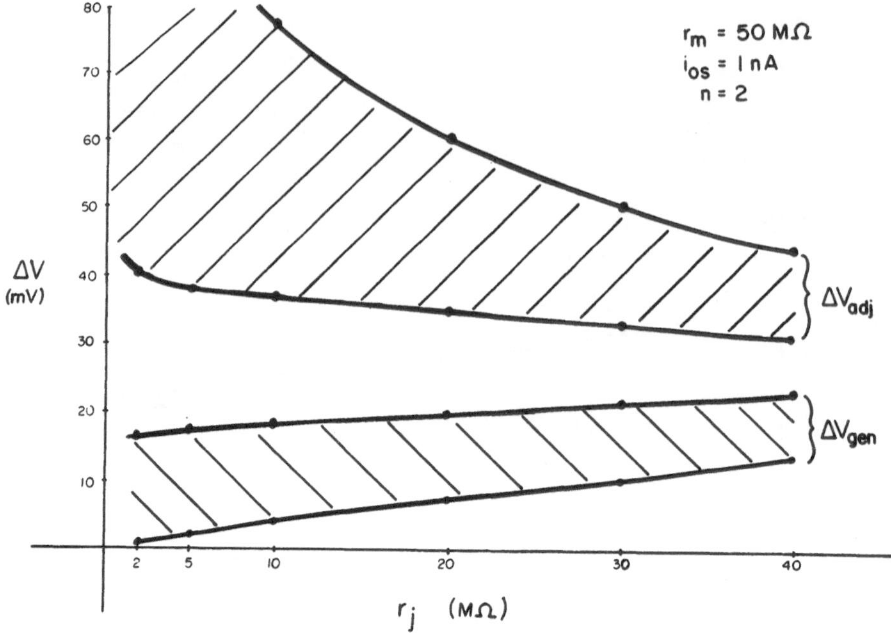

Figure 8. Same as Figure 7 except that r_m was increased to 50 MΩ to simulate r_m measured in modified Tyrode's solution.

inward oscillatory currents. Therefore, i_{os} is assigned a value of 4 nA, the maximum magnitude of depolarization-induced inward current we observed in isolated myocytes following ouabain intoxication. In this case, we assume that $n = 4$, a value suggested by indirect experimental data for the average number of junctions between cells under normal conditions [30].

Figure 9 analyzes the behavior of ΔV_{gen} and ΔV_{adj} when r_m is 15 MΩ, the normal value. Because i_{os} is larger, the range of values of ΔV_{gen} begins to exceed 20 mV at r_j of about 15 MΩ. Thus, even when the membrane resistance is normal, the voltage deflections caused by large depolarization-induced oscillatory currents might reach threshold, and therefore cause action potentials in the generator cell, if the junctional resistance is moderately elevated. However, in this case, the value of ΔV_{adj} falls below 20 mV as r_j exceeds 20 MΩ. This value is lower than in Figures 7 or 8 because increasing n reduces the value of r_{in} in the adjacent resting cell. Thus, if coupling resistances are extremely high, the action potential elicited by i_{os} in the generator cell will fail to propagate.

Finally, the curves in Figure 10 were calculated with the same parameters as Figure 9 except that r_m increased to 50 MΩ, an abnormally high value. In this case, even with low r_j, the range of ΔV_{gen} far exceeds values required to bring the membrane potential to threshold. Furthermore, the range of values of ΔV_{adj} remains above 20 mV for all r_j below 40 MΩ. Thus, increasing membrane resistance in the range of potentials between the resting potential and the threshold potential will increase significantly the likelihood that a small group of cells, or

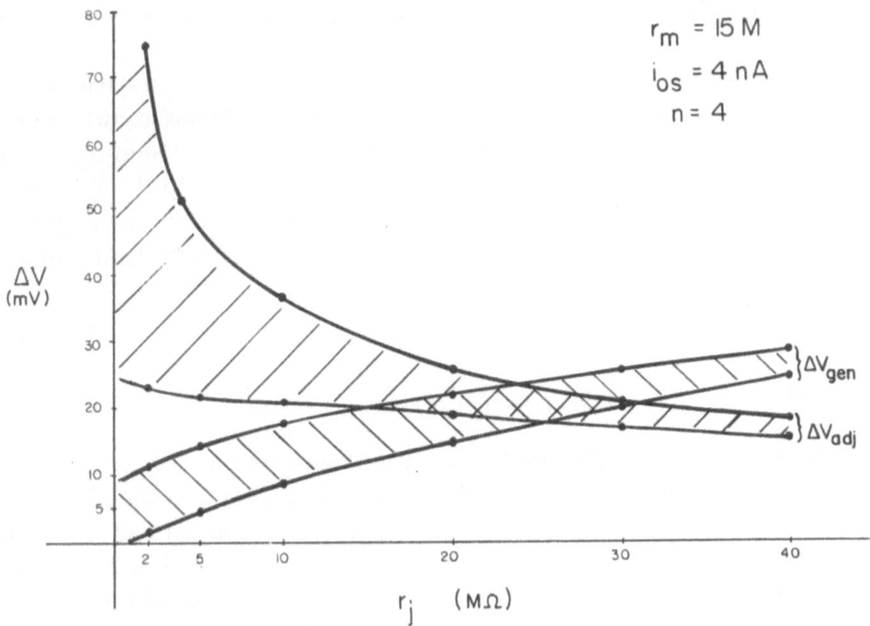

Figure 9. Same as Figure 7 except that i_{os} was increased to 4 nA to simulate the larger magnitude of i_{os} observed in ouabain and n was increased to 4.

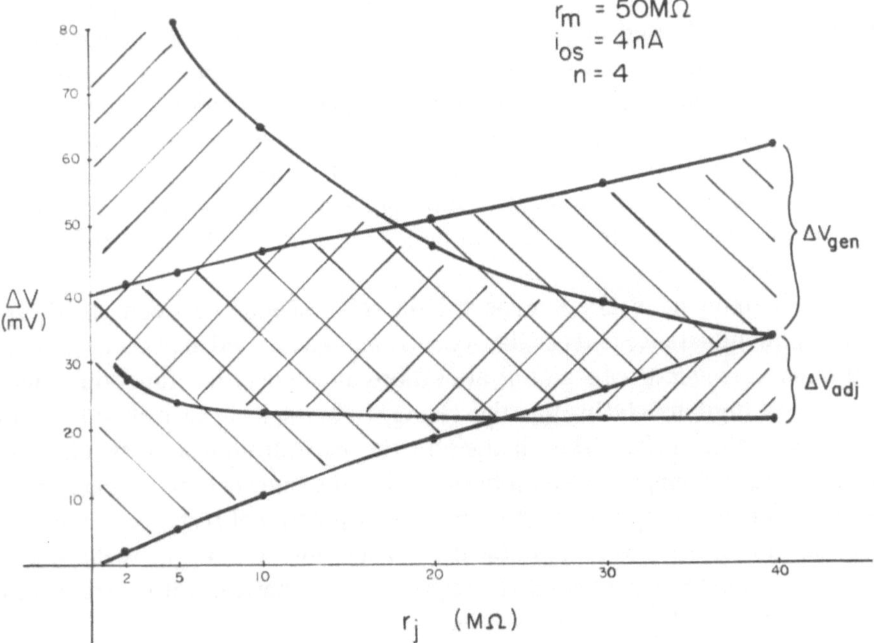

Figure 10. Same as Figure 9 except that r_m was increased to 50 MΩ to simulate r_m measured in modified Tyrode's solution.

even one cell, will be able to transform depolarization-induced inward currents into triggered action potentials.

Our preliminary modeling, therefore, suggests that if one or a small number of cells develop large, depolarization-induced transient oscillations in current of the magnitude shown in Figure 5C, such cells may, under certain conditions, generate non-driven triggered action potentials which propagate to the myocardial syncytium. Furthermore, the model demonstrates that reducing the membrane conductance may be crucial in allowing such cells to generate ventricular tachycardia.

Discussion

The experiments we have described clearly demonstrate that isolated myocytes can be used to study the current and voltage alterations associated with the development of recurrent, non-driven action potentials in cardiac ventricular muscle. Thus, the isolated myocytes develop self-sustained and, in some cases, apparently self-initiated action potentials after exposure to modified Tyrode's solution. The isolated cells also develop delayed after-depolarizations and triggered activity which are similar to these electrical events after digitalis intoxication in intact preparations of cardiac tissue [31–34].

In control solution, the myocytes did not develop delayed after-depolarizations following trains of rapid stimulation, and had a normal current-voltage relationship without oscillatory current at the zero-current intercept. These characteristics show that the myocytes were not damaged by isolation or impalement. Furthermore, the development of spontaneous action potentials in modified Tyrode's solution, or triggered action potentials in the presence of ouabain, could be reversed by reexposure to control solution. Thus, the development of oscillatory phenomena in the myocytes can be ascribed to the effects of the solution changes alone.

Data obtained in isolated myocytes on relationships between steady-state membrane conductance and oscillatory currents can be used in two ways. First, in conditions associated with global alterations in myocardial function, such as exposure to digitalis glycosides, the changes obtained in an isolated myocyte should accurately reflect the changes in the myocardium as a whole. More precisely, the current per unit membrane will be the same in both preparations. In this situation, it can be shown that changes in junctional restance will have no effect on the resulting voltage deflections if the inward current oscillations are coordinated temporally, as would be expected with phasic inward currents of the type that underlie delayed after-depolarizations.

Secondly, the information can be used to reconstruct the behavior of inhomogeneous myocardial syncytia in which the electrophysiological characteristics of one or a small group of cells may be different from the normal population. For this problem, the myocardium can be considered as an electrical network, with each cell representing a branch node between other cells and ground. Modeling techniques should yield valuable information on the behavior of myocardium with such heterogeneities. In this context, the quantitative information obtained from isolated myocytes under conditions associated with the development of nondriven action potentials is crucial to any realistic approach to modeling. The simple model we have developed confirms that ventricular tachycardia can be initiated under certain conditions if one or a small number of cells develop large, depolarization-induced current oscillations. Furthermore, the model demonstrates that the steady-state current-voltage relationship and the value of junctional resistance play a critical role in determining whether or not nondriven action potentials will develop and propagate from such regions.

Data from isolated cardiac myocytes should therefore serve as a major source for quantitative information that can be used in more sophisticated assessments of electrical behavior in regions of myocardium known to be associated with the development of ventricular tachycardia.

Acknowledgment

Supported by NIH grants HL-32688, HL-07071, and HHL-21993. Dr Nordin is the recipient of the Richard Rogers Investigator Award from the New York Heart Association. We gratefully acknowledge the technical assistance of Nadine Stram in the preparation of the isolated myocytes, and the secretarial assistance of Desiree Ditizio in the preparation of the manuscript.

References

1. Lederer WJ, Tsien RW (1976): Transient inward current underlying arrhythmogenic effects of cardiotonic steroids in Purkinje fibers. J Physiol 263: 73–100.
2. Aronson RS, Gelles JM (1977): The effect of ouabain, lithium, and dinitrophenol on the pacemaker current in sheep cardiac Purkinje fibers. Circ Res 40: 517–524.
3. Kass R, Lederer J, Tsien R, Weingart R (1978): Role of Calcium ions in transient inward currents and after-depolarizations induced by strophanthidin in cardiac Purkinje fibers. J Physiol 281: 187–208.
4. Vassalle M, Mugelli A (1981): An oscillatory current in sheep cardiac Purkinje fibers. Circ Res 48: 618–631.
6. Matsuda H, Noma A, Kurachi Y, Irisawa H (1982): Transient depolarizations and spontaneous voltage fluctuation in isolated single cells from guinea pig ventricles. Circ Res 51: 142–151.
7. Mehdi T, Sachs F (1978): Voltage clamp of isolated cardiac Purkinje cells. Biophys J 21: 167a.
8. Kass RS, Tsien RW (1982): Fluctuations in membrane current driven by intracellular calcium in cardiac Purkinje fibers. Biophys J 38: 259–269.
9. Aronson R, Nordin C (1984): Oscillatory current in single myocytes isolated from rat ventricles. Fed Proc 43: 636.
10. Wier WG, Hess P (1984): Excitation-contraction coupling in cardiac Purkinje fibers. Effects of

cardiotonic steroids on the intracellular [Ca^{2+}] transient, membrane potential and contraction. J Gen Physiol 83: 395–415.

11. Allen DG, Eisner PA, Orchard CH (1984): Characterization of oscillations of intracellular calcium concentration in ferret ventricular muscle. J Physiol 352: 113–118.
12. Powell T, Farrar D, Twist V (1980): Electrical properties of individual cells isolated adult rat myocardium. J Physiol 302: 131–153.
13. Hayworth R, Hunter D, Birkoff H (1980): The isolation of Ca-resistant myocytes from the adult rat. J Mol Cell Card 12: 715–724.
14. Aronson RS, Nordin C (1984): Electrophysiological properties of hypertrophied myocytes isolated from rats with renal hypertension. Eur Heart J 5 (Suppl F): 339–345.
15. Reuter H, Seitz N (1968): The dependence of calcium efflux from cardiac muscle on temperature and external ion composition. J Physiol 195: 451–470.
16. Eisner DA, Lederer WJ (1979): The role of the sodium pump on the effects of potassium depleted solutions on mammalian cardiac muscle. J Physiol 294: 279–301.
17. Dudel J, Peper K, Rudel R, Trautwein (1967): The potassium component of membrane current in Purkinje fibers. Pflügers Archiv 296: 308–327.
18. Isenberg G (1976): Cardiac Purkinje fibers: cesium as a tool to block inward rectifying potassium currents. Pflügers Archiv 365: 99–106.
19. Kenyon JL, Gibbons WR(1979): Influence of chloride, potassium and tetraethylammonium on the early outward current of sheep cardiac Purkinje fibers. J Gen Physiol 73: 117–138.
20. Gilat E, Nordin C, Aronson RS (1985): Lidocaine inhibits triggered activity in guinea pig papillary muscles without blocking after-depolarizations. Clin Res 33: 518A.
21. Deck KA, Kern R, Trautwein W (1964): Voltage clamp technique in mammalian cardiac fibers. Pflügers Archiv 80: 50–62.
22. Brown A, Lee K, Powell T (1981): Voltage clamp and internal perfusion of single rat heart muscle cells. J Physiol 318: 455–477.
23. Trautwein W, McDonald TF (1978): Current-voltage relations in ventricular muscle preparations from different species. Pflügers Archiv 374: 79–89.
24. Beeler G, Reuter H (1970): Voltage clamp experiments on ventricular myocardial fibres. J Physiol 207: 165–190.
25. Isenberg G, Klockner U (1982): Calcium currents in isolated bovine ventricular myocytes are fast and of large amplitude. Pflügers Archiv 395: 30–41.
26. Kameyama M (1983): Electrical coupling between ventricular paired cells isolated from guinea pig heart. J Physiol 336: 345–367.
27. White R, Mazer D, Spray D, Carvalho A, Wittenberg B, Bennett M (1983): Gap junction between isolated adult rat myocytes: Electrophysiological properties and morphologic changes. Circulation 68 (Suppl III): 24.
28. Nordin C, Aronson RS (1984): Spontaneous initiation and propagation of action potentials between cardiac cells with high coupling resistances. Circulation 70 (Suppl II): 342.
29. Nordin C, Gilat E, Aronson RS (1984): Intact structure influences electrical response of guinea pig ventricular myocardium to increased extracellular calcium. Circulation 70 (Suppl II): 73.
30. Clerc L (1976): Directional differences of impulse spread in trabecular muscle from mammalian heart. J Physiol 255: 335–346.
31. Ferrier GR (1977): Digitalis arrhythmias: Role of oscillatory afterpotentials. Prog Cardiovasc Dis 19: 459–474.
32. Gelles JM, Aronson RS, Hoffman BF (1975): Effects of transmembrane potentials on the manifestations of ouabain toxicity in sheep cardiac Purkinje fibers. Cardiovasc Res 9: 600–609.
33. Rosen MR, Danilo P (1980): Effects of tetrodotoxin, lidocaine, verapamil and AHR-2666 on ouabain-induced delayed after-depolarizations in canine Purkinje fibers. Circ Res 46: 117–124.
34. Karagueuzian HS, Katzung BG (1981): Relative inotropic and arrhythmogenic effects of five cardiac steroids in ventricular muscle: Oscillatory afterpotentials and the role of endogeneous catecholamines. J Pharmacol Exp Therap 218: 348–356.

9. General discussion

A. WIT, Moderator

Wit: I will give a short overview of the first session which dealt with impulse propagation and try to provoke some comments from those who participated in that session. The presentations were mostly concerned with the factors that govern propagation of electrical activity through the heart as exemplified by Dan Adam's beautiful model of excitation of the heart. We can divide these factors that govern propagation into two different subdivisions: one deals with the active processes in the cell membrane; that is, the membrane currents that govern depolarization and repolarization. Dr Clark presented some very nice simulation data on the currents that control the action potentials in the sinus node, and others have simulated the membrane currents responsible for propagation in ventricular tissues. The second very important factor that governs propagation of the cardiac impulse concerns the passive electrical properties, which affect current flow between myocardial cells, and we had a number of presentations concerning the factors that influence current flow. Dr Rudy, Dr Plonsey, Dr Sperelakis and Dr Spach talked about passive properties of myocardial cells. The reason that we are interested in both the active and passive properties is that abnormalities in both of them can cause cardiac arrhythmias. When we think about propagation, we are mainly interested in a type of arrhythmia mechanism called reentrant excitation. Prior concepts have put a great deal of emphasis on changes in the active membrane currents as a cause of reentrant excitation. But, as can be seen from the subjects presented here, more emphasis should be placed on changes in the passive properties of cardiac cells as a major factor responsible for cardiac arrhythmias. My feeling is that too much emphasis has been placed on changes in inward currents as a cause of slow conduction and not enough emphasis has been placed on the changes in passive properties as a cause of slow conduction, particularly in the case of cardiac ischemia and myocardial infarction.

Dr Spach has shown very nice data which indicate how structure can affect conduction in the cardiac muscle. In particular, he has shown that, with the aging process, the growth of connective tissue and the separation of cardiac cells can lead to slow conduction, which is probably a result of diminished coupling between cells. I've been interested in that work because our laboratory is studying the factors that govern propagation in myocardial infarcts. The healing infarct has a structure that is simular to Dr Spach's aging atrial tissue; that is, there is an ingrowth of connective tissue that separates cardiac cells during the healing process. And even though cells may have normal transmembrane action potentials, the separation of the surviving myocardial cells caused by the connective tissue can lead to the slow conduction that results in cardiac arrhythmias.

Dr Rudy's presentation shows how an increase in disk resistance can lead to the slow conduction that might cause reentrant excitation. This concept is more than just of academic interest, because it has great implications concerning the anti-arrhythmic therapy of reentrant excitation in healing myocardial infarcts. The tendency now in the development of anti-arrhythmic drugs is for an emphasis on pharmacological agents that affect inward currents that govern propagation, with the goal being to markedly diminish the depolarizing currents and cause conduction block which would abolish reentrant excitation. The fact that many of these types of agents do not work suggests that the role of diminished inward currents might be less important than previously thought and the role of altered passive properties in governing conduction may be more important in the setting of healed infarction. Maybe the emphasis on pharmacological therapy of certain types of reentry arrhythmias should be on drugs that affect passive properties and coupling between cardiac cells rather than drugs that affect inward current and conduction caused by the active properties of cardiac cells.

The other presentations were also very important in leading to concepts concerning the importance of cell coupling on conduction and the importance of abnormal cell coupling in the genesis of arrhythmias. Finally, I would like to ask Dr Rudy a question. I was very intrigued by his model showing how changes in coupling between cells could cause the slow conduction that is likely to result in reentrant excitation. The validity of models can only be proven if we can gather real experimental data that demonstrate that the models are correct. I was wondering whether he has any thoughts about how one could experimentally evaluate leakage resistance versus disk resistance to try to obtain data that might be used in his model.

Rudy: Trying to measure and separate the leakage is a very difficult experimental adventure. To try and separate the leakage resistance from the increase in disc resistance, and even to try and measure changes that are confined to the disc resistance alone, would be difficult. As you know, most of the preparations that look at the increase in disc resistance use drugs that also affect the membrane, so there is really no clear clean way of affecting or separating the disc from the membrane effects. The purpose of the model was to separate the disc from the membrane in a model that permits that. However, one way to do it is to compare the effects on the resistivity in the longitudinal and transverse direction. For example, an intervention with ouabain, a metabolic blocker that blocks the sodium pump, results in calcium accumulation in the cell and calcium accumulation causes decoupling. Consider the directional increase in intracellular resistance, assuming that the membrane action potential is the same in all directions and is affected by the oubain the same in all directions. Then, in the comparative study in the longitudial and transverse directions, assuming that the anisotropy results from the number of discs to be traversed by an activation front, you're only looking at changes. You isolate changes due to the disc if the membrane effects in all directions are the same. We do not think of the anisotropy as resulting from membrane properties. It only reflects the structure and distribution of discs. This is one way to separate discs from a membrane in an experimental set up. Other ways may not involve the use of drugs but may somehow increase the calcium concentration within the cell in a direct way. I do not know how you do it. One way to modulate the leakage resistance is to try and separate the discs, or the two opposing sides of the gap junction, by a hypertonic solution that has the effect of greatly decreasing leakage resistance values and increasing the leakage current. The increase in leakage current is an important factor. The results of the model show that the most important effect of the disc resistance is to cause discontinuous seltatory propagation, decremental conduction, and reduction in conduction velocity. On the other hand, the major effect of the leakage current is reduction in duration of the action potential and therefore creation of conditions of nonuniformity in refractory periods, which increase the vulnerability to arrhythmias. One of these factors can lead to decremental conduction and conduction block and therefore to reentrant tachycardia; the other can do the same thing, but by changing the refractory periods in a nonuniform way. These are two different mechanisms that you could look at. The model differentiates them clearly. Experimentally, it's a challenge!

Wit: Dr Sperelakis probably disagrees with at least some of the statements I have made. The audience should be aware that there are some controversies concerning the role of the disc in propagation, and I presented a viewpoint where the disc is a connection between cardiac cells, that has a low resistance in the normal state and disc resistance increases during pathological events such as ischemia or infarction. According to what Dr Sperelakis presented, the disc may normally have a relatively high resistance and therefore, perhaps, my hypotheses does not sit well with him.

Sperelakis: Dr Wit gave a very nice summary, and I have no problems with it. I was very happy with what was covered by Dr Rudy and Dr Wit. I wanted just to take one step further, introducing the possibility of a high-resistance interaction between cells. That is, our model does not require low-resistance connections. That would apply in the normal myocardium, and also might apply in various pathophysiological circumstances, like in infarction or in number of other conditions in which the cells might become uncoupled. As Dr Rudy said earlier, there are a number of things that will uncouple, such as acidosis or high internal calcium. Can that heart still propagate in the cases where it is supposedly uncoupled? I tried to make my hypothesis a little more general so that it can apply either in normal physiological circumstances or in the pathophysiological circumstances.

I alluded in my talk that I was very happy with Dr Rudy's calculations and also with the findings of Dr Spach on saltatory conduction. The saltatory conduction exactly fits the hypothesis I've been working with for a number of years, namely that the heart consists of a series of truncated cables with high-resistance junctions between cells. Cardiac muscle is not one long cable like a skeletal muscle fiber or a nerve fiber. In fact, saltatory conduction leads me to believe that something very special is going on at those intercalated discs, and it is a very labile junction. Of course, in cardiac arrhythmias, the changes in the so-called coupling resistance between the cells could be very important.

I tried to get across the message that I do not know whether our electric field model applies biologically, but given the circumstances of the morphology of the cells, where cells are very close together with a very narrow gap at the junction, like say a hundred Å, I do not see how it could not apply. The key requirement of our model is that the intercalated disc junctional membranes be excitable membranes. That is a reasonable assumption, because even the T-tubules of skeletal muscles, which are very narrow tubules about 300 Å in diameter, are excitable. They do fire sodium-dependent, TTX-sensitive action potentials. The burden of proof should be on those who want to say that the junctional membranes of cardiac muscle are not excitable. If they are excitable, then an electric field is developed in the narrow cleft between the cells, which I'll call the cleft potential. The cleft potential will depolarize the post-junctional membrane by an equal value. It is the equivalent of a patch-clamp experiment, where you change the outside reference potential with respect to the inside potential. Thus, the inside potential of the post-junctional membrane stays at, say, $-80\,mV$. The outside potential, which at rest is $0\,mV$ with respect to ground, becomes about $-40\,mV$ during the cleft potential. This depolarizes the post-junctional membrane by about $40\,mV$. That would take it beyond its threshold, and it would fire an action potential. This, in turn, would fire the surface membrane. Because the cell is a truncated cable, the entire cell will explode almost simultaneously. That would account for the discontinuous or saltatory propagation.

Thus, most of propagation time in the heart is consumed in the very narrow intercalated disc, which is, say, about 100 Å in width. In contrast, much less propagation time is consumed down the body of the cell which is about $150\,\mu m$ long. I tried to show in my talk that there is a junctional potential. In cardiac muscle, compared to a true cable like skeletal muscle, there is an extra component, the so-called step on the rising phase of the action potential. Somehow or other we have to explain that step. In cases of impeded propagation, in which propagation velocity is slowed down by a number of mechanisms, the step becomes much more prominent and sometimes there is failure of propagation. In such cases, one can observe the step in isolation, which then decays without triggering an action potential. I think that step really reflects the post-junctional membrane firing of an action potential. What you see with your microelectrode in the center of that cell is that action potential generated at the post-junctional membrane.

To summarize, what I tried to do is to propose an alternative hypothesis that can allow for bi-directional propagation, electrical in nature, which does not require low-resistance junctions. K^+ ion accumulation in the junctional clefts could be an accessory factor that could be involved which would facilitate this junctional transmission process.

Clark: One important piece of evidence that has been used in the past to support low resistance junctions has been the length constant, λ, measured by external application of current or some tracer. What I tried to show in the theoretical analysis is that you just can not deduct from that type of experiment what is the resistivity of the intercalated disc. In other words, it may turn out to be low resistance, but you cannot prove it, or even conclude from it, based on that type of measurement. The purpose of the last part of my talk was to show that, because of the anisotropic nature of the bundles of cardiac muscle, you just cannot do it that way in the cable analysis.

Bassingthwaighte: One of the models that I would suggest to support Dr Sperelakis' hypothesis is the olfactory nerve of the pike, where there is coordinated conduction along the nerve fiber bundle. At the front of the wave of depolarization following a multineuronal stimulus, the larger high velocity axons partially depolarize their smaller neighbors, which are trailing behind the front, and bring their axonal velocities up to those of the fast neurons, so that they all propagate uniformly within the bundle.This is purely capacitance coupling without any other effect. I still do not believe that what Dr Sperelakis is saying applies to the normal myocyte membrane. I think his hypothesis should be extended to include current transport across the intercalated disc, which is highly permeable. According to the studies of Weidman (J Physiol (London) 187: 323–342, 1960) potassium transport across the disc is quite rapid. Similar evidence is seen in the studies of procion yellow (Mol. Weight less than a 1,000) which moves from cell to cell across the disc. Now, taking that back to Dr Wit's question to Dr Rudy: why not look at the passive properties in the sense of looking at the length constant, which encompasses several cells? The passive electrical properties of the myocardial syncytium are such that the length constant for a minor depolarization would be expected to be longer in the parallel direction of the fibers than perpendicular to them. In both cases, the length constant should be a few cells long. This demonstrates the communication between the cells. Without such a communication, the length constant can not exceed one cell length. I suggest that this communication can be included in Dr Sperelakis' model.

Sperelakis: If you inject current (I_0) intracellularly in a slab of tissue through one microelectrode and record membrane potential with that same microelectrode ($\triangle V_1$) and with a second intracellular microelectrode ($\triangle V_2$), then you don't get any evidence of interaction between the two microelectrodes ($\Delta V_2/\Delta V_1$ approaches zero), unless the two electrodes are in the same cell. Several Japanese groups, like Matsuda, Tomita, and others, confirm our results. However, they find a long length constant λ of about 0.8–1.6 mm when they inject current extracellularly. The point that I want to make is the fact that the bundle of parallel fibers acts as a cable. This fact would account for their obtaining a λ value of several cell lengths. Therefore, one of the main messages of my talk is that one cannot use λ determinations from extracellular application of current to determine the resistive properties of the cell junctions.

Another point relates to Dr Norton's results. His data in the isolated single adult cardiac myocyte shows that the input resistance varies between 10 and 20 MΩ, with a typical value of 15 MΩ. That fact actually supports strongly the argument that cells are not electrically coupled by low-resistance connections. We have measured and published for many years the fact that input resistance measurements in intact cardiac muscle vary between about 3 MΩ up to about 15 MΩ. For a long time, this finding was debated. Some investigators, e.g., Johnson & Tille and Woodbury & Crill, thought that the input resistance was only 30–50 KΩ. Now, I think, everybody accepts the fact that the input resistance is about 3, 4 or 5 MΩ. An isolated single cell has an input resistance of only 15 MΩ. If you had a three-dimensional low-resistance syncytium, then the input resistance of one cell would have to be about 1000 to 2000 MΩ in order to allow free electrical connections between all of those neighboring cells. The fact that isolated single cell has an input resistance of only 15 MΩ, which approaches the value you get in an intact slab of tissue, like a papillary muscle, strongly supports the view that it can't be electrically coupled by low-resistance tunnels.

Sperelakis: The point showed was that in some double impalements, where the two electrodes were in one cell, there was good electrical coupling. In one such double impalement of one cell, a fortuitous thing happened. At the beginning, there was good electrical coupling. The resting potentials were low because of the fact that when two electrodes are in the same cell, some injury is produced. Then, with the subsequent contraction resulting from stimulation of an action potential, the one electrode spontaneously left that cell and went into a neighboring cell. Since the interelectrode distance was 11 μm, the neighboring cell could not be more than 11 μm away. You saw that when this happened, electrotonic interaction was not evident. That is, there was a change from good electrical coupling to no electrical coupling.

Bassingthwaighte: If you take two electrodes and depolarize one with a current impulse, you see that signal on the electrode half a millimeter away, and that's several cell lengths.

Wit: This argument points out that there are not just disagreements among those studying heart failure but there are also some controversies in the field of electrophysiology.

Lab: I feel as if I am out on a limb now. We went to a play last night and one of the

things that came across was that reality was a collective hunch. In other words, somewhere there is always a truth between two controversies. What I'd like to do is ask the audience where the particular observation that I have fits in . . .
I'm interesting in the reverse of excitation-contraction coupling, that is, some kind of mechanical to electrical coupling. One of my figures (Fig. 3b & c) demonstrated one possible manifestation of this coupling: an alternation in action potential height and duration associated with a mechanical alternation. We have consistently observed an electrical alternans at some stage during ischemia, quite often leading to arrhythmia. A striking observation is that the mechano-electric alternans can increase to reach a crescendo just before ventricular fibrillation. This observation is important. Perhaps not all present here realize that this type of arrhythmia is the number one cause of sudden death in the Western world. My first question is: can those who study passive electrophysiological properties provide other mechanisms for mechano-electric feedback and this alternans to the calcium one I propose? There is another striking feature that I'd like to comment on. An ectopic beat can switch the alternans both 'off' and 'on'. It looks as if there are two stable states in the myocardium. The question to the 'modelers' is: can there be a dynamic state built into a particular control modeling system which can be switched between two stable states; or lose its feedback control mechanism totally and result in complete instability – in ventricular fibrillation?
Sperelakis: I can not answer the question of Dr Lab, but I have three comments. One is that we showed a long time ago that the propagation in two directions in cardiac muscle, like papillary muscle, is not identical. The action potential duration, of a single cell impaled near the middle of the length of the muscle, often will be different with the direction of propagation. Thus, this might be an important factor. A second factor just mentioned is potassium accumulation that can have important effects on action potential duration. The third thing I want to mention is that we showed that the T-tubules of cardiac muscle have big effects on the waveshape that is recorded. If these tubules get pinched off with contraction, and it sometimes happens in the case of skeletal muscle, then this will have an effect on the recorded action potential duration.
Palsson: I would like to address the question of Dr Lab concerning the switch between the two stable states. When you analyze the nonlinear properties of coupled kinetic models, like the ones Dr Lab has shown here, it is quite common that you do find multiplicity of stable steady states under the same boundary conditions. You can even have a stable steady and stable oscillatory behavior. By shocking the system you can force it from one pattern to the other. We have observed this type of dynamic behavior in simple feedback loops, like those you see in metabolism in the biosynthetic pathways, and even in some cases you can see two stable oscillatory solutions. By pushing the system by an external disturbance or a shock, you can switch it from one periodic pattern to another. The answer to your last question, or your challenge to the modelers, is yes: you can achieve these models with nonlinear feedback coupling.

Sperelakis: One link that was not discussed here at all was the regulation of the myocardial calcium slow channels, which, in turn, control the force of contraction of the heart. We didn't hear anything in this conference dealing with the regulation of the calcium influx into the cell via these pathways. It turns out that they are metabolically dependent and are regulated by cyclic nucleotides. We and others have provided evidence that the Ca^{2+} slow channel protein, or an associated regulatory-type protein, must be phosphorylated by a cAMP-dependent protein kinase in order for the channel to be available for voltage activation (upon depolarization). Another way to view this is that phosphorylation increases the probability of opening of the slow channel at any voltage. We also have demonstrated that cGMP exerts an effect opposite to that of cAMP, namely inhibition of the Ca^{2+} slow channels. Finally, I wish to point out that acidosis selectively blocks the Ca^{2+} slow channels, and that this might be important in ischemic and hypoxic conditions.

Sideman: I would like to add the need for a macro-scale model which tries to follow the metabolic, mechanic and pathologic interactions with electrical interactions and define the physical boundaries which define the mathematical boundary conditions which will eventually lead us to describe, or maybe anticipate, arrhythmia. Eventually, that is what we would like to have.

Electrical and mechanical interactions

10. Influence of pacing site on ventricular mechanics

D. BURKHOFF and W.L. MAUGHAN

Abstract

We investigated the influence of pacing site on several aspects of left ventricular (LV) performance to test the hypothesis that the 'effective ventricular muscle mass' is reduced with direct ventricular pacing. All studies were performed on isolated supported canine hearts which were constrained to contract isovolumically. We observed significant influence of pacing site on the magnitude, but not the time course of isovolumic ventricular pressure waves. Pacing from different sites of the ventricle resulted in different chamber contractile strengths. There was a linear inverse relation between changes in QRS duration and changes in contractile strength. The decreased chamber contractility manifests itself as a decrease in the slope (E_{es}) and a small increase in the volume-axis intercept (V_0) of the end-systolic pressure-volume relation. The relation between ventricular oxygen consumption and pressure-volume area was independent of pacing site. These results are consistent with the hypothesis that the effective mass of muscle which participates in the generation of active contractile strength is reduced when the pacing site is moved from the atrium to the ventricle.

Introduction

Lewis and Rothchild, in 1915, were the first to investigate the influence of pacing site on the spread of electrical activation over the ventricle [1]. They showed that with normal supra-ventricular pacing, the activation front travels through the heart's rapid conduction system providing for relatively synchronous muscle contraction throughout the chamber. With direct ventricular pacing, however, the activation front travels slowly through the muscle around the pacing site until it reaches a branch of the conduction system, after which time, activation is dispersed through the conduction system (in an aberrent way), rapidly exciting the remaining muscle. Thus, with direct ventricular pacing the activation wavefront initially spreads via 'muscle conduction', and then via the specialized rapid conduction system. Guided by these electrophysiologic data, Carl Wiggers (1925) reasoned that with direct ventricular pacing, dyssynchrony of muscle activation would lead to dyssynchrony of muscle contraction, which will ultimately result in a less effective (weaker) contraction of the ventricle [2]. He further hypothesized an inverse relation between the amount of muscle activated by 'muscle conduction' and the strength of ventricular contraction. The data that he presented in his 1925 paper were consistent with, but did not prove, these hypotheses.

The influence of pacing site on ventricular mechanics has since been investigated in several studies. The conclusions of the majority of these studies are in accordance with those of Wiggers [3–9]. Lister et al. [8] experimentally varified an inverse relationship between the amount of muscle activated by 'muscle conduction' and ventricular contractile strength. Further evidence has been provided by Badke et al. [10] who demonstrated alterations in muscle shortening patterns with direct ventricular pacing indicative of dyssynchronous muscle contraction. However, the results of a few studies suggest no influence of pacing site on the strength of ventricular contraction [11–15].

Using the theories presented above as our basis, we generated a model which makes more detailed predictions than previously on the influence of pacing site on ventricular mechanics. We tested these predictions in an isolated canine heart preparation in which ventricular volume can be measured and controlled and baroreflexes are nonexistent. The experimental results of the present study have been presented in detail previously [16]. In this article we will review these results, but focus on the generation of the model and on an understanding of its predictions.

Model development

A schematic diagram of the left ventricle in cross-section is presented in the left panel of Fig. 1. The conduction system lines the circumference of the intraventricular chamber and sends off branches which penetrate through the ventricular wall at several places. As discussed above, with supraventricular pacing the activation front travels through the conduction system exciting the muscle nearly simultaneously; in the canine heart it is estimated in reality that there is an approximately 30 to 40 ms difference between the earliest and latest activated muscle fibers [17]. When pacing is from the epicardium, however, the activation wavefront propagates slowly through the muscle (as depicted in the figure) until reaching the conduction system (marked by an '*' in the figure). After reaching the conduction system, propagation is rapid. To illustrate the possible influence of this dyssynchrony of excitation on muscle contraction, assume that the ventricular wall is divided into two layers as shown in the top panel on the right side of Fig. 1. For the following discussion, let us consider only isovolumic contractions,

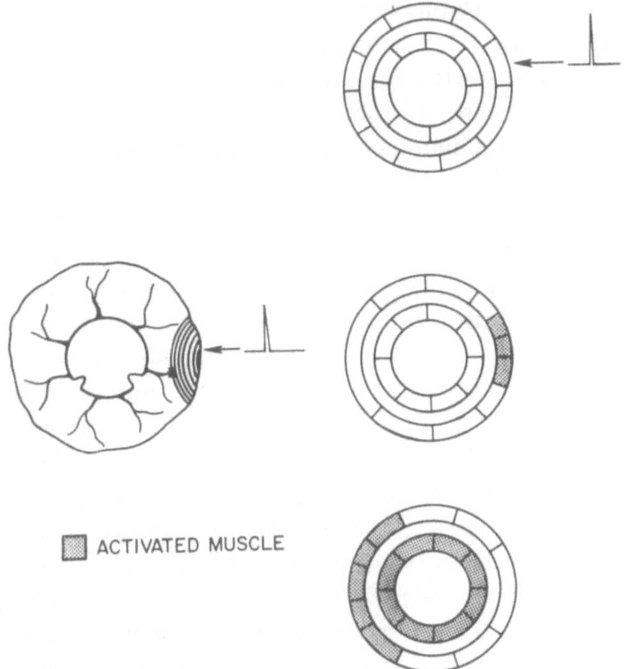

Figure 1. Left panel: schematic representation of the left ventricle in cross section which includes the specialized rapid conduction system. The heart is paced from an epicardial site and conduction spreads by 'muscle conduction' until it reaches the conduction system, marked by the '*'. Top right panel: the heart in its relaxed, diastolic state. The ventricular wall is divided into inner and outer layers. Middle right panel: with epicardial pacing, the muscles in the outer layer near the pacing site are activated. These muscles shorten at the expense of lengthening of the distant muscles in the same layer. Bottom right panel: the activation front reaches the conduction system and rapidly activates the remaining muscle. The inner core contracts normally. The muscles in the outer core near the pacing site are stretched by the distant muscles in the same layer.

so that the total circumference of each layer is assumed to be a constant throughout the cardiac cycle. The outer layer consists of the muscle activated by 'muscle conduction' *and* the muscle fibers with which they are confluent around the circumference of the heart. All the muscle of the inner layer is activated by the rapid conduction system. As shown in the middle right panel of Fig. 1, when an electrical impulse is applied to the epicardium, the muscle near the pacing site is activated and begins its contraction cycle (we will refer to these muscles as 'A' muscles); at this point the remainder of the muscles in the outer layer (which we will refer to as 'B' muscles) are in their diastolic, relaxed state. Thus, the activated 'A' muscles shorten at the expense of lengthening of the nonactivated 'B' muscles; remember that the total circumference of the circle is constrained to remain constant. As illustrated in the bottom panel on the right side of Fig. 1, once the activation front reaches the conduction system, the remainder of the muscle in the outer layer (i.e. the 'B' muscles) and all the muscle of the inner layer contract nearly simultaneously. In the outer layer, the 'A' muscles are far along their cycle, and may be stretched by the now activated 'B' muscles; this lengthening of the 'A' muscles is at the expense of shortening of the 'B' muscles. The muscles of the inner layer contract simultaneously with no shortening or lengthening of the muscle fibers.

According to this sequence of events, the force generated by the muscle in the inner layer will be the same with ventricular and supraventricular pacing (note that synchronicity of excitation provides for isometric contractions under the imposed constraint of isovolumic contraction). In contrast, it is easily appreciated that due to the alternate shortening and lengthening of the 'A' and 'B' muscles that the tension developed in the outer layer of muscle will be greatly reduced below that which would have existed had all the muscles contracted simultaneously (and isometrically). Thus, these outer-layer muscles undergo unloaded contractions (i.e., they shorten but generate little force).

With this simple 'layer model' of the ventricle, intraventricular pressure would be related to the tension in each layer of the wall and the relative thickness of each layer (e.g., by Laplace's law). Therefore, because the outer layer muscles generate little force, these fibers may not contribute significantly to the generation of pressure in the ventricle. In essence, this hypothesis predicts that pacing from a ventricular site reduces the effective mass of muscle which contributes to the generation of active contractile strength in the ventricular chamber.

Limitations

The model as presented above is, at best, an oversimplification of the real situation. The model assumes that the ventricular wall can be separated into layers which act independently. Due to extensive mechanical cell-to-cell coupling such a discrete separation of muscle is unrealistic. Also, in the extreme case, we assume that the wall tension generated in the outer, dyssynchronously contracting muscle layer is negligible compared to that of the inner layer. This assertion would be difficult to substantiate experimentally. Nevertheless, this model provides a simple way of predicting the influence of pacing site on ventricular contraction. Therefore, we will outline the model predictions below and experimentally test whether the real heart behaves in accordance with those predictions.

Model predictions

In order to test the model directly, it would be required that we be able to measure muscle tension at different depths within the ventricular wall. Existing technologies do not allow for this. However, there are at least five model predictions of how ventricular chamber properties would be influenced by pacing site which can be tested readily in an isolated heart preparation.

1. Contractile strength. First, ventricular chamber contractile strength should be different when pacing is from different ventricular sites. This is because the amount of muscle activated by 'muscle conduction' will depend on the distance from the pacing site to the conduction system. Thus, the percent of the total wall thickness which makes up the outer 'ineffective' layer in Fig. 1 will depend on pacing site.

2. Time course of contraction. The contribution of the outer layer to intraventricular pressure is hypothesized to be negligible. Therefore the shape of the isovolumic pressure wave will be determined by the time course of contractions of the inner layer which, as stated above, is determined by the rapid conduction system and thus independent of pacing site. Thus, despite changes in absolute contractile strength with myocardial pacing, the time course of ventricular pressure generation should be independent of pacing site.

3. Relation between contractility and QRS duration. There should be a negative correlation between chamber contractile strength and the dispersion of ventricular electrical activity which can be measured by the duration of the QRS complex. This follows from 1 above. The longer the activation front takes to get to the conduction system, the more muscle activated by 'muscle conduction'; the more muscle activated this way, the weaker the contraction *and* the longer will it take for excitation to spread to all the muscles of the heart.

4. End-systolic pressure-volume relationship (ESPVR). There are many determinants of E_{es}, the slope of the ESPVR: for example, the underlying contractility of muscle, amount of muscle, chamber geometry and fiber arrangement in the ventricular wall. With ventricular pacing we hypothesize a reduction in the effective mass of muscle; with a constant muscle contractility, chamber geometry and fiber arrangement, reduced muscle mass would result in a decrease in E_{es}. V_o, the volume axis intercept of the ESPVR, is predominantly determined by ventricular structure; since pacing site does not alter the physical structure of the heart, this parameter should not be significantly influenced.

5. MVO_2-PVA relationship. According to the model, the muscles in the outer layer undergo unloaded contractions with ventricular pacing as compared to isometric contractions with supraventricular pacing. When a muscle contracts against no load, the amount of oxygen it comsumes is less than when it contracts isometrically. Thus, because a certain fraction of the muscle will be consuming less oxygen with dircet myocardial pacing than normal, there should be an overall reduction in total ventricular oxygen consumption with ventricular pacing which is in proportion to the reduction in mechanical strength.

Methods

We employed a standard isolated heart preparation. These methods have been described in detail previously by Suga and Sagawa [18]. Briefly, a pair of mongrel dogs (approximate weight, 20 kg each) was anesthetized with pentobarbital sodium (30 mg/kg iv). A heart isolated from the 'donor' dog was metabolically supported by arterial blood from the second 'support' dog. A water filled balloon positioned inside the left ventricular chamber of the isolated heart, connected to a volume servo-system, was used to control and measure ventricular volume. Details of the design and performance of this volume servo-system have been reported by Suga and Sagawa [19] and Sunagawa et al. [20].

In all experiments the coronary perfusion pressure was maintained between 80 and 100 mm Hg by a servo controlled finger pump (Harvard Apparatus, model 1215). The temperature of the perfusate was maintained between 37 and 39° C.

Measurement of oxygen consumption

The coronary blood flow was estimated by canulation of the coronary sinus and measurement of venous outflow with an electromagnetic flow meter (Narco Biosystems, model RT-400). The difference between arterial and venous oxygen content (A-VO_2 difference) was continuously measured by an A-VOX meter (A-VOX Systems [21]). Oxygen consumption was determined by multiplying mean coronary sinus out-flow by A-VO_2 difference.

Electrical stimulation

Pacing leads were placed at 5 different sites on the heart: the atrium, right ventricular endocardial septum, right ventricular epicardial free wall, left ventricular apex and left ventricular epicardial free wall. The hearts were paced with square pulses of duration between 1 and 2 ms long and of amplitude approximately twice threshold. The site of pacing was changed using a manually controlled multiplexing switch box.

An A.C. coupled bipolar epicardial electrogram was measured between one electrode placed on the left ventricular free wall and another on the right ventricular free wall. The duration of the QRS complex of this electrogram was used as a rough measure of the degree of electrical dyssynchrony over the heart while pacing from different sites. The QRS duration was defined as the time interval between the Q and S wave inflection points.

Data collection

All signals were recorded on an 8-channel pen recorder (Gould 2800), and digitized on-line at a rate of 200 Hz and analyzed off-line.

Protocols and data analysis

The aforementioned 5 predictions were tested using two basic protocols, described below.

In the first series of measurements, the hearts were paced at a constant rate of 130 beats/min. The pacing site was switched from one site to the next in a random order while maintaining ventricular volume at a constant value of approximately 25 ml. Representative pressure waves and ECG signals for each pacing site were digitized. From these, we determined the peak developed pressures, the duration of the pressure wave at a level of 10% peak developed pressure, and the duration of the QRS complex as defined above, obtained with each pacing site in each of 9 ventricles.

In order to determine the influence of pacing site on the time course of chamber stiffening and relaxation, we compared the *shapes* of the isovolumic pressure waves. For each heart, a steady-state pressure wave (P(t)) was measured while pacing from each of the 5 pacing sites. Each of these 5 pressure waves was normalized in amplitude according to the following equation:

$$P^*(t) = \frac{P(t) - P_{min}}{P_{max}} \times 100\ (\%), \tag{1}$$

where t is time, P(t) is the directly measured isovolumic pressure wave, P_{min} is the minimum pressure and P_{max} is the maximum developed pressure attained during the beat. Then, each of the 5 curves obtained from a given heart were aligned in time at the point when P*(t) was equal to 50%. The shapes of the resulting normalized, time-shifted curves were quantitatively compared by determining the root-mean square difference, D_{rms}, between each curve obtained with ventricular pacing and that obtained with atrial pacing (i.e., atrial pacing was considered the 'control' curve to which all the others were compared).

In the second series of experiments, the ESPVRs measured with atrial and right ventricular free wall pacing were compared. At a given volume, the peak isovolumic pressure was determined while pacing from each of the two sites. The volume was then changed in a random manner and the pacing site variation repeated. In each heart studied, the volume was varied between approximately 5 and 35 ml at 5 ml increments. Linear regression analysis was used to determine the slope, E_{es}, and volume-axis intercept, V_o, of the relations between the end-systolic pressures and volumes measured with each pacing site. E_{es} and V_o obtained with atrial and right ventricular free wall pacing were compared.

Ventricular oxygen consumption was measured at each of the volumes for both pacing sites. For each series, myocardial oxygen consumption (VO_2) was plotted as a function of the total 'pressure-volume area' (PVA) which is defined by Suga et al. [22]. This relation between VO_2 and PVA has been described in detail [22] and has been found to be linear and independent of ventricular loading conditions. The PVA-VO_2 relation obtained from a given heart with both pacing sites were compared by analysis of covariance.

Results

Influence of pacing site on peak systolic pressure and duration of contraction

The pacing site dependence of peak developed pressure was studied in 8 hearts and the average results are presented in Fig. 2A. The peak pressures obtained with each site were compared using one-way repeated measures analysis of variance; multiple comparisons of group means was accomplished by the Dunckan multiple ranges test. The symbols, explained in the figure legend, summarize the results of this analysis which indicated that pacing from different myocardial sites generally resulted in significantly different developed peak pressures.

Next we determined the influence of pacing site on the duration of the pressure waves at a level of 10% maximum developed pressure. The results of this analysis are presented in Fig. 2B. Associated with an approximately 25% decrease in peak isovolumic pressure when pacing site was moved from the atrium to the ventricular free wall (Fig. 2A) was an average of only 12.5 ms increase in the duration of contraction. Statistical analysis indicated that in general this difference was not statistically significant.

Influence of pacing site on the time course of pressure development

Representative computer-reconstructed pressure curves obtained from a single heart with each of the five pacing sites are presented in Fig. 3A. The peak pressure decreased with ventricular pacing as described above, and there was no influence on minimum pressure. For this plot, the starting time (i.e., $t = 0$) was arbitrarily chosen for each beat. To compare the shapes of these pressure waves, they were rescaled in amplitude and aligned in time (see Methods) as shown in Fig. 3B. When this was done, all five curves were virtually superimposable during the rising phase of the pressure tracings up to t_{max}, and there were only small

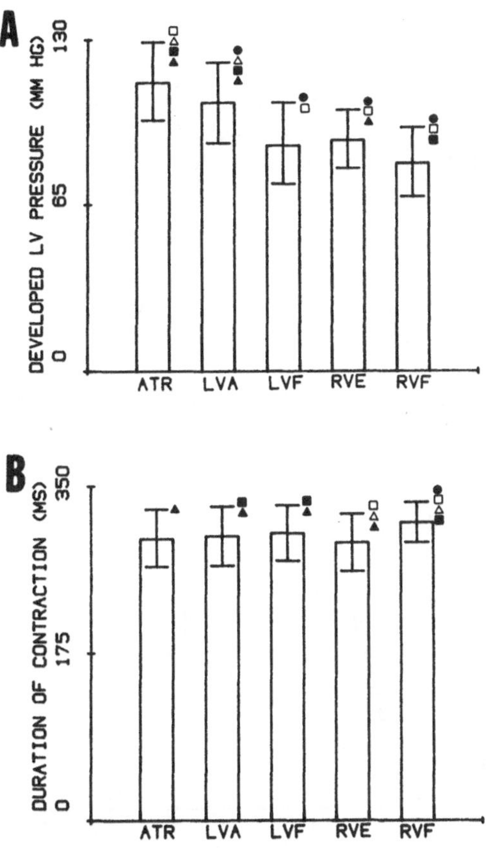

Figure 2. Average results obtained from 9 ventricles. Influence of pacing site (A) on peak isovolumic pressure and (B) on the duration of contraction at a level of 10% developed pressure. Statistical significance of inter-group differences were determined by repeated measures analysis of variance in combination with the Dunken test. The different symbols indicate statistically significant differences ($p<0.05$) between the means of two groups: ● = different than with ATR pacing, □ = different than with LVA pacing, △ = different than with RVE pacing, ■ = different than with LVF pacing, ▲ = different than with RVF pacing. From Burkhoff et al. [16], with permission of the authors.

differences between them for the remainder of the cardiac cycle. The similarity of these curves was quantified by determing the root-mean squared difference from the atrial curve (D_{rms}) as outlined in Methods. All of the normalized pressure waves obtained with ventricular pacing were equally similar to that obtained with atrial pacing and therefore the average results of this analysis from each heart are reported. When this analysis was carried out for the example of Fig. 3 it was found on average that D_{rms} was only 1.5% up to the time of t_{max} and 4.1% after t_{max}. This pacing site independence of the shape of the pressure wave was observed in all 8 hearts studied in this series, and the results are summarized in Table 1.

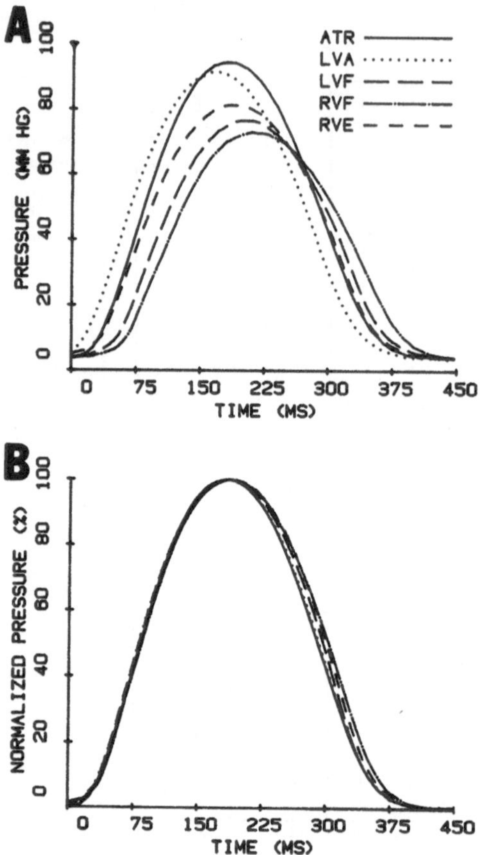

Figure 3. Influence of pacing site on the time course of pressure generation. A: computer reconstructed pressure waves from an isovolumically contracting left ventricle while paced from each site as indicated. B: the curves of Panel A were offset, rescaled in amplitude and shifted in time to reveal that the time course of pressure generation was independent of pacing site up to the time of peak pressure. The average root-mean difference between the normalized curves obtained with ventricular pacing as compared to the curve obtained with atrial pacing was 1.46% up to t_{max} and 4.08% from t_{max} to the end of contraction. These curves also illustrate the small changes in the duration of contraction. From Burkhoff et al. [16], with permission of the authors.

Correlation of peak pressure and epicardial QRS duration

When the heart was paced from the atrium the pressure development was maximal and the QRS complex was short in duration. With ventricular pacing the pressure development was less and the QRS duration was longer. The relationship between pressure development and QRS duration measured in each of the 8 hearts studied is presented in Fig. 4. As indicated in the figure, there was a negative correlation between these two parameters which was roughly linear in

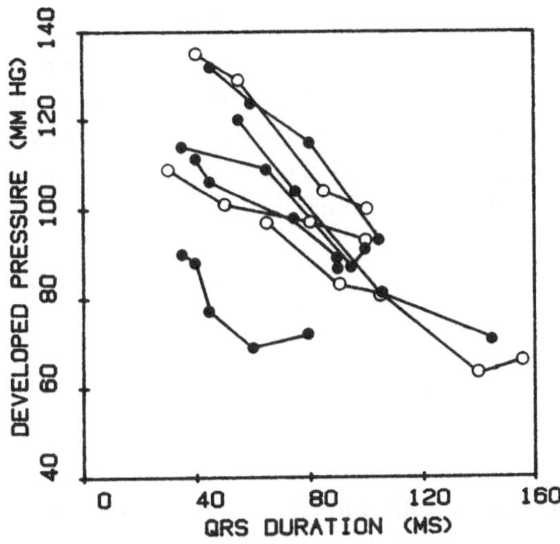

Figure 4. Summary of results from 8 ventricles on the relation between developed pressure and the duration of the QRS complex of an epicardial electrogram (different symbols used for clarity). In each heart this relation was linear with average (± SD) regression coefficients (slope) −0.51 ± 0.19 and correlation coefficient r = 0.971 ± 0.029. From Burkhoff et al. [16], with permission of the authors.

all hearts studied. The mean (± SD) slope was −0.51 (± 0.19) mm Hg/ms and the average correlation coefficient (r) was 0.971 (± 0.029).

Dependence of E_{es} and V_o on pacing site

Results of a typical experiment are illustrated in Fig. 5A. The linearity of the end-systolic pressure-volume relationship (ESPVR) was not altered by pacing from

Table 1. Root-mean square difference (D_{rms}) between normalized pressure waves obtained with ventricular pacing and atrial pacing.

Exp.	Time interval	
	0 to t_{max}	t_{max} to 460 ms
1	1.43 ± 0.12	3.60 ± 1.34
2	1.50 ± 0.25	2.18 ± 1.09
3	0.87 ± 0.12	1.80 ± 1.06
4	1.70 ± 0.19	5.38 ± 1.68
5	1.57 ± 0.61	5.03 ± 2.10
6	1.46 ± 0.33	4.08 ± 1.55
7	1.41 ± 0.80	1.92 ± 1.38
8	1.90 ± 0.59	1.73 ± 0.50

the RVF. The pacing site dependence of E_{es} (the slope of the ESPVR) was similar to the pacing site dependence of P_{max} at a constant volume. In this case, E_{es} decreased from 4.9 to 4.3 mm Hg/ml (a decrease of 12.2%) and V_0 increased from 0.3 to 1 ml. The results of experiments performed in 6 hearts are presented in Table 2 (data in Fig. 5A are Exp. 4). The data were compared by Student's paired t-test which indicated that the changes in both E_{es} and V_0 were statistically significant at the 1% level.

Oxygen consumption

When pacing site was switched from atrium to RVF, there was a decrease in arterial-venous oxygen content (A-VO_2) difference despite a relatively constant coronary sinus out-flow. This indicates that associated with the decrease in contractile performance associated with pacing site was a decrease in the amount of oxygen consumed by the ventricle. The magnitude of changes in these signals between pacing sites were small and oxygen consumption was determined accurately by digitizing all signals and averaging several seconds of data by computer.

In order to evaluate the influence of pacing site on the balance between ventricular energy consumption and total mechanical work performed by the ventricle, we determined the relation between the total pressure-volume area (PVA) and oxygen consumption per beat (VO_2) (see Methods). A typical result is presented in Fig. 5B for which the changes in the pressure-volume relation is presented in Panel A (discussed above). As illustrated, despite the fact that both

Table 2. Comparison of E_{es} and V_0 obtained with atrial pacing (Atr) and right ventricular free wall pacing (RVF).

Exp	Pacing site			
	ATR		RVF	
	E_{es}	V_0	E_{es}	V_0
1	4.2	0.0	3.6	2.4
2	4.0	8.5	3.6	10.6
3	6.2	11.5	5.1	12.1
4	4.9	0.3	4.3	1.0
5	6.0	15.0	4.6	15.0
6	4.2	8.5	3.9	9.6
Mean	4.9	7.3	4.2[a]	8.5[a]
SD	0.97	5.5	0.60	5.1

[a] Statistically significant difference between results obtained with atrial and RVF pacing at $p<0.01$ by Student's paired T-test.

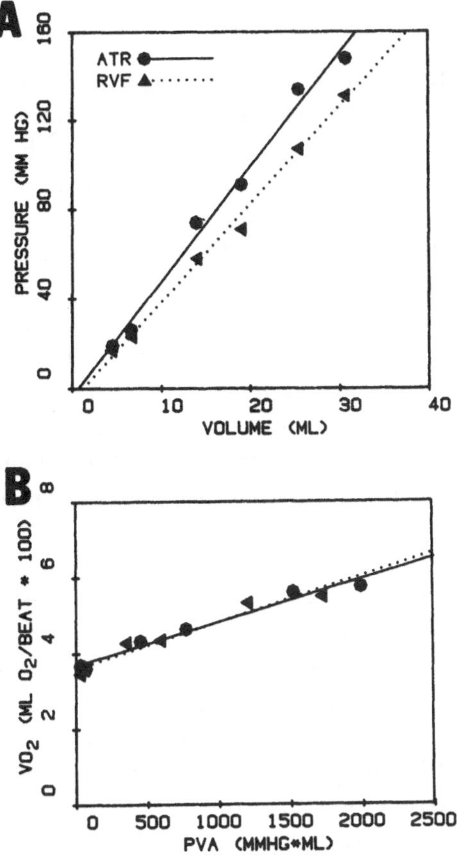

Figure 5. A: end-systolic pressure-volume relation obtained from a single heart first with atrial pacing and then with right ventricular free wall pacing. B: ventricular oxygen consumption, VO_2, and the corresponding total pressure-volume area, PVA, were measured for each loading condition and pacing site of Panel A. Pacing site influenced both PVA and VO_2 but did not alter the PVA-VO_2 relation. From Burkhoff et al. [16], with permission of the authors.

PVA and VO_2 changed when the pacing site was changed, the relation between these two was the same with both pacing sites. The PVA-VO_2 relation was quantified by its slope and y-axis intercept determined by linear regression analysis applied seperately to the data obtained from the two pacing sites. The two regression lines were compared by analysis of covariance. The results from 5 hearts studied in this series, summarized in Table 3, indicated that in 4 of the 5 hearts there was no statistically significant difference in the PVA-VO_2 relation. In one heart there was a statistical difference at the 1% significance level; however, the magnitude of this difference was small.

Discussion

We tested the hypothesis that with myocardial pacing the effective mass of muscle which contributes to active ventricular pressure generation is reduced below that which exists when pacing is from the atrium. This hypothesis was derived from a model generated from information available in the literature [1, 2, 8, 10]. Five predictions of the hypothesis were validated in isovolumically contracting canine left ventricles. The theoretical basis for each of these predictions has been discussed in detail (see Introduction).

First, consistent with previous studies, peak isovolumic pressures were smaller with ventricular pacing than with atrial pacing. Furthermore, pacing from different myocardial sites produced different levels of contractile strength; atrially paced beats were strongest, followed by (in the order of weakening contractile strengths) left ventricular apical pacing, right ventricular endocardial pacing, and finally right and left ventricular free wall pacing which produced the weakest contractions.

Second, despite the marked influences on ventricular contractile strength and electrical dispersion, there was relatively little influence on the duration of contraction or on the time-course of chamber stiffening and relaxation as judged by the similarity of the shapes of the isovolumic pressure waves.

Third, with a change of pacing site in a given heart, there was a highly significant, linear, negative correlation between peak isovolumic pressure and the duration of the QRS complex of an epicardial surface electrogram.

Fourth, the end-systolic pressure-volume relation (ESPVR) measured with RVF pacing had a lower slope, E_{es}, and a small increase in volume-axis intercept, V_o, as compared to that measured with atrial pacing.

Table 3. Influence of pacing site on the slope, A (ml O_2/mm Hg · ml/ beat), and y-intercept, B (ml O_2/ beat), of the regression of VO_2 on total pressure-volume area.

Exp.	Pacing site			
	Atrium		RV free wall	
	A ml O_2/beat mm Hg · ml	B ml O_2 beat	A ml O_2/beat mm Hg · ml	B ml O_2 beat
1	2.10×10^{-5}	0.035	1.90×10^{-5}	0.038
2	2.36×10^{-5}	0.035	2.30×10^{-5}	0.032
3	3.18×10^{-5}	0.020	3.11×10^{-5}	0.021
4	3.64×10^{-5}	0.011	3.60×10^{-5}	0.012
5[a]	2.96×10^{-5}	0.025	2.79×10^{-5}	0.031

[a] Statistically significant difference in regression lines by analysis of covariance, $p<0.01$.

Finally, reduced ventricular strength created by ventricular pacing was associated with decreased oxygen consumption such that the relation between the total pressure-volume area and oxygen consumption (PVA-VO_2) with atrial and RVF pacing was not effected.

While the results of some studies have suggested relatively little or no influence of pacing site on systolic ventricular performance [11–15] most studies have clearly demonstrated, as in the present study, a reduction in ventricular chamber 'contractility' with myocardial pacing [2–9]. These studies have been discussed in the Introduction and in greater detail in our original manuscript [16].

Most recently, Park et al. [9] very carefully studied the influence of pacing site on the ESPVR of closed chest chronically instrumented dogs. Their data differ from ours in that they found a significant increase in V_o with no significant influence on E_{es} when pacing is switch from atrium to myocardium. There are many methodologic differences between our study and theirs, making direct comparison difficult. Because the isolated heart preparation allows for direct measurement of volume and strict control of loading conditions and coronary perfusion pressure, we believe that the changes in the ESPVR we observed reflect direct effects of pacing site on ventricular mechanical properties. In contrast, the changes detected in a closed chest dog preparation may reflect the responses of the more complex in situ cardiovascular system in which influences of autonomic reflexes and changes in coronary perfusion pressure may be present. Additionally, the ESPVR is measured by *transient* vena caval occlusion in the closed chest dog, and in the isolated heart by *step-wise* decreases in ventricular volume allowing establishment of a steady mechanical state at each volume setting; there are definite differences in the ESPVRs measured by these two methods. However, it is possible, though it seems unlikely, that the difference may result from some altered properties of the electrical activation system created when the heart is studied in isolation.

One result we wish to discuss in greater detail here is the observed shape invarience of the isovolumic pressure wave which has an interesting physiologic implication pertinent to the 'time-varying elastance' theory of ventricular contraction [18]. According to this theory, under isovolumic conditions, instantaneous pressure (P(t)) and volume (V(t)) are related by the equation:

$$P(t) = E(t)\,[V(t) - V_o], \tag{2}$$

where E(t) is the time-varying volume elastance of the ventricle, and V_o is the volume at which the peak systolic pressure is 0 mm Hg. E(t) can be expressed as follows:

$$E(t) = E_{es} \times e(t) + E_{min}, \tag{3}$$

where E_{min} is the minimum elastance, E_{es} is the maximum developed elastance attained at end systole, and e(t) describes the time course of change of elastance (i.e., the time course of stiffening and relaxation) and has a value of 0 at end diastole and a value of 1 at end-systole. Under isovolumic conditions, (i.e., V(t) = constant in (2)), the shape of the pressure wave (P*(t) in (1)) is determined by the shape of the elastance curve, which as defined in (3) is described by e(t); that is, e(t) = P*(t). Thus, the relative shape invarience of the isovolumic pressure wave suggests that the asynchronously contracting 'ineffective' mass of muscle created by direct myocardial stimulation does not contribute significantly to the total elastance of the ventricle during the period of synchronous activation of the 'effective' muscle mass. Any such influence, if it does exist, was beyond the sensitivity of our measurements. The only consistent alteration in the pressure waves with pacing site was that observed during relaxation, i.e., the significant prolongation of contraction. This observation suggests that the contribution of the 'ineffective' muscle mass to overall chamber elastance may not be negligible during the relaxation phase of the cardiac cycle.

This concept of how pacing site alters the time-varying elastance representation of left ventricular contraction is summarized by the electric analog in Fig. 6, which consists of two capacitors and is derived from the model presented in Fig. 1. Each capacitor represents one layer in the model of Fig. 1.

E_{norm} represents the normal time course of ventricular volume-elastance had the ventricle been paced from the atrium. $E_{ineffective}$ represents the time varying elastance that would occur if the entire thickness of the ventricular wall was contracting 'ineffectively'. The quantity '*r*' is a weighting factor which represents the fraction of the total ventricular wall which is considered to be contained in the outer 'ineffectively' contracting layer (*r* has a value between 0 and 1.0); $(1 - r)$ is therefore the fraction of the wall represented by the inner layer. The value of r is different for different pacing sites, having a value of 0 for atrial pacing and, from the data of the present study, approximately 0.25 with right ventricular free wall pacing.

In summary, we observed significant influence of pacing site on the magnitude, but not the time course of isovolumic ventricular pressure waves. Pacing from different sites of the ventricle resulted in different chamber contractile strenghts. There was a linear inverse relation between changes in QRS duration and changes in contractile strength. The decreased chamber contractility manifests itself as a decrease in E_{es} and a small increase in V_0. The relation between ventricular oxygen consumption and pressure-volume area was independent of pacing site. These results are consistent with the hypothesis that the effective mass of muscle which participates in the generation of active contractile strength is reduced when the pacing site is moved from the atrium to the ventricle.

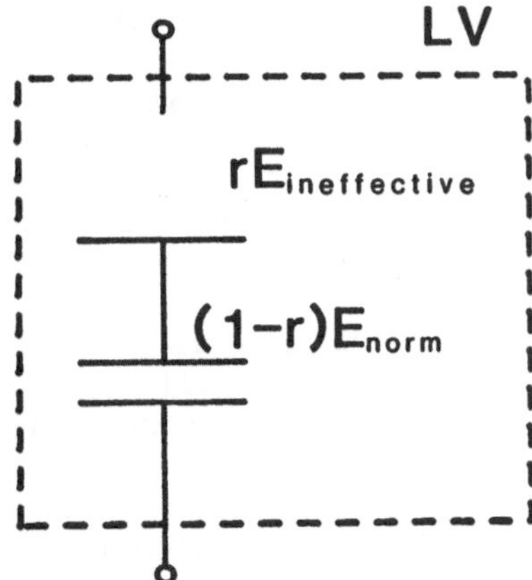

Figure 6. Electric analog of the model presented in Fig. 1. E_{norm} is the *normal* time-varying ventricular volume-elastance function. $E_{ineffective}$ is the time-varying ventricular volume-elastance if the entire wall thickness had been activated by muscle conduction. *r* represents the percentage of the wall which contracts asynchronously. The resulting global left ventricular (LV) time-varying elastance $E_{LV}(t)$ is the weighted sum of these two elastances: $E_{LV}(t) = rE_{ineffective} + (1 - r)E_{norm}$.

Acknowledgments

We are grateful to Dr A. Kimball for his advise on statistical methods. We are also grateful to Mr Kenneth Rent for his excellent technical assistance throughout this series of experiments. This work was supported by US NIH Research Grant HL-14903. D. Burkhoff was supported by NIH Biomedical Engineering Training Grant 5T32GM07057.

References

1. Lewis T, Rothschild MA (1915): The excitatory process in the dog's heart. Part II. The ventricles. Phil Trans Roy Soc London 206: 181–223.
2. Wiggers CJ (1925): The muscular reactions of the mammalian ventricles to artificial surface stimuli. Am J Physiol 73: 346–378.
3. Abildskov JA, Eich RH, Kenichi H, Smulyan H (1965): Observation of the relation between ventricular activation sequence and the hemodynamic state. Circ Res 17: 236–247.
4. Boerth RC, Covell JW (1971): Mechanical performance and efficiency of the left ventricle during ventricular stimulation. Am J Physiol 221: 1686–1691.
5. Dagget WM, Bianco JA, Powell J, Austen G (1970): Relative contributions of the atrial systole-ventricular systole interval and of patterns of ventricular activation to ventricular function during electrical pacing of the dog heart. Circ Res 27: 69–79.
6. Finney JO (1965): Hemodynamic alterations in left ventricular function consequent to ventricular pacing. Am J. Physiol 208: 275–282.
7. Gilmore JP, Sarnoff SJ, Mitchell JH, Linden RJ (1963): Synchronicity of ventricular contraction:

observations comparing hemodynamic effects of atrial and ventricular pacing. Br Heart J 25: 299–307.

8. Lister JW, Klotz DH, Jomain SL, Stuckey JH, Hoffman BF (1964): Effect of pacemaker site on cardiac output and ventricular activation in dogs with complete heart block. Am J Cardiol 14: 494–503.
9. Park RC, Little WC, O'Rourke RA (1985): Effect of alteration of left ventricular activation sequence on the left ventricular end-systolic pressure-volume relation in closed chest dogs. Circ Res 57: 706–717.
10. Fletcher FW, Theilen EO, Lawrence MS, Evans JW (1963): Effect of pacemaker location on cardiac function in complete A-V heart block. Am J Physiol 205: 1232–1234.
11. Grover M, Glanz SA (1983): Endocardial pacing site affects left ventricular performance in the intact anesthetized dog. Circ Res 53: 72–85.
12. Starzl TE, Gaertner RA, Webb RC Jr (1955): The effects of repetitive electric cardiac stimulation in dogs with normal hearts, complete heart block and experimental cardiac arrest. Circulation 2: 952–962.
13. Tsagarix TJ, Sutton RB, Kuida H (1977): Hemodynamic effects of varying pacemaker sites. Am J Psysiol 218: 246–250.
14. William-Olsson G, Andersen MN (1963): The effect of pacemaker electrode site on cardiac output. J Thorac Cardiovasc Surg 45: 618–621.
15. Badke FR, Boinay P, Covell JW (1980): Effects of ventricular pacing on regional left ventricular performance in the dog. Am J Physiol 238: H858–H867.
16. Burkhoff D, Oikawa RY, Sagawa K (1986): Influence of pacing site on ventricular contraction. Am J Physiol (in press).
17. Scher AM, Young AC (1955): Spread of excitation during premature ventricular systoles. Circ Res 3: 535–542.
18. Suga H, Sagawa K (1974): Instantaneous pressure-volume relationships and their ratio in the excised, supported canine left ventricle. Circ Res 35: 117–126.
19. Suga H, Sagawa K (1977): End-diastolic and end-systolic ventricular volume clamper for isolated canine heart. Am J Physiol 233: H718–722.
20. Sunagawa K, Lim KO, Burkhoff D, Sagawa K (1982): Microprocessor control of a ventricular volume servo-pump. Ann Biomed Eng 10: 145–159.
21. Shephard AP, Burgen CG (1977): A solid state arteriovenous oxygen difference analyzer for flowing whole blood. Am J Physiol 232: H434–H440.
22. Suga H, Hisano R, Goto Y, Yamada O, Igarashi Y (1983): Effect of positive inotropic agents on the relation between oxygen consumption and systolic pressure volume area in canine left ventricle. Circ Res 53: 306–318.

Discussion

Marcus: With the model you have been employing, utilizing implanted clips and biplane angiograms, you should be able to show directly the precise location and magnitude of abnormalities in regional ventricular function. Have you actually done that?
Maughan: We had hoped to have one or two experiments of that type done before this symposium but it has not been done yet. It would provide another piece of confirmating data.
Downey: A comment concerning the segment length data we saw earlier. It behaves almost like an infarct when you have this segment activated late in the cycle with the rest of the heart contracting dysynchronously. This causes the end-systolic pressure volume relationship to become very nonlinear in regional ischemia. Do you see anything like that in your model?
Maughan: Dr Little's paper will show phenomena similar to regional ischemia. We calculate a slope change rather than an intercept change and we do not detect a nonlinearity but the changes here are relatively small. Within the limitations that we make, we can't really make a judgement as to whether there is a parallel, or slope, change. We would like to do that because there are fundamental differences in the way they shift.
Marcus: The myocardial oxygen consumption measurement that you are making reflects an imprecise index of total left ventricular oxygen consumption. This could be very misleading in predicting myocardial oxygen consumption in specific regions that are functioning in a heterogeneous fashion. Is that correct?
Maughan: The ideal would be to measure blood from that portion of the myocardium that is involved in direct myocardial activation. We would then expect the degree of unloading in the portion of the myocardium to be proportional to the decrease in the developed pressure. We were not able to do this so we cannot be certain that the decrease in MVO_2 takes place in the earliest activated segments.
Weisfeldt: I may amplity what Dr Maughan said about conditions of an intact circulation being different than the isolated model. Some years ago, in Bill Daggett's laboratory, we studied a similar issue in a working intact circulation and we were able to show rather distinctly that abnormalities in the site of pacing would induce mitral regurgitation rather easily. This was particularly true in a volume loaded heart or in a heart that was abnormal for some other reason. One could even take a normal heart and bring it up high on its Frank Starling curve, and then induce abnormal pacing and measure mitral regurgitation occuring. If you are looking at overall pump function, you are impressed at the extent at which pump function is diminished when in fact what you are doing is inducing mitral regurgation by virtue of the lack of proper timing of the papilary muscle contraction. Was there a comparison of ventricular volume change with forward stroke volume?
Lab: When you look at your timing in your superimposed pressure curves, you

found a 10% difference when you look at 50% developed tension, or developed force. But if you look at the same level during relaxation your differences in force rather than time are quite high. This is deceptive. If you draw a line straight up, it looks to me as if it is about 30–40%.

Maughan: Actually we did that and the differences are pretty small. I think that in that particular illustration, the difference might have appeared exagerated but in fact the difference was less than 20%.

11. Effect of alterations of the left ventricular activation sequence on left ventricular performance

W.C. LITTLE, R.C. PARK and G.L. FREEMAN

Abstract

It is difficult to determine the effect of ventricular pacing on left ventricular (LV) performance using isovolumic or ejection phase indices, because ventricular pacing also produces changes in loading conditions. Accordingly, we investigated the effect of pacing from the atrium and various ventricular sites on the LV end-systolic pressure-volume relation, a relatively load-independent measure of LV performance. Studies were performed following autonomic blockade in dogs chronically instrumented to measure left ventricular pressure and determine left ventricular volume from three ultrasonic endocardial dimensions. During ventricular pacing, left ventricular end-diastolic volume, stroke volume, and end-systolic pressure were decreased, while the end-systolic volume was relatively unchanged. LV end-systolic pressure-volume relations were generated by vena caval occlusions during pacing at a constant rate from atrial and ventricular sites. Compared to atrial pacing, the LV end-systolic pressure-volume relations were shifted to the right during pacing from ventricular sites. The volume intercept of the LV end-systolic pressure-volume relation increased during ventricular pacing, while the slope of the LV end-systolic pressure-volume relation changed only slightly. We concluded that alterations of the normal activation sequence produced by ventricular pacing depress LV pumping function, independent of loading conditions, as indicated by a rightward shift of the LV end-systolic pressure-volume relation. The decreased stroke volume during ventricular pacing is due both to a decreased end-diastolic volume (decreased preload) and the rightward shift of the end-systolic pressure-volume relation (decreased pump function).

Introduction

During atrial pacing the ventricles are rapidly and nearly synchronously (within 60 msec) activated through the rapidly conducting His-Purkinje system. In contrast, the rate and pattern of activation during ventricular pacing are markedly different as depolarization spreads through the more slowly conducting ventricular myocardium. During ventricular pacing, the delay between the early and late activated areas of the left ventricle may be greater than 120 msec [1]. Since mechanical activity follows electrical activation, ventricular pacing produces dyssynchronous ventricular contraction which might be expected to impair left ventricular systolic performance [2].

Previous studies have evaluated the effects of ventricular pacing on the rate of LV pressure development, stroke volume, stroke work, cardiac output, and arterial blood pressure. While most studies have shown a depression of these parameters when ventricular pacing is compared with sinus rhythm or atrial pacing [3–8], some studies have noted little or no change in one or more of these parameters [9]. The interpretation of these observations is complicated by the fact that each of these parameters may also be influenced by the presence or absence of atrial contraction, as well as by loading conditions, heart rate, and autonomic reflexes, all of which may be altered by ventricular pacing. Furthermore, whether the site of ventricular pacing influences LV systolic performance has remained controversial [5, 10, 11].

The LV end-systolic pressure-volume relation is a sensitive index of LV systolic performance that is relatively independent of loading conditions. The relation is linear in normally contracting isolated canine hearts [12–14], conscious dogs [15], and man [16]. The slope of the relation is sensitive to changes in ventricular performance resulting from global interventions, increasing in response to positive inotropic interventions and decreasing with negative inotropic interventions, whereas the volume axis intercept is relatively unchanged (Figure 1). Acute regional ischemia produced by coronary occlusion in isolated, isovolumic canine hearts [17], and in chronically instrumented dogs [18] results in a rightward shift of the end-systolic pressure-volume relation (an increase in the volume axis intercept with little change in the slope) (Figure 2). This rightward shift of the LV end-systolic pressure-volume relation indicates that at a constant end-diastolic volume (preload) and end-systolic pressure (afterload) the stroke volume will be reduced. Since the LV end-systolic pressure-volume relation reflects both global and regional changes in LV performance and is relatively unaffected by loading conditions, it seemed to be ideally suited to the evaluation of the influence of ventricular pacing on LV pump performance. Consequently, we recently studied the effect of alterations of the activation sequence of LV performance using the end-systolic pressure-volume relation [19].

Methods

The studies were performed on adult mongrel dogs instrumented with a micromanometer pressure transducer and three pairs of ultrasonic crystals (5 MHz)

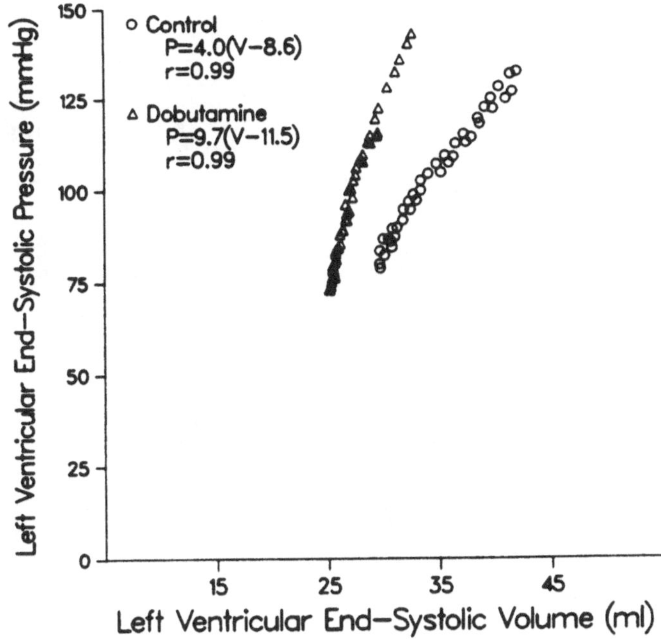

Figure 1. LV end-systolic pressure-volume relations generated by caval occlusions in a closed chest dog. Positive inotropic stimulation with dobutamine increases the slope and shifts the relation to the right. The regression equations are shown. P = end-systolic pressure, V = end-systolic volume and r = correlation coefficient. Reproduced from Little [20] with permission of the American Heart Association.

implanted in the endocardium of the LV to measure the anterior-posterior, septal-lateral, and base-apex (long axis) dimensions of the left ventricle. LV volume was calculated from the three LV dimensions as we have previously described [19–21]. Pairs of bipolar pacing electrodes were sutured to the epicardium of the left atrial appendage, the right ventricular free wall, the right ventricular apex, and the LV free wall.

After full recovery from the thoracotomy, the dogs were sedated with fentanyl in combination with droperidol sufficient to allow intubation. In four dogs, endocardial bipolar pacing catheters were inserted percutaneously via the jugular vein and positioned in the right ventricular apex and right ventricular outflow tract. To prevent reflex autonomic changes, the dogs were treated with atropine sulfate (0.2 mg/kg, iv) and propranolol (2 mg/kg, iv). The dogs were ventilated with room air. To minimize the effect of fluctuations in intrathoracic pressure, all data were recorded during 12-second periods while the dogs were apneic, with the glottis held open by the endotracheal tube [21].

The hearts were paced using 0.5-msec pulses at threshold levels at the minimum rate (128 ± 8/min epicardial and 131 ± 16/min endocardial) which ensured

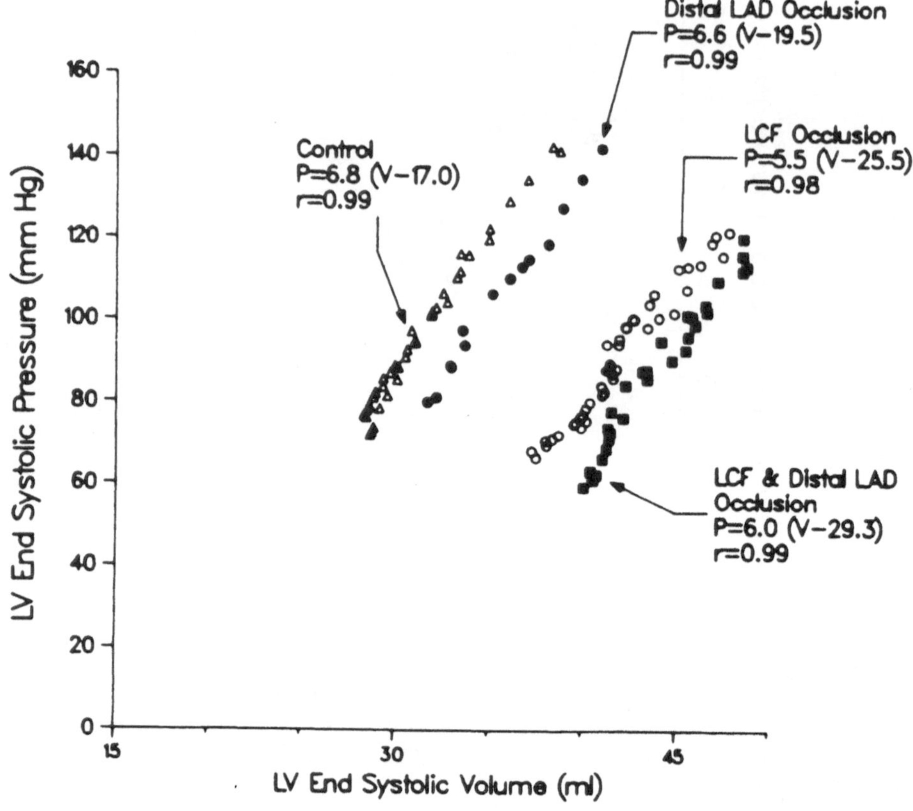

Figure 2. LV end-systolic pressure-volume relations generated by caval occlusion in a closed chest dog. Occlusion of progressively more branches of the left coronary artery results in rightward shifts of the LV end-systolic pressure-volume relation. Reproduced from Little and O'Rourke [18] with permission of the American College of Cardiology.

complete capture from each of the pacing sites. This rate was held constant throughout the study. The heart of each animal was initially paced from the atrium, followed by pacing from each of the ventricular epicardial and/or endocardial sites in random order. At the conclusion of the study, atrial pacing was repeated to confirm that there had been no change in the preparation. During ventricular pacing, the atria were paced simultaneously with the ventricle to prevent atrial echo beats and intermittent capture of the ventricle by atrial impulses. Pacing at each site was performed until all hemodynamic parameters were stable. The end-systolic pressure-volume relation then was generated by sudden transient occlusions of the inferior vena cava using a previously implanted hydraulic occluder. This caused a progressive fall of left ventricular end-systolic pressure and volume over the 12-second recording period allowing definition of the LV end-systolic pressure-volume relation.

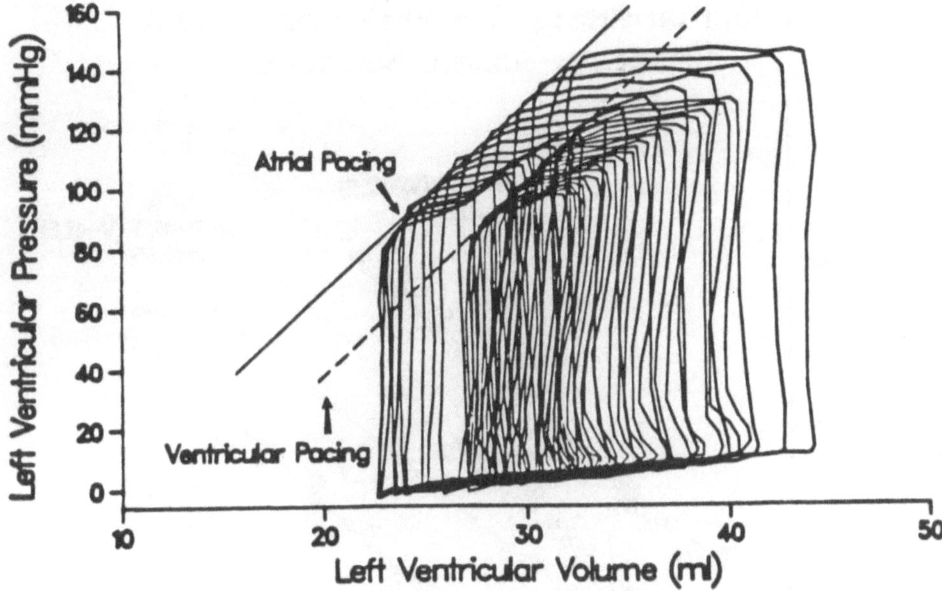

Figure 3. Representative pressure-volume loops generated by vena caval occlusion during pacing from the atrium and the right ventricular free wall. The upper lefthand corner of the pressure-volume loops (end-systole) describes the end-systolic pressure-volume relation during pacing from each site. Note that ventricular pacing produces a rightward shift of the LV end-systolic pressure-volume relation. Reproduced from Park et al. [19], with permission of the American Heart Association.

Results and discussion

We found that during pacing from right or left ventricular endocardial sites that the LV end-systolic pressure-volume relation remains linear, but compared to atrial pacing the end-systolic pressure-volume relation is shifted rightward, with an increase in the volume axis intercept but with no consistent change in the slope (Figure 3–5). A similar shift of the end-systolic pressure-volume relation occurred during pacing from the right ventricular endocardium (Figure 6). This rightward shift of the LV end-systolic pressure-volume relation indicates a depression of LV pumping performance during ventricular pacing that occurs independent of changes in preload.

In agreement with previous studies [9, 23], both ventricular epicardial and endocardial pacing resulted in a decrease in LV end-diastolic volume and stroke volume (Figure 7), whereas end-systolic volume was relatively unchanged. Our study indicates that the stroke volume falls during ventricular pacing for two reasons. First, left ventricular preload as measured by the end-diastolic volume is decreased. Second, ventricular pacing depresses LV pumping function independent of the fall in end-diastolic volume, as indicated by the rightward shift of the LV end-systolic pressure-volume relation. This shift indicates that the stroke

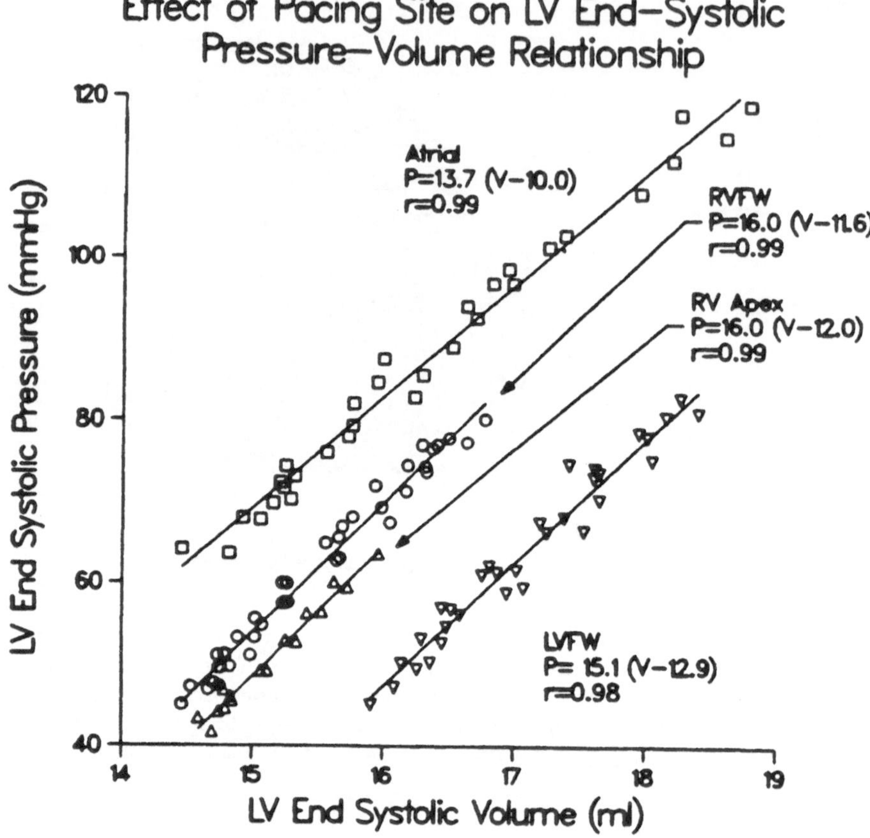

Figure 4. LV end-systolic pressure-volume relations produced by caval occlusions in one animal during pacing from the left atrium (atrial), epicardium of the right ventricular free wall (RVFW), the right ventricular apex (RV Apex), and LV free wall (LVFW). Reproduced from Park et al. [19] with permission of the American Heart Association.

volume is reduced for any given end-diastolic volume and end-systolic pressure. Our findings are consistent with some previous studies using different measures which also suggested that LV performance is decreased during ventricular pacing [4–8, 22, 23].

Grover and Glantz [9] observed a decrease in stroke volume during pacing from the endocardium of the right ventricular apex in closed-chest dogs due to a fall in end-diastolic volume, whereas end-systolic volume remained relatively constant. Since LV end-systolic pressure was not significantly changed, they speculated that the left ventricular end-systolic pressure-volume relation and systolic pumping performance were not altered by ventricular pacing. However, the end-systolic pressure-volume relation was not directly determined in their study. We directly determined the LV end-systolic pressure-volume relation and

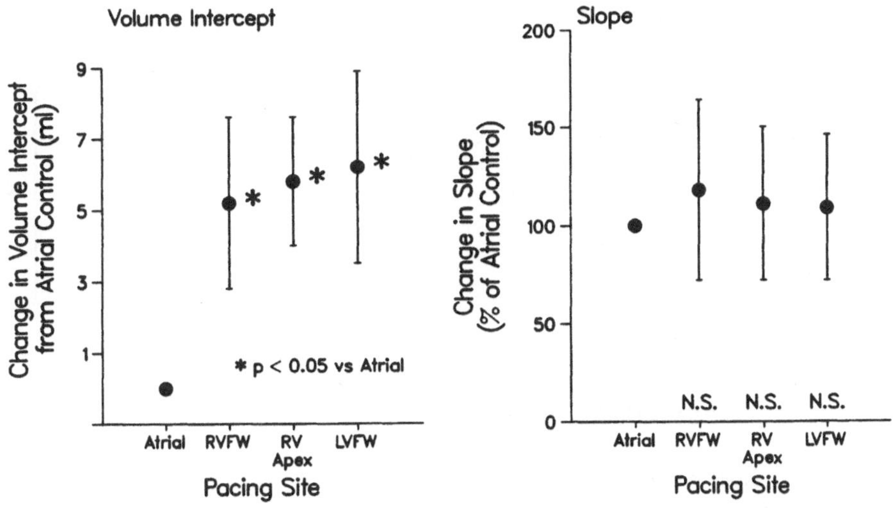

Figure 5. Effect of ventricular pacing on the slope and volume intercept of the end-systolic pressure-volume relation. Mean ± SD of 8 animals.

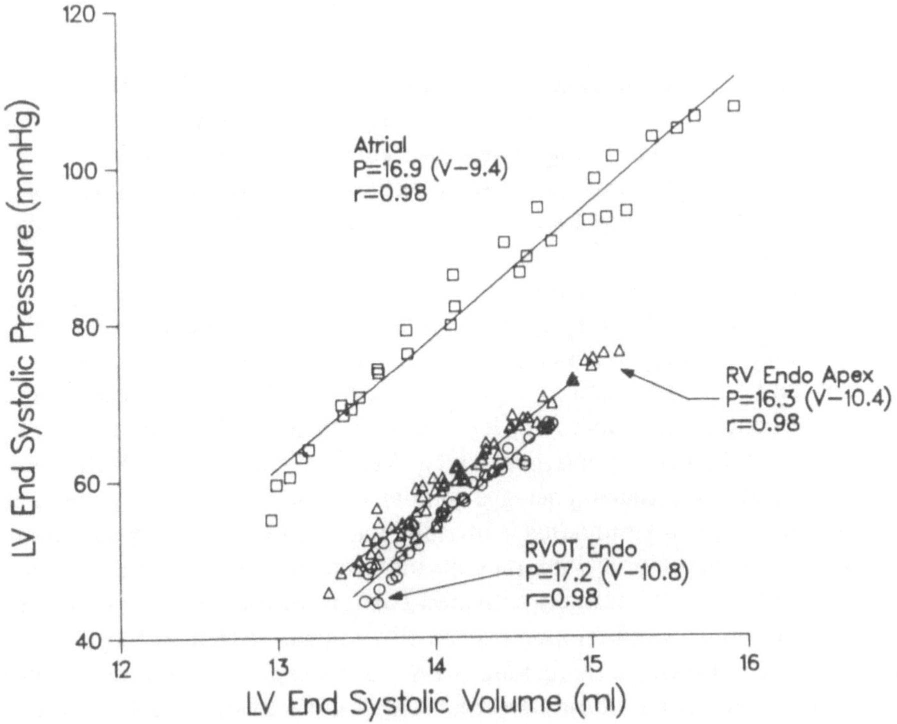

Figure 6. End-systolic pressure-volume relations produced by vena caval occlusion during pacing from the atrium (atrial), and the endocardium of the right ventricular outflow tract (RVOT), and right ventricular apex (RV Apex) are shown. Reproduced from Park et al. [19] with permission of the American Heart Association.

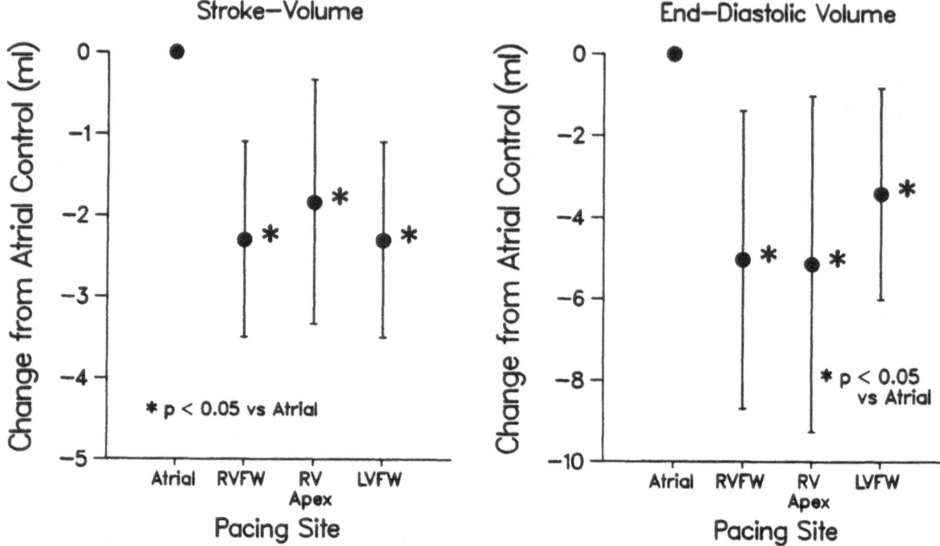

Figure 7. Ventricular pacing decreases left ventricular stroke volume and end-diastolic volume. Mean ± SD of 8 animals.

found that pacing from the ventricular endocardium or epicardium shifted the end-systolic pressure-volume relation to the right. The study of Grover and Glantz [9] was performed in dogs with intact autonomic reflexes. It is possible that, in their study, a reflex increase in contractility may have compensated for a rightward shift of the end-systolic pressure-volume relation during ventricular pacing.

Why does ventricular pacing produce a rightward shift of the LV end-systolic pressure-volume relation? This shift is similar to the parallel rightward shift of the LV end-systolic pressure-volume relation that occurs when contraction of a portion of the LV is prevented by regional ischemia in the isolated, isovolumic dog heart [17] and in the intact dog [18]. During ischemia the magnitude of the shift is related to the size of the ischemic area. Regional end-systolic LV dysfunction produced by ventricular pacing is similar, in some respects, to regional ischemia. Badke et al. [8] found that ventricular pacing produced dyssynchronous LV contraction with reciprocal interactions between the early and late activated areas. At end systole, the initially activated portions of the LV were no longer contracting, and thus, would not be expected to contribute to the generation of end-systolic LV pressure. In agreement with this concept, several investigators [23–25] have observed that, during dyssynchronous LV activation, early activated areas of the LV bulge paradoxically in late systole, displaying a motion similar to that observed when ischemic dysfunction prevents regional contraction.

Because of these similarities, a slight modification of the model of Sunagawa et al. [17] of the regionally ischemic ventricle may also account for the rightward

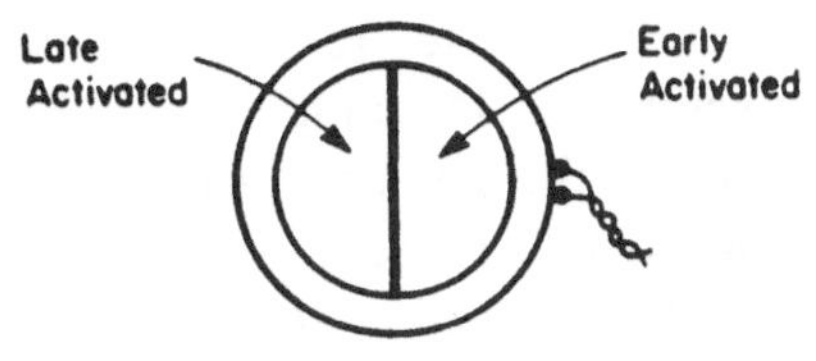

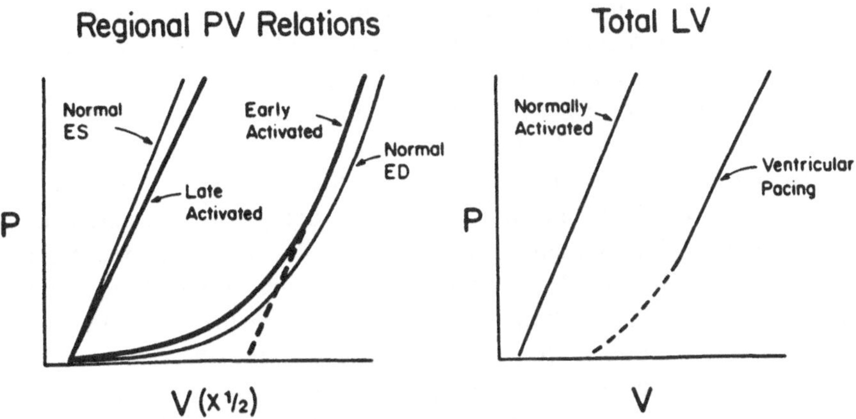

Figure 8. A schematic model of the left ventricle during ventricular pacing. The LV is considered to be composed of two compartments, an early activated region and a late activated region. The regional end-systolic ES) pressure (P)-volume (V) relations are shown on the left for each compartment. At end-systole, the early activated region is relaxing and has exponential ES P-V relation similar to the normal end-diastolic P-V relation. Whereas the ES P-V relation of the late activated region is similar to the normal ES P-V relation. The resulting ES P-V relation of the entire LV (the sum of the two regional ES P-V relations) is shown on the right for ventricular pacing compared to a normally activated LV. See text for discussion. Reproduced from Park et al. [19] with permission of the American Heart Association.

shift of the end-systolic pressure-volume relation we observed during ventricular pacing. The ventricle is considered to be composed of two compartments: an early activated region and a late activated region (Figure 8). The LV end-systolic pressure-volume relation is the sum of the relations of these two compartments. By end-systole of the entire ventricle, the early activated area is relaxing, and thus, may have a curvilinear pressure-volume relation similar to that seen in diastole. The pressure-volume relation of the late activated portion of the ventricle is similar to normal. At end-systole, the later activated region has displaced blood into the relaxing, early activated compartment. This increased volume in the early activated area moves it up to a relatively steep portion of its regional pressure-volume relation where the slope (or elastance) may be similar to the normal systolic value. In agreement with our observations, this model predicts that the resulting pressure-volume relation of the entire ventricle, in the range in which we studied, will be shifted to the right during ventricular pacing without much change in the slope. The magnitude of the shift will be equal to the volume of blood displaced into the early activated region, and, thus, proportional to the degree of dyssynchronous activation. This model does not take into account other factors that may also influence the LV end-systolic pressure-volume relation during dyssynchronous contraction. These may include ventricular interdependence [25], and the effect of the interaction of the dyssynchronously contracting fibers on their individual length-tension relations [26].

In two animals, we measured the time required for LV endocardial activation from bipolar electrograms recorded from the six endocardial crystals located in the endocardium of the apex, base, interventricular septum, lateral wall, anterior wall, and posterior wall of the LV [9]. The time from the onset of the first left ventricular electrogram to the last electrogram (the LV activation time) was measured. The shift of the volume intercept of the end-systolic pressure-volume relation during ventricular pacing correlated roughly with the extent of dyssynchronous activation as estimated by the ventricular activation time (Figure 9). In agreement with the model, this suggests that the magnitude of the shift of the LV end-systolic pressure-volume relation depends on the amount of dyssynchronous activation. Consistent with this hypothesis is the observation of Grover and Glantz [9] that pacing from sites near distal portions of the conduction system produced greater depressions of hemodynamic parameters than pacing from septal sites that result in a more normal pattern of ventricular activation.

Whether pacing from right or LV sites produces greater depression of LV systolic performance is controversial. Some studies have shown right ventricular [10] or left ventricular [1, 3, 11] sites to be superior hemodynamically, whereas others have found that the site of ventricular stimulation does not influence LV systolic performance [5, 6, 27–29]. We found that pacing from a right ventricular site produced the largest shift of the LV end-systolic pressure-volume relation in some animals, whereas LV pacing produced the greatest shift in others [19]. These variations in the relative effect of pacing from right or LV sites that we and others have observed may be due to differences in the degree of dyssynchronous activation depending on the location of the pacing site and its relation to the normal conduction system.

In our study, we quantified the shift of the left ventricular end-systolic pressure-volume relation using the extrapolated volume axis intercept, V_O [19]. Since this is an extrapolated value, it may be influenced by alterations in the slope and the degree of extrapolation required. Although the volume axis intercept was not measured directly, we [15, 18, 20, 30] and others [12–14, 31] have found that the end-systolic pressure-volume relation is described well by a straight line in the pressure range studied. Thus, the volume axis intercept should be a reliable index of the relative position of the relation and should be adequate to quantify relative shifts of the end-systolic pressure-volume relation during ventricular pacing. In addition, the shift of the end-systolic pressure-volume relation we observed during ventricular pacing was apparent not only as an increase in the volume axis intercept, but also by a greater end-systolic volume at each matched end-systolic

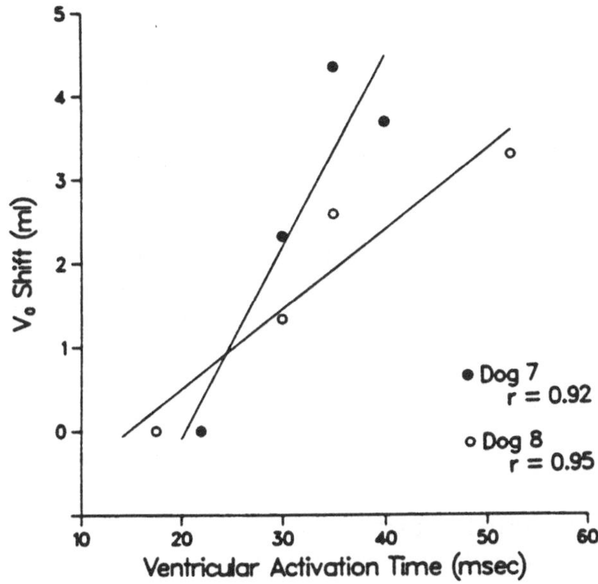

Figure 9. The shift in the volume intercept (V_0) of the end-systolic pressure-volume relation from the V_0 during atrial pacing is plotted against the time for left ventricular activation determined from six endocardial bipolar electrograms (ventricular activation time) in the two dogs in which it was measured. An increasing V_0 correlated roughly with an increasing LV activation time ($P = 0.08$, SEE = 0.95 ml in dog 7 and $P<0.05$, SEE = 0.55 ml in dog 8). Reproduced from Park et al. [19] with permission of the American Heart Association.

pressure during ventricular pacing (Figures 5–8).

Marked alterations in arterial input impedance may produce parallel shifts of the LV end-systolic pressure-volume relation [15, 20, 31]. All observations in this study were performed following autonomic blockade; thus, although the baseline aortic pressure was different during atrial and ventricular pacing, the vascular tone and arterial input impedance should not have been markedly altered. Any reflex increase in arterial tone, in response to the decreased arterial pressure during ventricular pacing, would tend to shift the LV pressure-volume relation to the left, thus, a rightward shift in response to ventricular pacing could not be attributed to changes in vascular tone.

This study has several clinical implications. First, any disturbance of ventricular activation due to ventricular pacing or conduction system abnormalities (i.e., left bundle branch block) should be considered when interpreting the left ventricular end-systolic pressure-volume relation. Second, ventricular pacing appears to depress left ventricular pumping performance in addition to the impairment of ventricular diastolic filling that usually results from the loss of a properly timed atrial systole and possibly other factors [9]. Thus, in patients with impaired ventricular performance, attempts to maintain the normal ventricular activation sequence, in addition to preserving a properly timed atrial systole, may be important in order to optimize left ventricular pumping performance.

Conclusions

1. alterations of the normal left ventricular activation sequence depress left ventricular systolic pumping function, as manifest by a rightward shift of the left ventricular end-systolic pressure-volume relation;
2. the extent of the rightward shift of the pressure-volume relation appears to be related to the degree of dyssynchronous activation of the left ventricle; and
3. the decrease in stroke volume during ventricular pacing results from both a decrease in left ventricular end-diastolic volume (decreased preload) and a rightward shift of the left ventricular end-systolic pressure-volume relation (decreased pump function).

Acknowledgment

This study was supported in part by the National Institutes of Health (1R01-37324) and a grant-in-aid from the American Heart Association with funds contributed by the Texas Affiliate.

References

1. Lister JW, Klotz DH, Jomain SL, Stuckey JH, Hoffman BF (1964): Effect of pacemaker site on cardiac output and ventricular activation in dogs with complete heart block. Am J Cardiol 14: 494–503.
2. Hotta S (1967): The sequence of mechanical activation of the ventricle. Jpn Circ J 31: 1568–1575.
3. Finney JO (1965): Hemodynamic alterations in left ventricular function consequent to ventricular pacing. Am J Physiol 208: 275–282.
4. Boerth RC, Covell JW (1971): Mechanical performance and efficiency of the left ventricle during ventricular stimulation. Am J Physiol 221: 1686–1691.
5. Walston A, Starr JW, Greenfield JC (1973): Effect of different epicardial ventricular pacing sites on left ventricular function in awake dogs. Am J Cardiol 32: 291–294.
6. Miyazawa K, Shirato K, Haneda T, Honna T, Arai T, Nakajima T (1976): Effects of varying pacemaker sites on left ventricular performance. Tohoku J Exp Med 120: 301–308.
7. Heyndrickx GR, Vilaine J-P, Knight DR, Vatner SF (1985): Effects of altered site of electrical activation on myocardial performance during inotropic stimulation. Circulation 71: 1010–1016.
8. Badke FR, Boinay P, Covell JW (1980): Effects of ventricular pacing on regional left ventricular performance in the dog. Am J Physiol 238: H858–H867.
9. Grover M, Glantz SA (1983): Endocardial pacing site affects left ventricular end-diastolic volume and performance in the intact anesthetized dog. Circ Res 53: 72–85.
10. Meijler FL, Wieberdink J, Durrer D (1962): L'importance de la position des électrodes stimulatrices au cours de traitement d'un bloc auriculoventriculaire postoperatif total. Arch Mal Coeur 55: 690–698.
11. Daggett WM, Bianco JA, Powell WJ, Austen WG (1970): Relative contributions of the atrial systole interval and of patterns of ventricular activation to ventricular function during electrical pacing of the dog heart. Circ Res 27: 69–79.
12. Sagawa K (1978): The ventricular pressure-volume diagram revisited. Circ Res 43: 677–683.

13. Sagawa K (1981): The end-systolic pressure-volume relation of the ventricle: Definition, modification and clinical use. Circulation 63: 1223–1227.
14. Suga H, Sagawa K (1974): Instantaneous pressure-volume relationships in the excised supported canine left ventricle. Circ Res 35: 117–128.
15. Sodums MT, Badke FR, Starling MR, Little WC, O'Rourke RA (1984): Evaluation of left ventricular contractile performance utilizing end-systolic pressure-volume relationships in conscious dogs. Circ Res 54: 731–739.
16. Grossman W, Braunwald E, Mann T, McLaurin LP, Green LH (1977): Contractile state of the left ventricle in man as evaluated from end-systolic pressure-volume relations. Circulation 56: 845–852.
17. Sunagawa K, Maughan WL, Sagawa K (1983): Effect of regional ischemia on the left ventricular end-systolic pressure-volume relationship of isolated canine hearts. Circ Res 52: 170–178.
18. Little WC, O'Rourke RA (1985): Effect of regional ischemia on the left ventricular end-systolic pressure-volume relation in closed chest dogs. J Am Coll Cardiol 5: 297–302.
19. Park RC, Little WC, O'Rourke RA (1985): Effect of alteration of the left ventricular activation sequence on the left ventricular end-systolic pressure-volume relation in closed-chest dogs. Circ Res 57: 706–717.
20. Little WC (1985): The left ventricular dP/dt_{max}-end-diastolic volume relation in closed-chest dogs. Circ Res 56: 808–815.
21. Little WC, Badke FR, O'Rourke RA (1984): Effect of right ventricular pressure on the end-diastolic left ventricular pressure-volume relationship before and after chronic right ventricular pressure overload in dogs without pericardia. Circ Res 54: 719–730.
22. Gilmore JP, Sarnoff SJ, Mitchell JH, Linden RJ (1963): Synchronicity of ventricular contraction: Observations comparing hemodynamic effects of atrial and ventricular pacing. Br Heart J 25: 299–307.
23. Miyazawa K, Arai T, Shirato K, Haneda T, Ikeda S, Honna T, Nakajima T, Miura T (1977): Regional contraction patterns of the left ventricle during ventricular pacing. Tohoku J Exp Med 124: 261–266.
24. Hood WB Jr, Joison J, Abelmann WH, Norman JC (1969): Asynchronous contraction due to late systolic bulging at left ventricular pacing sites. Am J Physiol 217: 215–221.
25. Little WC, Reeves RC, Arciniegas J, Katholi RE, Rogers EW (1982): Mechanism of abnormal interventricular septal motion during delayed left ventricular activation. Circulation 65: 1486–1491.
26. Tyberg JV, Parmley WW, Sonnenblick EH (1969): In vitro studies of myocardial asynchrony and regional hypoxia. Circ Res 45: 569–579.
27. Starzl TE, Gaertner RA, Webb RC Jr (1955): The effects of repetitive electric cardiac stimulation in dogs with normal hearts, complete heart block and experimental cardiac arrest. Circulation 11: 952–962.
28. William-Olsson G, Anderson MN (1963): The effect of pacemaker electrode site on cardiac output. J Thorac Cardiovasc Surg 45: 618–621.
29. Tsagaris TJ, Sutton RB, Kuida H (1970): Hemodynamic effects of varying pacemaker sites. Am J Physiol 218: 246–250.
30. Little WC, Freeman GL, O'Rourke RA (1985): Simultaneous determination of left ventricular end-systolic pressure-volume and pressure-dimension relationships in closed-chest dogs. Circulation 71: 1304–1308.
31. Maughan WL, Sunagawa K, Burkhoff D, Sagawa K (1984): Effect of arterial impedance changes on the end-systolic pressure-volume relation. Circ Res 54: 595–602.

Discussion

Beyar: The striking difference between what you and Dr Maughan have presented here is that you show a shift in the end-systolic pressure-volume relationship, whereas Dr Maughan has shown, predominantly, a decrease in the slope of the relation with ventricular pacing. I suggest that the shift that you observed may be due to your use of an ejecting ventricle whereas in Dr Maughan's preparation the ventricle was contracting isovolumically. We know that if you calculate the slope of the end-systolic pressure-volume relation using higher volumes, you may get a lower slope, which does not fully support the statement that the slope, or E_{max}, is independent of loading conditions. This may explain the difference between your two studies.
Little: It is correct that the slope of the end-systolic pressure-volume relation is only relatively independent of loading conditions, as used in our study; ejecting beats only approximate the isovolumic end-systolic pressure-volume relation. Both Dr Maughan's study and ours show that during ventricular pacing the end-systolic pressure-volume relation is shifted to the right. The difference is that they report a decrease in the slope and also an increase in the volume intercept, while we find only an increase in the volume intercept. In both studies the relation was shifted to the right and thus, the pumping performance of the left ventricle is decreased. Their studies of the isolated heart use a much more carefully controlled preparation, whereas our studies of the intact ejecting heart are less carefully controlled but more physiological. As you point out, our study was done using ejecting beats while Dr Maughan's study used isovolumic beats. It is possible that the interactions between different parts of the ventricle during pacing may be different when the ventricle is allowed to eject, as opposed to when it is isovolumic.
Kass: Did you find that the rightwards shift of the end-systolic pressure volume relationship that you report during epicardial pacing is similar to the shifts seen with endocardial pacing?
Little: The shift is qualitatively the same during both endocardial and epicardial pacing. Quantitatively, the shift is somewhat smaller during endocardial pacing than during epicardial pacing.
Kass: Aren't these results, with a smaller shift during endocardial pacing than during epicardial pacing, consistent with the model that Dr Maughan proposes?
Little: Maughan's model of the dyssynchronously contracting ventricle considers it to be a series capacitance. Our model is a parallel capacitance. A parallel capacitance is needed to account for the increase in the volume intercept that we both observed. A series capacitance, as they propose, is needed to account for the decrease in the slope that they observed. I think the best description is a combination of both a parallel and series capacitance. Such a model explains all the observations of both studies.
Marcus: Did mitral regurgitation occur during ventricular pacing and did this

possibly influence the results?
Little: We found no evidence of significant mitral regurgitation during ventricular pacing.
Hoffman: How good was your calibration of the end-systolic volume?
Little: We calibrated our volume measurements using the left ventricular stroke volume. Since ventricular pacing does not alter the ventricular end-diastolic configuration, but does alter the end-systolic configuration, we thought that if we have a consistent measure of the difference between the two, we also have a consistent measure of end-systolic volume. In other studies, we have also calibrated our volumes using radionuclide angiograms. We find that in any one animal, our calculated volumes give a consistent measure of the true left ventricular volume despite changes in the activation sequence.
Weisfeldt: What was the state of the pericardium?
Little: In our study in the animals the pericardium was opened for instrumentation and not reapproximated.
Weisfeldt: Was there a functional pericardium in the preparation?
Little: I am sure that there is a functional pericardium in our preparation because the pericardium scars over at the point in which the chest is closed. We do not close the pericardium for fear of producing functional restriction.
Weisfeldt: I wonder if the difference between Dr Maughan's studies and these studies is the fact that there is a functioning pericardium when you do ventricular pacing. There may be a change that occurs in right sided hemodynamics that may in fact shift the pressure-volume relationship in the same way as Dr Maughan shows for primary loading of the right ventricle. Dr Ritman and Dr Tyberg might also feel that external restraint in the left ventricle was present with the pericardium present. Changing from atrial to ventricular pacing might alter left ventricular geometry sufficiently to change end-systolic pressure relationships in this way.

12. Effect of the thyroid state on ventricular action potential characteristics in the mammalian heart

O. BINAH, I. RUBINSTEIN and Y. SWEED

Abstract

Certain ventricular action potential characteristics such as action potential duration and amplitude vary considerably among mammalian species. As previous studies showed that changes in the thyroid state are associated with alterations in action potential duration, we tested the hypothesis that these variations might be related to differences in the thyroid state of the species. Ventricular action potential characteristics from several species were studied, encompassing a wide range of metabolic rates. The species were dog, guinea pig, mole rat, rat, mouse, and shrew. Resting membrane potential and action potential amplitude, and area were found to be inversely correlated with heart rate, body mass, and metabolic rate, expressed as oxygen consumption of the species. Modification of the thyroid state in guinea pigs and rats by the administration of thyroxine (T_4) or propylthiouracil, yielded alterations in ventricular action potential characteristics. Hyperthyroidism was found to be associated with a reduction in action potential duration and a faster rate of repolarization, whereas hypothyroidism was associated with a marked increase in action potential duration.

Preliminary experiments, using the patch electrode to record action potentials from ventricular myocytes isolated from euthyroid, hypo- and hyperthyroid guinea pig hearts, showed that changes in the thyroid state were associated with alterations in the electrophysiological properties of ventricular myocytes, similar to those seen in multicellular preparations. The time course of thyroid hormone effects on ventricular action potential characteristics were also studied. Other preliminary experiments showed that the action potential duration was markedly reduced 4–6 hr after T_4 administration, whereas recovery towards control values occurred within 10–20 days.

Although the mechanisms are yet to be determined, the experiments suggest that thyroid hormones have an important role as modulators of the cardiac electrophysiological properties.

Introduction

Electrophysiological properties of the mammalian heart have been known to vary considerably among different mammalian species [1–4]; however, the variations have not been analyzed quantitatively, and the mechanisms responsible for these variations have not been determined.

The purpose of this paper is to present experimental evidence suggesting that thyroid hormones may have an important role as modulators of electrophysiological properties of the mammalian heart.

Methods and procedure

Animals

Throughout the studies reported here, we used six different mammalian species:
1. adult mongrel dogs, weighing 15–20 kg;
2. guinea pigs, weighing 300–400 g;
3. Sprague-Dawley rats, weighing 300–400 g;
4. mole rats (*Spalax ehrenbergi*), weighing 180–220 g;
5. laboratory mice, weighing 30–35 g; and
6. shrews (*Crocidura russula*), weighing 7–8 g.

Measurement of transmembrane potentials from multicellular preparations

The animals were anesthetized (dogs i.v. and other species i.p.) with sodium pentobarbital, 30–40 mg/kg. The hearts were rapidly removed and the right ventricles excised and placed in cold Tyrode's solution gassed with 95% O_2–5% CO_2. Ventricular preparations were mounted in a Lucite tissue bath and superfused at a rate of 11 ml/min with Tyrode's solution gassed with 95% O_2–5% CO_2 and warmed to 36.5° C. The Tyrode's solution contained (mM): NaCl, 131; $NaHCO_3$, 18; NaH_2PO_4, 1.8; $MgCl_2$, 0.5; $CaCl_2$, 2.7; dextrose, 5.5; and KCl, 4.0. The preparations were stimulated with rectangular pulses by means of bipolar silver electrodes insulated to their tips with Teflon.

Transmembrane action potentials were recorded from right ventricular papillary muscles using 3 M KCl-filled glass microelectrodes and standard microelectrode techniques.

Procedures for electrophysiological studies in isolated myocytes

Preparation of single myocytes

Single ventricular myocytes were prepared from guinea pigs [5–7]. The animals were anesthetized with pentobarbital sodium (30 mg/kg). The heart was rapidly removed and the aorta cannulated and perfused with Tyrode's solution in a Langendorff apparatus. After the blood was washed out, the heart was perfused with 50 ml of Ca^{2+}-free Tyrode's solution. Subsequently, 50 ml of Ca^{2+}-free Tyrode's solution containing 40 mg collagenase (Type 1; Sigma, St. Louis, MO, USA) were circulated for about 30 min. Thereafter, the heart was perfused with 50 ml of 'KB medium' containing high K^+ and low Cl^- concentrations. All solutions were oxygenated and warmed to 36° C. Finally, the ventricle was removed from the cannula, minced, filtered, and stored for 1–2 hr in KB medium at room temperature.

Solutions

The Tyrode's solution contained (mM): NaCl, 140; KCl, 4; $CaCl_2$, 1.8; $MgCl_2$, 1; glucose, 10; and HEPES, 5. Ca^{2+}-free Tyrode's was prepared by omitting $CaCl_2$ from the Tyrode's solution. pH was adjusted to 7.4 by 1 N NaOH. The KB medium contained (mM): KCl, 70; KH_2PO_4, 30; $MgSo_4$, 5; $CaCl_2$, 0.12; glucose, 20; taurine, 20; succinic acid, 5; pyruvic acid, 5; creatine, 5; Na_2ATP, 5; and EGTA, 0.5. pH was adjusted to 7.4 by 1 N KOH. The electrode solution contained (mM): K-aspartate, 100; KCl, 20; $MgCl_2$, 3.5; KH_2PO_4, 20; Na_2ATP, 3; and EGTA, 1. pH was adjusted to 7.4 by 1 N KOH.

Electrophysiological procedures

A small volume (0.5 ml) of KB medium containing myocytes was transferred to a recording chamber, which was mounted on the stage of an inverted microscope. The chamber was superfused at a rate of 1 ml/min with Tyrode's solution warmed to 24.5° C. For recording action potentials from single myocytes, we used the whole-cell recording technique [7], the principles of which are shown in Figure 1. Once the myocytes settle on the bottom of the chamber, a 'patch electrode' (1–2 mΩ) is advanced towards the cell until a contact is made. Subsequently, moderate suction is applied, which usually results in a tight seal ($10\text{–}100 \times 10^9\,\Omega$) between the electrode tip and the membrane. When a stronger suction pulse is then applied, the membrane under the electrode tip is ruptured, and a low resistance pathway is created for current and voltage-clamp recordings. Action potentials were recorded using List Medical patch-clamp amplifier L/M-EPC 7. Myocytes were stimulated through the patch electrode at a cycle length of 2000 msec.

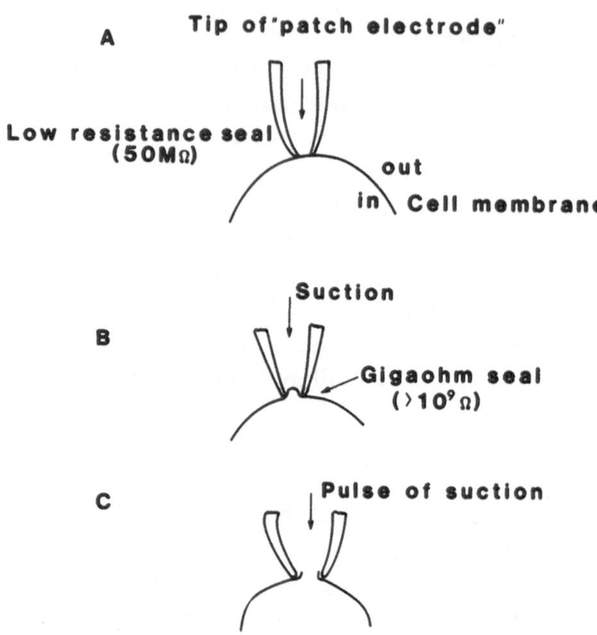

Figure 1. Schematic illustration of the principles of the whole-cell recording technique. A: micromanipulator-driven patch electrode is advanced towards the cell surface until contact is made. At this stage, the electrode resistance between the electrode and the membrane is in the order of $50 \times 10^6\,\Omega$ B: when moderate suction is applied, a tight seal (gigaseal) in the order of $10–100 \times 10^9$ is usually formed. C: thereafter, when a stronger suction pulse is applied, the membrane under the electrode tip is ruptured, and a low-resistance pathway is thereby available for current and voltage-clamp recordings.

Induction of hyper- and hypothyroidism

To induce hyperthyroidism in guinea pigs, two different protocols were used:

1. a single i.p. administration of L-thyroxine, 100 μg/kg, and
2. i.p. administration of L-thyroxine, 100 μg/kg, for 8–11 days. Hypothyroidism was induced by maintaining guinea pigs and rats on regular Purina chow and drinking water containing 0.05% propylthiouracil for 30–45 days. Both drugs were obtained from Sigma.

Statistical analysis

Linear regression analysis was used to determine the relationships between different action potential characteristics and heart rate, body mass, and oxygen consumption. To test the effects of hypo- and hyperthyroidism on action potential duration at different cycle lengths ANOVA was used.

Results

That ventricular action potential characteristics vary markedly among mammalian species, is illustrated in Figure 2. Although action potentials were recorded at identical experimental conditions, they differed in their overall configuration, in duration, and in rate of repolarization. To quantify some of these variations we analyzed the relationships between various action potential characteristics and the heart rate, body mass, and metabolic rate (expressed as oxygen consumption). In general, resting membrane potential and action potential amplitude, area, and duration were inversely correlated with heart rate, body mass, and oxygen consumption. For example, the correlation coefficients for the relationships between action potential amplitude, resting membrane potential, action potential duration at 50% repolarization, and action potential area (at cycle length = 1000 msec) and oxygen consumption were −0.78, −0.92, −0.91 and −0.92, respectively. $\dot{V}_{max}$ was poorly correlated with heart rate, body mass and oxygen consumption.

As several action potential characteristics correlated well with indices of the thyroid state, we reasoned that experimentally induced alterations in the thyroid state should alter these characteristics predictably. We therefore increased the thyroid state in guinea pigs by thyroxine (T_4) administration and decreased that of rats by propylthiouracil treatment, and studied the changes in the ventricular electrophysiological properties. Hyperthyroidism in guinea pigs was associated with a faster rate of repolarization and a reduction in action potential duration (Figure 3), whereas hypothyroidism in rats was associated with a marked increase in action potential duration (Figure 4).

Having found a close correlation between the thyroid state and the metabolic rate, and certain electrophysiological properties, we became interested in the mechanisms responsible for these relationships; as might be expected, thyroid hormones were chosen as the major candidates. The rationale for this selection is illustrated in Figure 5. As we have shown that resting membrane potential and action potential amplitude, area, and duration are inversely correlated with the metabolic rate and as, on the other hand, it is well known that thyroid hormone affects the metabolic rate, it was reasonable to suggest that these action potential characteristics are modulated either directly or indirectly by thyroid hormones.

In preliminary experiments, we studied the time course of thyroid hormone effect on ventricular action potential characteristics. In order to deal with this issue we injected guinea pigs with a single dose of T_4, 100 μg/kg, and studied action potential characteristics in animals sacrificed at various time intervals after T_4 administration. To our surprise, changes in action potential duration were

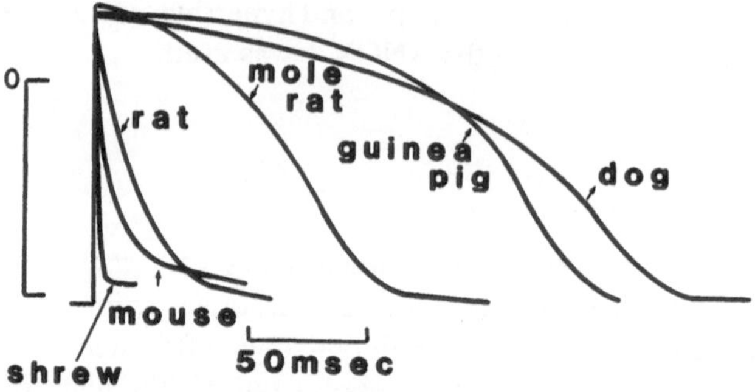

Figure 2. Typical action potentials from six mammalian species. The traces were reconstructed from the original action potential traces.

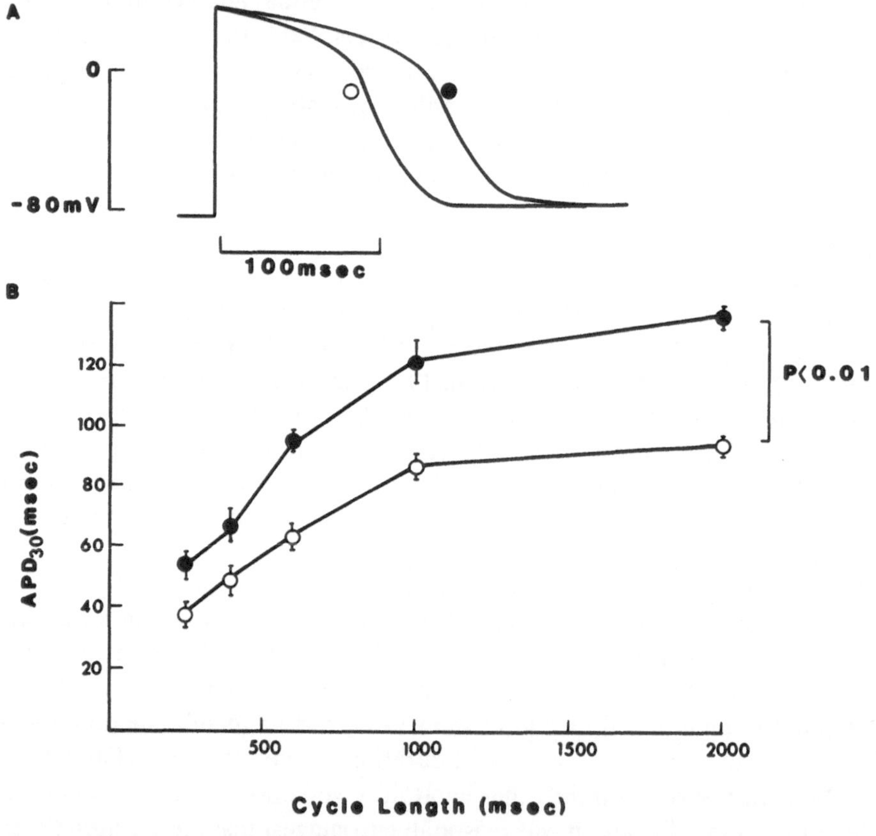

Figure 3. Effects of hyperthyroidism in guinea pigs on ventricular action potential. A: typical (reconstructed) action potentials from euthyroid (filled symbol) and hyperthyroid (open symbol) guinea pig ventricular muscle. Cycle length = 1000 msec. B: relationship between cycle length and action potential duration at 30% repolarization (APD_{30}) in euthyroid (filled symbols) and hyperthyroid (open symbols) ventricular muscle. (Modified from Figures 6 and 7 in Binah O, Arieli R, Beck R, Rosen MR and Palti Y. Modulation of ventricular electrophysiological properties by the metabolic rate. Submitted for publication.)

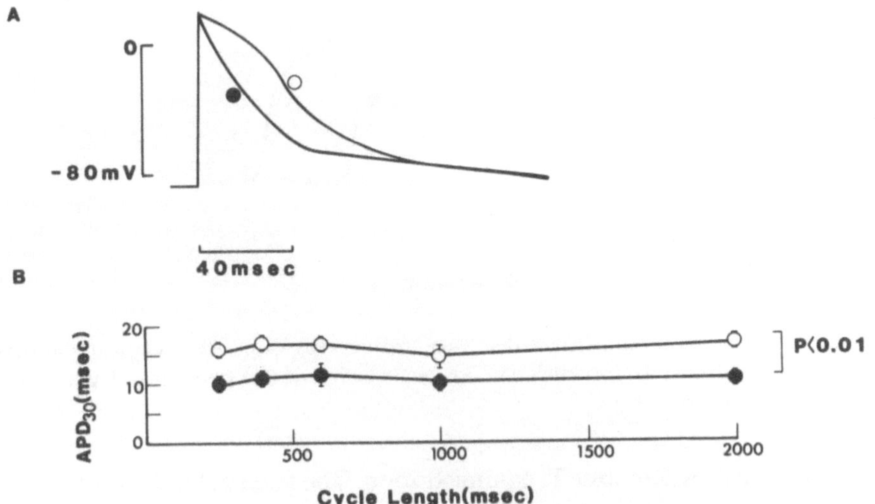

Figure 4. Effects of hypothyroidism in rats on ventricular action potential. A: typical (reconstructed) action potentials from euthyroid (filled symbols) and hypothyroid (open symbols) rat ventricular muscle. Cycle length = 1000 msec. B: relationship between cycle length and action potential duration at 30% repolarization (APD_{30}) in euthyroid (filled symbols) and hypothyroid (open symbols) ventricular muscle.

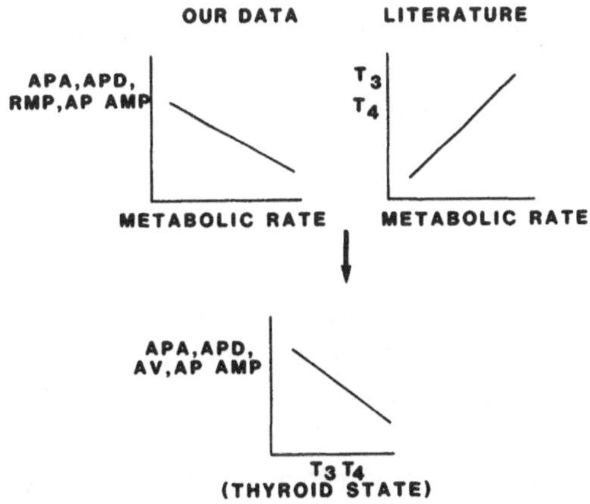

Figure 5. Rationale for investigating the role of thyroid hormones as modulators of the electrophysiological properties of the mammalian heart. We have shown that action potential area (APA), action potential duration (APD), resting membrane potential (RMP), and action potential amplitude (AP AMP) are inversely correlated with the metabolic rate of mammalian species. As the metabolic rate is, at least in part, determined by thyroid hormone action (not necessarily in a linear fashion), it is possible that the correlation between action potential characteristics and the metabolic rate results from the role of thyroid hormones as modulators (either directly or indirectly) of certain ventricular electrophysiological properties.

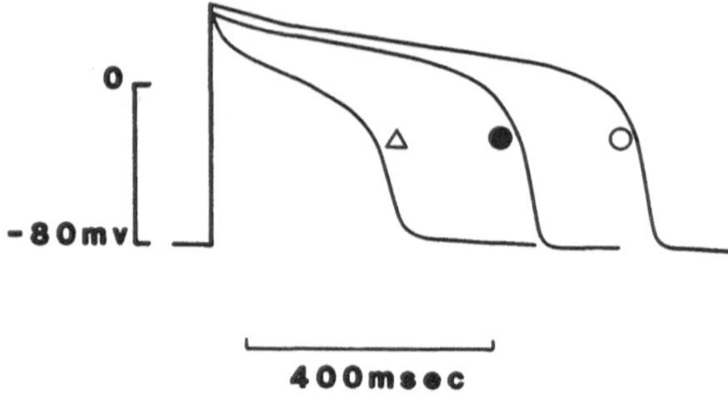

Figure 6. Typical action potentials recorded from enzymatically dissociated ventricular myocytes obtained from euthyroid (●), hyperthyroid (△), and hypothyroid (○) guinea pigs. Cycle length = 1000 msec. Temperature = 24.5° C.

observed as early as 2 hr after T_4 administration. The maximal reduction in action potential duration occurred at 4–6 hr, and from then onwards action potential duration recovered towards control values within 10–20 days.

In preliminary experiments we recorded action potentials from enzymatically dissociated ventricular myocytes isolated from euthyroid, hypo- and hyperthyroid guinea pigs. As can be seen in Figure 6, hyperthyroidism was associated with a shorter action potential and a faster rate of repolarization during the plateau, whereas hypothyroidism was associated with a marked increase in action potential duration. The fact that changes in the thyroid state were associated with similar electrophysiological effects in multicellular preparations and in ventricular myocytes renders the myocytes a very useful tool to study the effects of thyroid hormones on the electrical activity of the heart.

Discussion

The studies were designed to try to understand the physiological basis for the marked variations in cardiac electophysiological properties among mammalian species, and to determine the mechanisms that can be held responsible for these variations.

Studies of ventricular electrophysiological properties in species encompassing a wide range of metabolic rates (and thyroid states), showed close correlations between resting membrane potential and action potential amplitude, area and duration, heart rate, body mass, and oxygen consumption. Following these findings, we induced hyperthyroidism in guinea pigs and hypothyroidism in rats, and studied the changes in action potential characteristics [8]. The major findings were that hyperthyroidism was associated with a reduction in action potential duration and a faster rate of repolarization, whereas hypothyroidism was associated with a marked increase in action potential duration. Other preliminary results demonstrated that changes in action potential duration occur in guinea pigs as early as 2 hr after administering a single dose of T.

Conclusion

Based on these results, it is suggested that cardiac electrophysiological variations among mammalian species may result from differences in thyroid hormone action among these species. Moreover, it is suggested that thyroid hormone action in any one species can significantly affect, either directly or indirectly, cardiac electrophysiological properties and thereby may also modulate the mechanical performance of the heart.

References

1. Capasso JM, Aronson RS, Strobeck JE, Sonnenblick EH (1982): Effects of experimental phosphate deficiency on action potential characteristics and contractile performance of the rat myocardium. Cardiovasc Res 16: 71–79.
2. Elharrar V, Surawicz B (1983): Cycle length effect on restitution of action potential duration in dog cardiac fibers. Am J Physiol 244: H782–H792.
3. Gibbs CL, Johnson EA, Tille J (1963): A quantitative description of the relationship between the area of rabbit ventricular action potentials and the pattern of stimulation. Biophys J 3: 433–458.
4. McDonald TF, Pelzer D, Trautwein W (1984): Cat ventricular muscle treated with D600: effects on calcium and potassium currents. J Physiol (London) 352: 203–216.
5. Isenberg G, Klockner U (1982): Calcium-tolerant ventricular myocytes prepared by preincubation in a 'KB medium'. Pflügers Archiv 367: 6–18.
6. Taniguchi J, Kokubun S, Noma A, Irisawa H (1981): Spontaneously active cells from the sinoatrial and atrioventricular nodes of the rabbit heart. Jpn J Physiol 31: 547–558.
7. Hamill OP, Marty A, Neher E, Sakmann B, Sigworth J (1981): Improved patch-clamp techniques for high-resolution current recording from cells and cell-free membrane patches. Pflügers Archiv 391: 85–100.
8. Binah O, Arieli R, Beck R, Rosen MR, Palti Y (1985): Modulation of ventricular electrophysiological properties by metabolic rate [Abstract]. Circulation 72 (Suppl 3): 231.

Discussion

Weisfeldt: To what extent are the changes due to increased sensitivity to catecholamines in the hyperthyroid state?
Bina: When you apply 10^{-6} M adrenaline to a ventricular muscle, you observe a minor change in the plateau amplitude and in the rate of repolarization. I do not think that increased responsiveness to catecholamines in the hyperthyroid state is the major cause for the marked action potential shortening. Obviously, we are going to repeat these experiments in the presence of beta blockers.
Winegrad: Do you see any difference in the properties of the individual channels?
Bina: We don't have this data as yet.
Marcus: I am not clear about the rationale. We know that the action potential requires a tiny amount of energy utilization by the heart. Why then do you relate the action potential per se to the oxygen consumption? It has to be the mechanical activity rather than the electrical activity that is primarily responsible for the utilization of oxygen by the myocardium. The electrical activity, as shown long ago by Francis Klocke, accounts for only a very tiny fraction of total left ventricular myocardial oxygen consumption.
Bina: There is a paper by Josephson and his colleagues where they studied the basis for the differences between the guinea pig and the rat ventricular action potential. They showed that there were no changes in the amplitude of the slow inward current between the two species, but they found that the rate of inactivation was faster in the rat than in guinea pig ventricular myocytes.
Lab: The energy requirement of the action potential is indeed minute. If you take, as McLaud did, an anoxic preparation, both the action potential duration and the contractile phenomenon goes down. If you add glucose, the contraction does not come back but the action potential does.

13. Mechano-electric coupling in myocardium and its possible role in ischaemic arrhythmia

M.J. LAB

Abstract

The little-investigated reverse link to excitation-contraction coupling, mechano-electric coupling, was studied using electromechanical measurements in three types of preparation. First, in isolated superfused papillary muscle it was found that:

1. A change in one beat from isometric contraction to lightly loaded isotonic shortening curtailed mechanical activity, but prolonged the intracellular action potential.
2. Shortening late in systole produced an early afterdepolarization.
3. This was sometimes associated with apparant threshold excitation.

The second preparation, normal segments of the left ventricle in situ, regional electromechanical measurements (mechanical transducer and monophasic action potential) show comparable changes. Third, ischaemic segments of intact ventricle, regional electromechanical measurements also showed changes analogous to those in papillary muscle. These mechano-electric changes may contribute to arrhythmia, for it appears that ischaemic segments have monophasic action potentials with early afterdepolarizations and ectopic beats which sometimes precede ventricular fibrillation. Regional electromechanical alternans (alternation in action potential amplitude/duration and segment shortening) was also observed during ischaemia. The larger excursion was again associated with the longer action potential and mechano-electric coupling may contribute to this association. Intracellular calcium concentration, studied using aequorin which was microinjected into isolated papillary muscles, transiently increases with muscle shortening. Calcium can also demonstrate alternans when the muscle is rapidly stimulated. The calcium ion probably underlies the contractile dependent electrophysiological changes observed in mechano-electric coupling.

Introduction

Excitation-contraction coupling in myocardium has been extensively investigated (see for example other chapters in this book) but by comparison the reverse phenomenon, that of contraction-excitation coupling [1], has received little attention. The latter, mechano-electric coupling, obtains when an imposed or concurrent mechanical event influences transmembrane potentials, as opposed to the previously thought only-unidirectional process where membrane events influence contraction. Most of the studies that have been done in the reverse coupling field were carried out on isolated preparations [2–5] but some work on the intact heart is appearing [6–9]. There are several possible mechanisms to explain this phenomenon [1], and a calcium related possibility is currently favoured [10]. An important feature of mechano-electric coupling is its possible role in ischemic arrhythmia [1, 8, 9]. This chapter describes some circumstances in which this type of interaction occurs. The description includes comparisons of mechanoelectric records in isolated superfused myocardium, intact heart, and regional ischaemia. Some intracellular calcium concentration ($[Ca^{2+}]_i$) studies are also included.

Methods

Papillary muscles

Papillary muscles were dissected from the right ventricles of cats or ferrets which had been killed while anaesthetised with chloroform. The muscles were placed horizontally in a bath perfused with Tyrode's solution at 30° C and stimulated to contract at 0.2 to 0.33 Hz. One end of the muscle was attached to a force transducer and the other to a lever which was under feedback control. The lever could be used to produce isometric contractions, lightly-loaded contractions in which shortening occurred, or contractions with rapid length changes.

The action potentials were either recorded from individual cells using dangling microelectrodes or by sampling many cells with sucrose gap measurements [2, 4, 5]. The results were the same with both techniques.

$[Ca^{2+}]_i$ was measured with the calcium-sensitive protein aequorin [11] under comparable mechanical conditions. Aequorin was microinjected into 50–100 cells on the surface of the preparation [12, 13] and the resulting light emission (a function of $[Ca^{2+}]_i$) was monitored with a photomultiplier. The light collecting system was designed so that movements of the muscles did not significantly affect light collection [12, 14]. Aequorin records are intrinsically noisy and the signal-to-noise ratio was improved by signal averaging.

Intact hearts

Pigs of about 25 kg were anaesthetized with 1% halothane and a mixture of nitrous oxide and oxygen (1:1). The animals were ventilated using positive pressure. The chest was opened and a pericardial cradle fashioned to support the heart. A catheter was inserted through the apex of the ventricle and intraventricular pressure measured. Arterial pressure was measured via a catheter inserted into the proximal aorta. A pneumatically operated clamp was placed around the ascending aorta so that it could be occluded to produce isovolumic contraction of the left ventricle. The clamp could be suddenly applied, or released to allow ejection. A small branch of the left anterior descending branch of the left coronary artery was selected so that when a snare was tightened around the vessel a cyanotic area of about 1.5 cm × 2.5 cm was produced.

A tripodal device [16] was attached by vacuum through the legs to the area of epicardium to be made ischaemic. The device provided three outputs due to strains on gauges attached to the legs. The distance between each leg and the central point of the triangle they formed was about 7 mm. The movement of the legs along the axes from the centre to the corners of the triangular base plane was recorded and taken to represent length changes in the underlying segments of epicardium. This assumption depends on the compliance of the instrument which was less than 0.1 mm/g along the axis of movement of each leg. Little movement was possible in any other direction. Even though the device was somewhat stiffer than mercury-in-silastic gauges our results are similar to those obtained with these gauges and also to the results obtained from ultrasonic crystals [17, 18].

The three outputs from the legs of the tripod, representing mechanical changes in three directions over a small area produced a 'summed segment length' which was used to represent the mechanical behaviour of the underlying area of epicardium.

A monophasic action potential was obtained with a suction electrode which was capable of following slow changes in waveform [19], and changes in duration due to ischaemia [16]. The monophasic action potential was obtained either using one the suction legs of the tripod, or using a separate electrode from an area as close to the tripodal device as possible. All the signals was passed to a multichannel pen recorder and stored on magnetic tape for later analysis.

Results

Isolated papillary muscle

Figure 1 shows action potentials and contraction in the isolated superfused preparation under different loading conditions. In each panel the muscle contracted isometrically for several beats after which the load was changed. An

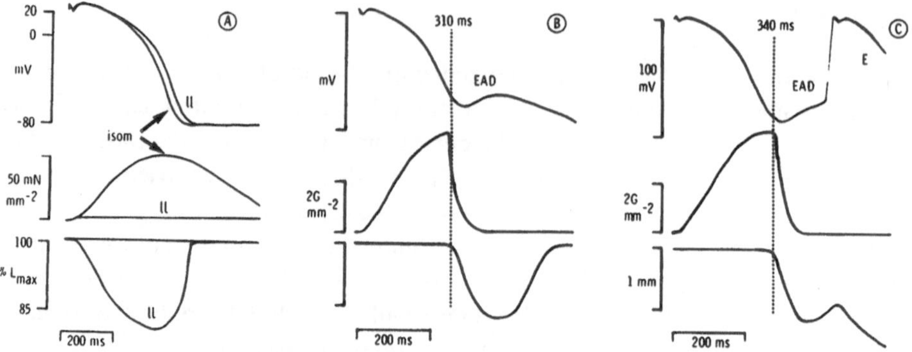

Figure 1. Superimposed records of action potentials (top trace) force (middle trace) and length (bottom trace) from cat papillary muscle [2, 4, 5]. Downward movement of length trace is shortening. A: a change in one beat from sometric contraction (isom) to lightly loaded shortening (11) abbreviates mechanical activity, contraction under isometric contraction continues for longer than that during isotonic contraction but the action potential is prolonged. Reproduced from [10] with permission. B: the muscle is allowed to shorten 310 ms after stimulation, just before peak isometric contraction. Force rapidly falls and the action potential shows an early afterdepolarization (EAD). C: slightly later shortening (340 ms) results in an non-driven action potential, presumably triggered by the EAD.

alteration from isometric contraction to lightly loaded isotonic shortening (Fig. 1A) reduced the duration of muscle activity [20], i.e. relaxation is complete before that seen in isometric contraction, but prolonged the action potential duration. When the shortening was delayed to 310 ms (Fig. 1B) the action potential also prolonged but the prolongation appeared as an early afterdepolarization (EAD) [21]. If the shortening was further delayed (Fig. IC) the EAD seemed to reach threshold and trigger an action potential.

Intact normal hearts

Analogous studies to those above were carried out in the intact pig heart in situ (Fig. 2). The electrophysiological recording was the monophasic action potential, and the mechanical recording was regional segment motion. An ejecting left ventricle was equivalent to lightly loaded isotonic contraction, whereas occlusion of the outflow tract resulted in the heavy afterload: the aortic snare was applied to produce an isovolumic contraction (Fig. 2). This does not cause *isometric* contraction throughout the ventricular wall, for there is an intramural rearrangement of fibre goemetry and fibre interaction. In this case the segment still shows some shortening, but of reduced amplitude. The clamp was subsequently quickly released to produce an ejecting beat. In consequence, segment shortening (eject – Fig. 2A) was increased in amplitude compared with the isovolumic contraction. The ejecting beat show segment relaxation starting at the time the isovolumic

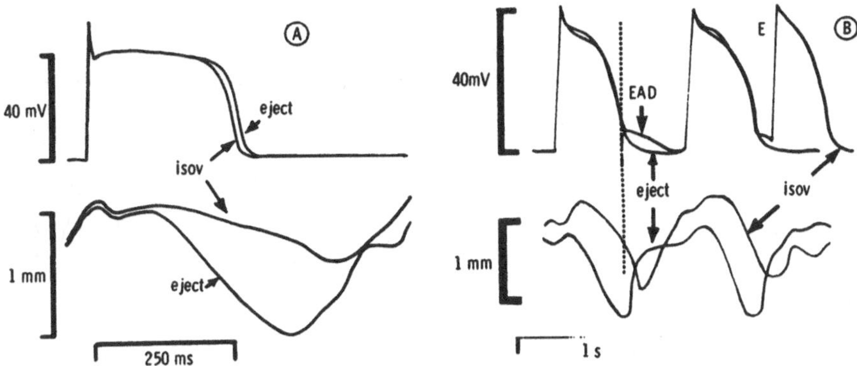

Figure 2. Superimposed monophasic action potentials (top traces) and segment motion (length-bottom traces) from the left ventricule of intact pig heart in situ during isovolumic contraction (isov) and ejection (eject). Downward movement of the length trace is shortening. A: compared with isovolumic contraction, the ejecting ventricle is associated with a greater segment shortening, a shorter and faster contraction, and a prolonged action potential. B: isovolumic contraction shows the same type of initial slow time course of contraction as in A, but there is a late rapid shortening just before repolarization of the action potential is complete. At this stage an early afterdepolarization (EAD) appears, and in the next beat it is associated with a ventricular ectopic (E).

beat still shows segment contraction: an analogous findng to that in isolated papillary muscle (Fig. IAII). The ejecting beat was also associated with a prolongation of the monophasic action potential. In some preparations, when the aortic clamp was applied to produce isovolumic contraction, segment motion was markedly out of phase compared with that in an ejecting ventricle. Figure 2B is an example of isovolumic contraction in which, after a period of restricted segment shortening in a given beat, there was an accelerated late shortening. The vertical dotted line indicates when the segment during the ejecting beat started relaxation, but shows that at the equivalent time during the isovolumic beat the segment is still shortening. With the latter, the action potential inflected near completion of repolarization. That is, the mechanical manoeuvre was associated with an early afterdepolarization. In the following beat, an extrasystole accompanied the afterdepolarization. These are also analogous findings to those seen in the isolated papillary muscle (Fig. 1B, C).

Regional ischaemia

Occlusion of a branch of the coronary artery produced the well described changes in action potential [22, 23] but the present description will only include changes in repolarization phase of individual action potentials. The monophasic action potential duration was unchanged for the first two minutes or so but occasionally it briefly increased. Thereafter it steadily declined over the next 15 minutes,

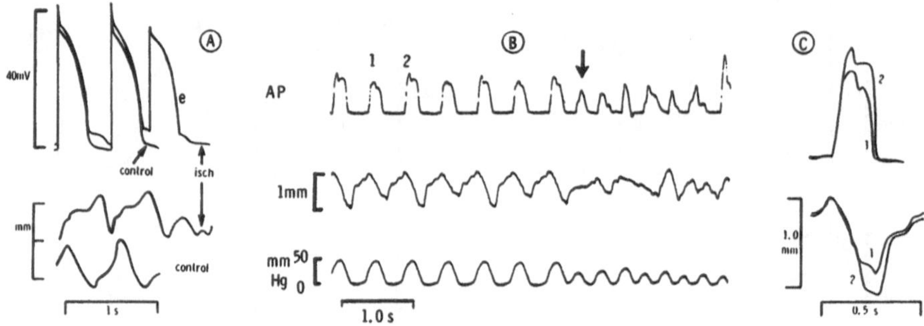

Figure 3. Action potentials and segment motion recorded just inside an ischaemic area of intact pig left ventricle in situ. A: superimposed control records with records after 5 minutes ischaemia (Isch). Top traces, action potentials; lower traces, segment motion. Control segment motion is normal – i.e. it shortens during systole. This corresponds with the normal configuration of the control action potential. During ischaemia the segment shows systolic lengthening followed by late systolic or diastolic shortening, and the action potential shows an early afterdepolarization. B: electromechanical alternans after 20 minutes ischaemia [25]. (Different preparation to that in A. Top trace – action potentials; middle trace – segment motion; bottom trace – intraventricular pressure. Both action potential and segment motion are alternating in amplitude despite the fact that the interbeat interval is constant. The mechanical alternans is not reflected in alternation of the intraventricular pressure. Ventricular tachycardia, followed shortly by fibrillation, began at the verticle arrow. C: superimposed electromechanical traces (1 and 2) from B. Top trace – action potentials; bottom trace – segment motion (downward is shortening). Compared with the electromechanical traces indicated by no 1, the no 2 trace show enhanced segment shortening with a prolonged action potential.

sometimes showing a temporary increase. During some of these stages the three features common to the preceding action potential changes could again be observed (Fig. 3). First, the early afterdepolarization could be seen in the early stages which could occasionally be accompanied by the second feature: ventricular ectopics (Fig. 3A). Wall motion went through the characteristic changes described in earlier studies [18]. The example in Figure 3A shows out of phase motion, with lengthening during early systole followed by late shortening. This is again analogous to some of the findings in Figures 1B, C and 2B. The stretch followed by shortening roughly coincided with the early afterdepolarization. It may be of significance that the early afterdepolarization and ectopics sometimes preceded ventricular fibrillation. The third feature, enhanced shortening with a prolongation of action potential duration was also observed. This occured during electrophysiological alternans (unchanged interstimulus interval but a beat to beat alternating action potential). Figure 3B, C is an example of this electrophysiological phenomenon which may be far more common than originally thought during ischaemia [22]. In addition, mechanical alternans was simultaneously seen. The electromechanical alternans in this case preceded ventricular fibrillation. Superimposition of a pair of alternating signals (Fig. 3C) shows once more that the long action potential is associated with the enhanced mechanical shortening. It is of interest that a second area, about 8 mm away showed brief

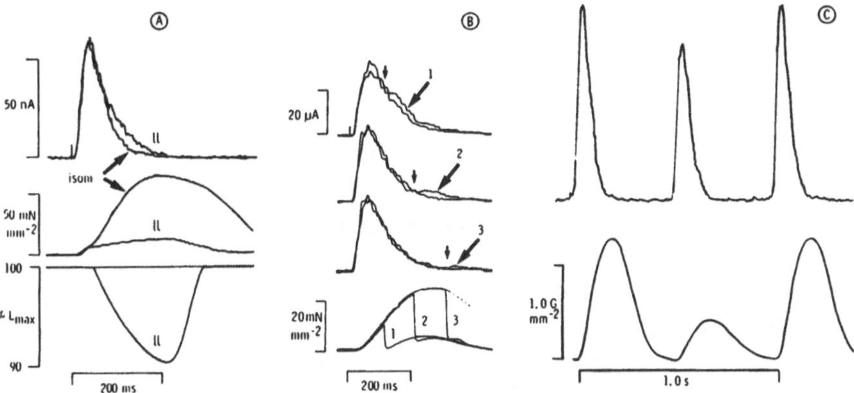

Figure 4. Intracellular $[Ca^{2+}]_i$ studies [10] in isolated papillary muscle. A: superimposed records of light, indicating $[Ca^{2+}]_i$ (upper traces), force (middle traces), and length (bottom trace – downward movement is shortening). Mechanical manoeuvres are the same as in Figure 1A. Compared with isometric contraction (isom), lightly loaded isotonic contraction (11) produces the same mechanical changes as in Figure 1A. These are associated with a prolongation of the time course of $[Ca^{2+}]_i$ (Ferret papillary muscle). Reproduced from [10] with permission. B: superimposed traces of light, $[Ca^{2+}]_i$ (top three traces) and force (bottom trace). The muscle first contracted isometrically (dotted line). In the next series of averaged beats the muscle was allowed three different delayed shortenings or releases [1, 2, and 3). Force immediately fell with each mechanical perturbation and each was associated with a transient rise in $[Ca^{2+}]_i$. Note that the $[Ca^{2+}]_i$ change in number 3 is in fact larger than it appears because of the non-linear conversion of light to $[Ca^{2+}]_i$ (Cat papillary muscle). Reproduced from [10] with permission. C: light transients $[Ca^{2+}]_i$ (top trace) and force (bottom trace) from ferret papillary muscle stimulated fast enough (3H2 in this case) to produce alternating large and small forces. The preparation shows alternation of $[Ca^{2+}]_i$ with the large light signal associated with the large force. (This record was obtained in collaboration with Dr D.G. Allen.)

periods of alternans where the behaviour of the action potential was out of phase with that of the first area.

Intracellular calcium studies ($[Ca^{2+}]_i$)

Calcium is involved in membrane and mechanical events, so intracellular calcium was studied in isolated papillary muscles under some of the preceding mechanical conditions [10]. $[Ca^{2+}]_i$ may in fact be almost instantaneously affected by the mechanical manoeuvres. In Figure 4A an identical manoeuvre to that in Figure 1A shows that by comparison with isometric contracting a lightly loaded muscle which shortens isotonically increases the duration of the calcium transient. Similarly, Figure 4B demonstrates that delayed shortening, as in Figure 1B, produces a 'bump' in the calcium transient. Finally, electromechanical alternans may be produced by stimulating isolated superfused muscle at high rates [26–29]. When $[Ca^{2+}]_i$ conditions calcium alternans is monitored under these conditions a calcium alternans (alternating amplitudes of $[Ca^{2+}]_i$ is also observed (Figure 4C).

Discussion

Concordance of the results and pitfalls in interpretation

In the current experiments isolated papillary muscle, intact heart in situ, and regionally ischaemic myocardium show common electromechanical relationships when viewed from a contraction-excitation feedback aspect.

1. By comparison with heavily loaded myocardium with reduced shortening, lightly loaded isotonic contraction (more shortening) produces earlier relaxation and a prolongation of action potential duration [2] (Figs 1A and 2A). Exaggerated shortening of ischaemic myocardium is also found with a prolonged action potential (Fig. 3C).
2. Within a given beat, initial heavily loaded contraction at a relatively long length followed by delayed shortening is associated with an early afterdepolarization (Figs 1B, 2B and 3A).
3. The afterdepolarization may be accompanied by threshold depolarisation and a non driven action potential (Figs 1C, 2B and 3A).

However the results with the monophasic action potential in the intact heart must be interpreted with caution. Although slow changes in membrane potential are faithfully reflected in the monophasic action potential [19] and any action potential duration changes observed in the latter are real, the early afterdepolarizations seen could conceivably be mechanically induced artefacts. However, the early afterdepolarizations in the intracellular action potential from the isolated preparation (Fig. 1B), the monophasic action potential from the intact heart (Fig. 2B), and regional ischaemia (Fig. 3A), are all comparable. Moreover, all three types of early afterdepolarizations can be accompanied by threshold depolarisations. If the early afterdepolarizations indeed reflect a real electrophysiological phenomenon, the question arises as to whether they have the same rate dependence as the early afterdepolarizations seen in isolated superfused preparations [30]. Preliminary results show that they do. Rises in heart rate reduce both the coupling interval and the amplitude of the early afterdepolarizations. Thus as with the action potential duration changes, the possibility that the afterdepolarisations in the monophasic action potential may also be the result of underlying membrane phenomena should be entertained.

Relationship to arrhythmia

Reentry, automaticity, triggered activity and afterdepolarizations have all been implicated in the cellular basis of ischaemic arrhythmia [31]. The results presented here suggest that one has to consider a mechanical component in the cellular mechanisms as well: in particular a mechano-electric interaction. The contribution could be via several pathways. One is through mechanically induced early afterdepolarizations which are capable of reaching threshold for ectopic impulse formation. However, apart from some isolated reports [32], early afterdepolarizations in ischaemic myocardium have escaped systematic observation using miroelectrodes. This may be due to the fact that these electrodes only sample one cell. Suction electrodes sample many. Moreover the suction electrode may conveniently be used to explore the myocardium and so find areas that show afterdepolarizations. It is of interest that phase I arrhythmias occur in the first hour of ischaemia and it is during this period that the myocardium is most compliant [33]. The compliance could enable the mechanical circumstances necessary for mechanically induced arrhythmia.

A second way in which a mechanoelectric interaction could promote arrhythmias is if this interaction contributes to local alternans, and thus dispersion of repolarization when compared with a nearby area. Enhanced dispersion has been observed when adjacent areas have each shown alternation in which the action potential duration changes have been going in opposite directions. This could result in the current flow which has been suggested to play a role in ectopic generation [23]. A third possibility is that the electrophysiological variability could also produce variations in refractory periods [8, 9], conduction velocities and reentry paths.

Possible mechanisms

The mechanical induced electrical changes in the isolated superfused preparation appear to be related to changes in $[Ca^{2+}]_i$. The action potential initiates calcium release from the sarcoplasmic reticulum (SR) and Ca quickly rises through calcium induced calcium release [34] to bind with troponin C and activate actin and myosin interaction. Muscle shortening reduces the affinity of troponin C for calcium and the unbuffered calcium increases to change the time course of the calcium transient [10]. This would affect the action potential either by an electrogenic Na/Ca exchange [36–38], or by a calcium activated inward current [39], to prolong the action potential duration or produce an afterdepolarization. A computer model of cardiac electrophysiology is able to simulate transient inward currents due to Na/Ca exchange consequent on transient rises of $[Ca^{2+}]_i$ [40]. This mechanism could also underly the observations in the intact heart. However, the precise force/length changes in a given area in intact ventricle are difficult to ascertain because of fibre interaction, and the difficulties are compounded in regional ischaemia where dyskinetic contraction is found. Moreover, passive stress/strain changes or changes in compartmentalised ionic concentrations could operate in intact heart in situ to affect membrane electrophysiology.

The electromechanical alternans in ischaemia may also have changes in $[Ca^{2+}]_i$ as its basis. Rapid stimulation of superfused myocardium may raise resting $[Ca^{2+}]_i$ and probably produces a reduction in oxygen supply/demand ratio. This could metabolically affect the rapid calcium cycling at the high heart rates. Beat-to-beat changes in cycling could produce the calcium alternans to affect alternate action potentials, perhaps also involving Ca-activated currents, but now outward [41]. High resting $[Ca^{2+}]_i$ is also conducive to $[Ca^{2+}]_i$ oscillations [42]. It is tempting to speculate that $[Ca^{2+}]_i$ oscillations, the membrane consequences of ischaemia [43], the metabolic consequences of ischaemia, and contraction-excitation coupling, all contribute to changes in $[Ca^{2+}]_i$ which could affect membrane electrophysiology to produce arrhythmia.

References

1. Lab MJ (1982): Contraction excitation feedback in myocardium: physiological basis and clinical relevance. Circ Res 50: 757–766.
2. Kaufmann R, Lab MJ, Hennekes R, Krause H (1971): Feedback interaction of mechanical and electrical events in the isolated ventricular myocardium (cat papillary muscle). Pflügers Arch 324: 100–123.
3. Hennekes R, Kaufmann R, Lab MJ, Steiner R (1977): Feedback loops involved in cardiac excitation contraction coupling: Evidence of two different pathways. J Mol Cell Cardiol 9: 669–713.
4. Hennekes R, Kaufmann R, Lab MJ 1981): The dependence of cardiac membrane excitation and contractile ability on active muscle shortening. Pflügers Archiv 392: 22–28.
5. Lab MJ (1980): Transient depolarization and action potential alterations following mechanical changes in isolated myocardium. Cardiovasc Res 14: 624–637.
6. Lab MJ (1978): Depolarization produced by mechanical changes in normal and abnormal myocardium. J Physiol (London) 143P–144P.
7. Covell JW, Lab MJ, Pavalec R (1981): Mechanical induction of paired action potentials in intact heart in situ. J Physiol (London) 320: 34P.
8. Bendit DG, Kriet JM, Tobler HG, Gornick CC, Baring LS, Detloff LS, Anderson RW (1985): Electrophysiological effects of transient aortic occlusion in intact canine heart. Am J Physiol 249: H1017–1023.
9. Lerman BB, Burkhoff D, Yue DT, Sagawa K (1985): Mechano-electrical feedback: independent role of preload and contractility in modulation of canine ventricular excitability. J Clin Invest 76: 1843–1850.
10. Lab MJ, Allen DG, Orchard CH (1984): The effects of shortening on myoplasmic calcium concentration and on the action potential in mammalian ventricular muscle. Circ Res 55: 825–829.
11. Blinks JR, Wier WG, Hess P, Prendergast FG (1982): Measurement of Ca concentrations in living cells. Prog Biophys Mol Biol 40: 1–114.
12. Allen DG, Blinks JR (1978): Calcium transients in aequorin-injected frog cardiac muscle. Nature 273: 509–513.
13. Allen DG, Kurihara S (1982): The effects of muscle length on intracellular calcium transients in mammalian cardiac muscle. J Physiol (London) 327: 79–94.
14. Cannel MB, Allen DG (1983): A photomultiplier tube assembly for the detection of low light levels. Pflügers Archiv 398: 165–168.
15. Woolard KV, Kingaby RO, Lab MJ, Cole AWG, Palmer NT (1981): Inosine as a selective inotropic agent on ischaemic myocardium. Cardiovasc Res 15: 659–667.
16. Lab MJ, Wollard KV (1978): Monophasic action potential, electrocardiograms and mechanical performance in normal and ischaemic epicardial segments of the pig ventricle in siu. Cardiovasc Res, 42: 519–528.

17. Bugge-aspheim B, Lerand S, Kiil GF (1969): Local dimensional changes of the myocardium measured by ultrasonic technique. Scand J of Lab Invest 24: 361–371.
18. Tyberg JV, Forester JS, Parmley W (1974): Altered segmental function and compliance in acute myocardial ischaemia. Eur J Cardiol 1: 307–317.
19. Hoffmann BF, Cranefield PF, Lepeschkin E, Surawicz B, Herrlich HC (1959): Comparison of cardiac action potentials recorded by intracellular and suction electrodes. Am J Physiol 196: 1296–1301.
20. Brady AJ (1965): Time and displacement-dependence of cardiac contractility: Problems in defining the active state and force-velocity relations. Fed Proc 24: 1410–1420.
21. Cranefield PF, Wit QL (1979): Cardiac arrhythmias. Ann Rev Physiol 41: 459–72.
22. Janse MJ, Kleber AG (1981): Electrophysiological changes and ventricular arrhythmias in the early phase of regional myocardial ischaemia. Circ Res 49: 1969–1081.
23. Janse MJ, van Capelle FJL, Morsink H, Kleber AG, Wilms-Schopman FW, Cardinal R, D'Alnoncourt CN, Durrer D (1980): Flow of 'injury' current and patterns of excitation during early ventricular arrhythmias in acute regional myocardial ischaemia in isolated porcine and canine hearts. Evidence for two different arrhythmogenic mechanisms. Circ Res 47: 151–165.
24. Russel D (1982): In Parrat J (ed) early arrhythmias resulting from myocardial ischaemia: mechanisms and prevention by drugs. MacMillan, London.
25. Dilly S, Lab MJ (1985): Is alternans ubiquitous in myocardial ischaemia. J Physiol 369: 129P.
26. Lu H, Lange G, Brooks C (1968): Comparative studies of electrical and mechanical alternation in heart cells. J Electrocardiol 1: 7–17.
27. Speare JF, Moore EN (1971): A comparison of alternation in myocardial action potentials and contractility. Am J Physiol 220: 1708–1716.
28. Boyett M, Jewell BR (1978): Analysis of effects of changes in rate and rhythm upon electrical activity in the heart. J Physiol (London) 285: 359–380.
29. Wohlfart B (1982): Analysis of mechanical alternans in rabbit papillary muscle. Acta Physiol Scand 115: 405–414.
30. Damiano BP, Rosen MR (1984): Effects of pacing on triggered activity induced by early afterdepolarization. Circulation 69: 1013–1025.
31. Hoffman BF, Rosen MR (1981): Cellular mechanisms for cardiac arrhythmias. Circ Res 49: 1–15.
32. Czarnecka M, Lewartowski B, Prokopczuk A (1973): Intracellular recording from the in situ working dog hearts in physiological conditions and during acute ischaemia and fibrillation. Acta Physiol Pol 24: 331–337.
33. Pirzada FA, Ekong EA, Vokonas PAS, Anstein CA, Hood WB (1976): Experimental infarction. XIII. Sequential changes in left ventricular pressure-length relationships in the acute phase. Circulation 53: 970–975.
34. Fabiato A, Fabiato F (1979): Calcium and cardiac excitation contraction coupling. Annu Rev Physiol 41: 473–484.
35. Housemans PK, Lee NK, Blinks JR (1983): Active shortening retards the decline of the intracellular calcium transient in mammalian heart muscle. Science 221: 159–161.
36. Mullins JJ (1979): The generation of electric currents in cardiac fibres by Na/Ca exchange. Am J Physiol 263: C103–110.
37. Kimura J, Norma A, Irisawa H (1986): Na-Ca exchange current in mammalian heart cells. Nature 319: 596–597.
38. Mechmann S, Pott L (1986): Identification of Na-Ca exchange current in single cardiac myocytes. Nature 319: 597–599.
39. Colquhoun D, Neher E, Reuter H, Stevens C (1981): Inward current channels activated by intracellular Ca^{2+} in cultured cardiac cells. Nature 294: 752–754.
40. Brown HF, Noble D, Noble SJ, Taupignon AI (1986): Relationship between the transient inward current and slow inward currents in the sino-atrial node of the rabbit. 370: 299–316.
41. Bassingthwaighte J, Fry C, McGuigan J (1976): Relationship between internal Ca^{2+} and outward

current in mammalian ventricular muscle. A mechanism for the control of the action potential duration. J Physiol (London) 262: 15–37.
42. Allen DG, Eisner DA, Orchard CH (1984): Characterization of oscillations of intracellular calcium concentration in ferret ventricular muscle. J Physiol 352: 113–128.
43. Coraboeuf E, Deroubaix E, Hoerter J (1976): Control of ionic permeabilities in normal and ischaemic heart. Circ Res [Suppl I]: 92–98.

Discussion

Yue: You showed a recording of potential and length in which the length was allowed to shorten very late in the potential, producing some kind of EAD (early after depot). Did you in the parallel experiments with aequorin see a blip in calcium augmentation for this late release?
Lab: Yes. Consistently so. It is small but exists. Since the aequorin/Ca is a non-linear relationship, the blip represents a significant but reproducible calcium bump with a late release.
Winegrad: How late do you go and still see a calcium bump?
Lab: This is as late as we have looked at.
Winegrad: You find a prolongation of action potential with isotonic contraction. Could this be the cause of the increase in intracellular Ca?
Lab: The answer is that it is not due to the prolongation of the action potential. If it were, then one would expect a higher force, which you do not see. An increase in calcium is actually associated with a drop in force. The second, and the more favoured hypothesis that the binding constant of calcium for troponin-C is reduced and it leaches off the actomyosin.
Beyar: You have shown that shortening prolongs the action potential; but data about relaxation shows that shortening enhances relaxation, makes it faster and earlier. Usually, longer action potentials are associated with longer mechanical contraction times. There is evidently a disparity between these statements. Could you explain it?
Lab: Yes. First, if the calcium is coming off actomyosin, then you get a reduction of the mechanical activity. So if fits (shortening does enhance relaxation). The other situation is where you get larger intracellular calcium associated with changes in construction with long time courses. These can give a long action potential and a high calcium transient.

14. Tetanization of intact hearts: a new strategy for studying the response of the contractile proteins to calcium

E. MARBAN, H. KUSUOKA and M.L. WEISFELDT

Abstract

Intact hearts of 8 to 14 week old ferrets were tetanized by perfusion with ryanodine, and used to study maximum force development and steady state behavior of the ventricle without the effect of relaxation. The maximal Ca^{2+}-activated pressure in the whole heart was studied in relationship to metabolic factors using phosphorus NMR to determine inorganic phosphate, creatine phosphate and ATP, and a comparison beween tetanus and normal twitch contractions is presented. Utilizing the simultaneously measured maximal Ca^{2+}-activated pressure, intracellular pH and phosphorus in the intact heart, the study indicates a major role of inorganic phosphate in the control of contractile function during the initial period of hypoxia.

Introduction

The heart normally contracts and relaxes during repetitive electrical stimulation, in contrast to skeletal muscle in which tension generation is maintained as a tetanus. After exposure to agents such as ryanodine and caffeine that interfere with the normal function of the sarcoplasmic reticulum, heart muscle can also be tetanized [1]. There are several reasons for interest in tetanus in heart muscle. Maximum force development, which can be measured using tetanization of heart muscle, provides a unique endpoint for the assessment of ventricular function and has even been equated with contractility [2]. Secondly, steady state behavior can be observed: one of the problems with measuring force during a single twitch is that it is influenced by relaxation as well as contractile parameters, whereas this ambiguity can be avoided by inducing tetanus.

There is considerable interest in measuring maximal Ca^{2+}-activated force, although until recently such measurements have been limited to skinned muscle preparations. As shown in such preparations, maximal Ca^{2+}-activated force is the peak point on the calcium concentration-response curve and represents the characteristics of the myofilaments when maximally stimulated. It remains controversial whether any positive inotropic agent can augment maximal Ca^{2+}-activated force as its mechanism of action [2]. If one could measure maximal force in intact muscle and intact heart, some of the ambiguities might be resolved. Finally, there is a great advantage to inducing tetanus and measuring maximal isovolumic pressure, or maximal Ca^{2+}-activated pressure in the intact heart, because such a preparation can be placed within a nuclear magnetic resonance system and the metabolic state of the heart measured on a moment-to-moment basis. Metabolic parameters can be correlated with this fundamental parameter of pump function in the intact perfused heart.

Experimental procedure

The approach that we have used to induce tetanus in intact hearts is as follows. Hearts from ferrets 8 to 14 weeks of age were Langendorff-perfused at 30° C with HEPES-buffered modified Tyrode solution containing sodium acetate [3]. The use of HEPES buffer allows an increase in the perfusate calcium concentration ($[Ca]_o$) without risk of precipitation of calcium salts. The hearts were perfused at a pressure of 65 mm Hg, and a latex balloon was inserted into the left ventricle. Isovolumic left ventricular pressure was measured at a balloon volume resulting in an end diastolic pressure of ~10 mm Hg, and the heart rate was either spontaneous (~1 Hz) or was controlled by pacing. To induce tetanus, the hearts were perfused for 20 minutes with 1–5 μM ryanodine, an inhibitor of calcium release by the sarcoplasmic reticulum [4]. Afterwards ryanodine can be removed from the perfusate, since the binding is essentially irreversible on this time scale. The hearts were then paced at a rapid rate (8 to 12 Hz). As shown in Figure 1, individual spontaneous beats, such as the one at the beginning of the record, generate approximately 90 mm Hg with an end diastolic pressure here of about 20 mm Hg. When rapid pacing is instituted (as indicated by the hash marks below the pressure record), we can induce a tetanus with the development of maximal pressure in this particular heart of 300 mm Hg. In 14 hearts, an average pressure of 290 mm Hg was developed during tetani elicited in 10–20 mM $[Ca]_o$. When the stimulus is terminated, developed pressure quickly decreases to baseline.

Results

The background for this work is based upon previous work of Yue, Marban and Wier [5] in isolated papillary muscles from ferrets under very similar conditions to those outlined for the perfused hearts. In the papillary muscles, they were able to use aequorin as an indicator of intracellular free calcium concentration ($[Ca^{2+}]_i$)

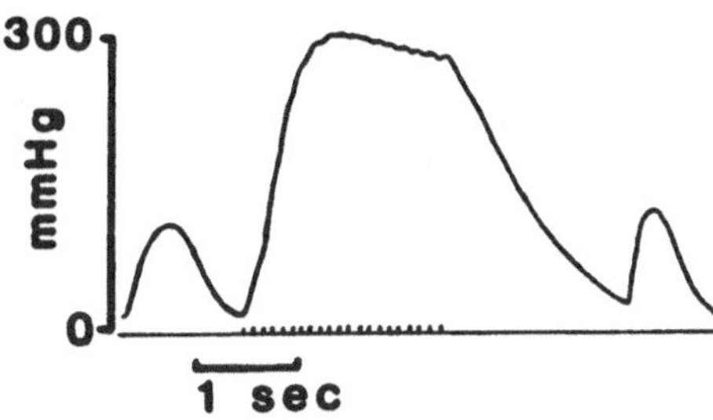

Figure 1. Left ventricular developed pressure during twitches and tetanus in a Langendorff-perfused ferret heart ($[Ca]_o = 15$ mM). Tetanus was induced by rapid pacing at the times indicated by the marks below the pressure record.

and thereby to demonstrate directly that maximal Ca^{2+}-activated force was indeed achieved. Saturation of tension as a function of increasing concentrations of calcium could easily be achieved at $[Ca]_o$ above 8 to 10 mM. Although there was no further increase in force, aequorin light progressively increased as $[Ca]_o$ was raised. Another indication that maximal force can be attained comes from results with the dihydropyridine Ca channel agonist Bay K 8644. In the papillary muscle and the whole heart, there is no further increase in tetanic tension when Bay K 8644 is added at high $[Ca]_o$, although in the papillary muscle the aequorin light signal does increase. Thus, maximal Ca^{2+}-activated force of cardiac muscle can be achieved with this method.

If we take the 300 mm Hg that we measured in the whole heart during tetanus and use a simple Laplace model for calculation of the maximum tension of the wall, we approximate very closely the level of papillary muscle tension that Yue, Marban and Wier found in the papillary muscle [3]. Thus, it is probable that in the isolated heart generating 300 mm Hg of sustained isovolumic pressure we are achieving maximum tension performance of this particular heart. Figure 2 shows the calcium concentration-response curves for the whole ferret ventricle. The developed pressures during twitches (△) and tetani (□) are shown as $[Ca]_o$ is increased from 0.5 mM to 20 mM. Developed pressure during twitches increases progressively as $[Ca]_o$ is increased, but during tetani peak pressure is maximal by 10 mM $[Ca]_o$. The rightmost points show the effect of adding Bay K 8644 to further augment $[Ca^{2+}]_i$ during both twitches and tetani. Even at 20 mM $[Ca]_o$, twitch pressure has not reached saturation, since there is a small further increase in tension with the addition of Bay K 8644. In contrast, tetanic pressure increases no further upon the addition of Bay K 8644, despite the increase in $[Ca^{2+}]_i$ that is predicted from the papillary muscle experiments. On the basis of these data we believe that in these hearts maximal Ca^{2+}-activated pressure is achieved during tetani in elevated $[Ca]_o$.

We can induce tetanus and can measure maximal Ca^{2+}-activated pressure in the whole heart in relationship to metabolic factors using phosphorus NMR [6]. We

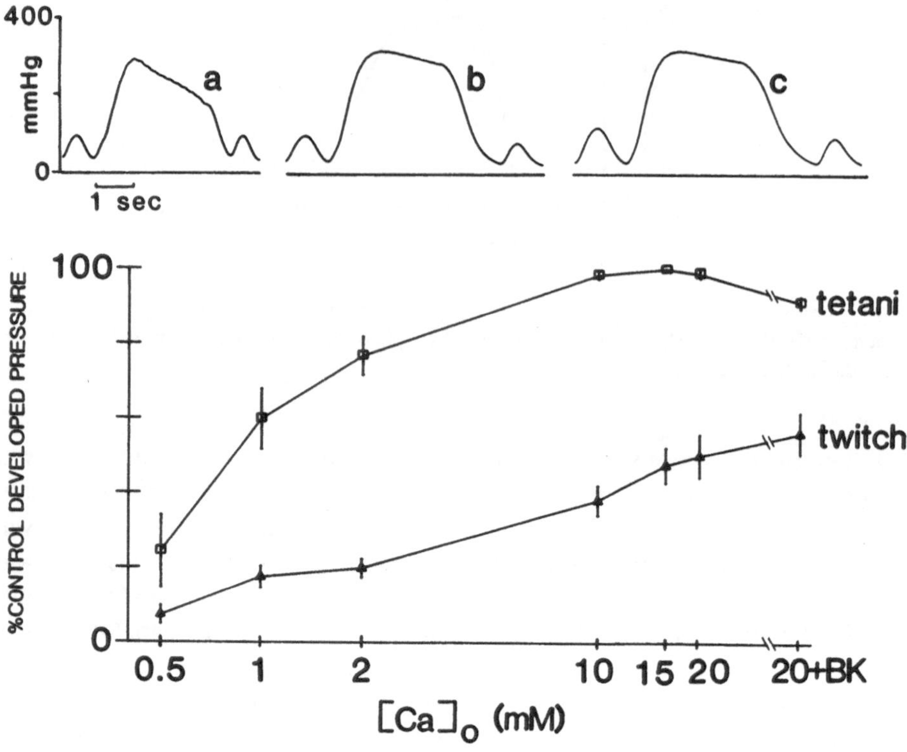

Figure 2. Calcium concentration-response curve in whole perfused hearts. In the upper panel, pressure recordings from a typical experiment at 2 mM, 10 mM and 15 mM $[Ca^{2+}]_o$ are shown. In the lower panel, the saturation of developed pressure during tetani (□) with respect to $[Ca]_o$ is obvious, whereas developed pressure during twitches (△) continues to increase as $[Ca]_o$ increases. Data were plotted as mean ± SEM of developed pressure as percent of the maximal pressure achieved in 15 mM $[Ca]_o$ in each experiment. Rightmost points illustrate data obtained in perfusate containing 20 mM $[Ca]_o$ and 300 nM Bay K 8644.

have taken these hearts and inserted them into the coil of an NMR spectrometer and obtained the spectra for phosphorus-containing metabolites. These spectra allow the determination of inorganic phosphate, creatine phosphate and ATP. A magnesium trimetaphosphate standard is placed in the balloon within the ventricle and is used in calibration. Intracellular pH is measured from the position of the inorganic phosphate resonance relative to that of creatine phosphate [7]. These measurements can be made during tetanus and during normal twitch contractions.

The initial interest was in whether tetanus itself made any major alteration in the metabolism of the heart, particularly as a result of the increased energy utilization that must occur during sustained active force generation. Figure 3 shows a spectrum taken one second after the onset of the tetanus (i.e., at or near peak pressure), and then a second spectrum taken 4.7 seconds later in the course

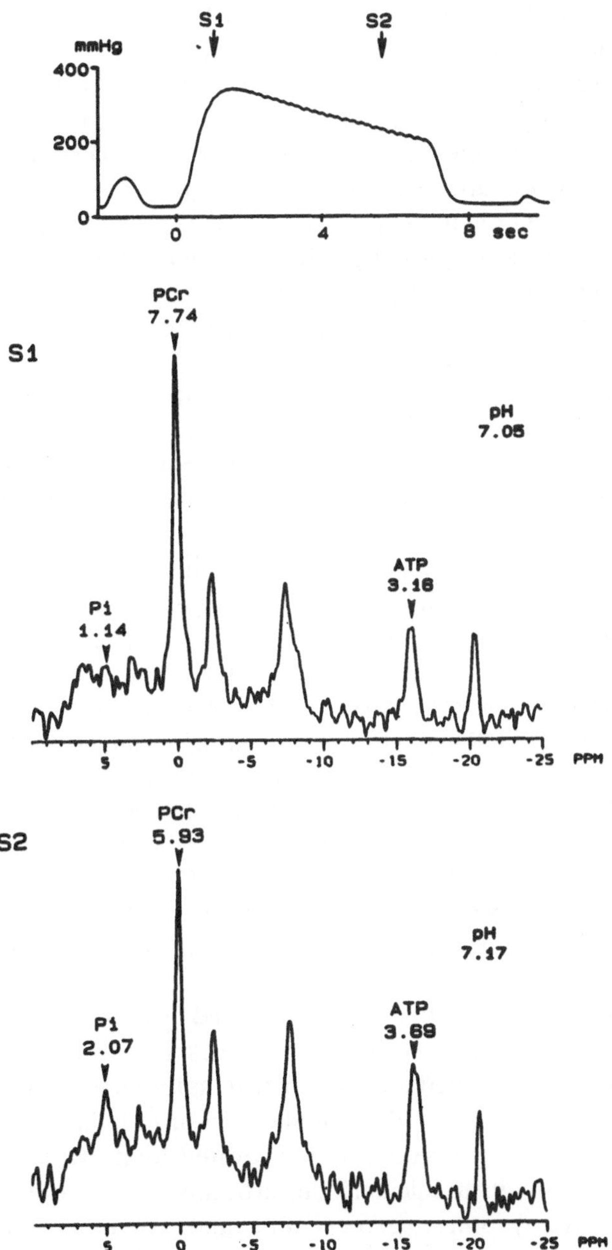

Figure 3. The phosphorus NMR spectra obtained during the early phase (S1) and the late phase (S2) of a tetanus. The upper panel shows the pressure record during a tetanus. The labels S1 and S2 indicate the timing of the pulses: the S1 spectrum was obtained 1 second after the start of tetanus, and S2 was obtained 4.7 seconds afterwards. The middle panel shows the spectrum at S1, and the lower panel shows the spectrum at S2. These spectra were obtained over 32 tetani repeated every 1–1.5 minutes. Pi: inorganic phosphate, PCr: phosphocreatine.

of the tetanus. Interestingly, the spectrum at 1 second (S1) is not significantly different from a control spectrum taken during spontaneous twitching (not shown). With sustained contraction, however, force begins to fatigue; the second spectrum (S2), obtained during fatigue, reveals an increase in inorganic phosphate, and a corresponding fall in creatine phosphate. These changes occurred consistently in eight hearts. The small increases in pH and in ATP seen in this particular experiment did not occur consistently. This is the kind of pattern that one would anticipate seeing in early ischemia, that is, a fall in creatine phosphate and a rise in inorganic phosphate. Such behavior is not unexpected during the course of a tetanus, since there is a pressure of 300 mm Hg in the ventricle with a coronary perfusion pressure of 65 mm Hg. Certainly there is decreased coronary perfusion during this period of time. The results suggest that the metabolic demands of the tetanus are not sufficient to induce ischemia or to modify function during the first second or so (S1 spectrum) but that as the tetanus goes on, the combination of ischemia and increased energy demand may modify function to a significant degree.

Recently we have concentrated on understanding the mechanism of the decrease in ventricular function that occurs during early ischemia and/or hypoxia [6]. It is well-established that hypoxia results in a fall in contractile function, despite the lack of any observable decrease in $[Ca^{2+}]_i$ [8]. There are some clues as to possible mechanisms for a decrease in contractile function in the work of others. The first is the fall in pH that occurs during an imbalance between supply and demand. In skinned cardiac cell preparations Fabiato and Fabiato [9] showed very clearly that there is a decrease in maximal Ca^{2+}-induced tension as the pH decreases. There is also a rightward shift in the curve, i.e. there is a decrease in sensitivity to calcium as a result of a fall in pH. One of the possibilities for the decrease in contractile function with hypoxia is that acidosis occurs and that this is the predominant factor responsible for the decrease in contractile function.

A second mechanism that has been suggested from experiments using skinned preparations by Herzig and his associates [10] and by Kentish [11] is that function declines as a result of an increase in inorganic phosphate. Kentish has shown very clearly in a chemically skinned preparation that, as the concentration of inorganic phosphate increases from 0 to 10 mM in the fluid surrounding the myofilaments, there is a marked fall in maximal Ca^{2+}-activated force. Kentish also found a decrease in the sensitivity to calcium induced by inorganic phosphate. Thus, there are two alternative hypotheses expressed by these experiments. One is that the drop in pH during hypoxia or ischemia decreases force by its effect on the calcium-tension relationship. The second is that inorganic phosphate (Pi) accumulates during hypoxia or ischemia and decreases the force by its effect on the calcium-tension relationship.

Because we are now able to measure maximal Ca^{2+}-activated pressure, pH and Pi simultaneously in the intact heart, we can obtain data during hypoxia that can be compared directly with the results from skinned preparations. In particular,

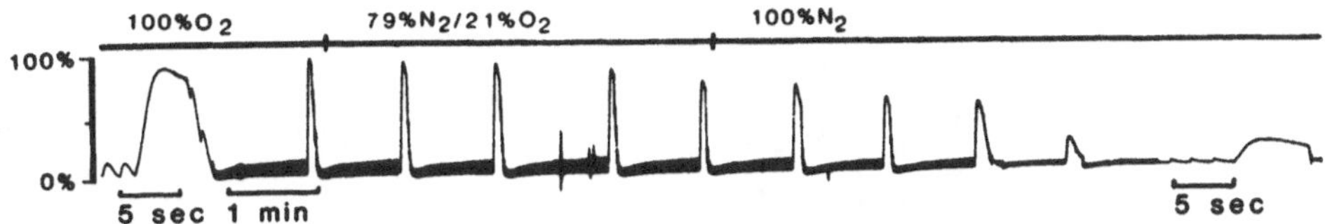

Figure 4. Change in maximal Ca^{2+}-activated pressure during hypoxia. The gas bubbling the perfusate was changed from 100% O_2 to 79% N_2/21% O_2 and finally to 100% N_2 as indicated in the bar above the pressure record. Tetani were elicited once a minute. The developed pressure was normalized by the pressure of the tetanus in the control period, i.e., the second tetanus in this figure.

we have used this preparation to distinguish the contributions of the two aforementioned mechanisms (pH and Pi). Figure 4 shows a continuous record of ventricular pressure. The first two tetani were obtained during perfusion with solution bubbled with 100% O_2. Subsequent tetani were recorded during hypoxia induced by equilibrating the perfusate with increasing amounts of nitrogen, as indicated above the pressure record. The maximal tetanic pressure decreases markedly during hypoxia.

We have simultaneously measured Pi and pH, and correlated these variables with the maximal pressure measured at different durations of hypoxia. The data presented in Figure 5 are from one heart during three interventions: hypoxia, the early and late (S1 and S2) tetani, and during rapid pacing to introduce a supply-demand imbalance. There is a very close correlation between the inorganic phosphate increase and the decline in pressure during all three of these interventions (A). In contrast, the correlation between intracellular pH and the decline in developed pressure (B) is quite poor.

Discussion

Table 1 summarizes the data from all of the hearts that were studied for the correlations between developed pressure and intracellular pH or inorganic phosphate. Developed pressure and inorganic phosphate had a mean correlation coefficient of 0.87 in a total of 12 hearts, contrasted with a mean correlation with pH of only 0.49. The correlation with pH reached statistical significance only for a few of the individual hearts. ATP similarly had no correlation. It is not surprising that the decline in creatine phosphate did correlate about as well as the increase in inorganic phosphate with the change in function. It is, of course, the decrease in creatine phosphate which leads to the increase in inorganic phosphate. In the studies of Kentish, a decrease in creatine phosphate in the bathing fluid for skinned fibers produced a slight increase, not decrease, in contractile function. Thus, the possibility that it is the decrease in creatine phosphate which controls developed pressure is unlikely. It is much more likely that the meaningful

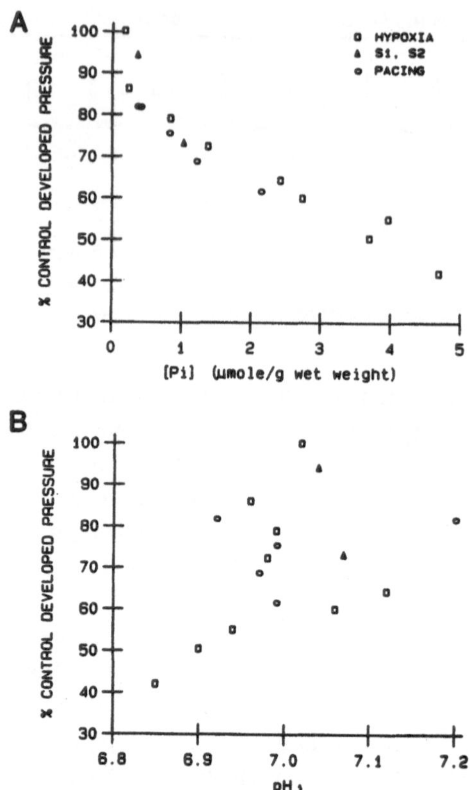

Figure 5. The relation between maximal Ca^{2+}-activated pressure and intramyocardial Pi (A) or intracellular pH (B). In both panels, the maximal Ca^{2+}-activated pressure was normalized by the developed pressure in the control period. A: maximal Ca^{2+}-activated pressure and Pi during hypoxia (□) and during pacing at various rates between tetani (○) show a strong correlation ($r = -0.945$, $P<0.001$, $n = 14$). The data obtained by comparing the early and late phases of tetani (△) are located within the 95% confidence range of the line regressed from the data obtained during hypoxia and pacing. B: maximal Ca^{2+}-activated pressure and pH_i during hypoxia (□) and during pacing (○) show no significant correlation ($r = 0.390$, $P>0.10$, $n = 14$). The change in pH_i during tetani (△) is noted to be in the opposite direction to the changes during hypoxia, despite the similarity of the changes in [Pi].

correlation here is between the increase in inorganic phosphate and the decline in function.

To ascertain that the small changes in intracellular pH that were measured were not causally related to the decline in pressure, we selectively changed intracellular pH by inducing either metabolic or respiratory acidosis, then measured the pH and function. Figure 6 shows the results of such an experiment. For levels of acidosis that result in pH changes between 6.7 and 7.1 there is essentially no change in maximal Ca^{2+}-activated pressure. It is only when the pH declines to less than 6.7 that there is a steep relationship between pH and developed pressure. In the studies of hypoxia, early contractile failure occurred at intracellu-

Table 1. Correlation coefficients between maximal Ca^{2+}-activated pressure and intramyocardial metabolites during hypoxia and pacing.

	n	DP-Pi	DP-PCr	DP-ATP	DP-pH_i
1	6	−0.939[b]	0.978[c]	0.808	0.683
2	9	−0.894[b]	0.877[b]	0.528	0.377
3	10	−0.956[c]	0.941[c]	0.413	0.629
4	8	−0.771[a]	0.883[b]	0.334	0.575
5	7	−0.989[b]	0.823[a]	0.272	0.366
6	12	−0.885[c]	0.892[c]	0.742[b]	0.080
7	17	−0.770[c]	0.660[b]	0.219	0.605[a]
8	14	−0.945[c]	0.876[c]	0.323	0.390
9	16	−0.872[c]	0.793[c]	−0.011	0.879[c]
10	16	−0.850[c]	0.795[c]	0.702[b]	0.317
11	17	−0.781[c]	0.946[c]	0.334	0.615[b]
12	16	−0.723[b]	0.787[c]	0.335	−0.143
	Mean	−0.870	0.860	0.410	0.491

n: the number of the data in each experiment, DP: maximal Ca^{2+}-activated pressure, Pi: inorganic phosphate, PCr: phosphocreatine, [a] $P<0.05$, [b] $P<0.01$, [c] $P<0.001$.

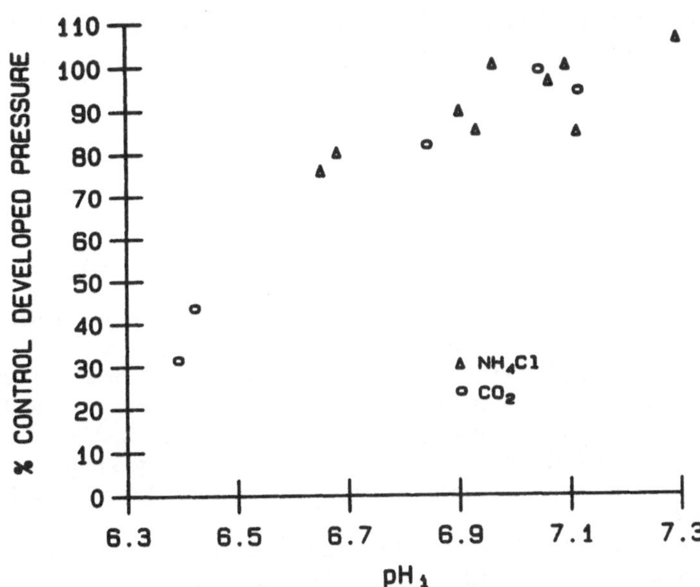

Figure 6. The relation between maximal Ca^{2+}-activated pressure and pH_i during acidosis. Maximal Ca^{2+}-activated pressure was normalized by the value during perfusion with control (15 mM $[Ca]_o$) solution. Results are included from two separate trials: 1. metabolic acidosis following exposure to 20 mM NH_4Cl (△), and 2. respiratory acidosis during perfusion with solution bubbled with 95% O_2/5% CO_2 (O).

lar pH values greater than 6.8. Thus, the pH changes that occurred during the supply-demand imbalances were entirely within the range in which pH, when it changes alone, has no significant effect on maximal Ca^{2+}-activated pressure. This supports the idea that pH is not the causal factor, and supports the conclusion that it is the rise in inorganic phosphate that is important, causing the initial decline in maximal force that results from hypoxia and ischemia.

Thus, the induction of tetanus after exposure to ryanodine enables the determination of maximal Ca^{2+}-activated pressure. Simultaneous measurements of metabolite concentrations along with tetanic pressure hold major promise in answering many questions about myocardial physiology and pathophysiology. Already it has allowed us to provide evidence for a major role of inorganic phosphate in the control of contractile function during the initial seconds to minutes of ischemia and hypoxia.

Acknowledgments

We thank David T. Yue and W. Gil Wier for helpful discussions. The figures are reproduced or modified from references 3 and 6, by permission of *Circulation Research.* This study was supported by Grant No. HL 17655-12, National Heart, Lung and Blood Institute. E. Marban is the recipient of a Research Career Development Award of the N.I.H. (K04 01872). H. Kusuoka was the recipient of a Fellowship for Japanese Scholars and Researchers to Study Abroad of the Japanese Ministry of Education, Science and Culture.

References

1. Strobeck JE, Krueger J, Sonnenblick EH (1980): Load and time considerations in the force-length relation of cardiac muscle. Fed Proc 39: 175–182.
2. Winegrad S (1984): Regulation of cardiac contractile proteins: correlations between physiology and biochemistry. Circ Res 55: 565–574.
3. Marban E, Kusuoka H, Yue DT, Weisfeldt ML, Wier WG (1986): Maximal Ca^{2+}-activated force elicited by tetanization of ferret papillary muscle and whole heart. Mechanism and characteristics of steady contractile activation in intact myocardium. Circ Res 59: 262–269.
4. Sutko J, Kenyon JL (1983): Ryanodine modification of cardiac muscle responses to potassium free solutions: evidence for inhibition of sarcoplasmic reticulum calcium release. J Gen Physiol 82: 385–404.
5. Yue DT, Marban E, Wier WG (1986): Relationship between force and intracellular $[Ca^{2+}]$ in tetanized mammalian heart muscle. J Gen Physiol 87: 223–242.
6. Kusuoka H, Weisfeldt ML, Zweier J, Jacobus WE, Marban E (1986): Mechanism of early contractile failure during hypoxia in intact ferret heart: evidence for modulation of maximal Ca^{2+}-activated force by inorganic phosphate. Circ Res 59: 270–282.
7. Jacobus WE, Pores IH, Lucas SK, Kallman CH, Weisfeldt ML, Flaherty JT (1982): The role of intracellular pH in the control of normal and ischemic myocardial contractility: a ^{31}P nuclear magnetic resonance and mass spectroscopy study. In Nuccitelli R, Deamer DW (eds) Intracellu-

lar pH: its measurement, regulation and utilization in cellular function., Alan R. Liss, Inc., New York, pp. 537–565.

8. Allen DG, Orchard CH (1983): Intracellular calcium concentration during hypoxia and metabolic inhibition in mammalian ventricular muscle. J Physiol (London) 339: 107–122.
9. Fabiato A, Fabiato F (1978): Effects of pH on the myofilaments and the sarcoplasmic reticulum of skinned cells from cardiac and skeletal muscles. J Physiol (London) 276: 233–255.
10. Herzig JW, Peterson JW, Ruegg JC, Solaro RJ (1981): Vanadate and phosphate ions reduce tension and increase cross-bridge kinetics in chemically skinned heart muscle. Biochim Biophys Acta 672: 191–196.
11. Kentish JC (1986): The effects of inorganic phosphate and creatine phosphate on force production in skinned muscles from rat ventricle. J Physiol (London) 370: 585–604.

Discussion

Lab: The increased phosphate sounds like an attractive hypothesis. Could there be a third hypothesis that you have an intracellular calcium overload, with random oscillatory calcium releases across the fiber, resulting in some kind of inhomogeneity of contraction? A particular segment might then be a series of elastic components.
Weisfeldt: If you take the hypoxic or ischemic heart and do the whole calcium concentration-response curve you find that there is a shift in the entire curve in the same direction as for the peak calcium. Thus, it is not likely that calcium overload, or the high calcium levels in the extracellular space are responsible for the changes that we have seen.
Yue: Also the experiments are performed after exposure to ryanodine, and it has been shown by numerous investigators that ryanodine interrupts spontaneous oscillations of intracellular calcium.
Sonnenblick: Some years ago we found that you could use tetanus to study mechanics [1].[a] One of the things that is different, and also shows up in the isolated muscle, is that the control twitches produce a pressure that is exceedingly low. If those are so low to start with, what is the metabolic setting that makes the heart so depressed that, when you tetanize it, it becomes non-depressed when your phosphate is normal to start with. I would think you would have to couple the twitch phenomena in the heart with the tetanus phenomena.
Weisfeldt: You are correct in your observation. What happens is that after you administer ryanodine and pace at a slow rate, or a modest rate, you see a fall in the systolic pressure and you see a decrease in the developed pressure. I would hypothesize that it is due to a decrease in activator calcium as a reflection of the blockade of calcium release mechanisms by ryanodine, and not a reflection of a more profound metabolic effect. I would support that notion by pointing out that during the tetanus, the generation of pressure is far in excess of what it was in the same heart before the ryanodine was given. Isolated perfused hearts at 2.0 mM calcium, generate about 110 mm Hg for an end-diastolic pressure of 10 mm Hg. Then you give the ryanodine and the peak pressure goes down to about 50 mm Hg. But when you start the rapid pacing, peak pressure goes up to 300 mm Hg. Furthermore, a decrease in activator calcium during twitches as a result of exposure to ryanodine has been confirmed in the aequorin experiments of Yue, Marban and Wier [5].
Hoffman: Why didn't you use more complex statistics in approaching the phosphate versus the pH question?
Weisfeldt: We have done more complex statistics (multiple regression analysis) and we have found that the pH has a minor additive effect to that of inorganic phosphate. That was, in part, the reason why we did the independent pH experiments to show that, within the pH range of interest, there was little or no change in maximal Ca^{2+}-activated pressure.

[a] Number relates to reference in the preceeding paper.

15. Modulation properties of myocardial contractile proteins

S. WINEGRAD, G. MCCLELLAN, L. E.R. LIN and S. WEINDLING

Abstract

The development of the active force in the cardiac muscle is related to β-adrenergic stimulation which controls the number of Ca responsible V_1 and V_3 force generators. The latter influences the amount of tension that can be produced and by altering the ratio of the V_1 and V_3 force generators, it regulates the kinetics of the contraction.

Introduction

Development of active force by striated muscle is initiated by the binding of calcium to troponin in the thin contractile filament following an increase in the concentration of calcium ions. This binding produces a movement of the protein, tropomyosin, in the thin filament from a position that blocks the interaction between actin and myosin, and allows the force generating reaction to occur. Relaxation follows a decrease in the concentration of calcium ions, release of calcium from troponin, and restoration of tropomyosin to its blocking position. Because of this change between a relaxed state with the calcium-control site on troponin unsaturated and a contracted state with the calcium control site saturated, the cardiac contractile system has been considered to have only two physiological states: relaxed and contracted.

Calcium sensitivity

Variation of the calcium requirements for activating contraction (defined as calcium sensitivity) can occur under physiological conditions. After Cole and Perry [1] and Grand et al. [2] had found that a cAMP-sensitive protein kinase could produce phosphorylation of the inhibitory component of both isolated cardiac and skeletal troponin (TNI), England [3–5] showed that this reaction was a physiologically meaningful one as much as it was produced by perfusing isolated hearts with β-adrenergic agonists. Following the appearance of a positive inotropic effect, the hearts were quickly frozen, and the amount of phosphorylation of the isolated contractile proteins was determined. The degree of phosphorylation of TNI and the concentration of the β-adrenergic agonist in the perfusion medium were related. Although, initially, both the time course and the extent of the increase in contractile force correlated well with the degree of phosphorylation of TNI, the two could be dissociated [4]. Contractility, as judged by the maximum force developed, was not altered by the phosphorylation of TNI, nor was the maximum actin-activated myosin ATPase activity. What changed, however, was the concentration of calcium ions that was necessary to produce a given percentage of maximum ATPase activity. Phosphorylation of TNI approximately doubled the concentration of calcium necessary for a given level of activation. This correlation has been observed in several different laboratories and is now generally accepted [6, 7]. During exposure to β-adrenergic agonists a decrease in calcium sensitivity has been detected with intracellular calcium-sensitive microelectrodes [8].

It has been possible to show direct correlation between the degree of phosphorylation of TNI and the calcium sensitivity of force generation in the same mammalian cardiac cells by first making the sarcolemma permeable to small molecules and ions with EGTA [6]. These hyperpermeable cells have properties that make them well suited for studies of the contractile proteins. The membrane has been shown to be permeable to calcium, EGTA, ATP, ADP, creatine phosphate, and inorganic phosphate, but at the same time the membrane retains a functional β-receptor, α-receptor, cholinergic receptor, adenylate cyclase, and phosphodiesterase [6, 9]. The ability to generate force is high, and it remains stable over hours. In these hyperpermeable cells, the concentrations of calcium necessary for production of half maximum tension is closely correlated with the percentage of TNI that has been phosphorylated [6]. The degree of TNI phosphorylation can be modified by cAMP, cGMP, and by activation of the β-adrenergic system. In this preparation, the range over which calcium sensitivity varies is 5-fold, which is over twice that observed with isolated proteins. Regulation of calcium sensitivity over a 2- to 3-fold range by cyclic nucleotides has been seen in Lubrol-treated pig heart cells [10, 11].

Dephosphorylation of TNI and increase in calcium sensitivity does not occur simply by the withdrawal of cAMP stimulation of the protein kinase, either in the intact or the hyperpermeable cell [4, 12]. In the hyperpermeable cells, dephosphorylation is due to a cGMP-regulated reaction, presumably catalyzed by a phosphatase [6]. cGMP with a phosphodiesterase inhibitor decreases TNI phosphorylation, but in the absence of TNI phosphorylation, cGMP has no effect on calcium sensitivity. Dephosphorylation through cGMP may be controlled by the cholinergic system [13]. Although withdrawal of the β-agonist reverses the increased inotropic state of intact cells, it does not reverse TNI phosphorylation [5]. A cholinergic agent does, however, produce dephosphorylation. In hyperpermeable cardiac cells in which the level of calcium sensitivity is low, methacholine increases calcium sensitivity to its maximum, but it has no effect where calcium sensitivity is already maximal. Atropine blocks this effect of the cholinergic agonist. Since cholinergic agents increase the production of cGMP, it seems reasonable that cholinergic agents produce TNI dephosphorylation by stimulating the synthesis of cGMP [14, 15], and activating a phosphatase. Although the cholinergic agonist may also produce TNI dephosphorylation by inhibiting membrane adenylate cyclase [16], this probably is not the major mechanism for its effect, since withdrawal of the β-agonist activating adenylate cyclase does not, by itself, reverse TNI phosphorylation.

Control of maximum Ca-activated force

Recent experimental work indicates that the contractile system of hearts from small mammals can exist in three different physiological states:

1. relaxed and Ca unresponsive;
2. relaxed and Ca responsive; and
3. contracted due to calcium activation.

The existence of a second relaxed state in which force is not produced with Ca ions, has been demonstrated by studies that permit assessment of the properties of the contractile proteins without interference from other steps in the contractile process having the capability of modulating the contractile properties of the proteins. One set of experiments uses hyperpermeable cardiac cells for mechanical studies. In another type of study, thin section of hearts, which have been frozen quickly to preserve the in vivo state of the cells, have been used to study the enzymatic properties of myosin; both Ca and actin activated ATPase activities have been measured as indications of the state of myosin and its ability to interact with actin in the force producing reaction. As the sections are about 1/3 the thickness of a single cell, serial sections include parts of the same cells and provide the opportunity of comparing the responses of the same cell to two different treatments.

Since the membrane of the hyperpermeable cells is permeable to calcium ions and EGTA, intracellular calcium concentrations can be buffered at any desired value, permitting the detection of calcium-independent changes in the amount of force generated by the myofibrils. Activation of the β-adrenergic system at any step between the binding of the agonist to the receptor and the elevation of the concentration of cAMP increases the maximum Ca-activated force in hyperpermeable ventricle cells from hearts of young rats by an average of about 150%. In order to see this effect, a phosphodiesterase inhibitor must be present to prevent the breakdown of cAMP and a low concentration of a non-ionic detergent must be included to facilitate the release of the factor responsible for the increase in force from its bound position within an intracellular membrane.

Hearts from young rats contain three isozymes of myosin that are the homodimers and the heterodimer of two different heavy chains [17]. The α-heavy chain produces a myosin with 3 times the ATPase activity but the same force generating capability as myosin formed with the β-heavy chain. The two homodimers which predominate in rat hearts are called V_1 and V_3 according to whether the heavy chains are respectively α or β. The degree to which activation of the β-adrenergic system increases maximum Ca activated force depends on the relative amount of the V_1 isoform of myosin [18]. The β-adrenergically dependent system that increases force in a Ca independent manner appears to distinguish between the different isozymes of myosin and acts selectively on the fast isozyme V_1.

The calcium and actin activated ATPase activities of myosin are also increased by β-adrenergic stimulation. This has been shown in the intact animal, in the isolated perfused heart, and in sections from quickly frozen hearts [19]. Tyramine injection into rats increases myosin ATPase activity as does addition of a beta agonist to the medium perfusing an isolated heart. Similarly, the addition of cAMP to the medium bathing sections of frozen hearts increases ATPase activity; the extent of the increase is also related to the percentage of V_1 myosin present. Because the ATPase activity of V_3 is irreversibly inhibited by exposure to an alkaline pH that has little effect on V_1, another property of the system can be demonstrated [20]. This makes it possible to measure both total ATPase activity due to the sum of V_1 and V_3 (and the small amount of V_2) and the ATPase activity of V_1 alone in the same cell. From the two measurements and discounting any contribution of V_2, the ATPase activities of V_1 and V_3 can be estimated. Not only does cAMP increase the ATPase activity of V_1, but it also inhibits the ATPase activity of V_3. The consequence of stimulation with cAMP is an increase in the contribution of the existing V_1 isozyme of myosin to the generation of force at the expense of the V_3 isozyme.

The response of a third parameter of the contractile system, maximum velocity of shortening (V_{max}), to β-adrenergic stimulation has been measured by the slack length technique [21] in which the time for unloaded hyperpermeable cells to take up a precisely produced amount of slack length is measured (Weindling and Winegrad, unpublished results). In tissue containing only V_1, β-adrenergic activation did not significantly change V_{max} even though it increased maximum Ca activated force. In cells from other rats in which the isozyme content is almost entirely or entirely V_3, V_{max} is about 30% of the value found in the cells that contained only V_1. The failure of β-adrenergic stimulation to alter V_{max} even though it increased ATPase activity and maximum Ca activated force indicates that it probably is changing the number of Ca-responsive force generators rather than the properties of individual force generators.

These results indicate that in the presence of a mixture of myosin isozymes, β-adrenergic stimulation can increase not only the total number of force generators that are Ca responsive to alter force, but also modify the ratio of V_1 to V_3 force generators that are Ca responsive to regulate V_{max}. Since both maximum force and maximum velocity of shortening can be altered in cells, each cell is capable of functioning along many different force-velocity curves, depending upon the regulatory state of the myosin isozymes [22, 23]. This allows the heart to change its function in a way that skeletal muscle bundles can. The latter does it by selecting not which isozymes in each cell are Ca responsive but by selecting which cells are stimulated by the nervous system (most skeletal muscles contain cells with different kinds of myosin). In light of this type of regulation, it is interesting to note that during most of the active, vigorous part of the life span of the rat, its heart contains substantial amounts of both myosin isozymes, facilitating the regulation of V_{max} [24]. It is only during the first few weeks and the senescent periods of the rat's life that the heart is composed primarily or exclusively of one type of myosin isozyme.

The factor responsible for the change in the state of V_1 myosin from Ca unresponsive to Ca responsive may be a 21K dalton protein that is bound to an intracellular membrane [23]. Perfusion of the coronary circulation with cold solution containing 10 mM EGTA and no ATP extracts the activity from the heart. The activity can be detected by exposing a skinned fiber to the crude extract and then treating the skinned fiber briefly with a low concentration of a non-ionic detergent. The need for using detergent on the skinned fibers is eliminated by treating the crude extract with detergent and then removing the detergent with adsorbing beads.

Conclusion

The ventricular cells of rat and rabbit hearts contain a system capable of controlling the number of Ca responsible V_1 and V_3 force generators in response to β-adrenergic stimulation. By modifying the total number of Ca responsive force generators, it influences the amount of tension that can be produced and by altering the ratio V_1 to V_3 force generators it regulates the kinetics of the contraction. The regulatory factor may be a 21 K dalton protein that is bound through an anchor peptide to an intracellular membrane. β-adrenergic stimulation causes its release, not due to phosphorylation of the active protein but possibly through phosphorylation of the anchor peptide. Modification of the V_1 force generator appears to occur as a result of the binding by myosin of the active factor.

Acknowledgment

This study was supported by grants from the National Institute of Health HL 16010 and HL 15835 to Saul Winegrad.

References

1. Cole H, Perry SV (1975): The phosphorylation of troponin I from cardiac muscle. J Biochem 149: 525–533.
2. Grand RJ, Wilkinson JM, Mole EI (1976): The amino acid sequence of rabbit cardiac troponin I. Biochem J 159: 633–641.
3. England P (1975): Correlation between contraction and phosphorylation of the inhibitory subunit of troponin in perfused rat heart. FEBS Lett 50: 57–60.
4. England P (1976): Studies of the phosphorylation of the inhibitor subunit of troponin during modification of contraction in perfused rat heart. J Biochem 160: 295–304.
5. Ray KP, England P (1976): Phosphorylation of the inhibitory subunit of troponin and its effect on the calcium dependence of cardiac myofibril adenosine triphosphate. FEBS Lett 70: 11–17.
6. Mope L, McClellan G, Winegrad S (1980): Calcium sensitivity of the contractile system and phosphorylation of troponin in hyperpermeable cardiac cells. J Gen Physiol 75: 271–282.
7. Holroyde J, Small D, Howe E, Solaro J (1979): Isolation of cardiac myofibrils and myosin light chains with in vivo levels of light chain phosphorylation. Biochem Biophys Acta 587: 620–637.
8. Marban E, Rink T, Tsien RW, Tsien RY (1980): Free calcium in the heart at rest and during contraction measured with Ca sensitive electrodes. Nature 286: 845–850.
9. McClellan G, Winegrad S (1978): The regulation of calcium sensitivity of the contractile system in mammalian cardiac muscle. J Gen Physiol 72: 734–764.
10. Hertzig J, Kohler G, Pfitzer G, Ruegg C, Wolffle G (1981): cAMP inhibits contractility of detergent treated glycerol extracted cardiac muscle. Pflüger's Archiv 391: 208–212.
11. Pfitzer G, Ruegg C, Flockerzi V, Hofmann F (1981): cGMP dependent protein kinase decreases calcium sensitivity of skinned cardiac fibers. FEBS Lett 149: 171–175.
12. Weisberg A, McClellan G, Tucker M, Lin LE, Winegrad S (1983): Regulation of calcium sensitivity in perforated mammalian cardiac cells. J Gen Physiol 81: 195–211.
13. Lin LE, Winegrad S (1986): Isolation of a factor that modulates the contractility of rat heart. Biophys J 49: 450a.
13. Horowits R, Winegrad S (1984): Cholinergic regulation of calcium sensitivity in cardiac muscle. J Mol Cell Cardiol 16: 277–280.
14. George W, Polson J, O'Toole J, Goldberg N (1970): Evaluation of the guanosine 3'-5' cyclic phosphate in rat after perfusion with acetylocholine. Proc Nat Acad Sc (USA) 66: 398–403.
15. George W, Wilkerson R, Kadowitz P (1973): Influence of acetylcholine on contractile force and cyclic nucleotide levels in isolated perfused heart. J Pharm Exper Therap 184: 228–235.
16. Jakobs K, Altories K, Schultz G (1979): GTP dependent inhibition of cardiac adenylate cyclase by muscarinic cholinergic agonist. Naunyn Schmiedeberg's Arch Pharm 310: 113–119.
17. Hoh J, McGrath P, Hale P (1978): Electrophoretic analysis of multiple forms of rat cardiac myosin: Effects of hypophysectomy and thyroid treatment. J Mol Cell Cardiol 10: 1053–1076.
18 Winegrad S, McClellan G, Tucker M, Lin LE (1983): Cyclic AMP regulation of myosin isozymes in mammalian cardiac muscle. J Gen Physiol 81: 749–765.
19. Winegrad S, Weisberg A, McClellan G (1986): Adrenergic regulation of myosin adenosine triphosphatase activity. Circ Res 58: 83–95.
20. Yazaki Y, Raben M (1974): Cardiac myosin adenisine triphosphatase of rat and mouse. Distinctive enzymatic properties compared with rabbit and dog cardiac myosin. Circ Res 35: 15–23.
21. Edman P (1979): The velocity of unloaded shortening and its relation to sarcomere length and isometric force in vertebrate muscle fibers. J Physiol 291: 143–160.
22. Schwartz R, Lecarpentier Y, Martin J, Lompre A, Mercadier J, Swynghedauw B (1981): Myosin isozyme distribution correlates with speed of myocardial contraction. J Mol Cell Cardiol 13: 1071–1075.
23. Winegrad S (1984): Regulation of cardiac contractile problems. Correlations between physiology and biochemistry. Circ Res 55: 565–574.

24. Lompre A, Mercadier J, Wisnensky C, Bouveret P, Pantaloni C, d'Albis A, Schwartz K (1981): Species and age dependent changes in the relative amounts of cardiac myosin isozymes in mammals. Develop Biol 84: 286–290.

Discussion

Beyar: Does the different response of the slow and fast types of myosin to adrenalin activity, in terms of the maximum velocity of shortening or ATPhase/ activity, also express itself by a similar change in the force of contraction?
Winegrad: No. It's only the dynamics that is affected. The ability to generate forces is the same. Similar results are available from two other laboratories.
Beyar: Hypertrophy is known to be associated with high content of the slow myosin. Does the hypertrophic heart behave differently in response to adrenegic simulation as compared to a normal heart?
Winegrad: We have not looked at it. But when you look at it you must be aware that when you take the heart out of the animal you assume it represents a normal operating state. In fact, we do things which are abnormal and expose the heart to different hemodynamic conditions and the heart responds to these changes. Because of these phenomena, one cannot infer conclusions from the literature on this question.
Marcus: Could you comment on the differences in myosins in animals and humans?
Winegrad: The better the new techniques, the more fast myosins has been found in large animals, including humans. The figure for humans is now between 5–10% under the conditions in which the heart was removed, and this, almost certainly, is not a normal heart. Let me point out what happens if you change the relative amount of the fast myosin by a small amount. A 10% increase in this fast myosin will give you 2–2.5 fold increase in the maximum velocity of shortening. Although the amount in absolute terms has been considered small and insignificant, if you look at its effect you see that the same small amounts affect large changes in the kinetics of contraction.
Sideman: Would you say that there is a change in the distribution of myosin across the myocardium?
Winegrad: Yes. We and others have studied it in the rat heart. We established that the cross section of the myocardium is not absolutely uniform. In the subendocardial area, some 3–4 cells thick (50–100 μm), you generally see a higher concentration of the fast isomyosin. Then you see gentle difference which we have not succeeded to quantify, but we have no doubt that the endocardial layer has a higher concentration of the fast myosin.
Sideman: This is indeed interesting and consistent with our theoretical finding which indicates a 'need' for faster myosin in the endocardial layers due to the increased velocity of shortening of these layers.
Winegrad: You may indeed anticipate it.

16. Insight into excitation-contraction coupling of heart derived from studies of the force-interval relationship

D.T. YUE and K. SAGAWA

Abstract

Recent attempts to extend understanding of excitation-contraction coupling of mammalian myocardium through studies of the force-interval relationship are summarized. Initial experiments were performed with isolated, blood-perfused, canine ventricles. In this relatively intact preparation, we determined that restitution of the strength of contraction recovered with a monoexponential time course whose time constant was invariant. Further experiments with isolated papillary muscles confirmed this behavior in superfused muscle, so long as relatively 'physiological' conditions were maintained. The monoexponential nature of the recovery of strength enabled us to unify conceptually the description of the entire physiological force-interval relationship, and also led us to a simple and testable model of excitation-contraction coupling. Three predictions of the model were proved true by experiments involving isolated ventricles and ferret papillary muscles that had been microinjected with calcium indicator aequorin to enable monitoring of intracellular free $[Ca^{2+}]_i$. Most recently, the model has proved useful in providing insight into the clinical disease known as restrictive cardiomyopathy.

Introduction

Historical perspective

The beautifully ordered fashion in which the strength of contraction of mammalian cardiac muscle responds to changes in stimulation pattern has long engendered the hope that clarification of these phenomena, known as the force-interval relationship, would lead to understanding the fundamental mechanisms underlying cardiac contraction [1]. Until the mid 1960s, however, this hope remained largely unfulfilled, as lamented by Braveny and Kruta [2]:

Leur nature, en dépit de nombreuses recherches et de grand efforts, reste cependant toujours obscure.

At this point, the striking discovery was made that tension development was regulated by the binding of calcium to troponin [3]. Shortly thereafter, Wood and coworkers [4] were among the first to advance the hypothesis that alterations in tension development with changes in stimulation pattern were related directly to underlying changes in calcium supplied to the myofilaments. Direct observations of parallel fluctuations of tension and calcium followed with the use of aequorin as an intracellular indicator of free $[Ca^{2+}]$ ($[Ca^{2+}]_i$) [5, 6]. During this same period, a group of European investigators enhanced the early hypothesis by Wood and coworkers, and evolved a beautiful framework for understanding the force-interval relationship, based upon purported movements of intracellular calcium [7–9].

In the present paper, we summarize our own recent attempts to extend understanding of excitation-contraction coupling of the mammalian heart through studies of the force-interval relationship. Initial experiments were performed with isolated, blood-perfused, canine ventricles. Then, based upon insight garnered from this relatively physiological preparation, we proceeded to studies in superfused papillary muscles microinjected with the intracellular calcium indicator aequorin. Because our initial experiments were performed in a relatively intact preparation, we were able to discern a particularly simple pattern to the force-interval relationship that may be recognized more clearly under physiological conditions. The simplicity of the description led us to a simple and, to some extent, testable model of e-c coupling [10]. Three predictions of the model were borne out by experimental investigations. Most recently, we have found the model useful in making sense of the clinical disease entity known as restrictive cardiomyopathy [11].

Simple description of the force-interval relationship seen from the perspective of monoexponential restitution

For the new student of cardiac muscle physiology, or the physiologist only infrequently concerned with the cardiac force-interval relationship (FIR), the FIR may appear to be a bewildering amalgam of unrelated phenomena and obscure terminology. However, we stumbled across a crucial property of the FIR that not only formed the basis of an extremely simple framework for clarifying this amalgam, but also suggested to us a hypothesis as to its underlying mechanism. The property is that, over a broad physiological range, restitution of the strength of contraction proceeds according to a monoexponential time course with a time constant that is invariant [10, 12]. We explain this property below.

Restitution is defined as the recovery of the strength of a given contraction as the interval preceding that beat is lengthened. This phenomenon is illustrated by the original records shown in Figure 1, taken from an isolated, blood-perfused, canine ventricle that was contracting isovolumically. In each of the three frames, the ventricle has been paced during the 'priming period' at regularly-timed intervals of 460 ms until a steady state has been attained. As the interval (ESI) before the beat in question (denoted by the *) is lengthened, dP/dt and P of that beat increases. This recovery of the strength of contraction is restitution.

Based on previous studies of isolated muscle, we expected that the precise time course of restitution would be quite complex. In superfused muscle, restitution followed a monotonic time course (Fig. 9) at lower levels of inotropy, but proceeded with an oscillatory time course [14] at augmented levels of contractilty, often associated with spontaneous oscillations of $[Ca^{2+}]_i$.

Contrary to expectation, restitution in the blood-perfused ventricle always followed a monoexponential time course whose time constant was essentially the same *despite vastly different histories of stimulation pattern* [10, 12], as illustrated in Figure 2. Here the strength (maximum isovolumic dP/dt, dP/dt_{max}) of each test beat is normalized by that of the preceding steady-state contraction, and plotted as a function of the interval separating the two responses, ESI. The open circles are actual data points, the solid curve is a best-fitting monoexponential function. These show that restitution begins only after a certain dead time (t_0, at arrow in Fig. 2) has elapsed, coincident with repolarization of the membrane [10, 12]. Thereafter, restitution proceeds monoexponentially to a plateau. The remarkable finding is that the time constant of this recovery (~200 ms for the canine ventricle at 37° C) remains essentially constant, independent of the particular pacing pattern prior to determination of the curve in question. Thus, restitution for any given beat over the broad physiological range investigated could be described by the following single equation:

$$dP/dt_{max} = CR_{max}\,(1 - \exp\,[(ESI - t_o)/T]), \tag{1}$$

where CR_{max} is the fully-restituted strength of contraction, t_o is the interval after which restitution can proceed appreciably, and T is the time constant of restitution.

The beautiful feature of having studied restitution in the isolated, blood-perfused canine ventricle is that we could observe the nature of restitution under a broad range of relatively *physiological conditions*, while concurrently maintaining strict control of hemodynamic parameters. Thus, we could observe the simple, monoexponential nature of restitution (Eq. 1) most relevant to the physiological state, and recognize the more complex characteristics of restitution sometimes observed in isolated muscle as being relevant to the supraphysiological conditions under which a superfused muscle can be made to operate.

To confirm that monoexponential restitution with an invariant time constant was indeed a property of myocardium and could be observed in isolated muscles

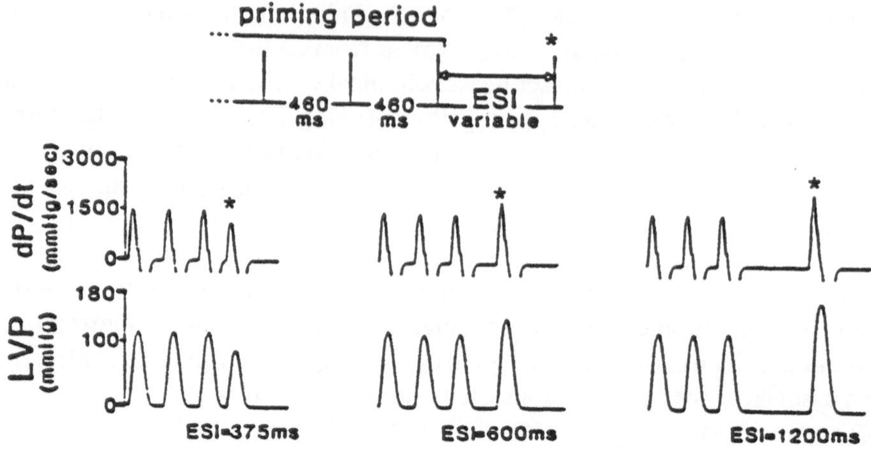

Figure 1. Original records of dP/dt and P from the left ventricle of an isovolumically beating, blood-perfused, canine heart. Each frame shows three steady state responses, an extrasystole and a post-extrasystole for the various stimulus intervals. Temperature was 37° C. Schematized stimulation pulses at the top illustrate the pacing pattern used to elicit the responses.

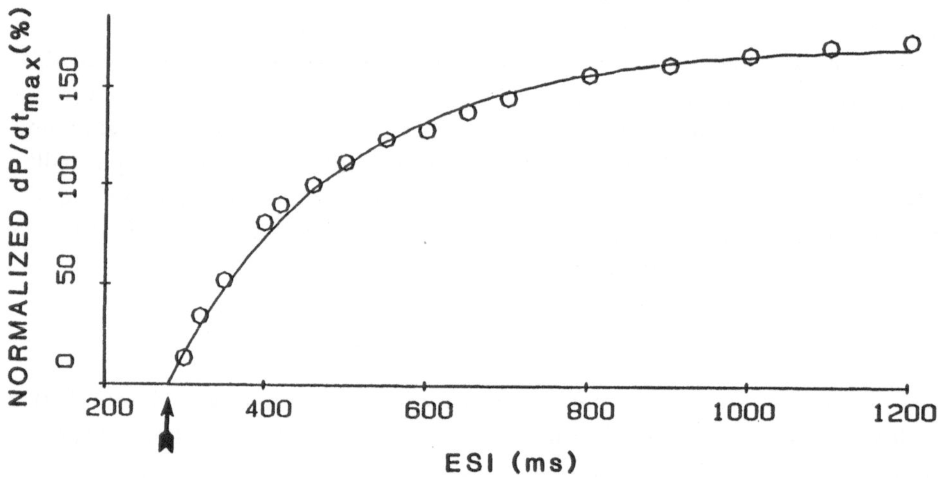

Figure 2. Mechanical restitution curve measured in an isovolumically beating, blood-perfused, canine left ventricle at 37° C.

under more physiological conditions, we measured restitution in isometrically contracting, isolated rabbit papillary muscles. Only when very long intervals (>10 sec) were considered, or very high levels of contractility obtained – conditions apparently not observed under blood-perfused conditions – were there deviations from the description in Eq. 1.

Thus, Eq. 1 can be used to unify conceptually not only the FIR of the ventricle per se, but also that of cardiac muscle in general, so long as physiological conditions are maintained. Aside from minor fluctuations in t_o, related to the duration of the action potential preceding a given beat, all the features of Eq. 1 are known, except for the precise value of CR_{max}. Then, if we could express CR_{max} as a function of prior pacing history, virtually the entire physiological FIR could be described by Eq. 1.

While we do not know the exact relation between CR_{max} and prior history of pacing, we do know enough to enable Eq. 1 to provide considerable intuitive predictive power regarding the FIR. Figure 3 summarizes schematically our understanding of the modulation of CR_{max} by prior history of pacing. If we stimulate at fixed, regularly-timed intervals, the response of the muscle or ventricle will soon become the same from one beat to the next. Under these steady state conditions, the relation between CR_{max} and steady heart rate is simple: as heart rate goes up, so does CR_{max} (open circles and solid line). If heart rate is abruptly changed, deviations from the steady state line do occur. For example, consider CR_{max} corresponding to a contraction '0' obtained at steady-state with heart rate ~60 min^{-1} (see 0 in Fig. 3). If stimulation rate is abruptly changed between beats 0 and 1 to 140 min^{-1}, the CR_{max} to which beat 1 can restitute will remain at the same level (see 1 in Fig. 3) as for beat 0 because CR_{max} depends on the *past* history of pacing. However, if the heart rate is maintained at 140 min^{-1} on a subsequent beat (no 2), CR_{max} will increase. Further maintenance of the increased heart rate on beats 3 and onward will result in a progressive approach of CR_{max} toward the steady-state value at 0*. A reciprocal course of events would occur if heart rate was to be abruptly reduced from 140 to 60 min^{-1} between beats 0* and 1* (0*→ in Fig. 3). Maintenance of the slowed heart rate would result in a gradual approach to the steady-state value for CR_{max} (1*→ 2*→ 3*→ ... →0 in Fig. 3). To summarize then, CR_{max} is related to prior pacing history by a unique, increasing steady state line, about which counterclockwise hysteretic loops are traversed during transient changes in stimulation frequency. The counterclockwise hysteretic loops reflect a 'memory' of myocardium for two or more intervals before the beat in question.

Taken together, Figure 2 (monoexponential time course of restitution with invariant time constant) and 3 (CR_{max} as a function of prior pacing history) allow us to predict, for the most part, the entire physiological FIR.

We illustrate this framework by describing the steady-state force-frequency relation, and postextrasystolic potentiation.

The well known steady state force-frequency relation, where greater force is produced in the steady state at shorter stimulus intervals, can be understood as follows. Fig. 4 shows four restitution curves obtained at steady state following priming period intervals, SSI, of 860, 600, 460, and 375 ms (greater plateau height with shorter interval). The plateau height of these curves (CR_{max}) correspond to the steady-state line in Figure 3. The strength of contraction of steady state responses at the different intervals are denoted by the filled circles labelled a-d. The strength of steady-state contractions increases with shortening of intervals

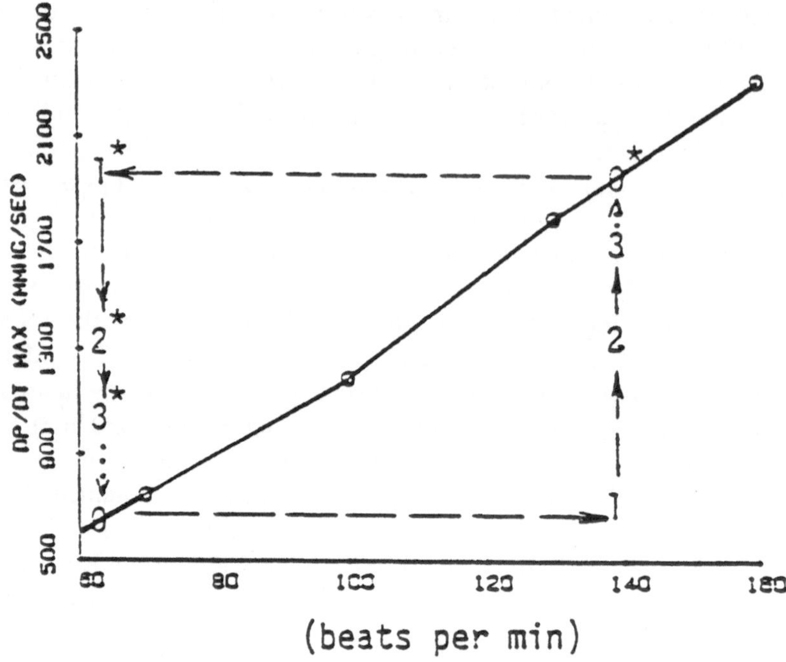

Figure 3. Relation between CR_{max} and stimulus frequency obtained from an isovolumically-contracting, isolated, blood-perfused canine left ventricle at 37° C. The open circles and solid curve depict the steady-state relationship between CR_{max} and stimulus frequency. The dashed path 0→ 1→ 2→ 3→ . . . → 0 shows the transient path that would be traced during an abrupt switch in frequency from 60 to 140 min^{-1}. The dashed path 0* → 1* → 2* → 3* → . . . → 0 displays the transient path that would be traced during an abrupt switch in frequency from 140 back to 60 min^{-1}.

(a<b<c≤d) because the plateau height of restitution increases to a large enough extent to offset the decreased time allowed for restitution at shorter intervals. That the strength of c approximates that of d illustrates that at very short intervals, the increase in plateau height of restitution does indeed become insufficient to overcome the progressively incomplete degree of restitution.

Figure 5 illustrates how postextrasystolic potentiation can be understood. The restitution curve comprised of open circles is obtained following steady pacing at intervals of 460 ms (analogous to Fig. 2). The strength of a steady-state response (0) is denoted by the solid circle labelled 0. If an extrasystole is stimulated after an altered interval (ESI not equal to 460 ms), a restitution curve measured for a subsequent contraction, the postextrasystole, will have a different plateau height (analogous to the hysteretic loop in Fig. 3, 0→ 1→ 2). The other three restitution curves in the figure were determined for postextrasystoles following different ESI as labelled. The shorter is ESI, the higher is CR_{max} for the subsequent postextrasystolic restitution curve. Consider the specific case illustrated by the pressure tracings in Fig. 5. The extrasystole (1) follows the steady state beat (0) by an interval ESI of 300 msec. The strength of the 'premature' extrasystole is dimin-

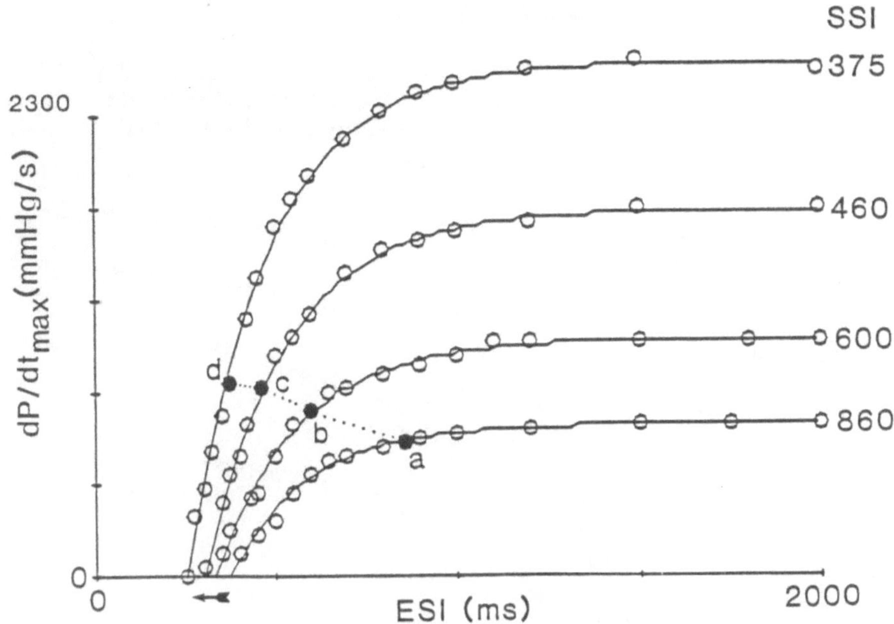

Figure 4. Mechanical restitution curves measured from variably-restituted extrasystoles in an isovolumically beating, blood-perfused, canine left ventricle at 37° C. The four curves were obtained following priming period intervals, SSI, of 375 through 860 ms as labelled. The solid curves are best fitting monoexponential functions with time constants ranging beween 217 and 232 ms. Filled circles labelled a through d are steady-state responses, and illustrate how the positive staircase represents the net effect of increasing CR_{max} counteracted by decreased degree of restitution with increased stimulus frequency. Arrow indicates how onset of restitution shifts to the left as action potential duration of steady state response decreased with diminished SSI.

ished, simply because there was less time for restitution to occur than on the steady state beat (see 0 and 1 on the curve in Fig. 5). Because ESI was less than 460 msec, the restitution curve pertaining to the ensuing postextrasystole (2) will have an augmented CR_{max} (see the height of the curve labelled ESI 300 ms). The postextrasystole is stimulated after a long period (PESI = 1200 msec) that allows for full expression of CR_{max} (see 2 on the curve in Fig. 5). Thus, the postextrasystole is augmented not only because PESI was sufficiently long to allow for full restitution, but also because the CR_{max} of restitution was augmented over the steady state since ESI was less than the steady state interval of 460 ms.

Model of excitation-contraction coupling derived from studies of the physiological FIR

The simplicity of the FIR seen from the perspective of monoexponential restitution enticed us into advancing the following model of excitation-contraction

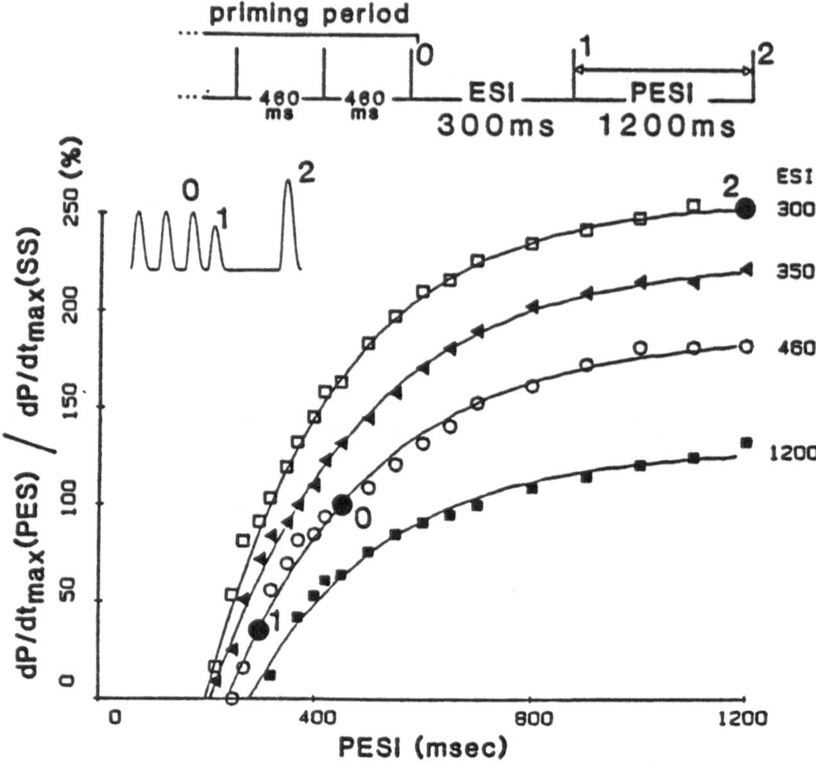

Figure 5. Four mechanical restitution curves measured for postextrasystoles following different ESI in an isovolumically beating, blood-perfused, canine ventricle at 37° C. Each curve corresponds to a given ESI as labelled. The solid curves are best fitting monoexponentials with time constants ranging betwen 243 and 278 msec. The stimulus pulse diagram at top, and the filled circles corresponding to beats 0–2, as labelled, illustrate how the variations in the strength of beats 0, 1 and 2 (note the pressure tracings) can be understood in terms of the restitution curve concept.

coupling. A more rigorous presentation of this model has appeared [10, 13].

The first feature of the model is that restitution is a reflection of the kinetics of the sarcoplasmic reticulum (SR). This postulate is based upon studies with skinned single cardiac cells [15] and voltage clamped cardiac preparations [16, 17] that suggest that most of the activator calcium for a given beat appears to come from SR. Calcium entering the cell across the sarcolemma appears to be taken up by the SR before it sees the myofilaments.

The second property of the model is that calcium sequestered by the SR on a given beat is only slowly made available for release on a subsequent beat. This property, then, accounts for restitution. Figure 6 represents this property in a functional sense by splitting the SR into two compartments: an uptake compartment (U) into which calcium is first sequestered but from which calcium cannot be released directly; and a release compartment (R), all of whose calcium

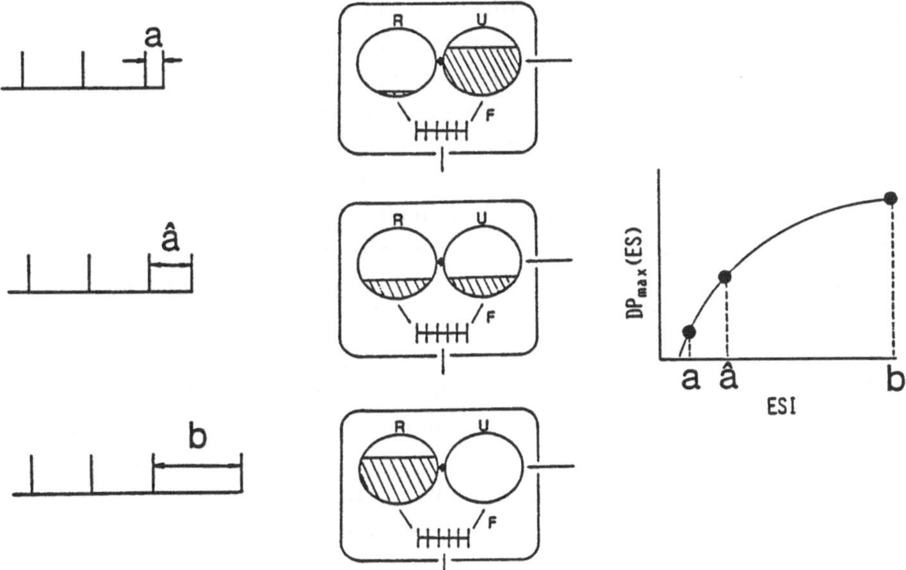

Figure 6. Cartoon of stimulation pulses (left), model cardiac myocyte (middle), and mechanical restitution curve (right). These illustrate the model concept of mechanical restitution.

contents are released upon stimulation. In the interim between beats, all the calcium in the U compartment can move slowly into the R compartment. Thus, as the interval is lengthened (a→ â→ b, leftmost third of Fig. 6) more and more calcium transfers to the R compartment (middle third of Fig. 6), so that the amount of calcium released and therefore the strength of contraction increases monotonically to a plateau level as shown in the schematic restitution curve at the right. Then, different plateau values, CR_{max}, imply different degrees of filling of the U store at the start of restitution. This depiction need not be taken in a literal, anatomical sense; a number of specific schemes boil down to the same functional representation.

To account for the monoexponential time course of restitution with invariant time constant, we propose that the transfer of calcium from U to R compartments (fat arrow in Fig. 6, middle third) proceeds according to first order kinetics with an invariant rate constant, $k = 1/T$. Thus,

$$dR/dt = k * U, \tag{2}$$

where U and R are the amounts of calcium in the R and U stores, respectively. Since restitution proceeds appreciably only after repolarization of the membrane, let k be 0 while the membrane is depolarized and let k take on an invariant, positive value upon membrane repolarization. Thus, any calcium still in the U store at the time of stimulation is trapped in there to contribute to the following contraction. Finally, in order that the solution to Eq. 2 be a single exponential function, we require that calcium sequestration by SR be substantially complete by the time of membrane repolarization, so that the only input/output of calcium to/from the U store be the U→ R transfer during the period when k is positive.

Fourthly, we assume that a constant fraction of the released calcium (F) be resequestered by the SR into the U store, after the notion of 'recirculation fraction' advanced by Morad and Goldman [18].

It is interesting to speculate on what the exact relation of this model to the mechanism of calcium-induced release of calcium [15] might be. One possibility is that calcium is first sequestered by the SR in a form that cannot exit directly through SR calcium channels. Two specific examples of this might be:
1. calcium is first sequestered as a free ion in a SR compartment that is anatomically separate from a compartment containing calcium channels through which escape of calcium from SR to myoplasm can occur, or 2. calcium is first bound to calsequestrin, and therefore cannot exit directly through calcium channels. With time, however, recently sequestered calcium could either move to the compartment with calcium channels, or dissociate from calsequestrin and thereby become available for direct exit through calcium channels. Either of these processes would proceed with first order kinetics in order to satisfy Eq. 2. The calcium that appears in a form that can leave the SR directly through calcium channels corresponds to the calcium in the R compartment of our model. Then, upon stimulation, calcium entering across the sarcolemma triggers SR calcium channels to open, allowing *all* of the calcium that can leave through the channels to be released. That all of the calcium in the R compartment can leave the SR implies that calcium inactivation of calcium channels in SR is lacking or insufficient to attenuate appreciably the amount of calcium that can be released. What keeps the SR from releasing all of its sequestered calcium with each contraction would not be calcium inactivation of calcium channels; rather it would be the limited time allowed for newly sequestered calcium to transform into a form that can be released through the channels. This notion differs somewhat from the classical ideas regarding the calcium-induced release of calcium from SR [15].

This model provided us with three predictions that we proceeded to test. The first of these was that there should be a roughly linear relation between amount of calcium released and the strength of contraction. It seemed implausible to us that a nonlinear Ca-tension relationship would be complemented by a non-monoexponential time course for the restitution of calcium release so as to fortuitously result in an overall monoexponential restitution of the strength of contraction with an invariant time constant. Nonetheless, the notion of a linear Ca-tension relationship for twitches seemed to go against previous results showing superposition of peak tension and peak $[Ca^{2+}]_i$ from twitches on the plot of steady state tension vs. $[Ca^{2+}]_i$ [19], the later plot well known to be markedly nonlinear.

Consistent with the first prediction are the results of Wier and Yue [13] that indicate a linear relationship in intact myocardium between either peak tension

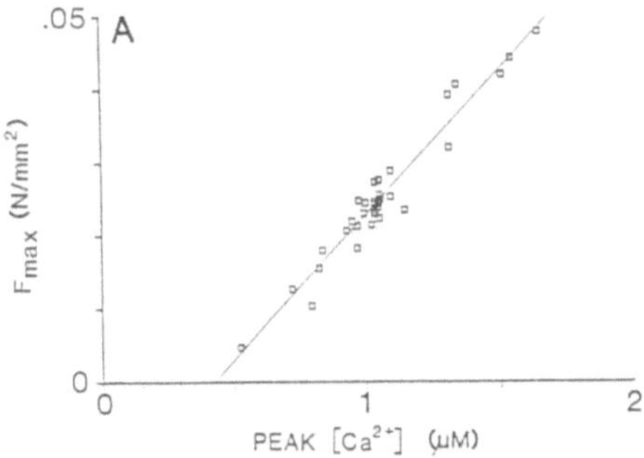

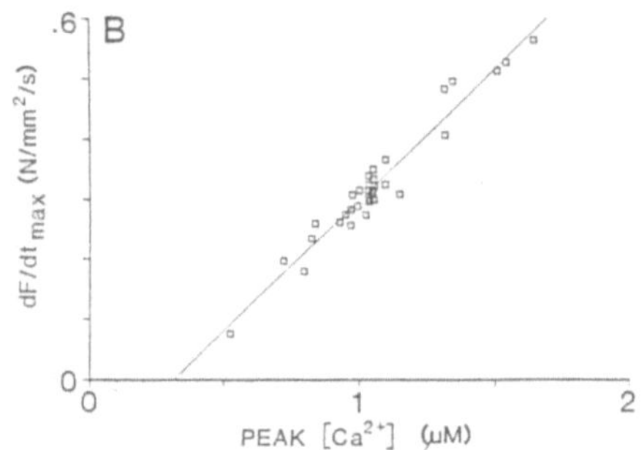

Figure 7. Relation between peak force (F_{max}) and peak $[Ca^{2+}]_i$ (A), and between peak rate of force development (dF/dt_{max}) and peak $[Ca^{2+}]_i$ (B) obtained from variably restituted and potentiated isometric twitches of a ferret papillary muscle. $[Ca^{2+}]_i$ estimated from the luminescence of aequorin that had been microinjected into the muscle. Temperature was 30° C. Straight lines are fitted by linear regression. Adapted from [13].

and peak $[Ca^{2+}]_i$ (Fig. 7A), or between peak rate of tension development and peak $[Ca^{2+}]_i$ (Fig. 7B) for variably restituted and potentiated isometric twitches in isolated, superfused ferret papillary muscles. This linear relation for twitches was distinct from the markedly nonlinear relation found between steady state force and $[Ca^{2+}]_i$ during tetanization of intact heart muscle [20]. In both of these studies, $[Ca^{2+}]_i$ was estimated from the luminescense emitted by aequorin that had been microinjected into the muscles.

A second prediction of our model regards the nature of postextrasystolic potentiation that derives from the 'conservation' properties of the U and R compartments. Figure 8 shows the mechanism of postextrasystolic potentiation as articulated through the model. For very premature extrasystoles (with a very short ESI = a, top frame), little time is allowed for restitution of the extrasystole so that virtually no calcium is available for release on the extrasystole. Still, there is calcium entry across the sarcolemma into the U compartment (dotted calcium) associated with the extrasystolic action potential. Then, given sufficient time for complete restitution of the ensuing postextrasystole, all of the calcium (dotted and hatched) moves to the R compartment to be released and produce a very strong postextrasystole. Accordingly, a very strong beat is registered on the graph of the strength of fully restituted postextrasystoles expressed as a function of ESI (Fig. 8 far right). For very 'postmature' extrasystoles (with long ESI = b, bottom frame), the extrasystole is fully restituted because all of the hatched calcium has had time to reach the R compartment. Only a portion (F * R = small hatched slice) of the released calcium is resequestered to contribute to the ensuing postextrasystole. The dotted amount of calcium entering across the sarcolemma also adds to the U compartment on the extrasystole to contribute to the postextrasystole. Then, on the ensuing fully restituted postextrasystole, only a very small amount of calcium (hatched plus dotted slices) is released, resulting in a

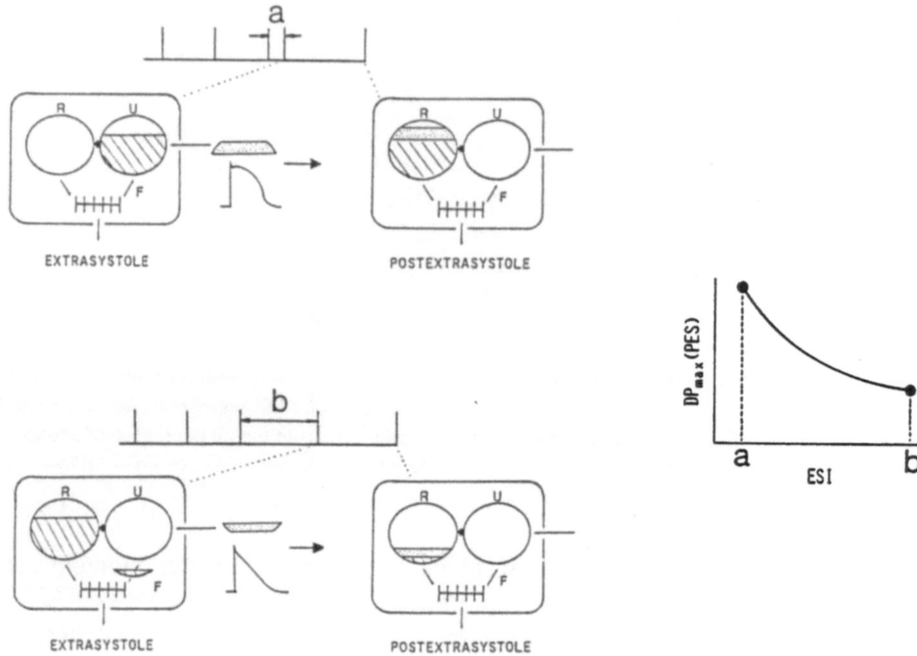

Figure 8. Cartoon of stimulation pulses and model cardiac cell (left), and plot of fully restituted strength of postextrasystoles as a function of ESI (right, known as 'postextrasystolic potentiation curve'). These illustrate the model concept of postextrasystolic potentiation, and the prediction that the plot at right should be a declining monoexponential function with time constant the same as for the mechanical restitution curve.

weak postextrasystole. Hence, a very small point is plotted on the graph at the right at ESI = b. Here, then, is the prediction: if the U and R compartments really 'conserve' calcium as we have been hypothesizing in this figure, a complete plot of the strength of fully restituted postextrasystoles vs. ESI (solid curve connecting the filled circles in Fig. 8, right) should be determined by the time course of the movement of calcium from U to R compartments. In other words, the solid curve in the figure should be a declining monoexponential, with time constant identical to that for restitution.

This second prediction also proved to be true, as illustrated by the results from isolated ferret papillary muscles shown in Figure 9. Restitution curves for extrasystoles, along with plots of the strength of fully restituted postextrasystoles expressed as a function of ESI, are shown (Panel A-D). Monoexponential functions were fit to the data, and the time constant for all of these curves were closely similar ($\simeq$700 ms) and statistically indistinguishable. The prediction also proved true in the isolated canine ventricle as well (Fig. 5 in [10]).

A third prediction of the model is that pharmacological interventions which render the SR incapable of contributing to the pool of activator calcium should

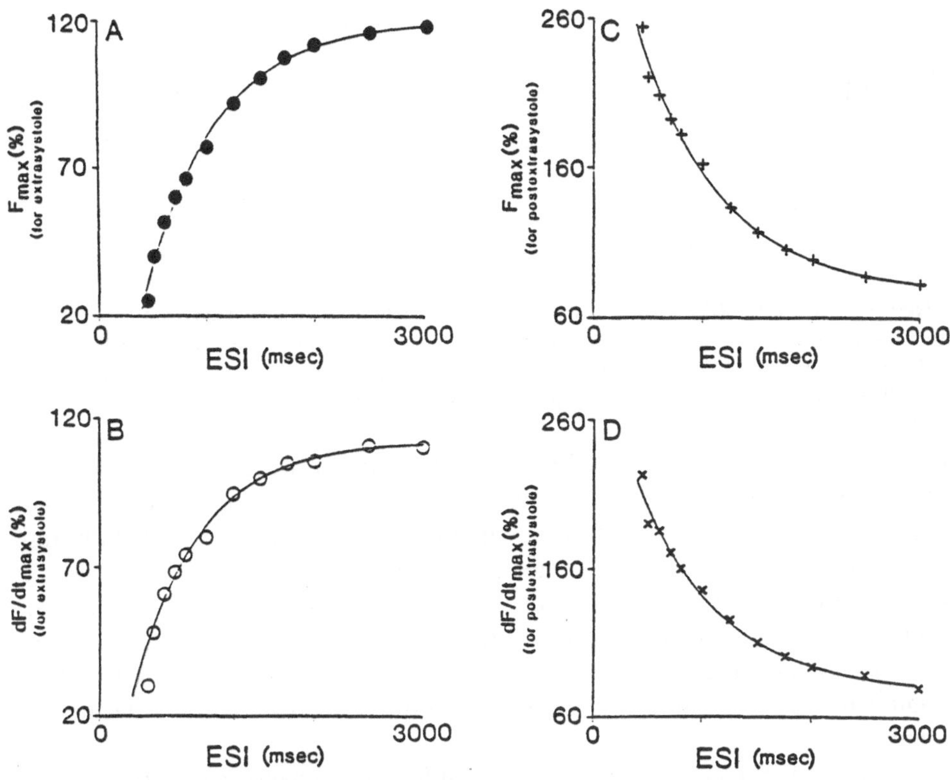

Figure 9. Restitution (A and B) and postextrasystolic potentiation (C and D) curves for peak tension (F_{max}) and peak rate of tension development (dF/dt_{max}), measured in an isometrically contracting, superfused ferret papillary muscle at 30° C. All responses have been normalized by their respective steady-state values and expressed as percentage. All postextrasystolic strengths are fully-restituted values. The continuous curves are best fitting monoexponential functions with time constant ranging between 626 and 753 ms. Adapted from [13].

accelerate restitution and abolish postextrasystolic potentiation. One such substance is ryanodine, a plant alkaloid believed to inhibit the release of calcium from SR [21]. If calcium release from SR is blocked, then in the steady state the SR can no longer take up calcium as well. Since contractions are still observed in muscle exposed to ryanodine, it must be that activator calcium is derived from calcium entry across the sarcolemma [13]. The time course of restitution would then reflect the very fast time course of recovery from inactivation of the sarcolemmal Ca channels (≃50 ms) [22]; thus, restitution in the presence of ryanodine should be greatly accelerated. Furthermore, the strength of postextrasystoles would reflect the magnitude of sarcolemmal Ca current during postextrasystoles. Given sufficient time to recover fully from inactivation, as would be the case for fully restituted postextrasystoles, Ca^{2+} conductance should not be a function of ESI; hence, the plot of the strength of fully restituted

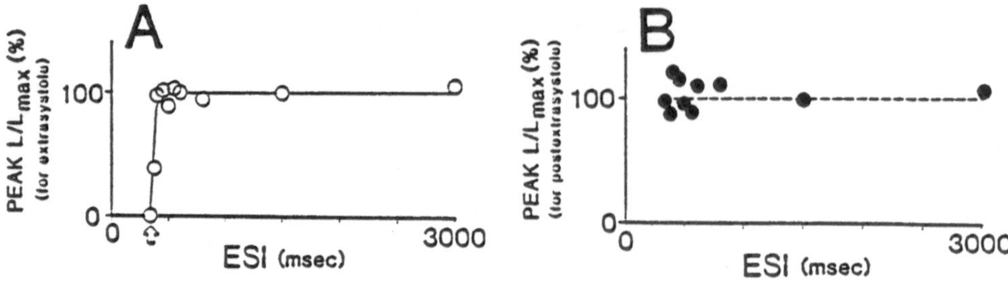

Figure 10. Restitution (A) and postextrasystolic potentiation (B) curves measured from an isometrically-contracting, superfused, ferret papillary muscle exposed to 5 μM ryanodine at 30° C. Curves were constructed from luminescence signals (L/L_{max}) derived from aequorin microinjected into the muscle. All postextrasystolic strengths are fully-restituted values.

postextrasystoles vs. ESI should be flat. These were precisely the observations made in isolated ferret papillary muscles [13]. These observations are displayed in Figure 10 which shows a restitution curve (Panel A) and strength of fully restituted postextrasystoles vs. ESI (Panel B) constructed with normalized aequorin luminescence (approximately proportional to $[Ca^{2+}]_i^{2.4}$). These show that restitution was essentially complete within the first 100 ms following the refractory period (A), and the postextrasystolic strength was independent of ESI (B). Similar results were obtained with exposure of rabbit papillary muscles to caffeine.

In summary, the monoexponential restitution phenomenon suggested to us an excitation-contraction coupling model, three of whose predictions appear to be holding up to experimental scrutiny.

Discussion: insight into restrictive cardiomyopathy in humans from the model of excitation-contraction coupling

Here we were able to use our model of excitation-contraction coupling to provide insight into a clinical disease known as restrictive cardiomyopathy (RCM) [11].

In restrictive cardiomyopathy, filling of the left ventricle is impeded by stiff diastolic pressure-volume characteristics, putatively due to fibrosis. Systolic function of the left ventricle is thought to be relatively intact. We had the fortune of studying restrictive cardiomyopathy in the explanted human heart of a heart transplant at the Johns Hopkins Hospital. Here we made the striking observation that the 'stiff' diastolic properties of the ventricle did not result from an altered diastolic pressure-volume relation relation per se, but rather was a reflection of slowed and therefore incomplete relaxation of active contraction due, apparently, to impaired SR function. One of the clues that suggested that SR function was impaired was that both the ventricle and trabecular muscle isolated from the ventricle failed to show postextrasystolic potentiation, just as the model would

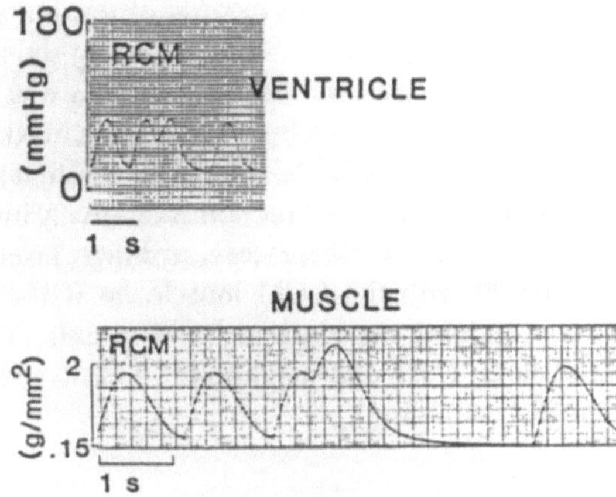

Figure 11. Original records of pressure (left) and tension (right) obtained from isovolumically contracting, blood-perfused, human left ventricle, and isometrically-contracting, superfused, human trabeculae from the same heart, respectively. The myocardium comes from a patient with restrictive cardiomyopathy (RCM). The records indicate an absence of postextrasystolic potentiation following the premature extrasystole.

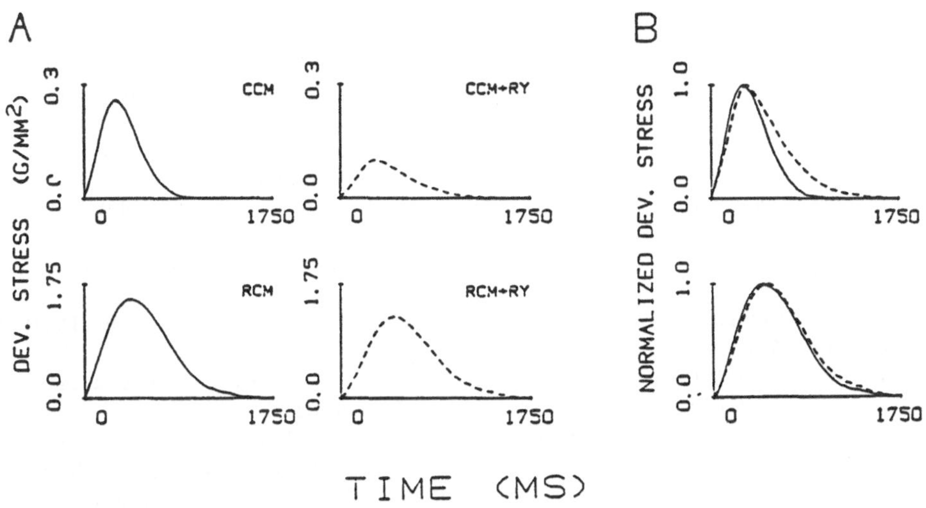

Figure 12. Records of tension obtained from congestive cardiomyopathic (CCM) and RCM human myocardium. Panel A shows tension wave forms before (solid curve) and after (dashed curve) exposure to 2 μM ryanodine (RY) for isometrically contracting, superfused CCM and RCM cardiac trabeculae, as labelled. Panel B replots the traces at left in Panel A after normalization for the same peak tension. These indicate the marked sensitivity of the time course of contraction to ryanodine in CCM, but not RCM muscle.

predict in Figure 10B. Figure 11 displays records of tension and pressure from RCM ventricle and muscle, respectively, demonstrating the absence of postextrasystolic potentiation. A second clue that SR function was impaired in RCM heart is shown in Fig. 12. Panel A shows traces of tension in RCM and congestive cardiomyopathic (CCM) trabeculae before and after (dashed lines in ryanodine) exposure to 2 μM ryanodine (RY) (SR function is relatively intact in CCM). The time course of contraction in the RCM muscle is strikingly insensitive to exposure to ryanodine as compared with the CCM muscle, as if the SR were already compromised before ryandoine exposure in RCM muscle. This observation is emphasized in Panel B in which the magnitude of contraction has been normalized (dashed lines in ryanodine).

Acknowledgment

We gratefully acknowledge the collaboration and support of Dr Daniel Burkhoff in the ventricular work, and that of Dr W. Gil Wier in the work with aequorin-injected papillary muscles. D.T. Yue was supported by Medical Scientist Training Program Grant 5T32GMO70309007. The work was supported by U.S. Public Health Service Research Grants RO1-HL-14903, HL-30552, and HL-29473-02.

References

1. Woodworth RS (1902): Maximal contraction, 'staircase' contraction, refractory period, and compensatory pause of the heart. Am J Physiol 8: 213–249.
2. Braveny P, Kruta B (1958): Dissociation de deux facteurs: Restitution et potentiation dans l'action de l'amplitude de la contraction du myocarde. Arch Int Physiol Biochim 66: 633–652.
3. Ebashi S, Endo M (1968): Calcium ion and muscle contraction. Prog Biophys Mol Biol 18: 123–183.
4. Wood EH, Heppner RL, Weidmann S (1969): Inotropic effects of electric currents. Circ Res 24: 409–445.
5. Allen DG, Kurihara S (1980): Calcium transients in mammalian ventricular muscle. Eur Heart J 1 (Suppl A): 5–15.
6. Wier WG (1980): Calcium transients during excitation-contraction coupling in mammalian heart: Aequorin signals of canine Purkinje fibers. Science 207: 1085–1087.
7. Tritthart H, Kaufmann R, Volkmer HP, Bayer R, Krause H (1973): Ca-movement controlling myocardial contractility. I. Voltage, current and time dependence of mechanical activity under voltage clamp conditions (cat papillary muscles and trabeculae). Pflügers Archiv 338: 207–231.
8. Edmand KAP, Johannsson M (1976): The contractile state of rabbit papillary muscle in relation to stimulation frequency. J Physiol (London) 254: 565–581.
9. Wohlfart B (1979): Relationship between peak force, action potential duration and stimulus interval in rabbit myocardium. Acta Physiol Scand 106: 395–409.
10. Yue DT, Burkhoff D, Franz MR, Hunter WC, Sagawa K (1985): Postextrasystolic potentiation of the isolated canine left ventricle: Relationship to mechanical restitution. Circ Res 56: 340–350.
11. Burkhoff D, Yue DT, Oikawa RY, Flaherty JT, Herskowitz A, Franz MR, Steward S,

Baumgartner WA, Schaefer J, Reitz BA, Sagawa K (1984): Insights into the pathophysiology of cardiomyopathy from studies of isolated supported human hearts (Abstract). Circulation 70 (Suppl II): 46.

12. Burkhoff D, Yue DT, Franz MR, Hunter WC, Sagawa K (1984): Mechanical restitution of isolated perfused canine left ventricles. Am J Physiol 246: H8–H16.
13. Wier WG, Yue DT (1986): Intracellular calcium transients underlying the short-term force-interval relationship in ferret ventricular myocardium. J Physiol (London) 376: 507–530.
14. Braveny P, Sumbera J, Kruta V (1966): Aftercontractions and restitution of contractility in the isolated guinea pig auricle. Arch Int Physiol Bioch 74: 169–178.
15. Fabiato A (1983): Calcium-induced release of calcium from cardiac sarcoplasmic reticulum. Am J Physiol 245: C1–C14.
16. Antoni H (1977): Elementary events in excitation-contraction coupling of the mammalian myocardium. Basic Res Cardiol 72: 140–146.
17. Trautwein W, McDonald TF, Tripathi O (1975): Calcium conductance and tension in mammalian ventricular muscle. Pflügers Archiv 534: 55–74.
18. Morad M, Goldman Y (1973): Excitation-contraction coupling in heart muscle: Membrane control of development of tension. Prog Biophys Mol Biol 27: 257–313.
19. Fabiato A (1981): Myoplasmic free calcium concentration reached during the twitch of an intact isolated cardiac cell and during calcium-induced release of calcium from the sarcoplasmic reticulum of a skinned cardiac cell from the adult rat or rabbit ventricle. J Gen Physiol 78: 457–497.
20. Yue DT, Marban E, Wier WG (1986): Relationship between force and intracellular [Ca^{2+}] in tetanized mammalian heart muscle. J Gen Physiol 87: 223–242.
21. Sutko JL, Kenyon JL (1983): Ryanodine modification of cardiac muscle responses to potassium-free solutions. Evidence for inhibition of sarcoplasmic reticulum release. J Gen Physiol 82: 385–404.
22. Kass RS, Sanguinetti MC (1984): Inactivation of calcium channel current in the calf cardiac Purkinje fiber. J Gen Physiol 84: 705–726.

Discussion

Beyar: How could the model that you presented account for the interspecies difference in the force-interval relationship? It is well known that different species behave differently in their force interval relationship: the rat heart and the dog heart are different. How can these models account for these differences?
Yue: The model that I presented is for a particular case of what we saw in the rabbit, the ferret and the dog. The rat is very different and one might explain it by changing what we call the recirculation fraction. This is one of the parameters in the model; it is the fraction of the calcium that is released and is taken up again, and not pumped out of the cell in that beat. As per the suggestion of Dr Wohlfart in a 1982 paper, if you make the recirculation fraction very high, the two compartment model that I have presented behaves somewhat like the rat.
Sonnenblick: One of the things that has always been very strange is that if you look at time to peak tension for the duration of the contraction, it is really quite fixed in the rabbit, and that is why your rate of force development and force are tightly coupled. Yet, in the rat the dP/dt does not change very much and the time to peak is variable; in the others you get a mixture between the two, so that the time to peak tension can also change from beat to beat, depending on the interval duration. You could change your model around to get two separate variables taking place: control of duration and control of greater tension development. Could you get an exponential relation between the two, depending on which is the variable that is modified in that particular species?
Yue: That is a very beautiful question. What turns out is that, as a rough approximation, there is not so much change in time to peak tension with the restitution protocol, in the rabbit, dog or ferret.Thus, peak tension and peak dF/dt show linear relationship. But in fact there are conditions where you can dissociate the two very distinctly, and we can show the change in this transient relationship between calcium and tension.
Sonnenblick: Some potential explanations have been offered. The dominant ones would be the rate of return from the longitudinal SR, the uptake site, to return it to the releasable site until there is that interchange. This is one of the governing things that Dr Yue is talking about. The other point is the reactivation time constant that Dr Wong will be talking about. Those two totally separate mechanisms offer you a great opportunity for species variation as well. Unfortunately, this indicates weakness of modelling as you can not tell how much is which, and that is why we need more experimental evidence.
Winegrad: In any model you get down to molecular basis for this. Most of the calcium in the reticulum is bound to calsequestrin and what you are dealing with then is the release of calcium. So if you have different counts of calsequestrin properties, as is actually known in different species, you would expect to have a different rate constant for releases of calcium. You can get data from the literature, because there are equilibrium constants available for binding the

counts of calsequestrin in different species. I would like to make a comment, again on a molecular basis. Three different kinds of studies indicate the release of calcium from the sarcoplastic reticulum is not a simple function of the amount of calcium in the reticulum, but the calcium in the reticulum seems to be in two forms; a releasable form and a non-releasable form. It appears that the capacity of those two are about similar. You can release up to about 50% of the total calcium and the amount that you release is the fraction of how much of the calcium above about 50% is present. That fits in very well with your model. There are semi-quantitative data to try and test this phenomena.

Yue: This gets back to the question of why calcium transients are so far ahead of the tension and what is the best way to relate fluctuating calcium to a developing tension. I'll say that there is roughly a linear relation between calcium released and peak $[Ca^{2+}]_i$. There is also a linear relation between peak calcium and peak rate of rise in tension. Further, under the conditions that I encountered, the shape of the calcium transient does not change so much so that peak force also tracks peak dF/dt. My feeling is that the truer relationship is really between calcium and peak dF/dt, and it is only by the fortutious nature of the fact that the calcium transient's shape does not change much that peak force is roughly linear to dF/dt. Here is an example where we have disassociated the change in dF/dt from the change in force. Consider Panel A*. You have tension, dF/dt, and estimated calcium from a control twitch. If you take this same muscle and expose it to ryanodine, you have tension, dF/dt, and calcium, but you slowed down the calcium transient tremendously and slowed down the time course of contraction. You see that peak tension is pretty high there, almost as high as in the control, but peak calcium and peak dF/dt go down. Thus there is a tighter correlation between peak calcium and peak dF/dt than between peak tension and peak calcium. So studies where people try to infer from a plot of peak force versus peak calcium whether there is a change in myofilament sensitivity are really not the best way to look at myofilament sensitivity. Now consider points on a line from extra-systoles, post-extra-systoles, and different steady-state frequencies of pacing. From these beats, it looks like there is a pretty tight correlation between peak calcium and peak force. When you add the ryanodine to slow the calcium transient way down, you get values which are way off the relationship, so that you might infer that there is some change in the calcium sensitivity of the myofilaments. In fact, if you look at a plot of dF/dt_{max} versus peak calcium, all those relationships, the slow one with ryanodine as well as for all the different sorts of pacing, fall on one relationship.

Sonnenblick: Still it will not work for the rat as the dF/dt stays the same and force goes down. I am not sure how that translates for the rat. The rat is always a special case.

Yue: The case where peak $[Ca^{2+}]_i$ remains constant, but the time course of the $[Ca^{2+}]_i$ transient decreases, may explain the situation in the rat.

* Fig. 8 in Yue, DT (1987): Intracellular $[Ca^{2+}]$ related to rate of force development in twitch contraction of heart. Am J Physiol 252 (in press).

17. Model of Ca release mechanism from the sarcoplasmic reticulum: Ca-mediated activation, inactivation and reactivation

A.Y.K. WONG, A. FABIATO and J.B. BASSINGTHWAIGHTE

Abstract

A model is developed to elucidate the mechanism of Ca release from the sarcoplasmic reticulum (SR) in cardiac cells. This model assumes that an increase of Ca^{2+} concentration at the outer surface (Ca_c) of the SR surface activates and inactivates this surface, triggering the release of Ca to the sarcoplasmic space from the 'releasable terminal' (RT) of the SR. The RT in turn is further activated and also inactivated by the increase of the sarcoplasmic Ca^{2+} (Ca_{sp}). The Ca^{2+} in the sarcoplasmic space is removed by the longitudinal SR (LSR). During the release process, Ca_e enters the SR by diffusion and bound by the binding substance. Free Ca^{2+} is released from the bound Ca. Both the free Ca from SR and LSR are transferred to the RT for subsequent release. After release, the rate and degree of reactivation of the RT is determined by Ca_c and Ca_{sp}. The activation, inactivation and reactivation obey Hodkin-Huxley kinetics.

The proposed model simulates the following events quantitatively similar to those observed in skinned Purkinje cell: cyclic release; Ca release at different concentration and rate of increase of trigger Ca^{2+}; effect of increasing trigger Ca^{2+} during the ascending and descending phase of Ca release; positive and negative staircase; removal of inactivation and the rate of inactivation of Ca^{2+} release from the SR.

Introduction

Excitation-contraction coupling (ECC) is an important process linking the electrical to the mechanical activity of cardiac muscle. Without an understanding of the sequence of events involved in ECC, it is difficult to elucidate the change of myocardial function either on a beat-to-beat basis in normal tissue or any basis in diseased tissue.

In most mammalian cardiac muscle, the activation of myofilaments requires

Ca^{2+}. The sources of Ca are:
1. the slow inward current, (I_s), mainly carried by Ca ion;
2. the calcium released from the sarcoplasmic reticulum (SR).

Fabiato and Fabiato [1, 2], using skinned cardiac cells, demonstrated a Ca-induced Ca release mechanism in SR. The contraction varied in size according to the quantity of the triggering Ca, suggesting that the Ca produced an amplifying effect.

Based on Fabiato's concept of Ca-induced Ca release, ECC models have been proposed [3–5]. The sequence of events proposed by these models are described in the following.

Upon excitation, Ca ions (I_s) enter the cell to the sarcoplasmic space surrounding the myofilaments. The increase of sarcoplasmic [Ca^{2+}] induces the release of Ca^{2+} from the SR, leading to the activation of the myofilaments and the development of the tension.

While these models are successful in simulating the voltage-current-tension relation [3, 4], strength-interval relationship [4, 5], they cannot explain the new experimental findings of Ca release in skinned Purkinje cell [6–8]. In addition, the past models are not able to explain the change in electrical and contractile events occurring in hypoxia in cardiac muscle [9, 10].

Fabiato's recent experimental data [6–8] clearly indicate that the activation and inactivation of the release mechanism is Ca-mediated. For this reason, we propose a model based on Fabiato's findings not only to elucidate the Ca release mechanism from the SR, but also to delineate the sequence of events involved in excitation-contraction coupling of mammalian cardiac muscle.

Assumptions of the proposed model

1. Upon excitation, Ca^{2+} ions (Ca current) enters the appositional space between the sarcolemma and the sarcoplasmic reticulum (SR).
2. The outer surface of the SR is activated and inactivated by the rapid increase of [Ca^{2+}] in the appositional space (Ca_c). The activation and inactivation are characterized by p(t), q(t) and $\bar{X}$ (t) which obeys the Hodgkin-Huxley kinetics and are functions of Ca_c.
3. Ca^{2+} enters the SR by diffusion and is bound by the binding substance in SR. The bound Ca releases free Ca^{2+} (Ca_f). The rate of free Ca released in SR is governed by the scheme of Bassingthwaighte and Reuter [11]. The exit of free Ca^{2+} out of SR (efflux) into the appositional space is by an exchange scheme of Wong and Bassingthwaighte [12].
4. The [free Ca^{2+}] in SR, i.e. Ca_f, is transferred to the 'releasable terminal' (RT), which differs from the SR only functionally. The rate of transfer is dependent on the apparent diffusion coefficient which is a function of the [free Ca^{2+}] in SR.
5. The release threshold in the releasable terminal is concentration-dependent [4,

13]. This assumption is based on the experimental data of Solaro [14] and the concept of fractional release hypothesis [1, 2].
6. The activation, inactivation and reactivation of the releasable terminal also obey the Hodgkin-Huxley kinetics. They are characterized by d(t), f(t) and x(t), being functions of the sarcoplasmic [Ca^{2+}].
7. Removal of sarcoplasmic Ca^{2+} is achieved by the longitudinal SR (LSR) which transfers the Ca to RT for subsequent release. The transfer rate is also dependent on the apparent diffusion coefficient which is a function of LSR [Ca^{2+}].

Description of the calcium movement in the model

The schematic diagram of the model is shown in Fig. 1. At resting state, the outer surface of the SR is inactivated, while the surface of the releasable terminal is slightly activated, but no Ca^{2+} is released. When the [Ca^{2+}] in the appositional space (Ca_e) increases, the outer surface of the SR is activated, Ca is released from RT, resulting in an increase of sarcoplasmic Ca^{2+}, i.e. Ca_{sp}. The elevation of Ca_{sp} further activates the RT surface, thus releasing more Ca. As the [Ca^{2+}] in RT is reduced, the release threshold increases, causing a reduction in the rate of release. The first contraction is, therefore, due to the initial [Ca^{2+}] in the releasable terminal.

At the time when Ca is being released from the RT, the free Ca in the SR is increased due to the diffusion of Ca^{2+} from the appositional space and the dissociation of Ca-binding substance complex (CaB). Part of the Ca_f is extruded into the appositional space through a Ca-Ca exchange (J_{ioCa}), and part of it is transferred to the RT. The LSR removes the Ca from sarcoplasmic space by an active process (J_{pump}) and transfers the Ca to the RT with a time constant of τ_{LSR}. The free Ca from SR and LSR becomes available for subsequent release.

Calcium variation within the cell

Based on the assumptions and the calcium movements shown in Fig 1, the following equations are formulated to describe the calcium variation within the cell.

Calcium concentration in the appositional space (Ca_e)

$$dCa_e/dt = J_{in} - J_{out} + (J_{ioCa} + J_{io}), \tag{1}$$

where J_{in} = calcium influx, J_{out} = calcium efflux, J_{ioCa} = calcium efflux from SR to appositional space, and J_{io} = calcium efflux from RT to appositional space.

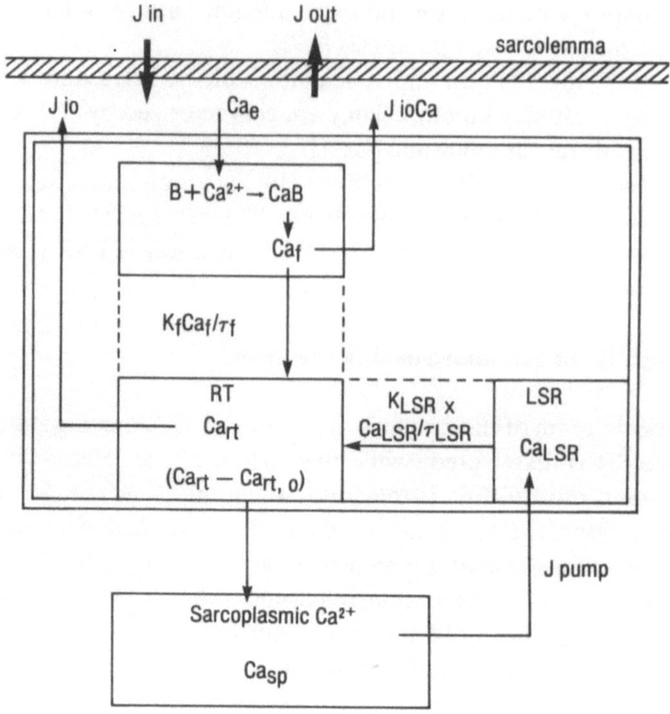

Figure 1. Schematic diagram of the model. The sarcoplasmic reticulum (SR) comprises of: a calcium binding region into which free Ca^{2+} entering from appositional space (Ca_e) by diffusion is bound by the binding substance B; a releasable terminal (RT) releasing Ca^{2+} to the sarcoplasmic space; the longitudinal SR sequesters Ca^{2+} from the sarcoplasmic space. Free Ca(Ca_f) from the binding region and from LSR(Ca_{LSR}) are transferred to the RT with time constants of τ_f and τ_{LSR}. J_{in} and J_{out} are the trans-sarcoleminal influx and efflux respectively. J_{ioCa}, J_{io} are Ca-Ca exchange between Ca_e and Ca_f, Ca_e and Ca^{2+} in RT (Ca_{rt}). Ca_{sp} is the sarcoplasmic Ca^{2+}.

In the case of skinned cell, the calcium sink is infinite; all efflux terms become insignificant. Therefore,

$$dCa_e/dt = J_{in}.$$

Free calcium concentration in SR (Ca_f)

$$\left.\begin{aligned} dCa_f/dt &= -K_1B \cdot Ca_f + K_2Ca \cdot B + J_{net}, \\ -dB/dt &= K_1B \cdot Ca_f - K_2Ca \cdot B, \end{aligned}\right\} \tag{2}$$

and

$$J_{net} = D(Ca_e - Ca_f) - J_{ioCa} - K_{fCaf}/\tau_f,$$

where B = concentration of binding substance, D = diffusion coefficient, and τ_f = time constant associated with the transfer process.

Binding is assumed at all times essentially at an equilibrium;

$$Ca_f \cdot B/Ca \cdot B = K_2/K_1 = K_a, \tag{3}$$

where K_a is a dissociation constant. Taking derivatives of (3) and substituting in (2) gives:

$$\frac{dCa_f}{dt} = J_{net}\left\{\frac{(K_a + Ca_f)^2}{(K_a + Ca_f)^2 + B_tK_a}\right\}, \tag{4}$$

where B_t is the total concentration of the binding substance, free and bound.

Calcium concentration in the releasable terminal (Ca_{rt})

$$\frac{dCa_{rt}}{dt} = K_fCa_f/\tau_f - \bar{g}_{Ca}p(t) \cdot q(t) \cdot r(t) \ [Ca_{rt} - Ca_{rt,o}] +$$

$$K_{LSR}Ca_{LSR}/\tau_{LSR} - J_{io}, \tag{5}$$

where

$$r(t) = d(t) \cdot f(t) - \bar{X}(t)x(t)$$
$$= 0 \text{ when } < 0.$$

The parameters p, g, d, f, $\bar{X}$, x are governed by the first order kinetic equation:

$$y(t) + t_y dy/dt = y_\infty;\ y = p, q, d, f, \bar{X}, x.$$

The steady state parameters p_∞, q_∞, $\bar{X}_\infty$ and the time constants τ_p, τ_q and τ_x. are function of Ca_e. Both τ_p and τ_q are also influenced by the rate of change of Ca_c, i.e.

$$\alpha = |dCa_e/dt|.$$

Thus:

$$\tau_p(\alpha, Ca_e) = \tau_p(Ca_e)/\alpha,$$
$$\tau_q(\alpha, Ca_e) = \alpha\tau_q(Ca_e).$$

The parameters d_∞, f_∞, x_∞ and the time constant τ_d, τ_f and τ_x are function of the sarcoplasmic calcium concentration.

The release threshold $C_{rt,\,o}$ is given by

$$Ca_{rt,\,o} = Ca_{rt}/\{1 + (Ca_{rt}/Ca_{ss})^{6(Ca_{ss}/Ca_{rt})}\},$$

where Ca_{ss} is constant.

The above equation indicates that the threshold is inversely related to the calcium concentration in the RT. As Ca_{rt} increases, the threshold is reduced. This equation is derived to fit the experimental data of Solaro and Briggs [14] and Solaro et al. [15] and to meet the requirements of mechanical alternans [13].

Calcium concentration in the sarcoplasmic space (Ca_{sp})

$$dCa_{sp}/dt = \bar{g}_{Ca}\, p(t) \cdot q(t) \cdot r(t)\, [Ca_{rt} - Ca_{rt,\,o}] - J_{pump}, \tag{6}$$

where

$$J_{pump} = \frac{x(t)V_{max}Ca^2_{sp}}{(K_m + Ca^2_{sp})} + \frac{f(t)V'_{max}Ca_{sp}}{K'_m + Ca_{sp}}.$$

As x(t) in the J_{pump} expression is a slow-varying function, Ca uptake by LSR starts near the end of Ca release. The second term accounts for the removal of Ca during relaxation phase of the cell.

Calcium concentration in longitudinal sarcoplasmic reticulum

$$dCa_{LSR}/dt = J_{pump} - K_{LSR}Ca_{LSR}/\tau_{LSR}. \tag{7}$$

Calcium efflux

J_{ioCa} is a Ca – Ca exchange between the free Ca_f and Ca_c. It is described as [12]

$$J_{ioCa} = \varphi(Na_o)\left[\frac{Ca_f}{k_1 + Ca_f}\right]\left[\frac{Ca_c}{k_2 + Ca_c}\right],$$

where $\varphi(Na_o)$ is a function [Na] in the appositional space; k, k_2 are constant. In this study, $k_1 = k_2 = 10\,\mu M$.

J_{io} is also a Ca – Ca exchange between Ca_{rt} and Ca_c. It is given as

$$J_{io} = K_{rt}\left[\frac{Ca_c}{10 + Ca_c}\right]\lambda(Ca_{rt}), \tag{8}$$

$$\lambda(Ca_{rt}) = \frac{1}{1 + \exp[2(8 - Ca_{rt})]}.$$

The function λ is an empirical, indicating that J_{io} is insignificant when Ca_{rt} is equal or below its resting value (4 μM), but increases exponentially with Ca_{rt} to prevent an unreasonable overloading of RT. The two time constants τ_f and τ_{LSR} associated with the transfer of Ca_f and Ca_{LSR} to the releasable terminal are assumed to be inversely proportional to the apparent diffusion coefficient for Ca. Based on the study of Safford and Bassingthwaighte [17], the apparent diffusion coefficient is related to the degree of binding of Ca^{2+} by the binding substance. Thus:

$$\tau_{LSR}, \tau_f \propto \left[\frac{(K_a + Ca_i)^2 + B_t K_a}{(K_a + Ca_i)^2}\right], \quad Ca_i = Ca_f, Ca_{LSR}. \tag{9}$$

Results

All model responses presented in this study were simulated by using the same set of steady state kinetic parameters and time constants as well as the following numerical constants:

Resting Ca_c, Ca_f, Ca_{sp}, $Ca_{LSR} = 0.0178\,\mu M$;
Resting $Ca_{rt} = 4\,\mu M$; $Ca_{ss} = 2\,\mu M$;
$D = 0.005/ms; \varphi(Na_o) = 0.5\,\mu M/ms$;
$K_f = 0.0052$; $K_{LSR} = 0.005$; $K_{rt} = 12.5\,\mu M/ms$; $K_m = 100\,\mu M^2$; $K'_m = 100\,\mu M$;
$\bar{g} = 0.2/ms$; V_{max}, $V'_{max} = 0.5\,\mu M/ms$;
$B_t = 50\,\mu M$, $K_a = 0.14$.

The above numerical values are chosen to produce an optimal performance of the model. The only variable in the model is the Ca^{2+} concentration at the outer surface of the SR and is empirically described by

$$Ca_c(t) = Ca_m\,[1 - \exp(-\alpha t)], \tag{10}$$

where Ca_m is the maximal Ca^{2+} concentration in μM and α is the rate (0.2/ms).

Kinetic parameters and time constants

Figure 2 depicts the steady state parameters as function of trigger Ca^{2+} and sarcoplasmic Ca^{2+}. The time constants as function of pCa is shown in Fig. 3. These functions are chosen after trial and error, and able to produce results qualitatively similar to those observed experimentally. It should be noted that $\bar{X}_\infty$

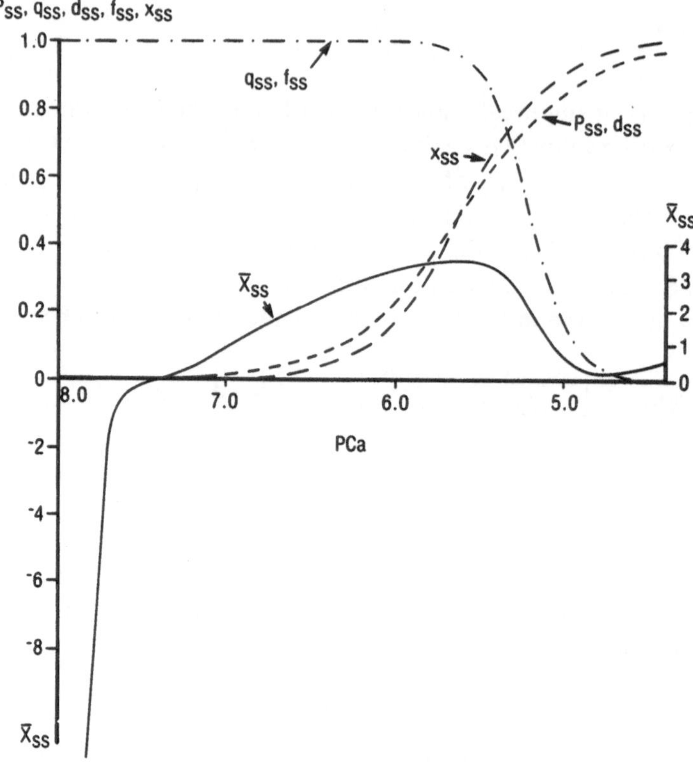

Figure 2. The steady state values for the activation (q_∞) and inactivation (p_∞, $\bar{X}$) parameters as functions of pCa at the outer SR surface. The activation (d_∞) and inactivation (f_∞, x_∞) parameters for the RT are function of pCa of the sarcoplasmic space.

can be considered as equivalent to $\hat{i}_{x1}$ in the action potential model of Beeler and Reuter [16].

Effect of increasing trigger Ca^{2+}

Figure 4 shows the effect of increasing the trigger Ca^{2+} (i.e. Ca_c) during the ascending and descending phase of the sarcoplasmic and Ca transient. An increase of Ca_c from 0.63 μM to 3.10 μM triggers additional Ca release from the releasable terminal due to a further increase of p(t)q(t), while $\bar{X}$ (t)x(t) is still small because of its slow-varying nature. During descending phase, $\bar{X}(t) \cdot x(t)$ has become significant; $(f \cdot d - \bar{X} \cdot x)$ is negative, the release threshold is elevated due to the reduction of Ca_{rt}. No Ca is released despite an increase of $p(t) \cdot q(t)$. However, when the high trigger Ca^{2+} is maintained at the outer surface of SR, a spontaneous Ca^{2+} release occurs after a delay (Fig. 5). Within the time delay, $\bar{X}(t) \cdot x(t)$ has decayed and the free Ca in SR is greatly increased. The free Ca from

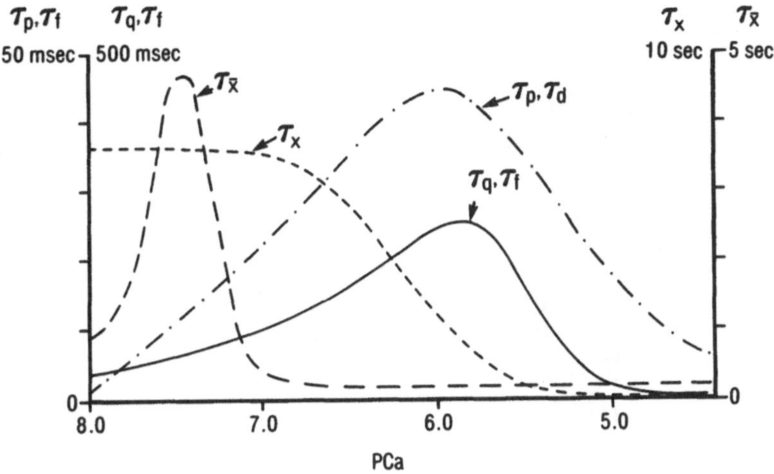

Figure 3. Time constants τ_p, τ_q, and $\tau_{\bar{x}}$ are functions of pCa of the outer SR surface; τ_f, τ_d, and τ_x are function of pCa of the sarcoplasmic space.

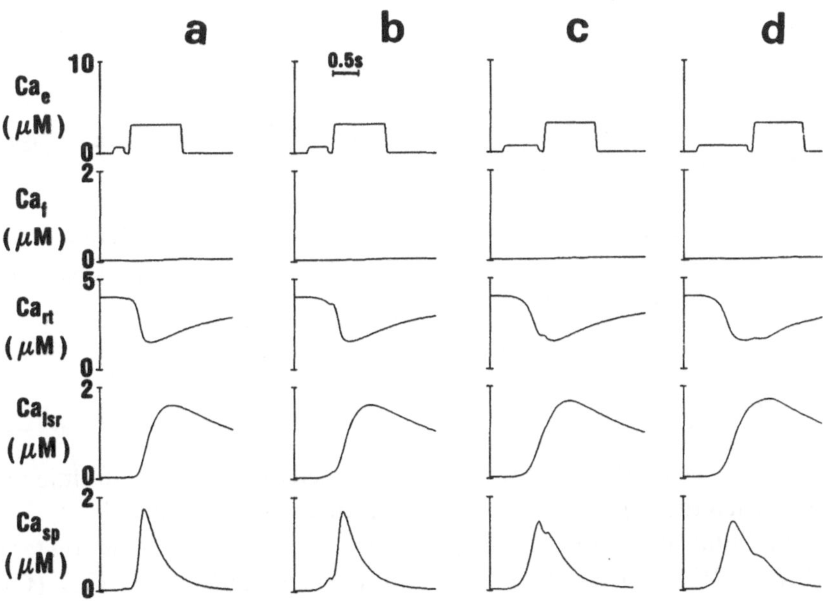

Figure 4. The model's response to the increase of trigger Ca^{2+} (Ca_e) at the outer SR surface from 1.0 μM to 6.3 μM during the ascending (a, b) and descending (c, d) phase of the Ca^{2+} transient in the sarcoplasmic space Ca_f is the free Ca^{2+} in the binding region of the SR, Ca_{rt} is the $[Ca^{2+}]$ in the releasable terminal, Ca_{LSR} is the $[Ca^{2+}]$ in the longitudinal SR and Ca_{sp}, the $[Ca^{2+}]$ in the sarcoplasmic space.

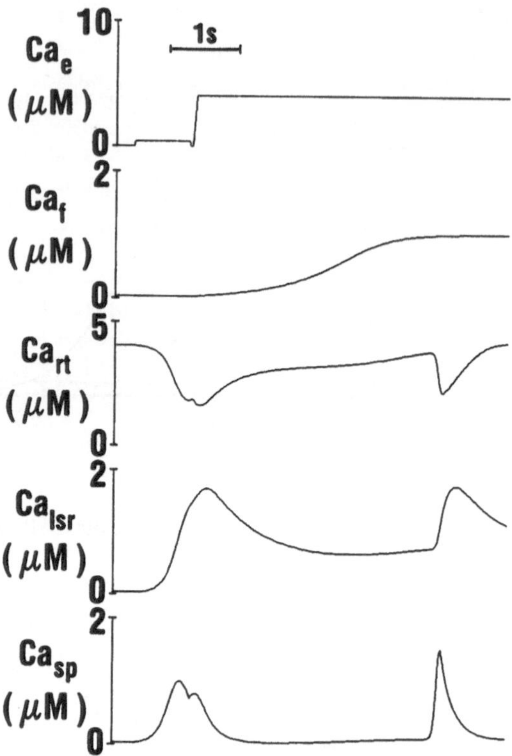

Figure 5. Model's response to the effect of increasing trigger Ca^{2+} transient. When the high Ca_e is maintained, a spontaneous Ca release occurs after a delay.

SR and LSR are transferred to fill and load the releasable terminal, thus reducing the release threshold. When the value of $p \cdot q(f \cdot d - \bar{X} \cdot x)$ $(Ca_{rt} - Ca_{rt.\,o})$ is just greater than zero, Ca^{2+} is released.

Cyclic release

Cyclic release of Ca from SR of skinned cardiac cell of rat [1] and Purkinje cell [7, 8] occurs when the trigger Ca^{2+} above a critical level is maintained.

The amplitude and frequency of the cyclic release depends on the trigger Ca^{2+} level (Fig. 6). With a trigger Ca^{2+} of 1.0 μM, the peak sarcoplasmic Ca^{2+} (Ca_{sp}) is 1.7 μM with a cycle period of 13.7 second. A trigger Ca^{2+} of 6.3 μM gives a peak Ca_{sp} of 1.6 μM and a period of 2.4 second. The underlying mechanism of cyclic release is the same as that in Fig. 5.

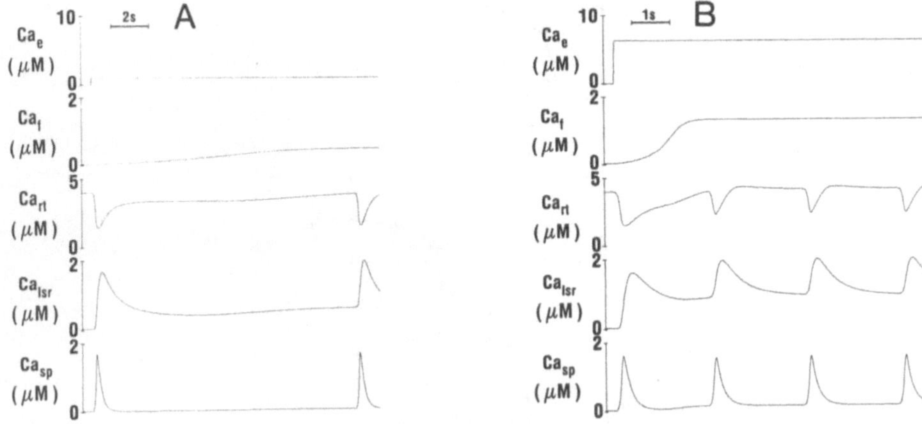

Figure 6. Simulated cyclic release of Ca at constant trigger Ca^{2+} (Ca_e). The cycle period is 13.7 sec at $Ca_e = 1.0\,\mu M$ in (A) and 2.4 sec at 6.3 μM in (B).

Effect of concentration and the rate of increase of trigger Ca^{2+} (Ca_e) on Ca release

The bell-shaped relationship between the trigger Ca^{2+} and peak sarcoplasmic Ca^{2+} (Fig. 7) is due to the activation q and inactivation p of the outer SR surface. This mechanism is equivalent to the kinetics of Ca current. The effect of the rate on Ca release is based on the assumption that the time constants of inactivation τ_p (pCa_e) and activation τ_q (pCa_e) are also determined by the rate (α) of rise of Ca_e, i.e. $\tau_p(\alpha, pCa_e) = \tau_p(Ca_e)/\alpha$, $\tau_q(\alpha, pCa_e) = \alpha\tau_q(pCa_e)$.

When Ca_e is increased slowly (α is small), the outer SR surface is slowly activated, but rapidly inactivated. Meanwhile, $\bar{X}(t) \cdot x(t)$ increases, inactivating the releasable terminal. Consequently, little or no Ca is released. The trigger Ca^{2+} however, enters the SR, raising the free Ca(Ca_f) to be transferred to the releasable terminal for subsequent release.

Rate of inactivation and of removal of inactivation

Fabiato's experiments [7] to demonstrate the rate of inactivation and of removal of inactivation were mimicked. The model response, shown in Fig. 8, is qualitatively similar to the experimental results. According to the model, the simulated results reflect the nature of $\bar{X}_\infty(pCa_e)$ rather than $p_\infty(PCa_e)$. Since $\bar{X}(t) \cdot x(t)$ is a slow-varying function, its value slowly decreases toward zero in 24 seconds before next triggering. When pCa_e of 7.9 is introduced at variable delay (τ) from the next triggering, $\bar{X}$ at the end of τ is:

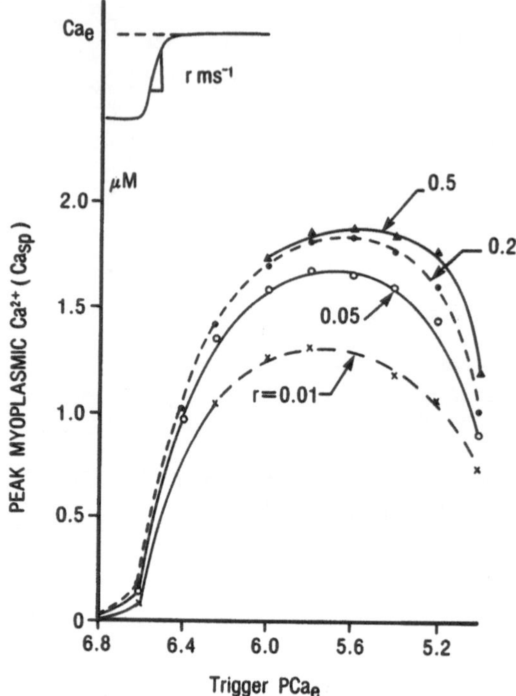

Figure 7. The relation between the pCa of the rate of rise of trigger Ca and the peak Ca^{2+} in the sarcoplasmic space. The number indicates the rate constant (r) of $Ca_e = Ca_m[1 - \exp(-rt)]$; the larger the number, the faster is the increase of Ca_e.

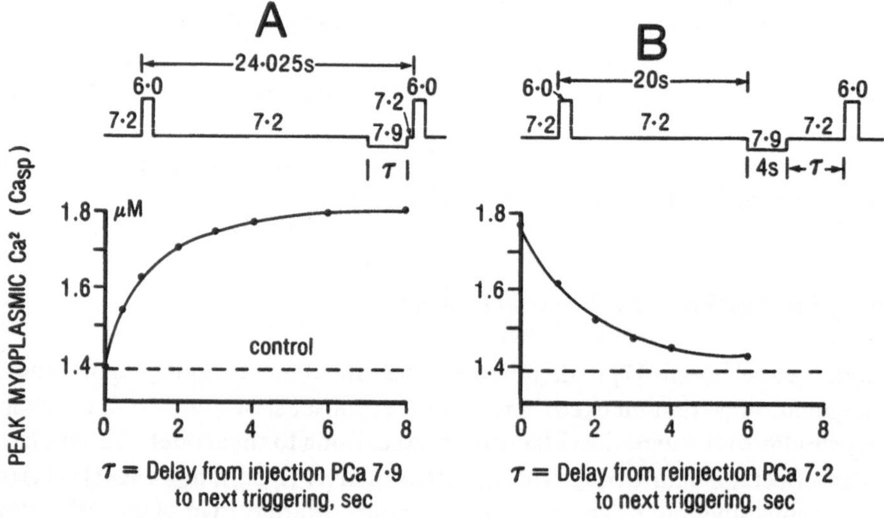

Figure 8. The simulated protocol (upper panel) and the model's results (lower panel) demonstrating the rate of removal of inactivation (A) and the rate of inactivation (B). The duration of trigger Ca at pCa = 6.0 is 500 ms.

$$\bar{X}(\tau) = \bar{X}_\infty(7.9) - [\bar{X}_\infty(7.9) - \bar{X}_\infty(24-\tau)]\exp(-\tau).$$

The activation of the releasable terminal $[f \cdot d - \bar{X}(\tau)x(\tau)]$ becomes positive as $\bar{X}_\infty$ (7.9) is negative. In other words, before next triggering, the releasable terminal is significantly activated, resulting larger amount of Ca released. The steady state peak sarcoplasmic Ca^{2+} in Fig. 8A represents the magnitude of $\bar{X}_\infty$ (7.9), and the rate, the time constant $\tau_{\bar{X}}$ (7.9).

Based on the model scheme, the rate of decay in Fig. 8B is a measure of the time constant $\tau_{\bar{X}}$ (7.2).

Discussion

In many aspects, the kinetics of the proposed Ca release mechanism is similar to that of cardiac action potential [16]. The kinetic parameters p, q, f and d can be considered equivalent to the activation and inactivation of inward currents $\bar{X} \cdot x$, the outward current. The rate of Ca released from the releasable terminal given as

$$\bar{g}Ca\,[\cdot p \cdot q(f \cdot d - \bar{X} \cdot x]\,[Ca_{rt} - Ca_{rt,\,o}]$$

differs little conceptually from the kinetics of ionic current: $I = g(E - E_r)$, in which g is the conductance and $(E - E_r)$, the driving force. The first term of the Ca release equation is equivalent to conductance, the second term, the driving force. The equilibrium potential E_r for Ca ions is not constant, but decreases with increasing intracellular Ca^{2+}. The release threshold also decreases with increasing Ca^{2+} in RT.

The expression for the J_{pump}, despite its empirical nature, has its physiological function. As x(t) is slow-varying and its value is small when Ca is being released, Ca uptake is not significant, thus allowing the increase of sarcoplasmic Ca^{2+} at a faster rate to activate the myofilaments. Near the end of release, x(t) has become relatively large, the sarcoplasmic Ca^{2+} is high, the Ca uptake is accelerated. This is an agreement with the experimental observation [7] that Ca uptake starts at the end of the release.

The delay of Ca uptake is physiologically meaningful. If release and uptake occurred simultaneously, more Ca^{2+} had to be released than necessary in order to be sufficient to activate the myofilaments; energy expenditure would be greater to keep the uptake process operating all the time.

An alternative and realistic scheme for J_{pump} is:

$$J_{pump} = K_{ATP}\,ATP \cdot Ca_{sp}^2 - K_{ADP}\,P_i \cdot ADP \cdot Ca_{LSR}^2$$

In this equation, ATP promotes Ca uptake while ADP, P_i inhibit it. If ATP is depleted early such as during hypoxia, or if there is an accumulation of P_i and ADP such as during moderate or severe hypoxia, the Ca accumulation by the LSR and the transport of Ca to the releasable terminal will be depressed. However, the variation of ATP, P_i and ADP with time on beat-to-beat basis is not clear.

Despite that the steady state kinetic parameters and the time constants are 'guessed' or speculated, the model is able to simulate many events qualitatively similar to those observed experimentally [6–8]. The kinetic parameters should be determined more realistically. The amplitudes and rate of rise of aequorin light data vs. trigger pCa [6, 7] can provide clues for estimating p, q, d, f, and their associated τ's. The $\bar{X}$, x and τ_x can be estimated from the periodicity and amplitude of the cycle release.

The aequorin data of loading SR with slow increasing or high trigger Ca and its subsequent release also provides clues for diffusion across the outer SR membrane and the Ca transfer process to the releasable terminal.

Acknowledgment

This work was supported by an MRC Program Grant and a grant from Nova Scotia Heart Foundation.

References

1. Fabiato A, Fabiato F (1975): Contractions induced by a calcium-triggered release of calcium from the sarcoplasmic reticulum of single skinned cardiac cell. J Physiol 249: 469–495.
2. Fabiato A, Fabiato F (1977): Calcium release from the sarcoplasmic reticulum. Circ Res 40: 119–129.
3. Kaufmann R, Bayar R, Furness T, Krause H, Tritthart H (1974): Calcium movement controlling cardiac contractility II. Analog computation of cardiac excitation-contraction coupling on the basis of calcium kinetics in multicompartment model. J Mol Cell Cardiol 6: 545–560.
4. Wong AYK (1981): A model of excitation contraction coupling of mammalian cardiac muscle. J Theor Biol 90: 37–61.
5. Adler D, Wong AYK, Mahler Y, Klassen GA (1985): Model of calcium movements in the mammalian myocardium: in interval-strength relationship. J Theor Biol 113: 379–394.
6. Fabiato A (1985): Rapid ionic modifications during the aequorin-detected calcium transient in a skinned canine cardiac Purkinje cell. J Gen Physiol 85: 189–246.
7. Fabiato A (1985): Time and calcium dependence of activation and inactivation of calcium-induced release of calcium from the sarcoplasmic reticulum of a skinned canine cardiac Purkinje cell. J Gen Physiol 85: 247–289.
8. Fabiato A (1985): Simulated calcium current can both cause calcium loading in and trigger calcium release from the sarcoplasmic reticulum of a skinned canine cardiac Purkinje cell. J Gen Physiol 85: 291–320.
9. McDonald TF, MacLeod DP (1971): Anoxia-recovery cycle in ventricular muscle: action potential duration contractility and ATP. Pflügers Archiv 325: 305–322.

10. Naylor WG, Poole-Wilson PA, Williams A (1979): Hypoxia and calcium. J Mol Cell Cardiol 11: 683–706.
11. Bassingthwaighte JB, Reuter H (1972): In DeMello WC (ed): Electrical phenomena in the heart. Academic Press, New York, pp. 353.
12. Wong AYK, Bassingthwaighte JB (1981): The kinetics of Ca-Na exchange in excitable tissue. Math Biosci. 53: 275–310.
13. Adler D, Wong AYK, Mahler Y (1985): Model of mechanical alternans in the mammalian myocardium. J Theor Biol In press.
14. Solaro RJ, Briggs FN (1974): Estimating the functional capabilities if sarcoplasmic reticulum in cardiac muscle: calcium binding. Circ Res 34: 531–540.
15. Solaro RJ, Wise RM, Shiver JS, Briggs FN (1974): Calcium requirements for cardiac myofibrillar activation. Circ Res 34: 525–530.
16. Beeler GW, Reuter H (1977): Reconstruction of the action potential of ventricular myocardiacl fibers. J Physiol 268: 177–210.
17. Safford RE, Bassingthwaighte JB (1977): Calcium diffusion in transient and steady states in muscle. Biophys J 20: 113–135.

Discussion

Lab: In one of your slides you showed that you could modify the frequency of your oscillations, if you had to modify one step in your equation, which step would be the most sensitive one to modify the frequency of your oscillation?
Wong: That would be the term $\bar{X} \cdot x$. Because this term determines how fast the SR is reactivated, bu this is a very slow varying function. For example, upon release, this term here becomes positive, so as a result, the term $(f \cdot d - \bar{X} \cdot x)$ is negative. According to the model you can not have negative release so I consider this to be zero. After a certain time, the $\bar{X} \cdot x$ term decays. If you can maintain the calcium concentration at the outer surface, that means the term $(p \cdot q)$ is always constant. This means that the release depends on how fast this term can decay to zero. When the calcium concentration at the outer surface is really high, the time constant is small. That is why the frequency is much higher. At low Ca concentration, because the time constant is very large, it takes a long time before the 'term' $(f \cdot d - \bar{X} \cdot x)$ can be reactivated.
Yue: How would you, without the equations, perhaps with diagrams, explain monoexponential restitution and potentiation phenomena? Is there any way that this would filter through this model and make sense?
Wong: Last year I published a paper together with David Adler which completely explained the phenomena you mentioned. Because the release threshold is not constant, and is inversely related to the amount of calcium available. For example, when after a regular beat you apply a premature beat this compartment cannot be filled to normal level because the time of resting is short, so that the calcium in this compartment is not as high as the normal case. This means that the amount of calcium available for release is reduced, and the release threshold is further increased. You would have less calcium available for release and, also, the release threshold increases. So as a result, you only have a little calcium released. What happens after the premature beat, if you go back to the normal or regular beat? Because of the little calcium release during the premature beat, more calcium remains in the releasable terminal of the SR. So the calcium available for release is higher than normal and the release threshold is greatly reduced. You have large amounts of calcium available and the release threshold is very small. As a result, the force developed during post-extrasystolic beat is high.

Microstructure and macroscale mechanics

18. A three-dimensional constitutive law for the passive myocardium based on a microstructural approach

A. HOROWITZ, Y. LANIR and M. PERL

Abstract

A three-dimensional constitutive law is proposed for the passive myocardium. The formulation is based on a structural approach, which considers the total strain energy of the myocardial tissue as equal to the sum of the strain energies of its constituents: the muscle fibers, the collagen fibers and the fluid matrix which embeds them. The ensuing material laws express the specific mechanical and structural properties of the tissue, namely, the stress-strain behavior of the comprising fibers, their spatial orientation, and their waviness in the unstressed state. After some functional form is assumed for the distribution of the fibers spatial orientation and waviness, the results of biaxial experiments serve for a preliminary estimation of the constants appearing in the constitutive equations. Finally, the advantages and the applicability of the structural material laws to the simulation of the cardiac mechanics are discussed.

Introduction

Specification of material laws for the myocardium is an essential part of the stress analysis in the heart. Several experimental and theoretical works were carried out to this end, resulting in various forms of stress-strains relations. Mostly, these have been uniaxial laws [1–4] and consequently their implementation in ventricular models required extension to two or three dimensions, which implicitly involves assumption of isotropy. However, recent biaxial experiments [5, 6] have shown that the myocardium is clearly anisotropic, and consequently two dimensional material laws were proposed [6].

Both the uniaxial laws, and the recently developed biaxial ones are based on a phenomenological approach in that they propose certain functional forms (usually exponential) for the stress-strain relations which seem to give the best fit to the experimental results.

As an alternative approach it is suggested here to formulate structural material laws which are based on the structure and mechanical properties of the actual constituents of the tissue. This approach follows the general structural theory for soft tissues [7], while considering the specific structural features of each fibrous network in the myocardium – the muscle fibers and the collagen fibers which connect them laterally [8]. Both fiber networks are embedded in a fluid matrix. The fibers carry tensile stresses, while the matrix transmits only hydrostatic pressure.

Having specified the stress-strain relations of each kind of fibers and having assumed some functional form for the distribution of their spatial orientation and for heir waviness in the unstressed state, a set of constitutive equations is derived. In order to allow estimation of the constants appearing in the equations, the constitutive laws are applied to the loading conditions of the above mentioned two-dimensional experiments. The results of these experiments serve for estimation of the material constants, using a nonlinear data fitting technique.

The structural material law presented here may be readily extended to the active state and may be also implemented in finite element models for the simulation of cardiac mechanics.

Formulation of the constitutive law

The proposed constitutive law is referred to the specific structure of the myocardial tissue. After this law is presented in a general manner, some more detailed form is formulated for the particular tissue considered here.

Histological considerations

The myocardium is basically a fibrous tissue. The myocytes are the prominent type of fibers occupying about 70% of the tissue volume. The remaining 30% consist of various interstitial components [9]. About 5% of the interstitial volume is occupied by collagen fibers [10]. These are organized in a spatial network, which laterally connects adjacent muscle fibers [8]. These two types of fibers considered here are the main structural elements of the tissue, their main mechanical role being the carrying of tensile stresses. The third is the interstitial fluid matrix, which occupies the remaining 25% of the tissue volume, and which transmits only hydrostatic pressures. Though a third kind of fibers has been identified, denoted as microthreads [11, 12], their structural contribution is not clear and due to their relatively low concentration they are considered here mechanically negligible in comparison to the collagen fibers.

General formulation of the structural constitutive law

Following the anatomic background, some additional basic assumption regarding the mechanical behavior of the myocardium are presented:

a. The fibers which comprise the myocardial tissue are relatively thin, and extensible. They do not resist any compressive stresses, and in the unstressed state of the tissue they may be undulated [8, 13], thus not demonstrating any resistance to stretching before being straightened.
b. The fluid matrix carries only hydrostatic pressure, which in turn is affected by length and configuration changes of the fibers. These cause pressure gradients which result in flow of the matrix. Nevertheless, the permeability of the tissue is low, and therefore the fluid flow within the tissue is negligible for the duration of the mechanical experiments considered (50 sec [6]). Thus, the myocardium may be treated as incompressible.
c. Numerous interconnections exist between the fibers. Therefore the uniaxial strain of each fiber may be obtained by a tensorial transformation of the overall strains (the affine deformation assumption).
d. The myocardial fiber defines an axis of symmetry for the spatial distribution of the collagen fibers which are connected to it (see Fig. 1).
e. The fiber interconnections are considered to be nodal inextensible points.

Considering these assumptions and supposing that the myocardium can be treated as a hyperelastic material which undergoes large deformations, the stress-strain relations for the tissue are subsequently formulated.

The contravariant Cauchy stress tensor components τ^{ij}, are derived from the strain energy function of the tissue, $W(\gamma^{ij})$, and from the hydrostatic pressure, P, by:

$$\tau^{ij} = \left(\frac{g}{G}\right)^{1/2} \frac{\partial W}{\partial \gamma_{ij}} + PG^{ij}, \tag{1}$$

where both the stress tensor τ as well a the Green-Lagrange strain tensor γ are referred to some global material coordinates ζ_i. The symbols g and G are the metric tensors before and after the deformation, respectively.

On the basis of the above assumptions it is proposed to adopt the structural theory for tissue in general and consider the total strain energy of the fiber networks in the myocardium as the sum of the strain energies of the muscle fibers, w_1, and of the collagen fibers, w_2.

Since not all fibers are necessarily straight at a given strain state, only a portion of the fibers contributes to the load bearing of the tissue at that state. In order to introduce this effect, a waviness distribution function $D_{k.\hat{n}}(x)$ is defined, such that for fibers of type k, passing through a plane defined by the normal $\hat{n}$, the portion of fibers having a straightening strain between x and x + x is $D_{k.\hat{n}}(x) \cdot \Delta x$. Also, since the fiber strain energy function is related to the fiber uniaxial strain, another

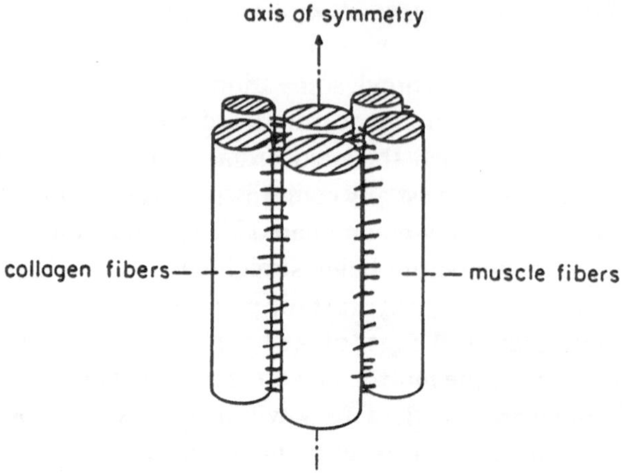

Figure 1. A scheme of the structure and interconnections of the constituent fibers in the myocardium.

coordinate system, ζ'_i, is defined in addition to the global system ζ_i, such that ζ'_1 coincides with the fiber direction. Thus, the uniaxial strain γ_{11} along the fiber axis is related to the global one, γ_{rs}, by the tensorial transformation:

$$\gamma'_{11} = \frac{\partial \zeta^r}{\partial \zeta'_1} \frac{\partial \zeta^s}{\partial \zeta'_1} \gamma_{rs}. \tag{2}$$

While the fiber uniaxial stress for an initially straight fiber is:

$$f_k(\gamma'_{11}) = \frac{\partial W_k}{\partial \gamma'_{11}}, \tag{3}$$

the uniaxial stress for a wavy fiber is given by:

$$f^*_k(\gamma'_{11}) = \int_0^{\gamma'_{11}} D_{k,\hat{n}}(x)\; f_k(\gamma'_{11t})\, dx, \tag{4}$$

where γ'_{11t} is the true fiber strain, related to the total fiber strain γ'_{11} by:

$$\gamma'_{11t} = \frac{\gamma'_{11} - x}{1 + 2x}\,. \tag{5}$$

Another structural feature of the myocardium is the spatial arrangements of the fibers. This arrangement can be stochastically described for each fiber type k by some density distribution function $R_{k\,(\hat{n})}$, so that the proportion of any fibers of type k which are confined within a given spatial sector $\Delta\Omega$ is:

$$p = \int_{\Delta\Omega} R_k(\theta, \varphi) \sin\varphi \, d\varphi \, d\theta, \tag{6}$$

where $R_{k(\theta,\varphi)}$ is defined in a spherical coordinate system (r, θ, φ). The strain energy of type k fibers in a volume unit is given by:

$$W_k = \int_{\Omega} S_k R_k(\theta, \varphi) \left[\int_0^{\gamma'_{11}} D_k(x)\, w_k(y'_{11t})\, dx \right] \sin\varphi \, d\varphi \, d\theta, \tag{7}$$

where S_k is the volumetric fraction of type k fibers. Carrying out the summation over k we obtain the total strain energy in a volume unit:

$$W = \sum_k \int_{\Omega} S_k R_k(\theta, \varphi) \left[\int_0^{\gamma'_{11}} D_k(x)\, w_k(\gamma'_{11t})\, dx \right] \sin\varphi \, d\varphi \, d\theta. \tag{8}$$

Consequently, the stresses in the tissue are obtained by employing (1) and (4):

$$\tau^{ij} = \left(\frac{g}{G}\right)^{1/2} \sum_k \int_{\Omega} S_k R_k(\theta, \varphi) \int_k^{*} (\gamma'_{11}) \frac{\partial \gamma'_{11}}{\partial \gamma_{ij}} \sin\varphi \, d\varphi \, d\theta + PG^{ij}. \tag{9}$$

Therefore, specification of the fibers waviness, spatial arrangement and stress-strain relations allows calculation of the stress as a function of the global strains of the tissue, up to the hydrostatic pressure P which has to be determined by the boundary conditions, and up to some yet unspecified material constants which may appear in the stress expressions.

Specification of the fibers' distribution functions and uniaxial material laws

Equation [9] is valid for fibrous tissues in general [7]. At this point it will be specialized to the myocardium by considering its specific structure. The distribution of the waviness of the muscle fibers and collagen fibers will be described by some density functions. The functions chosen here for both fiber types are normal distributions:

$$D_k(x) = \frac{1}{\sigma_k \sqrt{2\pi}} \exp\left[- \frac{(M_k - x)^2}{\sigma_k^2} \right], \tag{10}$$

where the mean, M_k, and the stanard deviation, σ_k, will generally be different for each fiber type.

The spatial orientation of the muscle fiber depends on the location in the ventricular wall of the segment under consideration, and may be determined by histologic inspection. The common approach, which is based on quantitative anatomic studies [14], assumes that the muscle fibers are parallel to the epicardial and endocardial surfaces and that their inclination angle varies gradually between +60° at the endocardium to −60° at the epicardium.

The availabe data on the spatial arrangement of collagen fibers [8] indicates that the collagen fibers are equally distributed around the muscle fiber (assumption (d) in *General formulation* above) and are mostly normal to them. If a spherical coordinate system (r, θ, φ) is defined such that the 0° polar angle coincides with the direction of the muscle fiber (Fig. 2), then the circumferential distribution is uniform and is given by:

$$\Theta(\theta) = \frac{1}{\pi}. \tag{11}$$

While most collagen fibers seem to be normal to the muscle fibers, some of them may deviate from the normal direction [8]. Since it is assumed here that the collagen fibers are equally distributed on both sides of the normal plane, a normal density distribution is chosen for the collagen fiber directions in the polar planes, with $\pi/2$ as mean:

$$\Phi(\varphi) = \frac{1}{\sigma_\Phi \sqrt{2\pi}} \exp\left[-\frac{(\pi/2-\varphi)^2}{2\sigma_\Phi^2}\right], \tag{12}$$

where σΦ is its standard deviation. Thus, the overall spatial arrangement of collagen fibers relative to muscle fibers is:

$$R_2(\theta,\varphi) = \Theta(\theta)\Phi(\varphi) = \frac{1}{\sigma_\Phi \pi \sqrt{2\pi}} \exp\left[-\frac{(\pi/2-\varphi)^2}{2\sigma^2\Phi}\right]. \tag{13}$$

In addition to the structural properties of the myocardium, the uniaxial stress-strain behavior of each of the two comprising fibers has also to be considered. Muscle fibers in the passive state exhibit exponential stress-strain relations under uniaxial tests [15, 16]. However, it is proposed here (on he basis of similar conclusions drawn for connective tissues [17] to attribute this exponential behavior to the gradual straightening of structural elements within the fiber (such as fibers in the sarcolemma [18, 19] or connectin fibers in the sarcomeres) and to ascribe to the straight fiber in the passive state a linear law:

$$f_1 = C_1 e_{1t}, \tag{14}$$

where e_{1t} is the fiber uniaxial true strain and C_1 is a constant coefficient corresponding to the slope of the steep part of the stress-strain curve. Experiments performed on hamster cardiac muscle fibers [16] yield values around 10^7 dyne/cm^2.

Elongation experiments with collagen fibers show a linear stress-strain relation:

$$f_2 = C_2 e_{2t}, \tag{15}$$

where C_2 is of the order of 1.0×10^{10} dyne/cm^2 and e_{2t} is the collagen fiber uniaxial true strain.

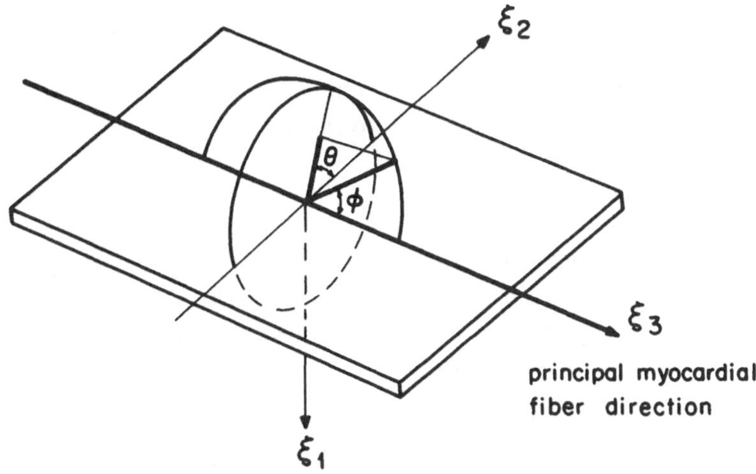

Figure 2. The alignment of the coordinate system relative to tissue sample.

Evaluation of material constants

In order to bring the structural constitutive laws to a concrete form, the still unspecified parameters must be determined by implementing the theory for the experimental results.

The data used here for this purpose is derived from biaxial stretch experiments. The material constants are estimated using a non-linear least square data fitting technique.

The experimental procedure and data

The data employed is derived from biaxial experiments carried out by Yin et al. on canine myocardium (for a detailed description of the experimental procedure see [6]).

The tissue samples, extracted from a subepicardial layer of the left ventricular wall, were square (4 cm × 4 cm) and thin (0.1 cm) and with the muscle fibers aligned in one direction, parallel to two of the edges.

The samples were subjected to several biaxial loading protocols, in each of which a constant ratio of the two normal strains, γ_{22} and γ_{33}, was maintained. The stress-strain curves obtained by these protocols serve here for the evaluation of the material constants.

Method of evaluation

Since the muscle fibers in the tissue sample are parallel and aligned in one direction, their distribution function is given by:

$$R_1(\theta, \varphi) = \delta(\varphi); \theta = 0, \tag{16}$$

where $\delta(\varphi)$ is Dirac's delta-function. The polar direction of the spherical coordinates (r, θ, φ) is chosen so as to coincide with the fibers direction (see Fig. 2). Having specified $R_1(\theta, \varphi)$, the general expressions for the overall stress in the tissue sample may be written as follows:

$$\tau^{ij} = \left(\frac{g}{G}\right)^{1/2} \left\{ S_1 \left[\int_0^{e_1} \int_1 (e_{1t})\, D_1(x)\, dx \right] \frac{\sigma e_1(\varphi)}{\sigma \gamma^{ij}} \Bigg|_{\varphi=0} + \right.$$

$$\left. S_2 \int_0^{\pi} \int_0^{\pi} \left[\int_0^{e_2} \int_2 (e_{2t})\, D_2(x)\, dx \right] \frac{\sigma e_2(\theta, \varphi)}{\sigma \gamma^{ij}} R_2(\theta, \varphi) \sin\varphi\, d\varphi\, d\theta \right\} + PG^{ij}. \tag{17}$$

Due to the disposition of the muscle fibers, e_1 is related to the global strains by:

$$e_1 = \gamma_{33}, \tag{18}$$

whereas the relation between the collagen fibers uniaxial strain and the global strain is given in general by:

$$e_2 = \gamma_{22} \cos^2\theta \sin^2\varphi + 2\gamma_{23} \cos\theta \sin\varphi \cos\varphi + \gamma_{33} \cos^2\varphi + \gamma_{11} \sin^2\theta \sin^2\varphi. \tag{19}$$

Bearing in mind that the tissue is incompressible we have:

$$\lambda_1 \lambda_2 \lambda_3 = |\underset{\sim}{G}| = 1, \tag{20}$$

where λ_i are the extension ratios. Since the present case involves only normal strains, it follows that:

$$\lambda_i^2 = 2\gamma_{ii} + 1, \tag{21}$$

(i is not summed) so that the thickness strain is dependent on the other two strains as:

$$\gamma_{11} = \frac{-2\gamma_{22}\gamma_{33} - \gamma_{22} - \gamma_{33}}{(2\gamma_{22} + 1)(2\gamma_{33} + 1)}. \tag{22}$$

This allows us to directly calculate the stresses, given the measured global strains γ_{22} and γ_{33}.

The parameters to be estimated are:

a. For the muscle fibers: the waviness parameters M_1 and σ_1, and the uniaxial stress-strain coefficient, C_1.
b. For the collagen fibers: the spatial distribution parameter σ_Φ, the waviness parameters M_2 and σ_2 and the uniaxial stress-strain coefficient C_2.

Further consideration has to be given to the contribution of the hydrostatic pressure in (17). Since the upper and lower faces of the tissue samples remained free of loading, it follows that at these faces:

$$\tau^{11} = \tau_f^{11} + PG^{11} = O, \tag{23}$$

where τ_f^{11} are the fibers' contributions.

Because the specimen is thin, τ_f^{11} may be assumed constant throughout the thickness, and since the muscle fibers are arranged in a planar array, only collagen fibers contribute to τ_f^{11}. By using (23), the stresses can be expressed solely by the contributions of the muscle and collagen fibers. The stress in the fiber direction is:

$$\tau^{33} = \tau_1^{33} + \tau_2^{33} + PG^{33}, \tag{24}$$

where τ_1^{33} is the muscle fibers' contribution and τ_2^{33} is the collagen fibers contribution. Using (23), τ^{33} is given by:

$$\tau^{33} = \tau_1^{33} + \tau_2^{33} - \frac{G^{33}}{G^{11}}\,\tau_2^{11}, \tag{25}$$

and similarily for the stress in the cross-fiber direction:

$$\tau^{22} = \tau_2^{22} - \frac{G^{22}}{G^{11}}\,\tau_2^{11}. \tag{26}$$

Results

Preliminary results for the parameters are hereafter presented. The values calculated for these parameters are based on the stress-strain data points obtained for the fiber and cross-fiber directions in a single experimental protocol performed by Yin et al. [6].

Because of the nonlinearity of the material laws (17) a nonlinear least squares data-fitting technique was used [22].

The seven parameters were simultaneously estimated by fitting the stress expressions for τ^{33} and τ^{22} to the measured values in the fiber and cross-fiber directions, respectively.

The least squares results (Figs 3 and 4) show a good fit to the experimental data points for the whole range of strains. The relative mean square errors were 0.077

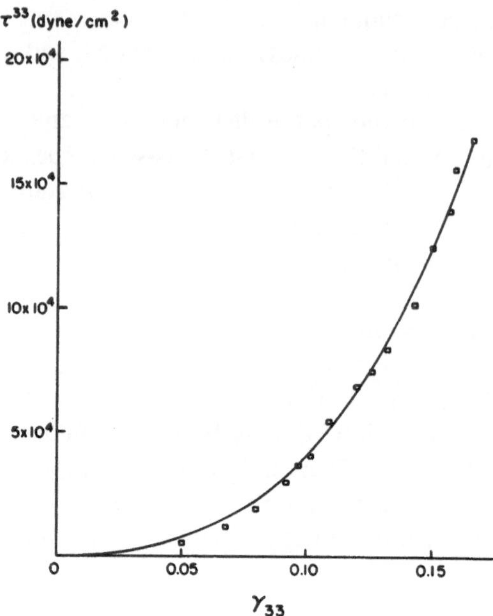

Figure 3. A comparison of the proposed model (solid line) to experimental points in the fiber direction. The values of the material constants are for the muscle fibers $C_1 = 4.7 \times 10^7$ dyne/cm^2, $M_1 = 0.304$, $\sigma_1 = 0.119$; for the collagen fibers $C_2 = 2.0 \times 10^9$ dyne/cm^2, $M_2 = 0.207$, $\sigma_2 = 0.070$, $\sigma_\Phi = 0.239$ rad. The relative mean square error is 0.134.

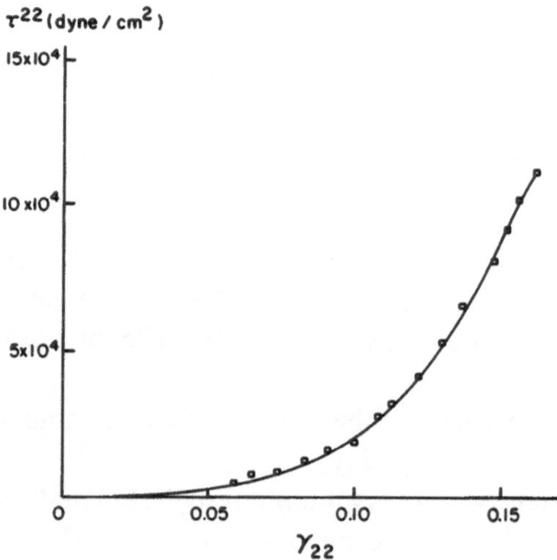

Figure 4. A comparison of the proposed model (solid line) to experimental points in the cross-fiber direction. The relative mean square error is 0.118.

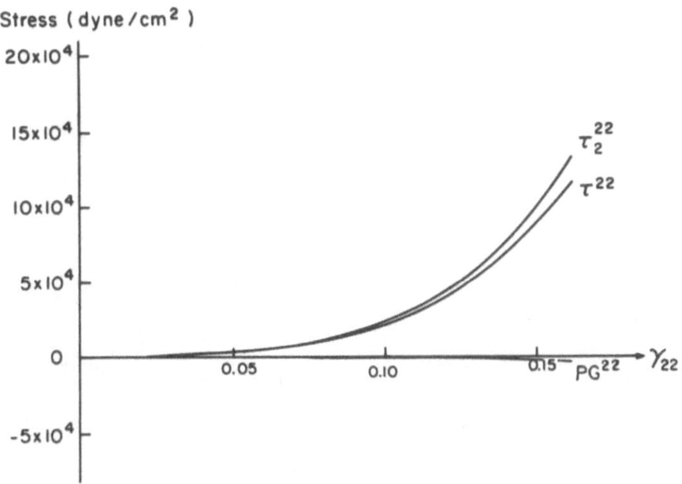

Figure 5. The contribution of the various tissue components to the total calculated stress in the muscle fiber direction. τ^{33} = the total stress, τ_1^{33} = the muscle fibers contribution, τ_2^{33} = the collagen fibers contribution, and $G^{33}P$ = the fluid matrix contribution.

and 0.139 for the fiber and the cross-fiber directions, respectively, for the following values of the parameters:
Muscle fibers: $C_1 = 5.6 \times 10^7$ dyne/cm², $M_1 = 0.366$, $\sigma_1 = 0.125$;
Collagen fibers: $C_2 = 2.3 \times 10^9$ dyne/cm², $M_2 = 0.193$, $\sigma_2 = 0.068$, $\sigma_\Phi = 0.149$ rad.

The calculated values of the material constants for the two fiber types are similar to those previously reported [16, 21], which are 1×10^7 dyne/cm² for muscle fibers and 1×10^{10} dyne/cm² for collagen fibers.

Both fiber types are found to be significantly slack in the unstressed state. This conclusion is in accordance with existing anatomical findings, regarding collagen fibers [8] and connectin fibers (the latter being probably responsible for a major portion of the muscle fibers behavior). Connectin fibers were found to be slack at strains below 0.25 [20].

The value of the standard deviation of the collagen fibers orientation distribution indicates a narrow distribution of the collagen fibers around the normal to the muscle fibers. This arrangement is also reflected in the contribution of each of the tissue constituents to the total calculated stress. Almost all the stress in the fiber direction is carried by the muscle fibers, while the collagen fibers carry less than 0.06 of the total stress (Fig. 5). The situation is reversed at the cross-fiber direction, where only collagen fibers carry tensile stresses (Fig. 6).

The contribution of the fluid-matrix is found to be negligible, accounting only for 1–2% of the total stress.

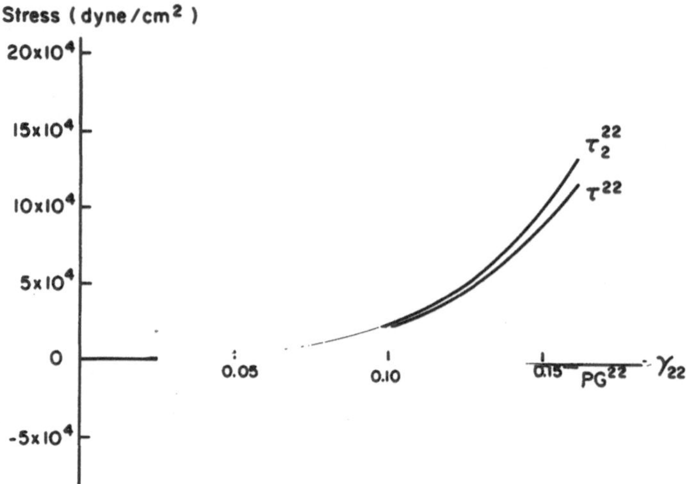

Figure 6. The contribution of the various tissue components to the total calculated stress in the cross-fiber direction. τ^{22} = the total stress, τ_2^{22} = the collagen fibers contribution, and $G^{22}P$ = the fluid matrix contribution.

Discussion

The constitutive law proposed here for the myocardium accounts for the mechanical behavior of the whole tissue by employing the mechanical properties, spatial distribution and waviness of its constituents. The distribution of the fibers orientations are responsible for the observed anisotropy of the myocardium, while the waviness of the fibers together with their orientation, result in nonlinear stress-strain relations.

The material constants appearing in the constitutive laws have direct physical meaning, being the coefficients of the uniaxial stress-strain relations of the fibers and the means and standard deviations of the waviness and orientation distributions. This is advantageous compared to existing material models based on a phenomenological approach, since it allows understanding of specific mechanisms and their effect on the tissue's mechanical response.

The calculated material constants presented here, though being preliminary, show a very good fit to the data from biaxial tests, and are of physically sound values. Moreover, these values provide insight into the mechanical behavior of the tissue, indicating that at physiological strain levels, the main load bearing elements in the passive state are the muscle fibers and the collagen fibers, while the fluid matrix has an insignificant role.

The present approach which is formulated for the passive state, may be extended to describe the active state, as well, since the distribution of the muscle fiber orientations coincides with the distribution of the directions of active forces. Both passive and active formulations may be implemented in finite element models, thus possibly providing an improved simulation of the mechanics of the heart. These aspects are currently being investigated.

References

1. Pinto JG, Fung YC (1973): Mechanical properties of the heart muscle in the passive state. J Biomech 6: 597–616.
2. Kitabatake A, Suga H (1978): Diastolic stress-strain relation of nonexcised blood perfused canine papillary muscle. Am J Physiol 234: 416–419.
3. Pao YC, Nagendra GK, Padiyar R, Ritman EL (1980): Derivation of myocardial fiber stiffness equation based on theory of laminated composite. J Biomech Eng 102: 252–257.
4. Capelo A, Comincioli V, Minelli R, Poggesi C, Reggiani C, Ricciardi L (1981): Study and parameters identification of a rheological model of excised quiescent cardiac muscle. J Biomech 14: 1–11.
5. Demer LL, Yin FCP (1983): Passive biaxial mechanical properties of isolated canine myocardium. J Physiol 339: 615–630.
6. Yin FCP, Strumpf RK, Chew PH, Zeger SL (1986): Quantification of the mechanical properties of noncontracting canine myocardium under simultaneous biaxial loading. J Biomech (in press).
7. Lanir Y (1983): Constitutive equations for fibrous connective tissues, J Biomech 16: 1–12.
8. Caulfield JB, Borg TK (1979): The collagen network of the heart. Lab Invest 40: 364–372.
9. Frank JS, Langer GA (1974): The myocardial interstitium: its structure and its role in ionic exchange. J Cell Biol 60: 596–601.
10. Caspari PG, Newcomb M, Gibson K, Harris P (1977): Collagen in the normal and hypertrophied human ventricle. Cardiovasc Res 11: 554–558.
11. Winegrad S, Robinson TF (1978): Force generation among cells in the relaxing heart. Eur J Cardiol 7 (Suppl): 63–70.
12. Lazarides E (1980): Intermediate filaments as mechanical integrators of cellular space. Nature 283: 249–256.
13. Gay WA, Johnson EA (1967): An anatomical evaluation of the myocardial length-tension diagram. Circ Res 21: 33–43.
14. Streeter DD, Hanna TH (1973): Engineering mechanics for successive states in canine left ventricular myocardium: II. Fiber angle and sarcomere length. Circ Res 33: 656–664.
15. Fabiato A, Fabiato F (1978): Myofilament-generated tension oscillation during partial calcium activation and activation dependence of the sarcomere length-tension relation of skinned cardiac cells. J Gen Physiol 72: 667–699.
16. Fish D, Orenstein J, Bloom S (1984): Passive stiffness of isolated cardiac and skeletal myocites in the hamster, Circ Res 54: 267–276.
17. Lanir Y (1979): A structural theory for the homogenous biaxial stress-strain relationship in fat collagenous tissues. J Biomech 12: 423–436.
18. Fields RW, Faber JJ (1970): Biophysical analysis of the mechanical properties of the sarcolemma. Can J Physiol Pharm 48: 394–404.
19. Orenstein J, Hogan D, Bloom S (1980): Surface cables of cardiac myocites. J Mol Cell Cardiol 12: 771–780.
20. Matsubara S, Maruyama K (1977): Role of connectin in the length-tension relation of skeletal and cardiac muscles. J Physiol 27: 589–600.
21. Viidik A (1973): Functional properties of collagenous tissue. In: Hall DA, Jackson DS (eds) International review of connective tissue research, Vol 5. Academic Press, New York/London, pp. 127–215.
22. Harwell Subroutine Library (subroutine VA05AD) Computer Science and Systems Division, Atomic Energy Research Establishment (1984). Harwell, Oxfordshire, England.

Discussion

Beyar: Is the passive myocardium in your calculations stiffer in the fiber direction or in the perpendicular direction?
Horowitz: It is stiffer in the fiber direction.
Bassingthwaighte: I am bothered by the assumption that the element is freely compressible in the fiber direction, i.e., there is no force maintaining the structural shape of the myocardium. If you take a ventricle and cut off the atrium, aorta, etc., and put it in water it would continue to contract and will jet around in the water for a considerable time, which means that there are restoring forces that regenerate the shape of the ventricle after its contraction. The force is real enough; you may consider it to be the equivalent of negative pressure. In the elastic sense, they are putting the ventricle back into shape. There is a restoring force there and when the ventricle contracts, it works against this elasticity. Should it not be accounted for in the model? The other point to note is your fiber direction. My electromicroscope observations on collagen fiber direction show that many fiber parallel the muscle fibers. You have the normal direction instead. I wonder if either scanning EM or transmission EM will give you the measurement of the directions of these fibers. It is your assumption that I am concerned about.
Horowitz: Indeed, we assume that most collagen fibers are normal to the muscle fibers, but not all of them, and some may be even parallel to muscle fibers.
Yellin: We know that a stimulated muscle will contract down below the slack length, therefore there must be some compressive forces.
Horowitz: We consider single fibers to have no resistance to compression, but the whole ensemble may resist compression due to interconnections between fibers and due to the hydrostatic pressure.
Lanir: Dr Bassingthwaighte is referring to the compressibility of the whole tissue, while the authors refer to specific elements and not to the whole structure. There is no contradiction here.

19. 3-D simulation of left ventricular contraction combining myocardial mechanics and electrical activation

H. AZHARI, R.BEYAR, E. BARTA, U. DINNAR and S. SIDEMAN

Abstract

A computerized 3-D temporal simulation of the left ventricle (LV) was developed and utilized to study the complex phenomena associated with the contraction of the LV during systole. The simulation utilizes helical coordinates and a procedure which yields a fast realistic approximation of the instantaneous 3-D geometry of the LV. The electrical activation delay time from end diastole (ED) is calculated, using a 3-D electrical activation procedure based on minimal orthogonal pathways. Local and global deformations of the LV account for the myocardial structure and spatial fiber angle distribution, the mechanics and dynamics of the sarcomeres and the time required for the electrical activation to reach the specific location within the myocardium. The simulation yields the instantaneous LV 3-D geometry (from 2-D echocardiographic cross-sections) and calculates the cavity pressure, volume and the aortic blood flow under various conditions. The model also yields the instantaneous sarcomere length and their angular distributon at any desired location within the myocardium. The calculated results define the elliptization characteristics of the LV contraction and are consistent with experimental data.

Introduction

Various models have been used in numerous attempts to simulate, describe and predict the complex phenomena of LV contraction [1–4]. These models can generally be classified as:

1. analytical models, and
2. finite element (FE) models.

In the analytical models, the LV is usually approximated by a simple geometrical structure such as a spheroid [5], a cylinder[6], or a set of rings [7], and simple contraction patterns (mostly uniform) are stipulated. Since the geometry is assumed to be invariant throughout the systole, the global deformation is calculated based on a single representative myocardial element. These models, despite their inherent inaccuracies, fit the physiologically measured global LV performance fairly wel and have the advantage of being defined by a set of equations that enable to use fast solvers.

FE models, on the other hand, relate to realistic LV geometries, and are capable of calculating local deformations as well as global LV performances. However, the FE models require complicated constitutive laws for the myocardium, usually represented by a nonphysiological analog such as set of rods [8], and involve very intensive calculations [9].

The present work utilizes a new approach to the description of 3-D geometries [10] and to the 3-D analysis of the LV performance which combines the advantages of exact equations and fast computation offered by the analytical models, with a realistic geometry and enables to calculate the local deformations as well as the global LV performance.

Methods and procedures

Geometrical considerations

Consider an imaginary cylinder which surrounds the LV, with a diameter (D) larger than the largest diameter of the LV (Fig. 1). The axis of the cylinder is parallel to the major axis of the LV. A unidimensional function $R(\xi)$ is obtained by moving along a helical passway located on the surface of the cylinder and measuring the external radial distance (R) from the helix to the endocardial surface. The function $R(\xi)$, which represents a helical curve wrapped around the endocardial surface, can be used to approximate the 3-D geometry of the LV cavity (Fig. 2). It is noted that the accurary of the geometrical approximation is inversely proportional to the helical pitch or, equivalently, proportional to the length of the wrapped helical 'curve'. Hence, in order to retain the geometrical information throughout the contraction, we allow the curvilinear coordinate ξ to deform vertically together with the LV. As shown in Fig. 3, the deformation is simulated by demanding that the vertical distance between two consecutive helical windings of ξ, $H(\xi)$, be the same as the vertical distance between the two corresponding (projected) points on the myocardium. Thus, the instantaneous geometry of the LV cavity ($\heartsuit(\xi,t)$) is defined by two functions:

$$\heartsuit(t,\xi) = \begin{cases} R(t,\xi) \\ H(t,\xi) \end{cases} . \tag{1}$$

Given the two instantaneous principle tangential deformations, $\varepsilon_{\varphi\varphi}$ and $\varepsilon_{\theta\theta}$ (Fig. 3) of a small myocardial element, the corresponding deformations, ε_R and ε_H can

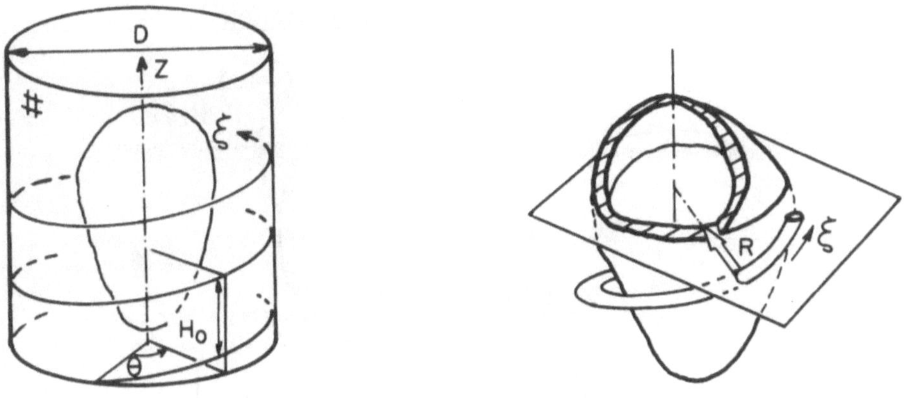

Figure 1. Schematics of the enclosing cylinder and the helical coordinate system used.

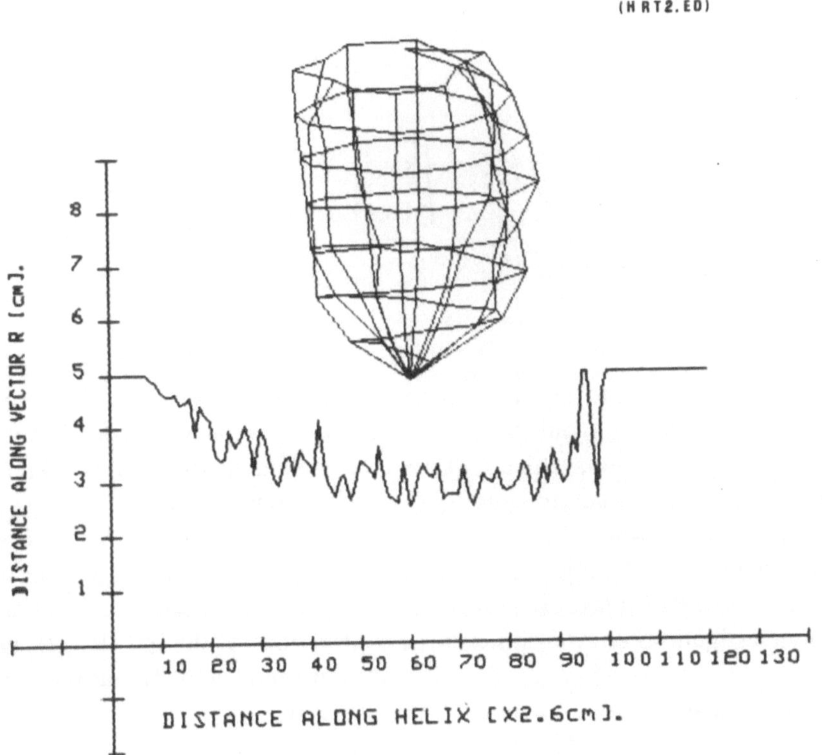

Figure 2. A typical function R(ξ) and its corresponding 3-D reconstruction. (Obtained by echocardiographic measurements [10]).

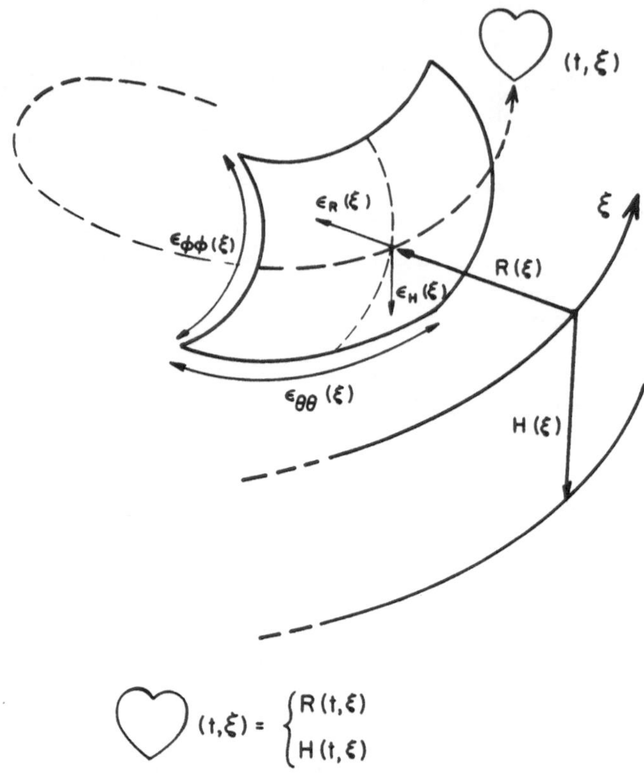

Figure 3. Relation between myocardial deformation and deformation of the helical coordinate system.

then be calculated and (1) utilized to describe the deformed LV geometry. However, in order to avoid the complexity of the myocardial constitutive laws and boundary conditions which require a finite element solution, two kinematic assumptions can be made to simplify the calculations involved.

The first assumption is that all the endocardial points on the LV cross-section perpendicular to the major axis deform radially with reference to the instantaneous centroid of this cross-section (see Fig. 4). This assumption is inherent in many investigations of two-dimensional contractions of the LV [11, 12]. Hence, the new instantaneous interception distance between vector R and the endocardial surface is given, as shown in Appendix A, by:

$$R_i' = R_i - \varepsilon_{\theta\theta i}\left[\frac{(D/2-R_i)^2 + R_{ci}^2 - a^2}{(D-2R_i)}\right], \tag{2}$$

where all the parameters are difined in Appendix A.

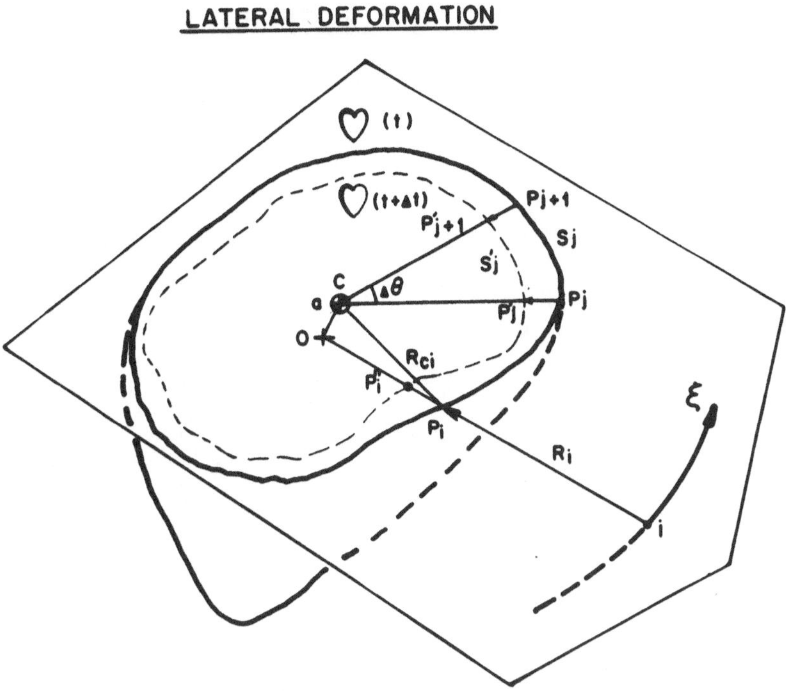

LATERAL DEFORMATION

$$R_I' = R_I - \mathcal{E}_{\theta\theta I}\left[\frac{(D/2-R_I)^2 + R_{CI}^2 - a^2}{(D-2R_I)}\right]$$

$$\mathcal{E}_{\theta\theta\, I} = (S_I' - S_I)/S_I$$

Figure 4. A cross section view perpendicular to the long (Z) axis, and the corresponding geometrical dimensions used for calculation of the lateral deformation.

The second assumption is that the radius of curvature $R_{\varphi\varphi}$, on a cross-section which includes the major axis (Fig. 5), is very large with respect to the associated instantaneous strain. Consequently, this radius can be assumed to be constant for a very short time interval. Thus, the 'new' vertical winding pitch $H'(t)$ for a point i on ξ is derived in Appendix B and is given by:

$$H' = H\left[1 + \varepsilon_{\varphi\varphi}\frac{S}{2R_{\varphi\varphi}\tan(S/2R_{\varphi\varphi})}\right], \qquad (3)$$

where S, the arch length, is defined in Fig. 5.

In order to describe the instantaneous 3-D geometry of the LV, the two instantaneous functions $R(t,\xi)$ and $H(t,\xi)$ in (1) must be determined for every value of ξ at the moment of interest. This requires the solution of the two local myocardial strains $\varepsilon_{\varphi\varphi}$ and $\varepsilon_{\theta\theta}$ for every myocardial element located along the

LONGITUDINAL – DEFORMATION

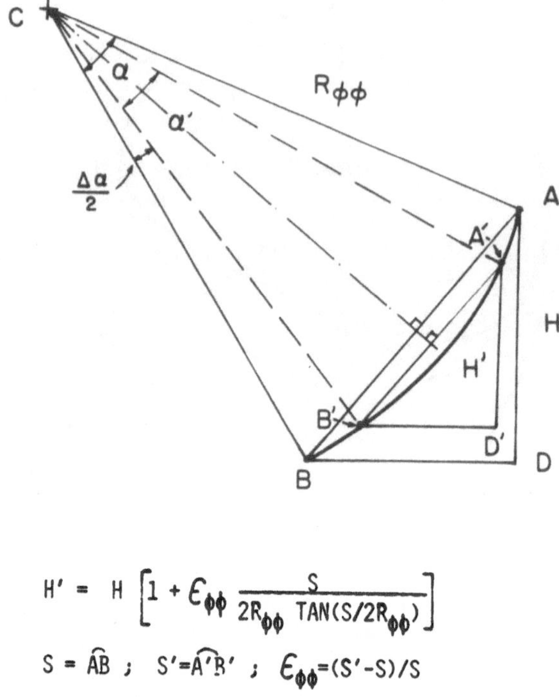

Figure 5. Geometrical dimensions used for calculation of longitudinal deformation.

wrapped helial curve. Following the suggestion that the myocardial deformation is rather uniform in the normal LV [13], it is expected that plotting the instantaneous strain (in any of the directions described above)as a function of the distance along ξ shall yield a very smooth and flat curve, Fig.6. Perturbations will occur only near locations where the myocardial properties deviate from normality. Consequently, it is possible to apply common sampling rules (Nyquist theorem, for instance) to the strain calculations and thus reduce the amount of calculations without losing any relevant information.

Myocardial structure

The LV muscle is divided into many (up to 120) small myocardial elements by sampling the function R(ED,ξ) at a rate of 12 points per one helical winding while maintaining the function H(ED,ξ) constant. As seen in Fig. 7, each myocardial element is represented by two radi of curvature $R_{\varphi\varphi}$, $R_{\theta\theta}$, and the wall thickness

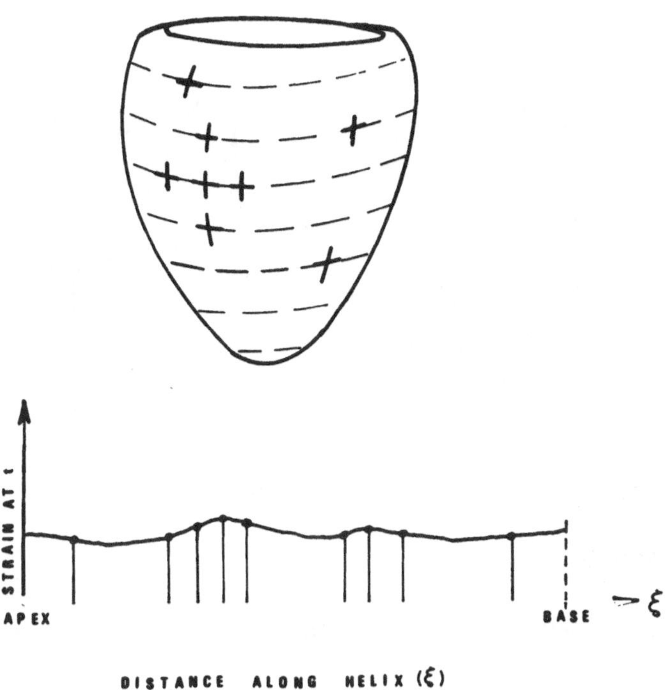

Figure 6. Demonstration of the sampled calculation concept.

W. The element is assumed to consist of 10 layers of fibers, where all the sarcomeres are parallel to each other and have the same angle of inclination from the horizontal plane. The ED angle of inclination in each of the layers is determined from the data published by Streeter et al. [14]. The sarcomeres' length in each layer is calculated utilizing the following equation which resembles the equation suggested by Wong et al. [15]:

$$SL_i = SL_{oi} + \ln[P/P_{oi} + 1]/K_i, \qquad (4)$$

where SL_i and SL_{oi}, are the sarcomeres' length in layer i, at ED pressure P and zero pressure, respectively, and P_{oi} and K_i are empirical constants, determined from the data of Yoran et al. [16]. Due to insufficient physiological information, the layers in the present work were divided into three groups, and the sarcomeres in each group were assigned the same ED length.

The ED pressure was determined by using the following passive pressure-

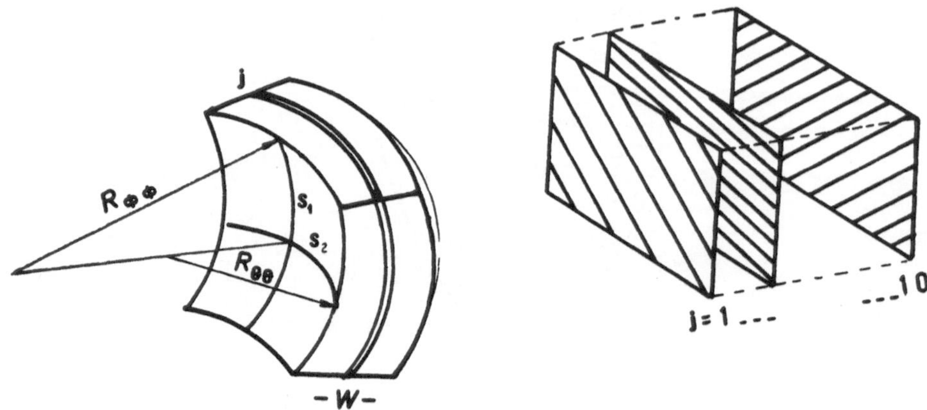

Figure 7. A myocardial element used in the present work.

volume (P-V) relation:

$$P_P = A[\mathrm{Exp}(-B(V/V_o)-1)) - 1], \tag{5}$$

Where P_P is the LV pressure obtained by the passive stretching of the LV due to a volume increase from zero pressure volume V_o, to the given instantaneous volume V. A and B are empirical constants, here obtained by curve fitting the data published by Spotnitz et al. [17].

The mass M_i of each myocardial element i is conserved throughout the LV contraction and is estimated by:

$$M_i = \varrho S_{1i} S_{2i} W_i. \tag{6}$$

S_{1i}, S_{2i} are the arc lengths (shown in Fig. 7), W_i is the wall thickness of the element and ϱ is the density of the muscle = 1.06 gr/cc [18].

Stress-strain relationship

The instantaneous strain rate of a myocardial element is detemined by the ratio of the resistive stresses σ induced on its walls (due to the internal pressure of the LV) and the active stresses applied by the activated fibers, σ_f. This relationship is defined by the familiar Hill's equation:

$$\dot{\varepsilon} = -b(1 - \sigma/\sigma_f)/(a + \sigma/\sigma_f), \tag{7}$$

where $\dot{\varepsilon}$ is the instantaneous strain rate, and a, b are empirical constants, here determined by curve fitting of the data published by Taylor et al. [19]. Equation (7) can be extended for normalized stresses ($\sigma/\sigma_f > 1$), by taking the antisymmetric function of (7) around $\sigma/\sigma_f = 1$, thus yielding curves similar to the data published by Mashima et al. [20].

The average active stresses applied to the walls of the myocardial elements (Fig. 7) are calculated by utilizing equations (C-1) to (C-4) in Appendix C. The resistive stresses due to the internal LV pressure are calculated utilizing (D-2) and (D-3) in appendix D.

Activation delay time

The time required for the electrical activation signal to reach a certain layer, l, inside a given myocardial element i from the closest point of excitation is calculated by the sum of the time intervals required for the electrical excitation wave to propagate first along the Purkinje network on the endocardial surface, and then, in the radial (transmural) direction, from the endocardium to the layer l under consideration. Thus the activation delay time for a layer in a myocardial element i, is given by:

$$\tau_{il} = S_i/Vp + W_{il}/Vr, \tag{8}$$

where the distance S_i is the minimal geodetic pathway on an ellipsoid (as calculated by Barta et al. [1]), Vp and Vr are the propagation velocities along the radial direction respectively, and W_{il} is the distance from the endocard to the layer l.

Isovolumic deformation

During isovolumic contraction the volume is kept constant to within 0.1 cc by an iterative calculation procedure.

Afterload

Afterload is simulated by a modified Windkessel model with an additional serial resistance, Ro. This modification yields a more realistic frequence response (see for instance O'Rourke et al. [21]) and the LV pressure during the ejection period is given by:

$$P(t) = e^{-1/Res \cdot Cap}\left[P_{AO} - \frac{1}{Cap}\int_0^t {}^{t/Res \cdot Cap}\, Q(t)dt\right] + R_o Q(t), \qquad (9)$$

where P(t) is the instantaneous LV pressure, P_{AO} is the aortic pressure at ED, Q(t) is the blood flow at time t, Res and Cap are the peripheral resistance and arterial capacitance respectively.

Computation procedure

The basic structure of the computation procedure is outlined in the 'flow-chart' shown in Fig. 8. It consists of three major computation loops, nested within each other. The most inner loop computes the sarcomeres lengths and angle of inclination for each of the ten fiber layers within each myocardial element. The external loop, which contains the previous two, performs calculations of the global LV performance, every 0.01 sec.

The simulation is initiated at ED for a given LV 3-D geometry. Activation delay times are computed independently and inserted as an input. Ejection is obtained once the LV pressure exceeds the aortic pressure. The simulation is terminated when the aortic blood flow becomes negative i.e. 'flows' towards the LV. Output data comprises of the LV 3-D ES geometry, LV pressure, LV volume and aortic blood flow as functions of time as well as the P-V loop, local strains, sarcomeres' lengths and angles of inclination for each of the layers of a pre-selected myocardial element. The instantaneous 3-D geometry can be continuously displayed on a graphic monitor.

ED geometry

Two ED geometries were utilized in the present study:

1. a truncated ellipsoidal shell of revolution with dimensions based on the data published by Streeter et al. [22] for a canine LV, and
2. a human LV reconstructed from six apical echocardiographic planes in vivo. The human LV shape was low-pass filtered in order to obtain a smooth 3-D geometry.

Results

Effect of changes in the preload

The preload is represented here by the LV ED volume. This change is associated with a change in the initial LV pressure through the passive P-V relation given by

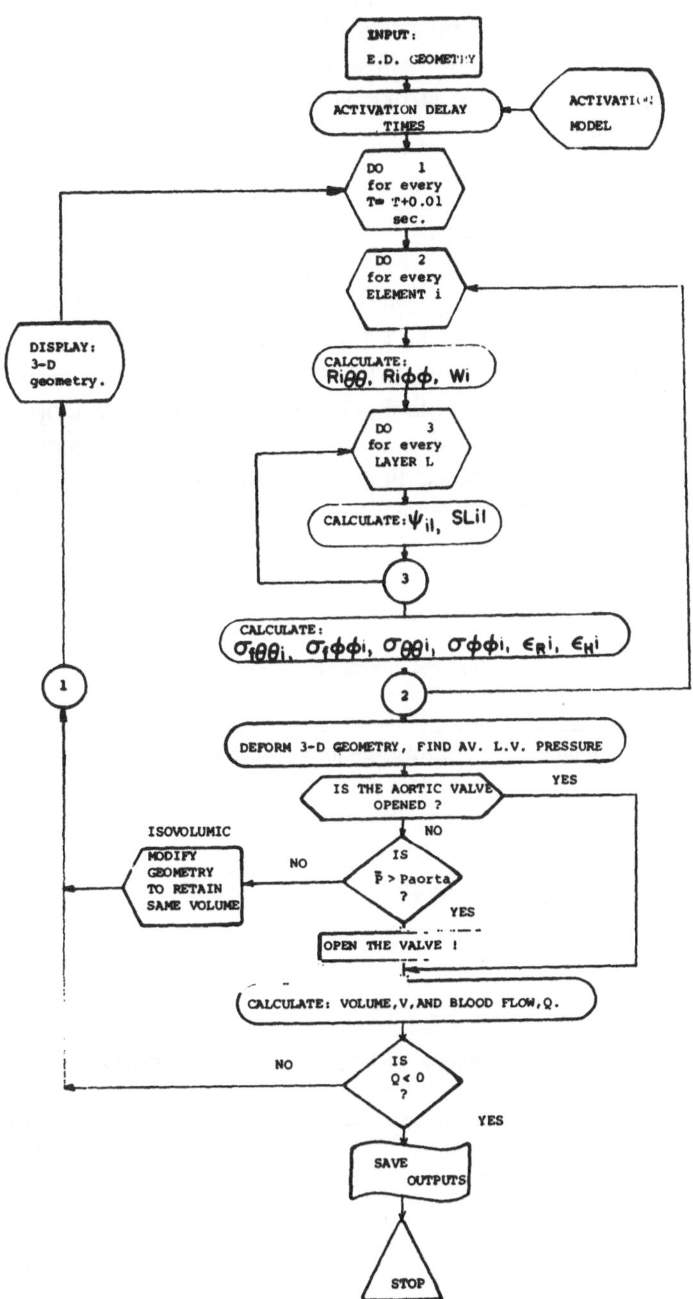

Figure 8. A flow chart of the computer program used for simulating the LV contraction.

(5). The performance of the LV is examined for 3 different ED volumes. The results obtained by the simulation are summarized in Table 1. The corresponding P-V loops, the LV volumes and the aortic blood flows as a function of time (from ED), are shown in Fig. 9. As can be observed, the classical Starling mechanism relating the dependence of the stroke volume on the ED volume is clearly demonstrated by these results.

Effect of changes in the afterload

The aortic pressure is used here to represent the afterload. The effect of changes in the afterloading conditions on the LV performance is studied by varying the ED aortic pressure along with the LV ED volume. The results obtained by the simulation are summarized in Table 2. The corresponding P-V loop curves are shown in Fig. 10. A linear regression analysis of the predicted ES pressures and volumes yielded the ES elastance line [23] with a correlation coefficient of $R = 0.99$ and a slope of 8.3 [mmHg/cc].

Table 1. Effect of different preloading conditions on LV performance. Aortic ED pressure = 80 mm Hg.

ED volume (ml)	ES volume (ml)	Stroke volume (ml)	Ejection fraction (%)	Max. press. (mm Hg)
42.6	22.7	19.9	46.7	103.4
53.2	25.4	27.8	52.2	113.7
63.9	27.0	36.9	57.7	125.1

Table 2. Effect of different loading conditions on LV performance. Simultaneous increase in preload and afterload.

ED volume (ml)	Aortic ED pressure (mm Hg)	ES volume (ml)	Stroke vol. (ml)	Ejection fraction (%)	ES pressure (mm Hg)
42.6	60	22.2	20.4	47.9	63.9
47.9	70	24.0	23.9	49.9	74.8
53.2	80	25.4	27.8	52.2	96.3
58.2	90	27.3	32.0	54.7	96.3
63.9	100	27.3	36.6	57.3	107.4

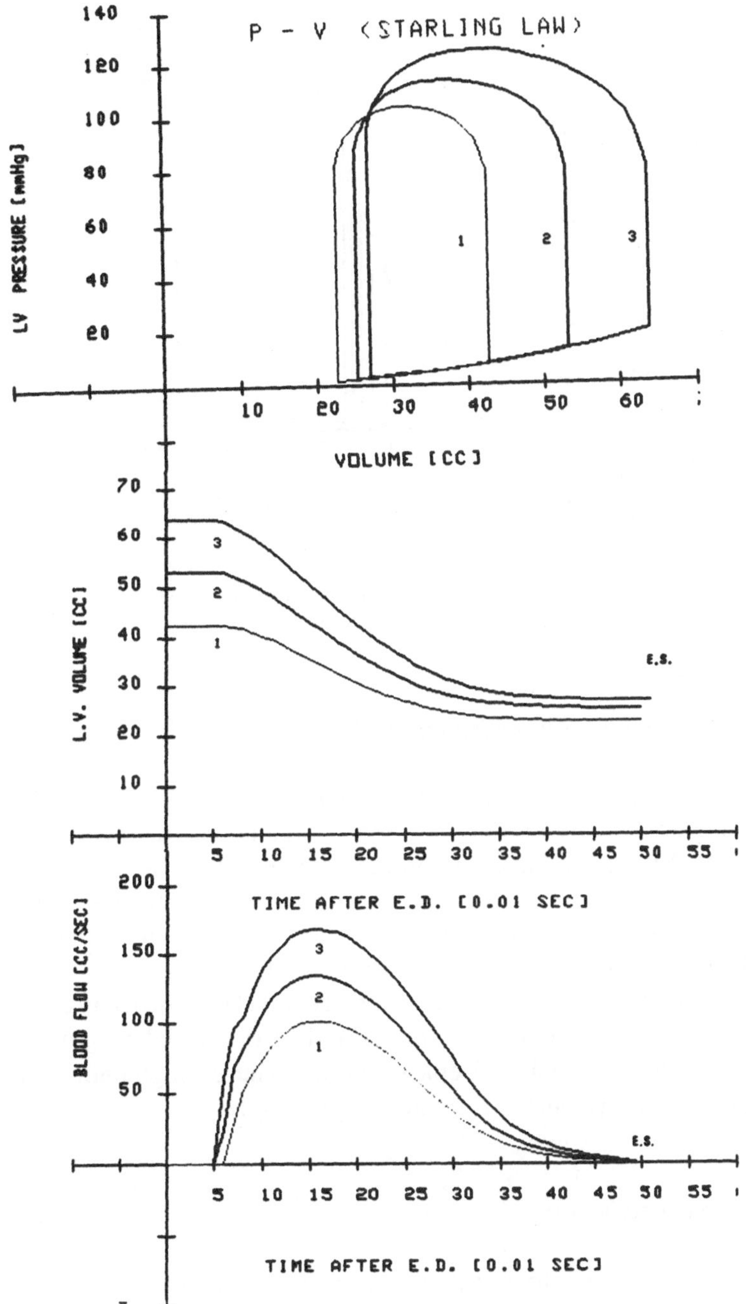

Figure 9. The performance curves of the LV for different preloading conditions (see table 1).

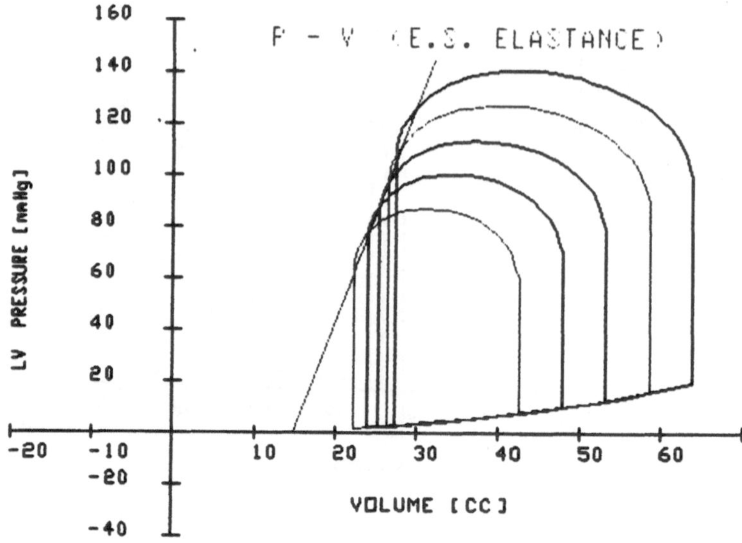

Figure 10. Pressure volume loops calculated for different loading conditions (see Table 2), and the corresponding ES elastance line.

Effect of the instantaneous activation of the endocardium

The geometrical manifestations of the instantaneous activation of the endocardium are presented here in the levels of the sarcomeres, the myocardial element and the global LV geometry. The predicted extension ratio, in the vertical (H) and lateral (R) directions as a function of time from ED for a myocardial element located at the mid LV height, is shown in Fig. 11. Note a slight shortening in the longitudinal direction followed by shortening after, roughly, 80 ms. The manifestations of this contraction at the sarcomeres level is shown in Fig. 12 and at the global 3-D geometry in fig. 13. It seems that the initial lengthening affects primarily the endocardial and epicardial sarcomere lengthening followed by contraction of all sarcomeres throughout the systole.

Effect of apical activation

The effect of an apex-initiated excitation wave on the extension ratio of three myocardial elements, located at 20%, 50% and 80% of the LV height, is demonstrated in Fig.14. Note that the apical segments demonstrate transient shortening and lengthening in the longitudinal direction whereas the basal segment shows only lengthening prior to the ejection shortening.

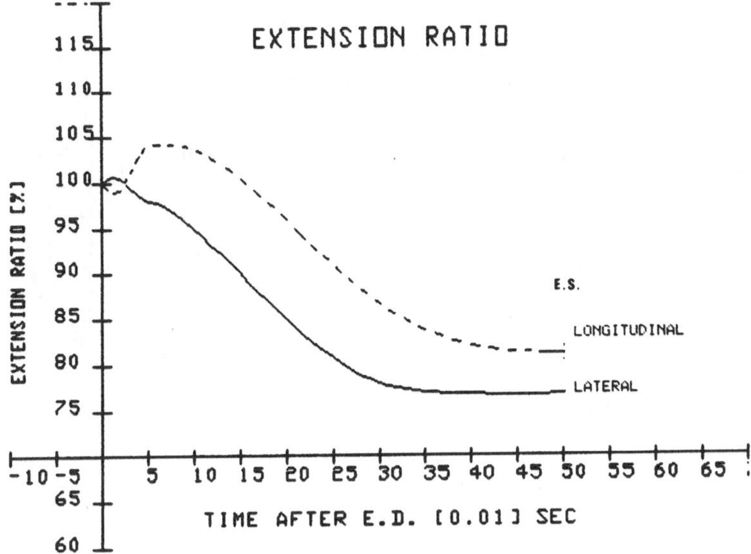

Figure 11. Calculated extension ratio in both the longitudinal and lateral directions, for an instantaneous excitation of the endocardium.

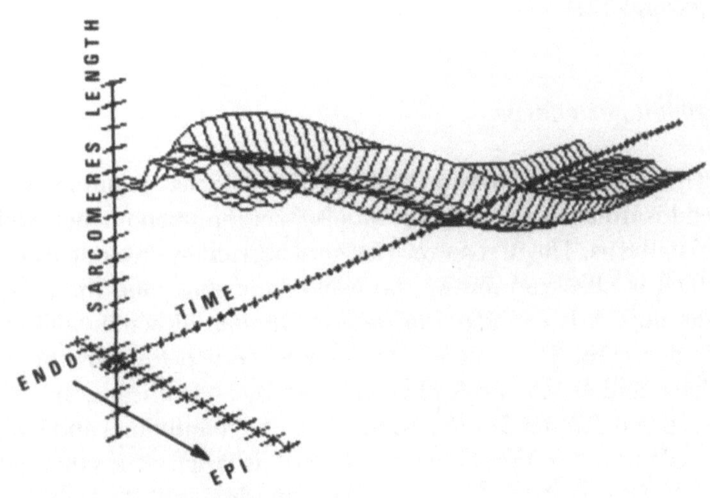

Figure 12. Sarcomeres' length as a function of time and the relative location within the myocardial wall.

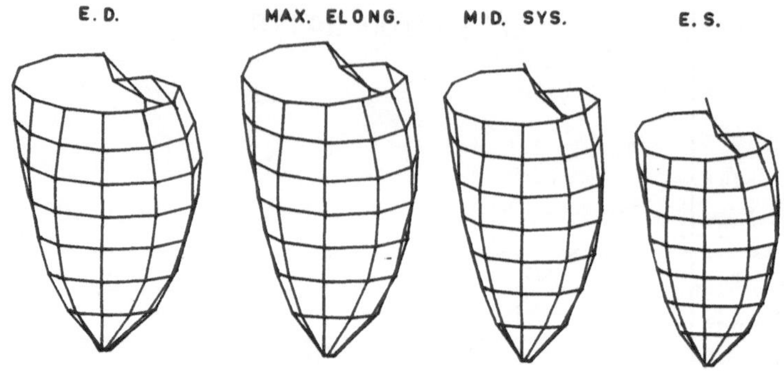

Figure 13. Calculated 3-D geometrical changes during systole.

Discussion

The capability of the suggested simulation to yield reliable predictions of the global LV performance under varying loading conditions has been clearly demonstrated here. As shown in Table 1 and Fig. 9, the manifestation of the Frank-Starling mechanism is evident from the reaction of the simulation to different preloading conditions. The corresponding temporal changes in LV volume and aortic blood flow are in good agreement with reported physiological measurements [24].

The ES elastance line obtained for different loading conditions by linear regression of the ES P-V values is consistent with the phenomena reported by Suga and Sawaga [23].

The elliptization phenomena

Examining the predicted extension ratio for a LV which is simultaneously excited from the endocardial surface reveals an elliptization phenomenon which is evident by two patterns. The first pattern is characterized by an elongation of the LV muscle, which is observed during the isovolumic stage and the early stage of ejection: the muscle is elongated in the longitudinal direction while the lateral dimensions decrease. The second pattern is observed towards the end of the ejection phase and at ES and is characterized by a significant, and rather constant, difference (of about 5% at ES) between the lingitudinal and lateral extension ratios. Clearly, the long-to-short axis ratio is larger at ES than at ED [25]. Note that both these patterns were observed experimentally by Rankin et al. [26].

The manifestation of the elliptization phenomena seems to be important in the level of the individual sarcomere and at the level of the global LV geometry. As seen in Fig. 12, the simulation predicts that the sarcomeres in the endocardial and

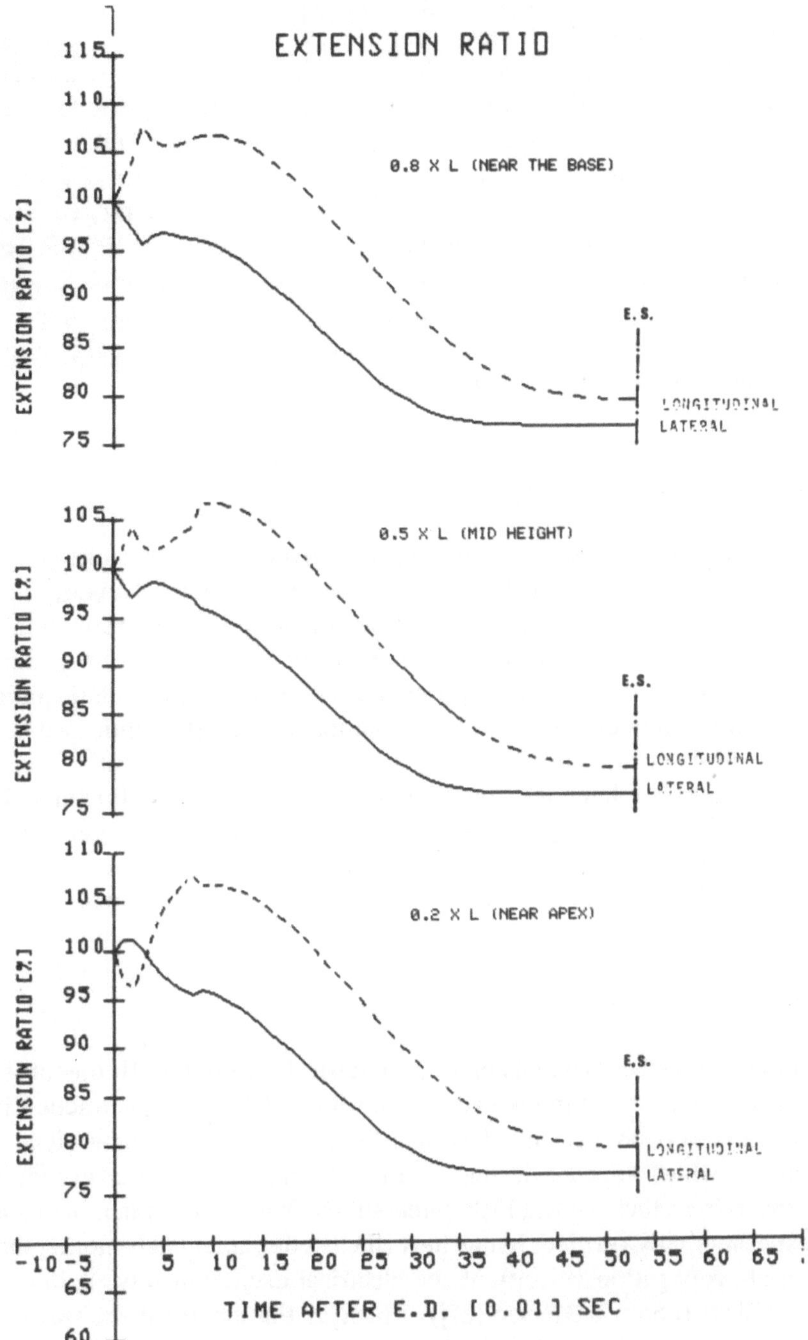

Figure 14. Calculated extension ratio for three myocardial elements located at 20%, 50% and 80% of the LV height. Electrical excitation is initiated at the apex.

epicardial layers which are more longitudinally oriented stretch more than the mid-wall layers during the initial systolic stages. However, the difference in sarcomeres lengths is minimal at ES. This stretching phenomena rearranges the sarcomeres lengths distribution so that the contraction in both the longitudinal and the lateral directions is uniform during the ejection phase. This is equivalent to the application of the Frank-Starling mechanism in the longitudinal direction which compensates for the smaller number of longitudinally arranged fibers.

The elliptization phenomena in the global 3-D level is seen in Fig. 13. The LV lateral diameters become shorter while the major axis becomes longer.It is suggested that the stretching of the long axis creates a 'catapult effect' which pushes the blood forward in a piston-like manner, thus improving the conditions for blood flow during the ejection period.

Electro-mechanical interaction

The combination of electrical excitation with myocardial mechanics presented here, provides a new theoretical tool for studying the mechanical manifestation of different activation configurations of LV. In the present study, activation delay times were calculated by using a simple model which is based on the assumption that the electrical excitation wave propagates along minimal geodetic pathways [1]. This simple model restricts the simulation to simple elliptic geometries. However, since it is not an inherent part of the simulation, realistic geometries can be studied by implementing more advanced electrical excitation models, (as an input), without changing anything in the simulation described here. Regardless of this limitation, the importance of the electro-mechanical interaction is well demonstrated by the prediction of the interesting 'vertical kick' phenomena.

'The vertical kick' phenomena

Examining the predicted extension ratio pattern shown in Fig. 11, one observes, in the very short interval immediately following ED, a rapid contraction in the longitudinal direction associated with a lateral increase in dimensions. This phenomena, which appears during the first 20 milliseconds after excitation, is referred herein as the 'vertical kick' phenomena. Though this phenomena is still to be experimentally verified, it may nevertheless be explained by noting that the transmural propagation velocity of the electrical excitation wave is finite, and relatively slow (about 0.3 m/sec [27]). Thus, as the electrical excitation wave propagates radially, the endocardial fibers are activated first while the mid wall layers are still in their passive state. Due to the fact that the endocardial fibers have angles of inclination which are closer to 90 degrees, the sarcomeres shortening will occur mainly in the longitudinal direction. The lateral increase of the dimensions is thus a constraint induced by the isovolumic state.

A similar phenomena is noted in Fig. 14 where the calculated patterns for three myocardial elements, located at different heights, is shown for the case of an apical excitation of the LV. Examining the myocardial element closest to the point of excitation (20% of the LV height, from the apex), identifies the 'vertical kick' phenomenon. However, as one approaches the LV base it is seen that the muscle is stretched longitudinally before performing the 'vertical kick'. The delay in the 'vertical kick' increases even more as one approaches the LV base. The explanation for this phenomena is as follows: as the myocardial muscle near the apex (which is the point of excitation) deform, the LV pressure increases. Unactivated zones of the LV muscle (closer to the base) deform passively due to the increase of the internal pressure. Passive elongation will occur since the radius of curvature in the longitudinal direction is larger (and the stress is greater) than the lateral one, and the deformations in both directions are related through the isovolumic constraint. The 'vertical kick' is produced when the excitation wave reaches the endocardial layers. Finally, the elliptization phenomena takes place once the muscle is fully activated.

Summary

A simulation procedure which combines myocardial mechanics with electrical excitation of the LV is introduced. The simulation is based on real 3-D LV geometry and is captable of predicting local phenomena in the sarcomeres and myocardial elements levels as well as global 3-D deformations. The simulation demonstrates reliable responses to various loading conditions and yields good agreement with reported experimental data. The model describes and explains the experimentally reported [26] and verified [27] elliptization phenomenon and relates the theories of electrical wave propagation and fiber structure to local myocardial deformations.

Acknowledgment

This study was supported by a grant from The Jack and Pauline Freeman Foundation and sponsored by the Women's Division, American Technion Society, USA and the British Technion Society, London, UK.

Appendix A: Lateral deformation

Lateral deformation is defined in the curvilinear coordinate system used here by the change in the length of the external radial distance Ri (see Fig. 4). This length represents the distance from point P_i on the coordinate ξ to the new point of intersection P_i' (on the vector $\bar{R}_i$ and the deformed endocardial surface, $M(t+dt)$). Since it is assumed that all endocardial points move radially with reference to the instantaneous centroid (point C) of the cross-section, the angular distance $\Delta\theta$ between any two sampled points P_j and P_{j+1} is the same before and after deformation. Thus, the arc length S_j at time t can be estimated by:

$$S_j = \int_0^{\Delta\theta} [R_{cj} + \frac{\Delta R_{cj}}{\Delta\theta}\theta]d\theta = \Delta\theta[R_{cj} + \Delta R_{cj}/2], \quad \text{(A-1)}$$

while the deformed arc length at time $t + dt$ is estimated by:

$$S_j' = \int_0^{\Delta\theta} [R_{cj}' + \frac{\Delta R_{cj}'}{\Delta\theta}\theta]d\theta = \Delta\theta[R_{cj}' + \Delta R_{cj}'/2], \quad \text{(A-2)}$$

where R_{cj} and R_{cj}' are the pre and post deformation distances from the centroid to the points P_j and P_j', respectively (R_{cj} is calculated from the given instantaneous geometry), and $\Delta R_{cj} \equiv R_{cj} - R_{cj}'$.

The myocardial strain $\varepsilon_{\theta\theta}$ is defined by:

$$\varepsilon_{\theta\theta j} = (S_j' - S_j)/S_j, \quad \text{(A-3)}$$

the strain along R_{cj} is defined by:

$$\varepsilon_{R\,cj} = (R_{cj}' - R_{cj})/R_{cj}, \quad \text{(A-4)}$$

and the new radial difference $\Delta R_{cj}'$ is estimated by:

$$\Delta R_{cj}' \cong \Delta R_{cj}[1 + \varepsilon_{R_{cj}} + \frac{\Delta\varepsilon_{R\,cj}}{\Delta\theta}\Delta\theta]. \quad \text{(A-5)}$$

Substituting all these relations into (A-3) yields:

$$\varepsilon_{\theta\theta j} = \varepsilon_{R_{cj}} + \Delta R_{cj}\, \Delta\varepsilon_{R_{cj}}/2[R_{cj} + \Delta R_{cj}/2], \quad \text{(A-6)}$$

where the second term may be neglected for all practical purposes. The distance between point O (the cylinder's axis) and point Pj is given by,

$$r_j = D/2 - R_j, \quad \text{(A-7)}$$

and the distance between point O and C, defined as a, is calculated from the given instantaneous geometry. Applying the cosine theorem to triangle OCPj the new value of Rj (marked R_j') can be estimated from:

$$R_j' = R_j - \varepsilon_{\theta\theta j}[(D/2 - R_j)^2 + R_{cj}^2 - a^2]/(D - 2R_j). \quad \text{(A-8)}$$

Appendix B: Longitudinal deformation

Consider two points, A and B, on a longitudinal cross-section of the endocardial (Fig. 5), for which the vertical distance is H and the arc length is S. These points deform into their new location A′ and B′, for which the vertical distance is H′ and the arc length is S′. It is assumed that the radius of curvature is very large with comparison to the deformation involved so that for a very short interval of time it may be taken as a constant and so is its center point C.

By definition all the following relations are given:

$$\varepsilon_{\varphi\varphi} = (S' - S)/S,$$
$$\alpha = S/R_{\varphi\varphi},$$
$$\alpha' = S'/R_{\varphi\varphi},$$
$$\Delta\alpha = \Delta S/R_{\varphi\varphi},$$
$$\overline{AB} = 2R_{\varphi\varphi}\mathrm{Sin}(\alpha/2),$$
$$\overline{A'B'} = 2R_{\varphi\varphi}\mathrm{Sin}(\alpha'/2).$$

Since the myocardinal element between A and B is rather small, it may be assumed that its deformation is homogeneous and symmetric as shown in Fig. 5. Thus two similar triangles may be built:

$$\Delta ABD \sim \Delta A'B'D',$$

so that:

$$\frac{A'B'}{AB} = \frac{H'}{H}, \tag{B-1}$$

or, equivalently,

$$\frac{\mathrm{Sin}\ (\alpha'/2)}{\mathrm{Sin}\ (\alpha/2)} = \frac{H'}{H}. \tag{B-2}$$

By definition,

$$H' = H + \Delta H = H(1 + \varepsilon_H), \tag{B-3}$$

therefore,

$$1 + \varepsilon_H = \frac{\mathrm{Sin}\ (\alpha'/2)}{\mathrm{Sin}\ (\alpha/2)},$$

$$\varepsilon_H = -1 + \frac{\mathrm{Sin}\ (\alpha'/2)}{\mathrm{Sin}\ (\alpha/2)}$$

$$= -1 + \frac{\text{Sin}\ (\alpha/2 + \frac{\Delta S}{2R_{\varphi\varphi}})}{\text{Sin}\ (\alpha/2)}$$

$$= -1 + \frac{\text{Sin}\ (\alpha/2)\cos(\frac{\Delta S}{2R_{\varphi\varphi}}) + \cos\ (\alpha/2\ \text{Sin}\ (\frac{\Delta S}{2R_{\varphi\varphi}})}{\text{Sin}\ (\alpha/2)}, \tag{B-4}$$

but $\Delta S \ll 2R_{\varphi\varphi}$, hence:

$$\varepsilon_H = -1 + \frac{\Delta S}{2R_{\varphi\varepsilon}} + \text{Sin}\ \frac{\Delta S}{2R_{\varphi\varphi}}/\text{Tan}\ (\alpha/2)$$

$$\simeq 1 - 1 + \frac{\Delta S}{2R_{\varphi\varphi}\ \text{Tan}\,(\alpha/2)} \tag{B-5}$$

Substituting for ΔS

$$\Delta S = \varepsilon_{\varphi\varphi} S$$

yields,

$$\varepsilon_H = \varepsilon_{\varphi\varphi} \frac{S}{2R_{\varphi\varphi}\text{Tan}\,(s/2R)}, \tag{B-6}$$

or, equivalently,

$$H' = H[1 + \varepsilon_{\varphi\varphi} \frac{S}{2R_{\varphi\varphi}\text{Tan}\,(s/2R_{\varphi\varphi})}]. \tag{B-7}$$

Appendix C: Average active stresses

Average active stresses $\bar{\sigma}_{f\theta\theta}$ and $\bar{\sigma}_{f\varphi\varphi}$ were calculated by integrating the projection of the active fiber stress σ_f of every layer of sarcomeres in the principle directions θ and φ (Fig. 15) and are given by:

$$\bar{\sigma}_{f\theta\theta} = \int_0^1 \sigma_f[t(\tau),\ SL(\eta)]\text{Cos}^2[\psi(\eta)]d\eta, \tag{C-1}$$

$$\bar{\sigma}_{f\varphi\varphi} = \int_0^1 \sigma_f[t(\tau),\ SL(\eta)]\text{Sin}^2[\psi(\eta)]d\eta, \tag{C-2}$$

where ψ is the angle of inclination for the fibers, η is the integration variable representing the normalized location along the LV wall, SL is the sacomeres length in the fiber, t is the time measured from ED and τ is the activation delay time, here calculated by [1].

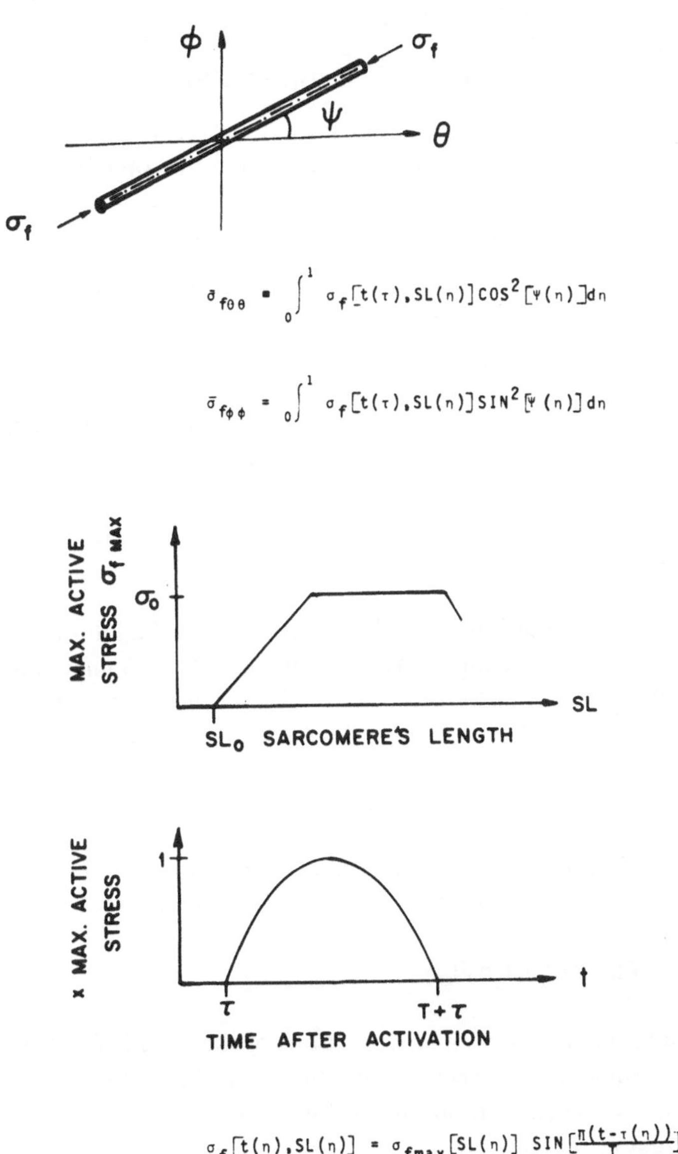

$$\bar{\sigma}_{f\theta\theta} = \int_0^1 \sigma_f[t(\tau), SL(n)]\cos^2[\psi(n)]dn$$

$$\bar{\sigma}_{f\phi\phi} = \int_0^1 \sigma_f[t(\tau), SL(n)]\sin^2[\psi(n)]dn$$

$$\sigma_f[t(n), SL(n)] = \sigma_{fmax}[SL(n)] \sin\left[\frac{\pi(t-\tau(n))}{T}\right]$$

$$= 0 \text{ for } t > T+\tau(n) \text{ or } \tau(n) > t$$

Figure 15. Relations used for calculating the average active stresses (see Appendix C).

The time-dependent stress function is approximated by a half sinusoidal function of the form [28]:

$$\sigma_f[t(\eta),SL(\eta)] = \begin{cases} \sigma_{f_{max}}[SL(\eta)]\ \mathrm{Sin}[\frac{\pi(t-\tau(\eta))}{T}] \\ 0 \text{ for } t > T + \tau(\eta) \text{ or } \tau(\eta) > t. \end{cases} \tag{C-3}$$

The relationship between the maximum normalized isometric stress at sarcomere length SL is calculated using the function provided by Pollack et al. [29]:

$$\sigma_{f_{max}} = \begin{cases} \frac{(SL - SL_o)\bar{\sigma}_o}{0.55}, & 1.65 < SL < 2.2\mu; \\ \bar{\sigma}_o, & 2.2 < SL < 2.4\mu; \\ \bar{\sigma}_o - \frac{(SL - 2.4)\bar{\sigma}_o}{0.55}, & SL > 2.4\mu, \end{cases} \tag{C-4}$$

Where $\bar{\sigma}_o$ is the maximum normalized isometric stress at sarcomere length SL and SL_o is the minimum sarcomere length required for active stress development.

Appendix D: Average resistive stresses

The resistive stresses induced in the LV muscle due to the internal pressure are calculated by taking a horizontal cross-section through the point of interest at the state of equilibrium, as shown in Fig. 16. First, the contribution of passive stretching is eliminated by subtracting the passive pressure:

$$Pa = P - P_P, \tag{D-1}$$

where Pa and P_P are the LV passive and active pressures respectively. The longitudial stresses are then calculated, assuming equilibrium by:

$$\bar{\sigma}_{\varphi\varphi} = Pa\, Ab/Am\, \mathrm{Cos}^2(\gamma), \tag{D-2}$$

where Ab and Am are the area cross-sections of the blood and muscle, respectively, and γ is the angle between $\sigma_{\varphi\varphi}$ and the vertical direction.

Applying the Laplace equation for a thin walled shell, the estimated lateral tangential stress $\bar{\sigma}_{\theta\theta}$ is given by:

$$\bar{\sigma}_{\theta\theta} = R_{\theta\theta}[\,Pa/W - \bar{\sigma}_{\varphi\varphi}/R_{\varphi\varphi}]. \tag{D-3}$$

resistive stresses

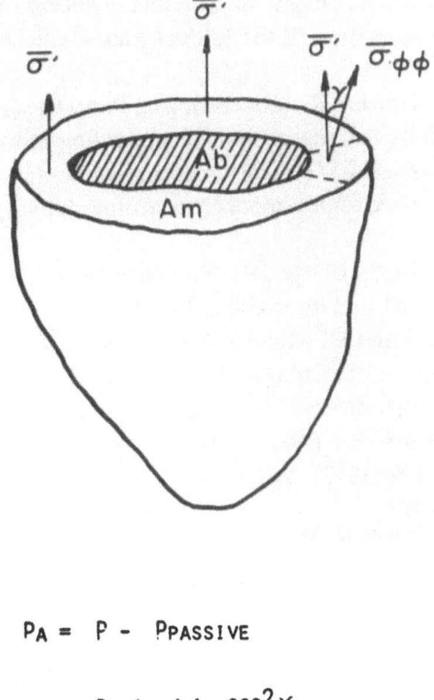

$$\sigma_{\phi\phi} = P_A A_B / A_M \cos^2\gamma$$

$$\sigma_{\theta\theta} = R_{\theta\theta}\left[P_A/W - \sigma_{\phi\phi}/R_{\phi\phi}\right]$$

Figure 16. Configuration used for calculating the average resistive stresses (see Appendix D).

References

1. Barta E, Adam D, Salant E, Sideman S (1987): 3-D ventricular myocardial electrical excitation: A minimal orthogonal pathways model. Annal Biomed Eng (in press).
2. Welkowitz W (1975): Indices of cardiac status. IEEE Trans Biomed Eng 28: 553–567.
3. Weber KT, Janicki JS (1979): The heart as a muscle pump system and the concept of heart failure. Am Heart J 98: 371–384.
4. Dewysen BA (1977): Parameter estimation of a simple model of the left ventricle and of the systemic vascular bed with particular attention to the physical meaning of left ventricular parameters. IEEE Trans Biomed Eng BME-24: 29–38.
5. Beyar R, Sideman S (1984): Model for left ventricular contraction combining the force length velocity relationship with the time varying elastance theory. Biophys J 45: 1167–1177.
6. Arts T, Reneman RS, Venstra PC (1979): A model of the mechanics of the left ventricle. Ann Biomed Eng 7: 299–318.
7. Arena DJ, Ohley WJ (1983): Analysis of left ventricular mechanics during filling isovolumic contraction and ejection. IEEE Trans Biomed Eng BME-30 1: 35–42.

8. Perl M, Horowitz A, Sideman S (1986): A comprehensive model for the simulation of left ventricle mechanics. IEEE Med and Biol Eng & Comput 24: 145–156.
9. Heethar RM, Pao YC, Ritman EL (1977): Computer aspects of three dimensional finite element analysis of the stresses and strains in the intact heart. Comp & Biomed Res 10: 271–285.
10. Azhari H, Beyar R, Gzenadier E, Dinnar U, Sideman S (1987): An analytical descriptor of 3-D geometry. Application to the analysis of the left ventricle shape and contraction. Trans Biomed Eng (in press).
11. Schnittger I, Fitzgerald PJ, Gordon P, Alderman EL, Popp RL (1984): Computerized quantitative analysis of wall motion by two dimensional echocardiography. Circulation 70(2): 242–254.
12. Moynihn PF, Parisi F, Feldman CL (1981): Quantitative detection of regional left ventricular contraction abnormalities by two dimensional echocardiography: 1) analysis of methods. Circulation 63(4): 752–760.
13. Walley KR, Grover M, Raff GL, Benge JW, Hannaford B, Glantz SA (1982): Left ventricular dynamic geometry in the intact and open chest dog. Circulation 50(4): 573–589.
14. Streeter DD, Spotnitz HM, Patel DP, Ross J, Sonnenblick EH (1969): Fiber orientation in the canine left ventricle during diastole and systole. Circ Res 24: 339–347.
15. Wong AYK (1973): Myocardial mechanics: application of sliding-filament theory to isovolumic concentration of the left ventricle. J Biomech 6: 565–581.
16. Yoran C, Covell JW, Ross J Jr (1973): Structural basis for the ascending limb of left ventricular function. Circ Res 32: 297–303.
17. Spotnitz HM, Sonnenblick EH, Spiro D (1966): Relation of ultrastructure to function in the intact heart: Sarcomere structure relative to pressure volume curves of the intact left ventricles of dog and cat. Circ Res 18: 49–65.
18. Hussy M (1975): Diagnostic ultrasound. Blackie & Son Ltd, Glasgow p. 148.
19. Taylor RR, Ross J, Covell JW, Sonnenblick EH (1967): A quantitative analysis of left ventricular myocardial function in the intact, sedated dog. Circ Res 21: 99–115.
20. Mashima H (1984): Force – velocity relation and contractility in striated muscles. Jpn J Physiol 34: 1–17.
21. O'Rourke MF, Yaginuma T, Avolio AP (1984): Physiological and pathological implications of ventricular/vascular coupling. Annals Biomed Eng 12: 119–134.
22. Streeter DD, Hanna WT (1973): Engineering mechanics for succesive states in canine left ventricular myocardium. 1 – Cavity and wall geometry. Circ Res 23: 639–655.
23. Suga H, Sagawa K (1974): Instantaneous pressure-volume relationships and their ratio in the exercised supported canine left ventricle. Circ Res 35: 117–126.
24. Vatner S (1986): personal communication.
25. Rushmer RF (1972): Organ physiology. Structure and function of the cardiovascular system. WB Saunders Comp, Philadelphia, PA, p. 53.
26. Rankin JS, McHale PA, Arentzen CE, Ling D, Greenfield JC, Anderson RW (1978): The three dimensional dynamic geometry of the left ventricle in the conscious dog. Circ Res 39: 304–313.
27. Berne RM, Levy MN (1967): Cardiovascular physiology. CV Mosby Publ, St Louis, Chapter 2, pp. 17–19.
28. Beyar R, Sideman S (1984): A computer study of the left ventricular performances based on fiber structure, sarcomere dynamics and transmural electrical propagation velocity. Circ Res 55: 358–375.
29. Pollack GH, Krueger JW (1978): Myocardial sarcomere mechanics: Some parallels with skeletal muscle. In: Baan Y, Noordergraaf A, Raines J (eds) Cardiovascular system dynamics. MIT Press, Cambridge, pp. 3–10.

Discussion

Arts: Do you introduce torsion into the model?

Beyar: It is possible to include the torsion into the model in these helical coordinates. Although the torsion is not shown here, it can be included in the calculation.

Marcus: What has been done to verify the results predicted by the model?

Azhari: Global LV performance has been verified as shown in the paper. It is also potentially possible to verify the 3-D geometrical prediction by quantitatively estimating the similarity of two 3-D geometries using the helical coordinate system. However, in order to do so, one has to supply accurate dynamic 3-D geometrical data obtained experimentally for a heart which is excited in a certain configuration. Should such data be available, the predicted LV 3-D geometry could be examined.

Bassingthwaighte: What can also be done is to test the model by attempting to fit data obtained under special or extreme conditions. Then you can see if the experiment matches the predictions.

Lab: If you had an infarct in the model it would affect excitability and you would also get mechanical dyskinesis. Would it be difficult to model this? Would it shift the pressure-volume relationship? This would be a very useful model if it did.

Azhari: It is possible to insert an infarct, or other abnormal myocardial properties, to the model. However, since the model utilizes a kinematic assumption regarding lateral contraction, one should check very carefully before doing so, and verify the validity of such an assumption to the abnormal heart.

20. The mechanical effects of the pericardium on the left ventricle

J.V. TYBERG

Abstract

Evidence is reviewed which shows that pericardial hydrostatic (liquid) pressure is an inappropriate and sometimes seriously inaccurate measure of the mechanical effect of the pericardium on left ventricular diastolic filling. The appropriate measure, so-called pericardial surface pressure, is approximately equal to right ventricular diastolic pressure under many circumstances. Thus, the constraint exerted by the pericardium is much more significant than previously appreciated. Studies also suggest that effective left ventricular preload (i.e., transmural end diastolic pressure) can be estimated by subtracting right ventricular from left ventricular diastolic pressure.

Introduction

The recent resurgence of interest in the role of the pericardium in health and disease is related to the magnitude of pericardial pressure. As recently as 1983 Spodick [1] succinctly summarized the consensus opinion in a special article for the inaugural issue of the *Journal of the American College of Cardiology*. He referred to the pericardium '... as a fluid-filled chamber at slightly subatmospheric pressure ...' and later stated that '... pericardial pressure is approximately equal to and varies with pleural pressure ...' and that '... the normally negative pericardial pressure produces a [LV] distending pressure that is higher than intracavitary pressure ...'. Although earlier physiologists had notably elucidated the physiology of the pericardium [2–5], the position most commonly supported was the interpretation resulting from the experiments of Kenner and Wood [6]. Using liquid-filled, open pericardial catheters in intact dogs they obstructed the pulmonary arterial outflow, raised right atrial pressure considerably ($\approx$30 mm Hg) and demonstrated that pericardial pressure remained near 0 mm Hg and did not change systematically as a function of right atrial pressure. Accordingly, the opinion developed that the size of the heart could be varied dramatically without making pericardial pressure different from the generally accepted value of pleural pressure. Thus, there seemed no reason to consider the effect of the pericardium in the hemodynamic analysis of congestive heart failure.

The objectives of this discussion are, first, to examine the newer evidence which brings the previously prevailing concensus position into question and, second, to consider some reinterpretations of the role of the pericardium if, indeed, pericardial pressure is sometimes much greater than heretofore appreciated.

Surface pressure vs. liquid pressure

The hemodynamic significance of the pericardium obviously depends upon the magnitude of pericardial pressure, as discussed above. The magnitude of pericardial pressure depends upon the techniques used to measure it and these, in turn, depend upon our concept of pericardial pressure.

A cardiologist or a cardiovascular physiologist generally assumes that 'pressure' can be measured with a liquid-filled catheter and a conventional pressure transducer, of course, for good reason. Pressure is a stress that is uniform in all directions [7], this relation being known as Pascal's Law. This definition is critical to our reasoning about the concept of pericardial pressure. While it is obvious from common experience and from experimental observations [6] that the pericardium is not normally distended, the possibility remains that there may be significant, radially-directed forces exerted between the ventricular epicardial surface and the pericardium. This possibility is, perhaps, best illustrated by a consideration of the human knee joint [8]. While the pressure of the liquid in the joint space has been found to be near atmospheric pressure [9], the average force per unit area of the common articular surface can be estimated to be equivalent to nearly 10 atmospheres. Obviously, the atmospheric pressure of the synovial fluid has no important relation to the mechanics of the joint. By analogy, I suggest that the pressure of the liquid in the pericardium may not be the most relevant parameter by which to assess the mechanical effect of the pericardium on ventricular diastolic filling.

A very similar problem was solved several years ago by Agostoni and Mead and their coworkers – the interaction between lung and chest wall [10, 11]. They defined the term 'surface pressure' and stated that it is equal to 'liquid pressure' (i.e., the conventionally measured pressure of a fluid) plus 'deformational forces' which can be taken as radially directed, compressive, contact stress. (This definition represents a significant semantic problem since 'surface pressure' does not fulfill the definition of pressure given above.) The evidence discussed below suggests that 'surface pressure' is the appropriate measure of the mechanical effect of the pericardium.

It was reasoned [12] that a static force balance could be constructed for the LV endocardial surface at end diastole (and at any other time when motion, and thus inertial and viscous forces, could be neglected) (see Figure 1). If this is true, effective pericardial pressure must be equal to the difference between LV intracavitary pressure and transmural pressure. Fortunately, if one assume that there

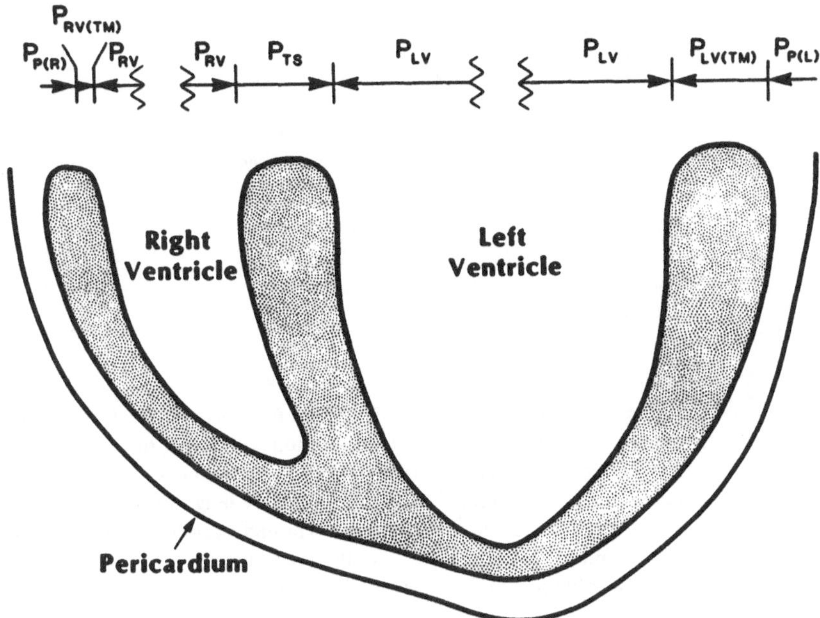

Figure 1. Static equilibria at end diastole. On the right, the LV intracavitary pressure (P_{LV}) is exactly opposed by the sum of the transmural pressure of the LV free wall ($P_{LV(TM)}$) and the effective pericardial pressure ($P_{P(L)}$). In the center, the LV intracavitary pressure is exactly opposed by the sum of the transseptal pressure (P_{TS}) and the RV intracavitary pressure (P_{RV}). On the left, the RV intracavitary pressure is exactly opposed by transmural pressure of the RV free wall ($P_{RV(TM)}$) and the effective pericardial pressure exerted on the surface of the RV ($P_{P(R)}$). (Reproduced with the permission of the publisher [12].)

is a constant relationship between ventricular transmural pressure and volume (i.e., that the distensibility of the ventricle is not changed by removing the pericardium) it is possible to directly measure LV transmural pressure as a function of volume after the pericardium has been removed [13]. Thus, the effective pericardial 'pressure' at any ventricular volume is equal to the difference between the end diastolic LV intracavitary pressure recorded when the pericardium is intact and that same pressure (at the identical volume) after the pericardium has been removed and any contact with the lungs prevented (see Figure 2).

We then undertook to compare two technical approaches to the measurement of pericardial pressure – an open, liquid-filled, multiple-side-hole catheter and a transducer consisting of a flat liquid-containing balloon connected to an external manometer [5] – to each other and, more importantly, to the effective pericardial pressure estimated by the rationale just described [13]. We showed that when all the liquid is removed from the pericardium the pressure measured with an open catheter is virtually zero while pericardial surface pressure (as measured with the balloon) can be very significant in relation to intracavitary pressure. Perhaps this

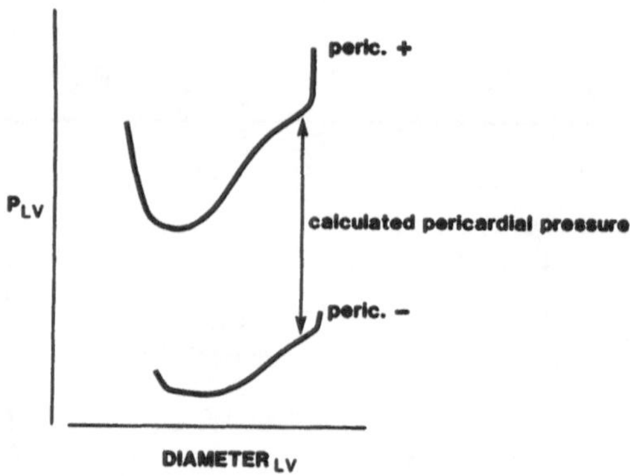

Figure 2. Schematic diagram indicating the means of calculating effective pericardial pressure over the free wall of the left ventricle. The top line represents the diastolic portion of the pressure-diameter (sonomicrometry) loop with the pericardium intact (peric. +). The bottom line represents the loop recorded after the pericardium had been removed (peric. −) and the lungs prevented from touching the heart. Note that the end diastolic diameters are identical. The end diastolic pressure of the bottom loop represents the LV transmural pressure. Therefore, the vertical distance between the two loops represents the effective pericardial pressure. (Compare Figure 1.) (Reproduced with permission of the American Heart Association [13].)

was best illustrated when, near the end of the experiment, we made several small incisions in the pericardium. The liquid (50 ml) escaped and pressure measured with the open catheter fell to zero. However, pericardial surface pressure remained significantly high (see Figure 3).

If pericardial surface pressure is equal to liquid pressure plus contact stress and if contact stress is different at different locations over the surface of the heart (as would seem obvious from *a priori* geometrical and mechanical considerations), it follows that pericardial surface pressure can vary over the surface of the heart. We recently demonstrated this by measuring pericardial surface pressure over the right and left ventricular free walls [14]. We compared the changes in these pressures during volume loading and during pulmonary artery constriction (cf. [6]). Whereas the change in right ventricular pericardial surface pressure was equal to that over the left ventricle when the heart was expanded rather symmetrically as a result of increasing the circulating blood volume, pulmonary artery constriction results in a large increase in RV pericardial surface pressure but an actual *decrease* in LV pericardial surface pressure. We offered two explanations:

1. pulmonary artery constriction decreases 'venous return' to the left ventricle (LV preload decreased) and
2. the mechanical attachments of the heart and pericardium may be sufficient to prevent leftward motion of the heart (which would allow the respective pericardial surface pressures to equalize).

More recently, LeWinter and his colleagues have confirmed that surface pressures vary in different locations [15].

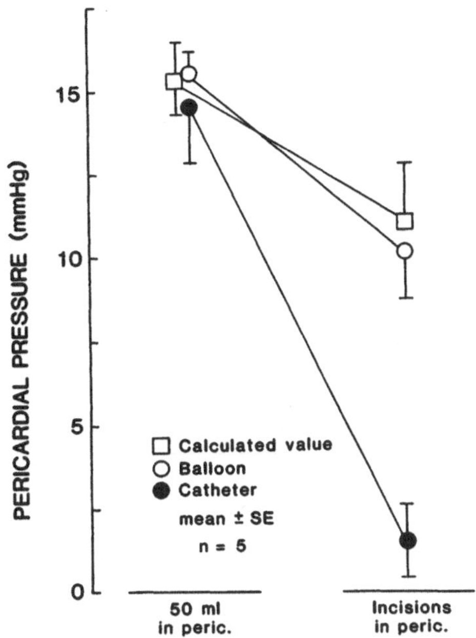

Figure 3. Data showing the effect on pericardial pressure of making several small incisions in pericardia originally containing 50 ml of saline. The LV end diastolic pressure at the beginning of the experiments was 20 ± 2 mm Hg. While pericardial liquid pressure (open catheter) was equal to pericardial surface pressure (balloon) and to calculated effective pericardial pressure at the beginning of the experiment, draining the pericardium caused pericardial liquid pressure to approach zero. Although manipulation of the heart caused pericardial surface pressure to decline it stayed equal to the calculated effective pressure, thus indicating that only a balloon or similar device can measure pericardial constraint in an unsealed pericardium. (Reproduced with permission of the American Heart Association [13].)

Thus, two comments must be made about the observations of Kenner and Wood [6]. First, in principle, pericardial constraint cannot be assessed with an open catheter and, if the pericardium does not contain sufficient liquid, the disparity between liquid pressure and surface pressure may be very significant hemodynamically. Second, an assymetrical expansion of one side of the heart (e.g., pulmonary artery constriction) may not increase the pericardial surface pressure over the contralateral ventricle.

As apparent in Figure 1, if the elastic properties of the interventricular septum are similar to that of the LV free wall and if the transmural pressure of the right ventricle is relatively small, right ventricular diastolic pressure must be approximately equal to pericardial pressure. In dogs we have shown that mean diastolic pericardial surface pressure over the left ventricular free wall is approximately equal to right ventricular mean diastolic (and right atrial) pressure [16]. Recently, we demonstrated a similar relationship in patients studied at the beginning of elective cardiac surgery [17]. As shown in Figure 4, in each case the change in

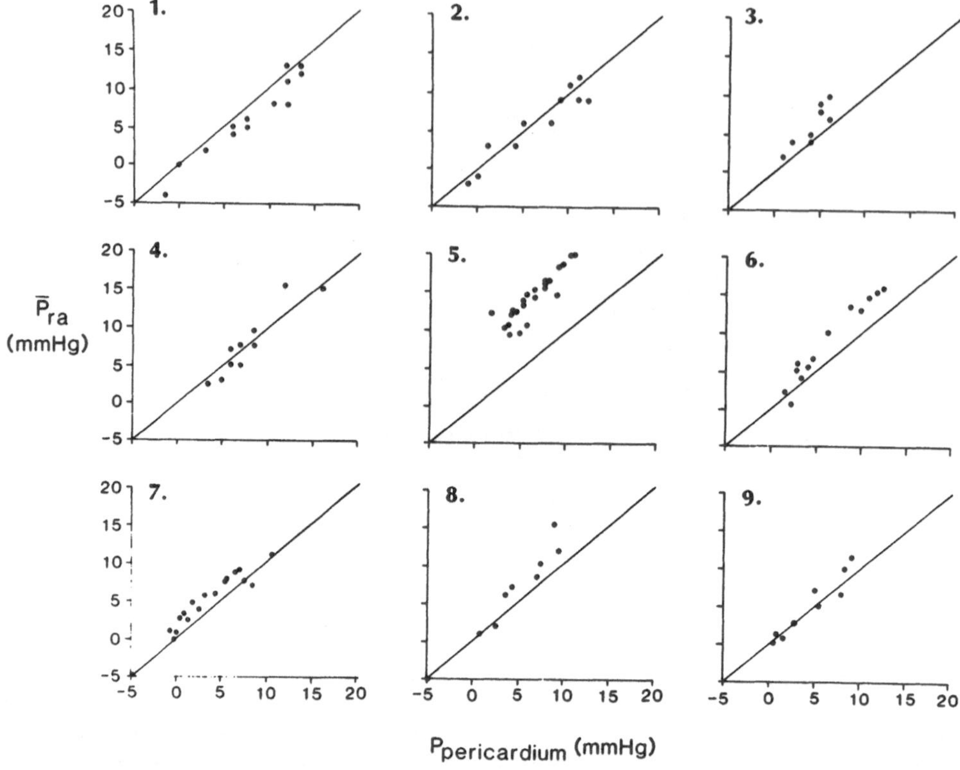

Figure 4. Mean right atrial pressure vs mean pericardial surface pressure recorded with a balloon placed between the LV lateral free wall and the parietal pericardium. In 9 patients the balloon was inserted through a 2 cm pericardial incision immediately after sternotomy and before intravenous saline infusion. In each patient the change in mean right atrial pressure was equal to the change in mean pericardial surface pressure. Furthermore, except in patient 5, mean right atrial presssure was approximately equal to the mean pericardial surface pressure. (Reproduced with permission of he American Heart Association [17].)

mean right atrial pressure was exactly the same as the change in mean pericardial surface pressure recorded from the LV lateral free wall. In addition, the absolute magnitudes seemed virtually identical.

These findings imply that RV transmural pressures are negligible over the range studied. This somewhat surprising finding requires further study. For example, the relationship between RA and pericardial pressure should be determined in patients with RV hypertrophy.

Thus, these observations in patients which confirm previous experimental work suggest a strategy to be tried in evaluating the cardiac performance of patients. If mean right atrial or right ventricular diastolic pressure is a useful indicator of the pressure external to the left ventricle, these quantities can be subtracted from left ventricular filling pressure to estimate transmural pressure, end diastolic transmural pressure being the best measure of preload. Of course, preload determines end diastolic volume which, in the absence of changes in contractility, predicts systolic performance according to the Frank-Starling Law.

Clinical implications

In the case of pericardial tamponade, pericardial liquid pressure (i.e., the pressure measured through the draining cannula) represents the effective external constraint to left ventricular diastolic filling. However, our recent work suggests that this is not always true as the effusion is drained [8]. As the pericardial (liquid) pressure falls below right atrial pressure others [18, 19] have shown that left ventricular performance no longer improves. We showed in dogs that when the pressures diverge pericardial surface pressure remains high and equal to right atrial pressure. Therefore, it seems that right atrial pressure is the best measure of effective pericardial pressure in the case of pericardial effusion as well. When the effusion is considerable, right atrial pressure is equal to pericardial liquid pressure (which is equal to surface pressure under these circumstances since, when the heart is suspended in a larger volume of liquid, the compressive contact stress is negligible). Most importantly, however, right atrial pressure continues to reflect effective pericardial constraint even after removal of fluid causes the pericardiocentesis catheter pressure to significantly underestimate pericardial surface pressure. These conclusions need to be verified in patients in which pressures, volumes and systolic performance are measured simultaneously.

While rate-related changes in diastolic 'compliance' [20] in the presence of ischemia [21] have been shown to be caused by very transient changes in the distensibility of the myocardium [22], the shifts in the diastolic pressure-volume relationships which are seen in patients with a degree of congestive heart failure and which follow the administration of certain vasoactive drugs [23, 24] have not been explained. Recently, we gave nitroglycerin and empirically employed the analysis outlined above in patients who were shown at cardiac catheterization to have minimally elevated end diastolic pressure [25]. We confirmed the earlier observations by demonstrating that nitroglycerin produced a statistically significant parallel downward shift in the LV diastolic pressure-volume relationship. However, when the estimated transmural diastolic pressure-volume relationships (i.e., transmural LV pressure $\approx$LV intracavitary pressure $-$RV pressure) were compared, there was no evidence of a shift in the pressure-volume relationship – early and late diastolic points both before and after nitroglycerin all appeared to fall on the same curve.

The fact that vasodilators such as nitroglycerin and nitroprusside can shift the left ventricular pressure-volume relation is important hemodynamically, regardless of whether or not this is caused by an unappreciated reduction in pericardial surface pressure. While the therapeutic benefit of agents which are effective in *both* lowering LV filling pressure *and* maintaining (sometimes increasing) cardiac output is universally appreciated, this was difficult to explain since it was assumed that the reduction in LV intracavitary diastolic pressure meant a decrease in preload which would diminish performance (on the basis of the Frank-Starling Law). The parallel downward shift in the diastolic pressure-volume relationship means that end diastolic volumes does not decrease nearly as much as would have been expected, assuming a single, unchanging curve. Thus, while the decreases in arteriolar resistance undoubtedly help to maintain output, the maintenance of preload perhaps caused by the reduction in pericardial constraint may play a critical role [26].

During the past several years much of the work related to the so-called diastolic function of the heart has focussed on abnormalities in isovolumic relaxation of the left ventricle. Much of that work has employed the original semilogarithmic analysis of Weiss and Weisfeldt [27] to characterize isovolumic relaxation by $t_{1/2}$, the half time of the pressure decline. Studies in patients with cardiomyopathy or congestive neart failure have indicated that $t_{1/2}$ is elevated from normal values of 40–50 msec to values of 60–80 msec and that agents which lower filling pressure tend to reduce $t_{1/2}$ toward normal. We have shown that as pericardial pressure is elevated by means of pericardial effusion $t_{1/2}$ (as calculated from the slope of the semilogarithmic pressure decay) falls [28]. This is intuitively predictable since the addition of a constant (e.g., pericardial pressure) must decrease the slope because of the fundamental non-linearity of the logarithmic relation. While we also showed that newer analytical approaches [29, 30] are statistically independent of changes in pericardial pressure, there was considerable scatter in these data. Assuming that pericardial surface pressure affects $t_{1/2}$ in a similar way, it may be necessary to re-evaluate this literature.

Conclusion

In summary, I have reviewed evidence which suggest that the hemodynamic role of the pericardium may be much greater than previously appreciated. This conclusion depends critically on our conception of pericardial pressure and, if one can assume a static balance of forces at end diastole, the previously accepted measurements of pericardial liquid pressure are, in principle, irrelevant and, in practice, inaccurate as indicators of the mechanical effect of the pericardium on left ventricular diastolic filling. Our early studies in patients have suggested that in order to reliably estimate changes in effective LV preload (i.e., transmural end diastolic pressure) pericardial constraint must be accounted for. The empirical, simple relation between right ventricular filling pressure and pericardial surface pressure may prove to be a valuable tool.

References

1. Spodick DH (1983): The normal and diseased pericardium: Current concepts of pericardial physiology, diagnosis and treatment. J Am Coll Cardiol 1: 240–251.
2. Kuno Y (1915): The significance of he pericardium. J Physiol (London) 50: 1–36.
3. Gibbon JH Jr, Churchill ED (1931): The mechanical influence of the pericardium upon cardiac function. Clin Invest 10: 405–422.
4. Sarnoff SJ, Berglund E (1954): Ventricular function. I. Starling's law of the heart studied by means of simultaneous right and left ventricular function curves in the dog. Circulation 9: 706–718.
5. Holt JP, Rhode EA, Kines H (1960): Pericardial and ventricular pressure. Circ Res 8: 1171–1181.
6. Kenner HM, Wood EH (1966): Intrapericardial, intrapleural, and intracardiac pressures during acute heart failure in dogs studied without thoracotomy. Circ Res 19: 1071–1079.
7. Moore WJ (1962): Physical chemistry, 3rd ed. Prentice-Hall, Inc., Englewood Cliffs, p. 8.
8. Smiseth OA, Frais MA, Kingma I, White AVM, Knudtson ML, Cohen JM, Manyari DE, Smith ER, Tyberg JV (1986): Assessment of pericardial constraint: The relation between right ventricular filling pressure and pericardial pressure measured after pericardiocentesis. J Am Coll Cardiol 7: 307–314.
9. Muller W (1929): Über den negativen Luftdruck in Gelenkraum. Dtsch Z Chir 218: 395–401.
10. Agostoni E (1972): Mechanics of the pleural space. Physiol Rev 52: 57–128.
11. Agostoni E, Mead J (1964): Statics of the respiratory system. In: Handbook of physiology; Respiration. Washington, D.C. American Physiological Society, Sec. 3, Vol. I, pp. 387–409.
12. Tyberg JV (1985): Ventricular interaction and the pericardium. In: Levine HJ, Gaasch WH (eds) The ventricle: basic and clinical aspects. Martinus Nijhoff, Dordrecht/Boston, pp. 171–184.
13. Smiseth OA, Frais MA, Kingma I, Smith ER, Tyberg JV (1985): Assessment of pericardial constraint in dogs. Circulation 71: 158–164.
14. Smiseth OA, Douglas NWS, Smith ER, Tyberg JV (1985): Non-uniformity of pericardial surface pressure in dogs. Circulation 72: III-297 (Abstract).
15. Hoit B, Lew W, LeWinter M (1986): Regional variation in pericardial contact pressure. J Am Coll Cardiol 7: 205A (Abstract).
16. Smiseth OA, Refusm H, Tyberg JV (1984): Pericardial pressure assessed by right atrial pressure: A basis for calculation of left ventricular transmural pressure. Am Heart J 108: 603–608.
17. Tyberg JV, Taichman GC, Smith ER, Douglas NWS, Smiseth OA, Keon WJ (1986): The relation between pericardial pressure and right atrial pressure: An intraoperative study. Circulation 73: 428–432.
18. Reddy PS, Curtiss EI, O'Toole JD, Shaver JA (1978): Cardiac tamponade: hemodynamic observations in man. Circulation 58: 265–272.
19. Grose R, Greenberg M, Steingart R, Cohen MV (1982): Left ventricular volume and function during relief of cardiac tamponade in man. Circulation 66: 149–155.
20. Braunwald E, Ross J Jr (1963): The ventricular end-diastolic pressure. Am J Med 34: 147–150 (Editorial).
21. Barry WH, Brooker JZ, Alderman EL, Harrison DC (1974): Changes in diastolic stiffness and tone of the left ventricle during angina pectoris. Circulation 49: 255–263.
22. Serizawa T, Carabello BA, Grossman W (1980): Effect of pacing-induced ischemia on left ventricular diastolic pressure-volume relations in dogs with coronary stenoses. Circ Res 46: 430–439.
23. Alderman EL, Glantz SA (1976): Acute hemodynamic interventions shift the diastolic pressure-volume curve in man. Circulation 54: 662–671.
24. Ludbrook PA, Byrne JD, Kurnik MS, McKnight RC (1977): Influence of reduction of preload and afterload by nitroglycerin on left ventricular diastolic pressure-volume relations and relaxation in man. Circulation 56: 937–943.

25. Kingma I, Smiseth OA, Belenkie I, Knudtson ML, MacDonald RPR, Tyberg JV, Smith ER (1986): A mechanism for the nitroglycerin-induced downward shift of the left ventricular diastolic pressure-diameter relationship of patients. Am J Cardiol 57: 673–677.
26. Tyberg JV, Misbach GA, Parmley WW, Glantz SA (1980): Effects of the pericardium on ventricular performance. In: Baan J, Yellin EL, Arntzenius AC (eds) Cardiac dynamics. Martinus Nijhoff, Dordrecht/Boston, pp. 159–168.
27. Weiss JL, Frederiksen JW, Weisfeldt ML (1976): Hemodynamic determinants of the time-course of fall in the canine left ventricular pressure. J Clin Invest 58: 751–760.
28. Frais MA, Kingma I, Groves G, Smith ER, Tyberg JV (1983): The dependance of the time constant of left ventricular relaxation on pericardial pressure. J Am Coll Cardiol 1: 627 (Abstract).
29. Craig WE, Murgo JP (1980): Evaluation of isovolumic relaxation in normal man during rest, exercise and isoproterenol infusion. Circulation 62 (Suppl III): III-22 (Abstract).
30. Thompson DS, Waldron CB, Juul SM, Naqvi N, Swanton RH, Coltart DJ, Jenkins BS, Webb-Peploe MM (1982): Analysis of left ventricular pressure during isovolumic relaxation in coronary artery disease. Circulation 65: 690–697.

Discussion

Welkowitz: Rather than relating the results to artificial pressures, you may want to use a multiple shell model. This approach is feasible since the left ventricle is a shell enclosing a varying liquid volume. The multiple shell structure is useful, at least for some geometries, to calculate the movement of the heart. These calculations can then be compared with measurements.

Tyberg: This certainly sounds like a plausible approach which should be tried.

Ritman: Are most of your measurements done in open chests? Your point regarding balloon pressure vs. fluid pressure are well made. I am concerned about the open chest because the heart changes volume, relative to the heart in the closed chest, and the loss of mechanical interaction between the heart and lungs should alter ventricle to atrium interaction.

Tyberg: Most of our measurement are done in acutely prepared, anesthetized dogs in which we reclose and seal the chest under suction. Certainly, these observations require confirmation in more intact preparation.

Perl: If I need to assume pressure distribution in the pericardium and outside wall, what would you suggest as a first approximation? Will it follow the atrial pressure at all times?

Tyberg: I suggest using right ventricular diastolic pressure [25] or mean right atrial pressure [17] as a first approximation for pericardial constraint since right ventricular filling pressure is approximately equal to mean pericardial surface 'pressure' over the free wall of the left ventricle. This surface 'pressure' may be different over different areas of the heart, as one might expect. However, important differences have been shown only under rather extreme, transient conditions (e.g., severe constriction of either the aorta or pulmonary artery). [14, 15].

Lanir: One way to estimate the effect of the pericardium will be to measure the deformation of the pericardium. This will give you the idea on the stresses that develop there and if you know the geometry, you can get some estimate of the forces exerted by the pericardium on the myocardium.

Tyberg: Of course, you are correct in principle. While we have chosen to make a more direct measurement (with its own intrinsic limitations) we would be very interested to compare the results of such a different but complementary approach.

21. Conversion of fiber stress to global left ventricular pump work

T. ARTS and R.S. RENEMAN

Abstract

In the present study, muscle fiber stress (T_f) and strain in the wall of the left ventricle is expressed as a function of left ventricular pressure (p_{lv}) and the ratio of cavity volume (V_{lv}) to wall volume (V_w). Muscle fiber stress is assumed to be homogeneously distributed within the wall. The left ventricle may be represented by a thick-walled cylinder as well as by a thick-walled sphere. For both cases: $T_f = 3\,p_{lv}/\ln(1 + V_w/V_{lv})$. From the latter equation, a relation is derived between cavity volume and fiber strain. The ratio of cavity to wall volume appears to be the only relevant geometric parameter. The real geometry of the left ventricle is close to an ellipsoid, which is in between a cylindric and a spherical geometry. So, the relation found may be valid for a wide variety of realistic cardiac shapes. Fiber stress calculated with the present model appears to be 1.5 to 2 times higher than circumferential stress calculated with existing models, depending on the assumed geometry. This difference is in agreement with our current understanding of fiber stress in relation to circumferential stress.

Introduction

The left ventricle is a cavity, enclosed by a muscular wall (Fig. 1). Contraction of the wall is triggered by depolarization of the myocardial tissue. Then stress in the muscle and, hence, left ventricular cavity pressure increases. When left ventricular pressure reaches the level of aortic pressure, the aortic valve opens and ejection of blood occurs. During the ejection phase the left ventricle generates pump work, as indicated by cavity pressure being positive while blood volume is expelled. This work is generated by the muscle fibers in the wall. The decrease of left ventricular cavity volume during ejection is directly related to shortening of the muscle fibers in the wall. So, during the ejection phase these fibers generate mechanical work, associated with a positive stress while the fibers shorten. After

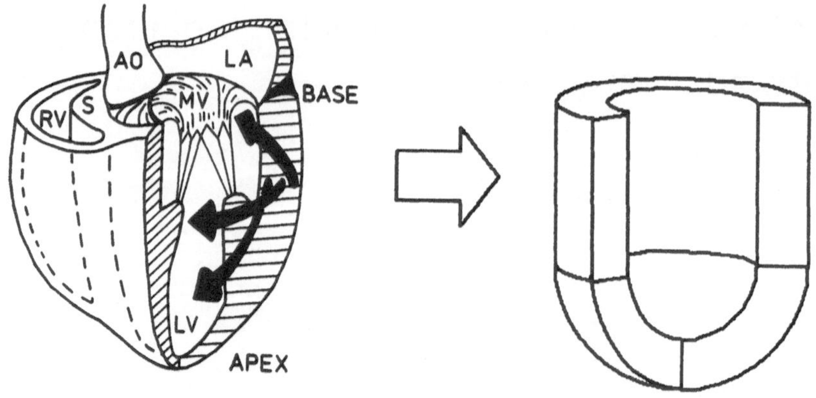

Figure 1. Schematical representation of the heart (left panel), and the simplification of the left ventricle (LV) to a cylinder attached to a half a sphere (right pannel). AO = aorta, RV = right ventricle, S = septum, MV = mitral valve. The arrows denote muscle fiber orientation.

ejection stops, the aortic valve closes and left ventricular pressure drops steeply to a low diastolic level. Filling of the left ventricle by mitral inflow is associated with much less work, because in this situation left ventricular pressure as well as muscle fiber stress are relatively low.

Understanding the mechanism of conversion of muscle work to pump work in a quantitative sense requires investigation of the relation between muscle fiber stress and strain on the one hand, and left ventricular cavity pressure and volume on the other. Because it is nearly impossible to measure muscle fiber stress directly, a variety of mathematical models have been developed to estimate stress in the wall. A review of such models was given by Yin [1]. In these models generally assumptions are made about geometry and material properties. The simplest models assume a thin-walled geometry obeying LaPlace's law [2]. A more realistic approach is the introduction of a thick wall, enabling the consideration of transmural differences in stress. A model, estimating mid-wall stress at the equator of a pressurized thick-walled prolate ellipsoid was developed by Sandler et al. [3] and improved by Falsetti et al. [4]. Recently, Kim et al. [5] described a solution for stresses everywhere in a thick-walled ellipsoid. A more accurate description of the geometry of the left ventricle required application of finite element analysis [6, 7, 8]. The above mentioned models predicted stress to be significantly higher in the subendocardial than in the subepicardial layers, often a factor of two or more. However, when introducing anisotropic properties of the myocardium, arranged according to anatomical findings on muscle fiber directions in the wall of the left ventricle [9, 10, 11], fiber stress appeared to be much more homogeneous. When adding freedom of torsion of the left ventricle around its long axis, a further decrease in stress inhomogeneities is observed [12, 13]. Taking into account loading of the left ventricle by the free wall of the right ventricle further diminishes these inhomogeneities [14].

The more realistic the simulations, the less arguments are left to assume that muscle fiber stress is inhomogeneously distributed over the various structures of the left ventricle. Deviations from the average are suggested to be less than ±10%.

In this study we take the average of muscle fiber stress and strain to be representative of the whole left ventricle. The relation between left ventricular pressure and volume on the one hand, and muscle fiber stress and strain on the other will be approached by considering anisotropy of the wall. An indication of the importance of geometrical factors is obtained by deriving the relation for a spherical as well as a cylindrical geometry. It is expected that the behavior of the more realistic prolate ellipsoidal geometry is somewhere in between these two extremes. Finally, experimental data are compared with some predictions of the model.

Fiber stress in a thin wall enclosing a pressurized cavity

In the model, myocardial material is considered to be a soft incompressible material, imbedding parallel muscle fibers. During systole when fiber stress is high, deviatoric stresses in the soft tissue may be neglected. Then for the principal stress component along the fiber direction (σ_1) and both components perpendicular this direction (σ_2 and σ_3), it holds:

$$\begin{aligned} \sigma_1 &= -p + \sigma_f, \\ \sigma_2 = \sigma_3 &= -p, \end{aligned} \tag{1}$$

where p represents hydrostatic pressure of the soft tissue and σ_f is the stress born by the fibers.

In a thin wall, the fibers are directed parallel to the surface. Let us assume the fibers to have an angle β with the circumferential direction, then for the circumferential (σ_{cc}) and the axial component (σ_{zz}) related to fiber stress, it holds:

$$\begin{aligned} \sigma_{cc} &= \sigma_f \cos^2 \beta, \\ \sigma_{zz} &= \sigma_f \sin^2 \beta. \end{aligned} \tag{2}$$

From (2) it follows by adding:

$$\sigma_f = \sigma_{cc} + \sigma_{zz}. \tag{3}$$

Thus, the sum of two perpendicular fiber stress components is always equal to fiber stress, independent of the actual fiber orientation.

In a thin-walled sphere with cavity V_c and wall volume V_{sh}, the two perpendicular stress components (σ_{cc}, σ_{zz}) in the wall depend on internal pressure (p_i) by:

$$\sigma_{cc} = \sigma_{zz} = p_i \frac{3\,V_c}{2\,V_{sh}}. \tag{4}$$

After substitution of (4) into (3), for fiber stress it follows:

$$\sigma_f = 3\,p_i \frac{V_c}{V_{sh}}. \tag{5}$$

Analogously, in a cylinder, the axial and circumferential stress is:

$$\sigma_{cc} = 2\,\sigma_{zz} = 2\,p_i \frac{V_c}{V_{sh}}. \tag{6}$$

After substitution of (6) into (3), the fiber stress (5), appears to hold.

Thus, for a sphere as well as for a cylinder, the ratio of fiber stress to internal pressure appears to be determined by the ratio of enclosed volume to shell volume, as expressed by (5). The shape of the left ventricle may be represented by a bullet, consisting of half a sphere attached to a cylinder with the same radius (Fig. 1). Because (5) holds for a sphere as well as a cylinder, it also holds for all combinations of both shapes. So, (5) might be quite universal and applicable to the left ventricle as well.

Fiber stress in a thick wall enclosing a pressurized cavity

The relation between muscle fiber stress and cavity pressure (p_{lv}) in a thick-walled left ventricle is found by integration of pressure increments associated with a sufficient number of thin-walled shells from the outer to the inner wall:

$$p_{lv} = \sigma_f \int_{V_{lv}}^{V_{lv}+V_w} \frac{dV}{3V}, \tag{7}$$

where V_{lv} and V_w represent left ventricular wall and cavity volume, respectively. After integration of (7) and rewriting for fiber stress it follows:

$$\sigma_f = 3\,p_{lv} \Big/ \ln\left(1 + \frac{V_w}{V_{lv}}\right). \tag{8}$$

Using the principle of conservation of energy, saying pump energy is equal to muscle fiber work in the wall, the following relation is found [14]:

$$V_w \frac{de_f}{dV_{lv}} = \frac{P_{lv}}{\sigma_f}, \tag{9}$$

where e_f represents muscle fiber strain. Substitution of the ratio of left ventricular pressure to fiber stress, as expressed by (8), into (9), followed by integration with respect to left ventricular volume, results in:

$$e_f = \frac{1}{3}\,[(1 + X)\ln(1 + X) - X\ln(X)], \tag{10}$$

where $X = V_{lv}/V_w$. Thus, muscle fiber mechanics in the wall of the left ventricle are related to left ventricular pressure and volume as described by (8) and (10). The related functions are shown in Figs 2 and 3, respectively.

In the present study epicardial muscle fiber strain, as measured directly, is compared to the value of this strain as calculated by (10) from the change in left ventricular volume during the ejection phase. Moreover, for a normal cardiac cycle as well as for an isovolumic contraction a fiber stress – fiber strain loop was calculated from a pressure – volume loop using (8) and (10).

Experimental set-up

The experiments were performed on 4 mongrel dogs weighing 25–34 kg. The animals were premedicated with Hypnorm (1 ml Hypnorm contains 10 mg fluanoson and 0.2 fentanyl base). Anesthesia was induced by pentobarbital sodium (10 mg/kg IV) and after endotracheal intubation was maintained by oxygen and nitrous oxide. Ventilation was kept constant with a positive pressure resperator (Pulmomat). The chest was opened through the left fifth intercostal space, and the heart was suspended in a pericardial cradle. Ascending aortic pressure was measured via the carotid artery with a catheter connected to a pressure transducer (Ailtech). Left ventricular pressure was measured with a catheter-tip micromanometer (Millar) inserted through the femoral artery. Deformation of the epicardial surface of the free wall of the left ventricle was measured with an inductive system using a triplet of coils as transducer system [15]. In this way recordings of circumferential strain (e_{cc}), base to apex strain (e_{zz}) and shear (e_{zc}) were obtained simultaneously.

During the experiment, various levels of hypervolumia were induced by administration of saline. Thereafter, various levels of hypovolumia were induced by venous bleeding. Isovolumic contractions were obtained by quick banding of the aorta during the preceding diastolic phase. The experiment was terminated by a letal dose of KCl. The heart was removed and the ventricles were dissected from the atria. Left ventricle and septum were separated from the right ventricular free wall and weighed separately.

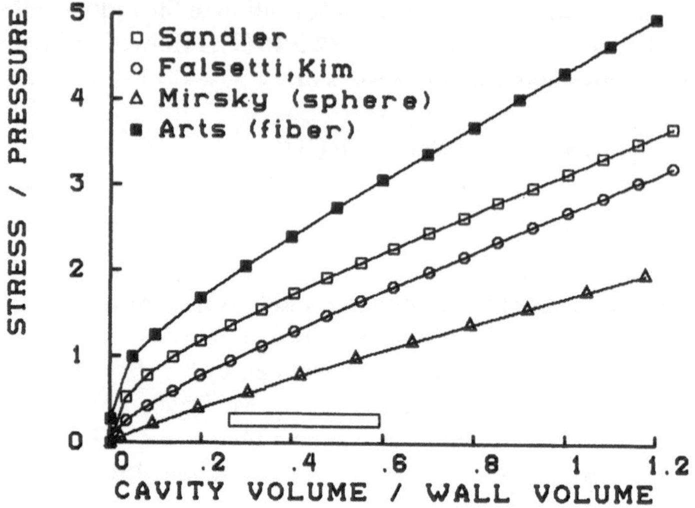

Figure 2. Stress in the wall, normalized to left ventricular pressure, plotted as a function of cavity volume, normalized to wall volume. The closed squares represent the result of our model (8). The open squares and cricles represent circumferential stress of a prolate ellipsoid (major/minor axis ratio 2:1), as calculated with the model of Sandler et al. [3], and of Falsetti et al. [4] and Kim et al. [5], respectively. The open triangles represent the results, as calculated for a thick-walled sphere [20]. The horizontal bar below indicates the normal range of volumes during a cardiac cycle.

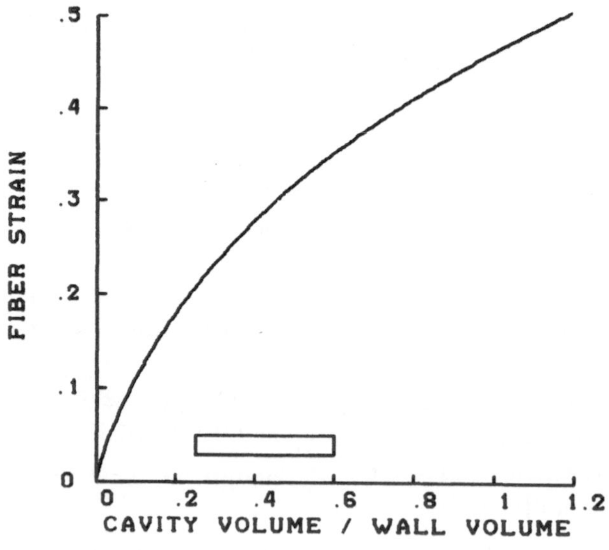

Figure 3. Model calculation (10) of fiber strain in the wall plotted as a function of cavity volume, as normalized to wall volume.

Data analysis

During the ejection phase muscle fiber strain at the epicardial surface $e_{f,cpi}$ can be determined by calculating strain along the direction with maximal shortening according to Prinzen et al. [16]:

$$e_{f,\,cpi} = \frac{1}{2}\,(e_{cc} + e_{zz} + \sqrt{(e_{cc} + e_{zz})^2 + e_{zc}{}^2}). \tag{11}$$

Assuming that, in the control situation, the end-diastolic left ventricular cavity volume ($V_{lv,\,ed}$) equals 54% of wall volume, the total volume enclosed by the epicardial surface of the left ventricle is equal to 1.54 times left ventricular weight divided by the specific tissue density. During the ejection phase this volume decreases. Assuming contraction of the free wall of the left ventricle to be representative of that of the whole ventricle, and wall volume to be constant, it holds [14]:

$$V_{lv} = (V_w + V_{lv,ed})\,\exp(e_v - e_{v,ed}) - V_w, \tag{12}$$

where $e_v = e_{zz} + 2e_{cc}$. The index ed denotes the end of diastole during the control situation.

To find average muscle fiber strain in the wall, the result of (12) was substituted into (10) for the beginning and the end of the ejection phase. Pressure volume curves associated with a cardiac cycle were constructed by application of (12). Fiber stress – fiber strain loops were obtained by applying (8) and (10). Using the observation that average sarcomere length in a passively inflated left ventricle at 12 mmHg is equal to 2.12 μm [17], a sarcomere length scale was plotted along the axis of fiber strain.

Results

Figure 4 illustrates typical recordings of a cardiac cycle with normal contraction (solid lines) and with isovolumic contraction (dotted line). The beginning of the ejection phase is indicated by the crossing of the aortic (dashed line) and left ventricular pressure (solid line) tracings. During the ejection phase, circumferential strain, base to apex strain and shear change gradually. During isovolumic relaxation, fast changes of the deformation parameters occur. During an isovolumic cardiac contraction (dotted line), deformation is less pronounced than during an ejective beat, and left ventricular pressure rises to a much higher level.

In Fig. 5 muscle fiber strain, as estimated from left ventricular volume using (10) is plotted as a function of muscle fiber strain as measured at the epicardium. Different symbols refer to different conditions of ventricular filling. The data

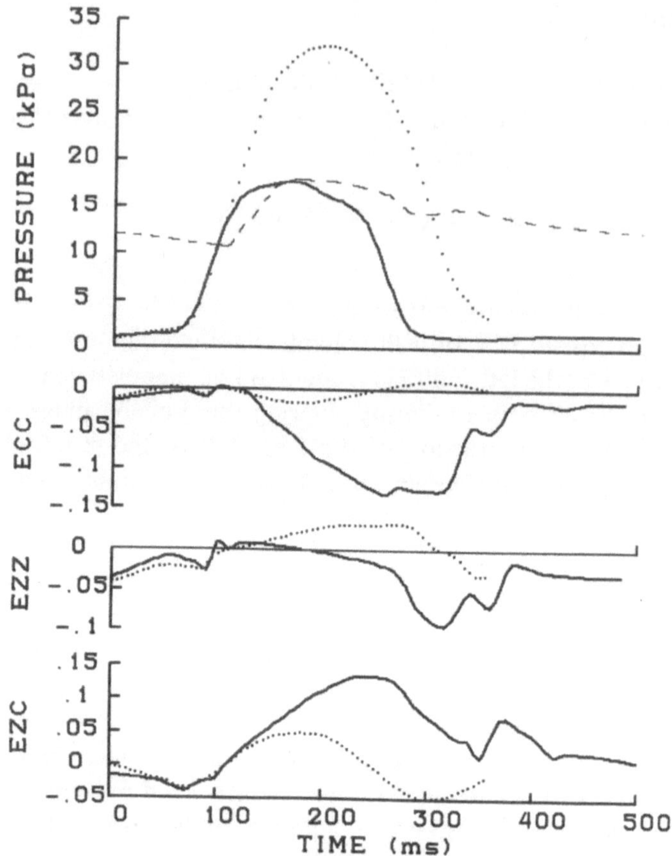

Figure 4. An example of measurements obtained during a normal cardiac cycle (solid lines) and during aortic occlusion (dotted lines). The upper panel shows left ventricular pressure and aortic pressure (dashed line). The lower three panels show circumferential strain (e_{cc}), base to apex strain (e_{zz}) and shear (e_{zc}).

cover a wide range and they are all close to the line of identity.

Figure 6 shows pressure volume loops derived from the tracings in Fig. 4, for a normal ejective beat (solid line) and an isovolumic contraction (dots). Figure 7 shows fiber stress – fiber strain plots of the same beat. Fiber stress during isovolumic contraction appears to be more than twice the maximum fiber stress during an ejective beat. The magnitude of fiber stress during isovolumic contraction is 97 kPa (9.7 g/mm^2) at an estimated sarcomere length of 2.1 μm. This value is close to the value found in isolated muscle during isometric contraction at that sarcomere length [18, 19]. During the ejection phase, fiber stress decreases approximately linearly with fiber strain, whereas left ventricular pressure is relatively independent of cavity volume. During isovolumic contraction and relaxation, changes in cavity volume and sarcomere length are visible.

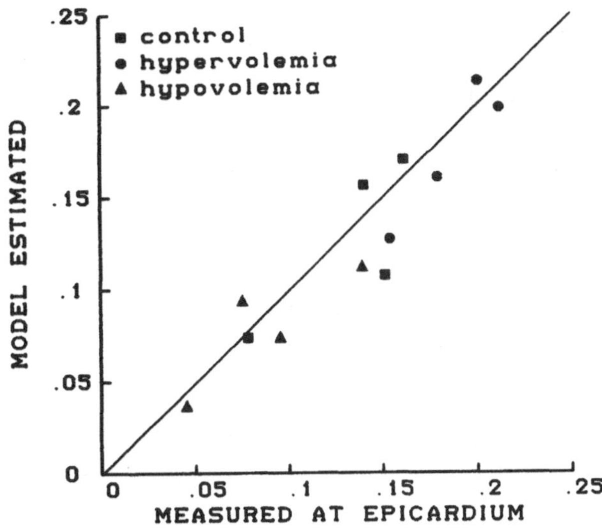

Figure 5. Fiber shortening as calculated from left ventricular volume by (10), plotted as a function of fiber shortening as measured directly at the epicardial surface of the anterior free wall of the left ventricle. During the experiments (N = 4) volume load of the left ventricle was varied. The diagonal indicates identity.

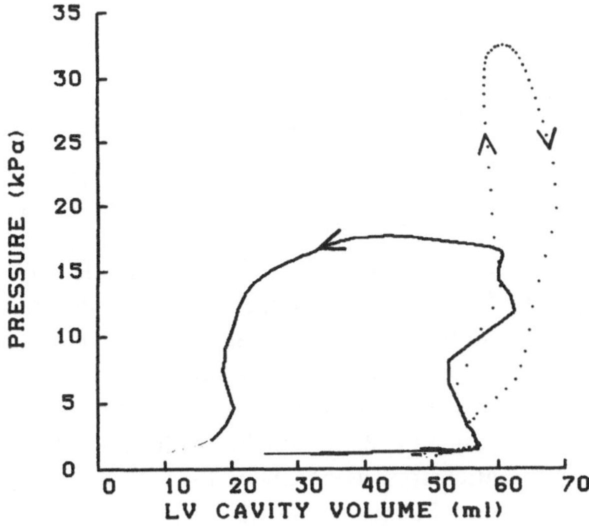

Figure 6. Pressure-volume plot of the left ventricle, during a normal cardiac cycle (solid line) and an isovolumic one (dotted line). These data are derived from the curves represented in Fig. 2. Volume was calculated from epicardial deformation by (12).

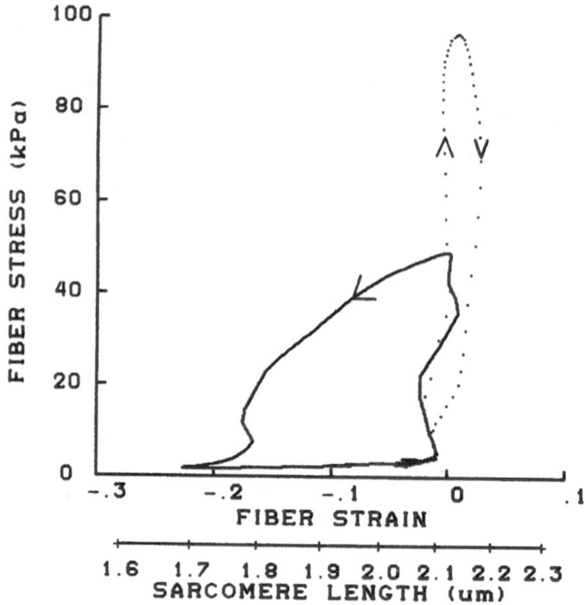

Figure 7. Fiber stress – fiber strain plot, as calculated for the wall of the left ventricle on the basis of the data presented in Figures 2 and 6, using (8) and (10). On the horizontal axis, calculated sarcomere length is also indicated.

Discussion

Several models have been developed to relate wall stress to cavity pressure. In Fig. 2 the results of these models are compared with the model described above. Sandler et al. [3] calculated circumferential wall stress in a prolate thick-walled ellipsoid at the equator. Falsetti et al. [4] improved the latter equation. Recently, for a prolate ellipsoid, Kim et al. [5] presented a more general equation. At the equator the latter equation simplifies to Falsetti's model of the ellipsoid. As shown by (3), (4) and (6) fiber stress is larger than circumferential stress, and the proportionality factor depends on the actual geometry. When assuming for the ratio of long axis length to short axis length a value of 2, the ratio of circumferential stress to wall stress is calculated to be 0.64, which value fits the ratio, as derived from the data in Fig. 2, reasonably well. The lower curve in Fig. 2 represents circumferential stress as calculated for a thick-walled sphere [20]. In a sphere, the circumferential stress equals half the fiber stress (4), and Mirsky's findings are also in reasonable agreement with those derived from our (8). Often, circumferential stress and muscle fiber stress are poorly distinguished. However, there is a considerable difference. Circumferential stress depends on the shape of the cavity as well as the ratio of cavity volume to wall volume, whereas muscle fiber stress appears to be independent of the actual shape of the cavity. Moreover, when investigating muscle mechanics, fiber stress is of much more interest than circumferential stress.

In the in vivo experiments, muscle fiber strain in the investigated area of the epicardium was considered to be representative of the epicardium everywhere. On this basis left ventricular volume was calculated from local epicardial deformation and in a next step average muscle fiber strain was calculated. In Fig. 4 it is shown that during the ejection phase this strain is in close agreement with the fiber strain, as measured directly at the epicardium. This finding suggests that the model presented is accurate and that calculated mean fiber strain equals epicardial fiber strain at the anterior free wall of the left ventricle. The finding that mean fiber strain is equal to fiber strain at an arbitrarely choosen area suggests homogeneity of muscle fiber strain in the whole wall of the left ventricle.

As shown by the data in Figs 4 and 6, during the isovolumic contraction and relaxation phases fast changes in epicardial deformation can be observed. Then calculated volume appears to change despite isovolumia of the whole left ventricle. This discrepancy is likely to be caused by asynchrony of contraction and relaxation in the wall, causing inhomogeneity of deformation during these phases. For instance during relaxation, calculated volume decreases fastly at low ventricular pressure. This may be explained by the fact that in the open chest preparation the exposed epicardial surface is cooler than the rest of the heart, resulting in a postponed relaxation especially of the epicardial fibers. As mentioned above, these phenomena appear to be of minor importance during the ejection phase.

Figures 6 and 7 show that pressure – volume loops can be converted to fiber stress – fiber strain loops. Normal values of left ventricular pressure appear to be associated with levels of fiber stress, normally found in experiments on isolated muscle. In this respect, the relatively high values of fiber stress, as calculated by our model, seems to be more realistic than the lower values of circumferential stress as calculated with other models.

Conclusion

Muscle fiber stress and fiber strain in the wall of the left ventricle is expressed as a function of left ventricular cavity pressure and the ratio of cavity volume to wall volume. This relation appears to be insensitive to the actual shape of the ventricle, which may be a sphere, a cylinder or a combination of these shapes. Fiber stress behaves like circumferential stress except for a scaling factor. The scaling factor for circmferential stress depends on the shape of the ventricle. The value of fiber stress, as calculated from left ventricular pressure and volume appears to match the values, obtained in in vitro experiments on isolated muscle.

References

1. Yin FCP (1981): Ventricular wall stress. Circ Res 49: 729–842.
2. Woods RH (1982): A few applications of a physical theorem to membranes in the human body in a state of tension. J Anat Physiol 26: 362–370.
3. Sandler H, Dodge HT (1963): Left ventricular tension and stress in man. Circ Res 13: 91–104.
4. Falsetti HL, Mates RE, Grant C, Greene DG, Bunnell IL (1970): Left ventricular wall stress calculated from one plane cineangiography – An approach to force-velocity analysis in man. Circ Res 26: 71–83.
5. Kim HC, Min BG, Lee MM, Seo JC, Lee YW, Han MC (1985): Estimation of local cardiac wall deformation and regional wall stress from biplane coronary cineangiograms. IEEE Trans BME 32: 503–511.
6. Janz RF, Grimm AF (1972): Finite element model for the mechanical behavior of the left ventricle. Circ Res 30: 224–252.
7. Pao YC, Ritman EL, Wood EH (1974): Finite-element analysis of left ventricular myocardial stresses. J Biomech 7: 469–477.
8. Yettram AL, Vinson CA, Gibson DG (1983): Effect of myocardial fiber architecture on the behavior of the human left ventricle in diastole. J Biomed Eng 5: 321–328.
9. Beyar R, Sideman S (1984): A computer study of left ventricular performance based on fiber structure, sarcomere dynamics and transmural electrical propagation velocity. Circ Res 55: 358–375.
10. Feith TS (1979): Diastolic pressure-volume relations and distribution of pressure and fiber extension across the wall of a model left ventricle. Biophys J 28: 143–166.
11. Streeter DD, Vaishnav RN, Patel DJ, Spotnitz HM, Ross J, Sonnenblick EH (1970): Stress distribution in the canine left ventricle during diastole and systole. Biophys J 10: 345–363.
12. Arts T, Veenstra PC, Reneman RS (1979): A model of the mechanics of the left ventricle. Ann Biom Engng 7: 299–318.
13. Chadwick RS (1982): Mechanics of the left ventricle. Biophys J 39: 358–375.
14. Arts T, Veenstra PC, Reneman RS (1982): Epicardial deformation and left ventricular wall mechanics during ejection in the dog. Am J Physiol 243: H379–H390.
15. Arts T, Reneman RS (1980): Measurement of deformation of canine epicardium in vivo during cardiac cycle. Am J Physiol 239: H432–H437.
16. Prinzen FW, Arts T, van der Vusse GJ, Reneman RS (1984): Fiber shortening in the inner layers of the left ventricular wall as assessed from epicardial deformation during normoxia and ischemia. J Biomech 17: 801–812.
17. Grimm AF, Lin HL, Grimm BR (1980): Left ventricular free wall and intraventricular pressure sarcomere length distributions. Am J Physiol 239: H101–H107.
18. Pollack GH, Krueger JW (1976): Sarcomere dynamics in intact cardiac muscle. Eur J Cardiol 4 (Suppl): 53–65.
19. Ter Keurs HEDJ, Rijnsburger WH, van Heyningen R, Nagelsmit MJ (1980): Tension development and sarcomere length in rat cardiac trabeaculae: Evidence of length-dependent activation. Circ Res 46: 703–714.
20. Mirsky I, Parmley WW (1973): Assessment of passive elastic stiffness for isolated heart muscle and the intact heart. Circ Res 33: 233–243.

Micro to macro coronary circulation

22. An analysis of a vascular arborization model for the microcirculation

C. ENG

Abstract

A model is constructed and analyzed where microspheres are conceptually used to measure regional blood flow as well as to form 'controlled' emboli in the branches and decrease regional blood flow. Depending on whether the ratio of branching numbers is greater or less than unity, the model predicts that the regional flows are related to the cumulative dose of emboli by convex or concave relationships, and linear for equal branching. The analysis also yields the regional density of the arterioles. Modifications and limitations are discussed.

Introduction

All circulations undergo extensive arborization from their origin in the aorta to the capillaries that supply the nutritional substrates for the cells. The arborization scheme is difficult to describe quantitatively. Qualitative ordering procedures have been applied to describe the bronchial tree and neural dendrites. The purpose of this preliminary communication is to describe methods in which anatomic information may be derived from macroscopic, physiological measurements, without recourse to stereology.

The two macroscopic tools required for the experimental study are:

1. a means to measure regional blood flow, and
2. an ideal embolic probe.

Regional blood flow can be measured with the microsphere technique using microspheres of 9–10 μm in diameter. The ideal probe can be a larger microsphere of a known size or diameter that can be embolized into the vascular bed, completely obstructing a certain number of arterioles. Regional blood flow will be decremented depending on the number of obstructed vessels. The procedure is then repeated. It is assumed that the sampled regions for blood flow measurement contain a large number of arterioles.

The analytical model

A vascular branching model is constructed as follows: in each region, there is a certain number of arterioles of a given size. This arteriolar density is designated, α_i. Each of these feeding arterioles give off a certain number of branches, β_i, the branching number index characteristic for the *ith* region. The total number of post-arteriolar vessels is simply $\alpha_i * \beta_i$. Thus the α, β, and $\alpha * \beta$ values can all vary for different regions. The first assumption is that the flow to a given region is proportional to the total post- arteriolar vascularity of the region. Thus, the flow to one region is: $f_i = k\alpha_i\beta_i$, where k is a proportionality constant that converts 'vascularity' to flow, and contains the driving pressure of the system (assumed to be constant during the experimental procedure). This constant is also assumed to be the same for the regions, but can also be modified. A bolus of emboli, $\triangle M$, is now injected into the circulation. These emboli lodge and obstruct arterioles of a similar diameter as the emboli.

The distribution of the dose of emboli to the different regions is assumed to be proportional to the relative flow received by the region. Thus, the proportion of the total flow going to the *ith* region is: f_i/(total flow). The number or density of emboli going to that region is: $\triangle M * f_i$/(total flow). These emboli obstruct the arterioles and remove them from further participation to blood flow in that region. Thus, a new arteriolar density in the region results after the bolus of emboli: $\alpha_i - \triangle M * f_i$/(total flow). With a new arteriolar density, a new regional flow can be calculated, based on the first assumption: $f'_i = k\alpha'_i\beta_i$, where f', α' are the new regional flow and arteriolar densities. This iterative process can be repeated for the next bolus of emboli. For small $\triangle M$, the process can be approximated by a series of coupled differential equations. It is recognized that the emboli are discrete and are not a continuous variable. For a two region model, the equations are:

$$df_1/dM = -k\beta_1 * (f_1/(f_1 + f_2)), \tag{1}$$

$$df_2/dM = -k\beta_2 * (f_2/(f_1 + f_2)). \tag{2}$$

The solutions of these differential equations are of the form:

$$M = M_{max} - (1/k\beta_1) * f_1 - (1/k\beta_2 A^{(\beta_2/\beta_1)}) * f_1^{(\beta_2/\beta_1)}, \tag{3}$$

$$M = M_{max} - (1/k\beta_2) * f_2 - (A/k\beta_1) * f_2^{(\beta_1/\beta_2)}, \tag{4}$$

where M_{max} is the maximum number of emboli needed to produce zero flow (i.e. obliterate the vascular bed) and A is a positive constant. Two terms are subtracted from M_{max}: a negative term that is linear with the regional flow, and another negative term that has the regional flow raised to a power, probably non integer. Depending on whether the ratio of branching numbers (β_1/β_2) is greater or less than unity, the solution of the model predicts that the regional flows are related to the cumulative dose of emboli by convex or concave relationships. If the branching numbers are equivalent in the two regions, the relationship is linear.

Another differential equation can be derived, by simply dividing the two coupled differential equations:

$$df_1/df_2 = (\beta_1/\beta_2)(f_1/f_2). \tag{5}$$

This differential equation which relates the two regional flows has a simple solution:

$$\ln f_1 = (\beta_1/\beta_2) * \ln f_2 + \text{constant}, \tag{6}$$

$$f_1 = A * f_2^{(\beta_1/\beta_2)}, \tag{7}$$

where A is a positive constant.

This particular solution of the model provides experimentally testable relationships. If the model and the assumptions are reasonably correct, then the logarithm of the regional flows should have a linear relationship. Furthermore, the slope of the linear relationship should yield the ratio of branching numbers for the two regions. This is an important anatomical insight provided by the model. Another prediction of model solution is that the regional flows should converge towards zero flow concomitantly at the end of the embolization process. Thus, one region cannot have zero flow and the other region have some residual flow. This is a testable prediction.

The density of arterioles in the different regions can be derived from the final density (M_{max}) of emboli (which can be radioactively labelled). With knowledge of the relative regional arteriolar density and the relative branching number, the relative total vascularity for the regions can be determined. Embolic probes of different sizes can be used to map out the arterial arborization scheme at other levels of the circulation using a similar analysis. Of course the validity of the assumptions in the model must be assessed at each level using the experimental data.

Modifications of the general approach can be made at several points in the analysis. As an example, a rheological factor can be readily accomodated. The embolic probes may not behave ideally where there may be preference of the emboli for a given region irrespective of the relative flow to the region. For the two layer model described above, the amount of emboli distributed to layer 1 would become:

$$\Delta M_1 = \varrho * (f_1/(f_1 + f_2))\, \Delta M, \tag{8}$$

where ϱ is a rheological factor that is bounded by $0 \leqslant \varrho \leqslant 1$. When $\varrho = 1$, the emboli would be distributed strictly according to the relative regional flow (ideal probes). Smaller values indicate a greater rheological influence. Since $\Delta M = \Delta M_1 + \Delta M_2$:

$$\Delta M_2 = (((1 - \varrho) * f_1 + f_2)/(f_1 + f_2))\ \Delta M. \tag{9}$$

The derivation of the differential equations follows a similar pattern. The solution of relationship between the regional flows is of the form:

$$f_2 = \text{constant} * f_1^{(r_{\beta/\varrho})} + ((r_\beta - r_\beta \varrho)/(\varrho - r_\beta)) * f_1, \tag{10}$$

where $r_\beta = \beta_2/\beta_1$. This solution indicates that if the rheological factor is important experimentally, the log-log relationship between the regional flows would be non-linear. This aspect can be readily tested experimentally.

Discussion

The indirect physiologically derived anatomic data should be viewed as complementary to more directly derived data. Although a morphometric confirmation is desirable, and may be viewed as the 'gold standard', there are several potential problems that must be resolved with such methods. The stereological treatment of a continuously tapered cylindrical structure has not been addressed from a theoretical viewpoint. It may be possible to approximate the vascular system as a concatenation of non-tapered cylindrical structures of various diameters. Thus, in oblique sections through vascular structures, the minor axis of the ellipse would represent the diameter of the vessel. However, important assumptions must be made with regards to the length of these cylindrical structures. They cannot be assumed to be infinitesimally short since the actual stereological results will be expressed in terms of 'length-density'.

Besides this theoretical problem, there is a practical problem of arbitrarily grouping the data into diameter ranges. A continuous diameter histogram would require an enormous amount of data measurements. The grouping interval must be consistent with the theoretical assumptions. The stereological data will yield regional length-densities with units of mm/cm^3. It should be appreciated that this result is not the same as frequency or density. The primary goal is to define how many vascular pathways of a specified diameter occur in a given volume of tissue. For ideal embolic probes, this is readily provided by M_{max}. Length density is a combination of both density and length of the vessels. Accordingly, the level of the vasculature with a specified diameter, but with very short path length prior to arborization, would yield values of length density that underestimate the actual frequency of these vessels. Thus, the combination of physiological and morphometric results are complementary. Both methods are subject to basic theoretical assumptions and experimental constraints.

Acknowledgment

This study was supported in part by National Institutes of Health Grants HL23171, HL27219, HL37412 and an Established Fellowship from the New York Heart Association.

Discussion

Bassingthwaighte: It is nice to see an attempt to get at the complexity of the branching relationships. Such conceptual approaches are greatly needed, together with data from anatomic studies on the branching angles, interbranch distances, diameters, etc. of the arteries that make up the myocardial network.
Becker: Your transmural flow distributions are rather unphysiological. Epicardial flow is considerably greater than endocardial flow at baseline. I wonder if this was caused by cannulation of the coronary artery. If so, could your results have been affected?
Eng: The control endo/epi flow ratio was 0.7. I think this is due to the relatively high heart rates in this study, about 145 beats/min.
Marcus: I wonder if they had it something to do with the cannulation of the coronary artery.
Eng: I don't think so. In a maximally dilated vascular bed, the endo/epi flow ratio is highly dependent on the heart rate. Bache and Cobb (Circ Res 41: 648–653, 1977) demonstrated this. Several other studies have endo/epi flow ratios during maximal dilation similar or lower than our values (Cobb et al., J Clin Invest 53: 1618–1625, 1974; Johannsen et al., Circ Res 50: 510–517, 1982).
Marcus: It seems to me that the results may be affected by the unphysiological state of anesthetized unconscious dogs
Eng: If you look at the second intermediate stage of embolization, the endo/epi flow ratio is now 1.2. You may consider this point as the 'beginning' of the experiment. The results still show that epicardial flow decrements much more rapidly than endocardial flow. I think the results are independent of the initial conditions.
Marcus: I think it is due to the fact that you cannulated the arteries that gave an intense maximal vasodilation.
In a normal awake dog, if you give an adenosine infusion, the endo/epi ratio will always be less than 1 (about 0.9).

23. Delineating coronary hemodynamic mechanisms by computer simulation

J.M. DOWNEY

Abstract

Simple computer models were used to gain insight into the complex hemodynamics of the coronary arterial system. Both the terminal arteries and the collateral vessels were examined. It was proposed that oscillations in tissue pressure as well as perfusion pressure would affect coronary flow through

1. vascular collapse when extravascular pressure exceeds intravascular pressure,
2. vascular capacitance when the transmural pressure in a vessel changes.

The role of each of these processes were clarified by producing a simple model of each system which could be solved using numerical methods on a computer. The models were then run under a wide variety of conditions to see if any model-specific responses could be identified. Once a model specific response was identified, appropriate animal experiments were performed to see if that response could be demonstrated. Failure to observe the response disproved the model, while observation supported it. A multi-leg vascular waterfall model predicted a unique pressure flow curve for the coronary circulation which was verified in the dog heart. Addition of a small vessel capacitance site near the capillaries and upstream of the waterfall collapse site allowed the model to duplicate phasic coronary flow under a wide variety of conditions. The collateral circulation was modeled as a slightly pressure dependent resistance running between the large branches which was unaffected by cardiac contraction. Behavior predicted from a load line analysis of this model was demonstrated in the dog heart.

Introduction

Two components contribute to the coronary resistance. These are conveniently classified as the intravascular and the extravascular components. The intravascular component results from smooth muscle tone in the coronary walls and is determined by the diameter of the patent coronary vessels. Intravascular resistance is under the influence of autoregulation and of the cardiac nerves. It can also be modulated by pharmacological agents such as nitroglycerine. The extravascular component derives from outside the coronary vessels and is the result of mechanical deformation of the coronary vessels as the heart contracts and relaxes. While changes in the intravascular resistance are usually purposeful and represent the effectors for the coronary control systems, the extravascular changes are inescapable perturbations which the control systems must overcome. Early physiologists thought that the rythmic contractions of the heart might act to propel blood through the coronaries by a muscle pump mechanism [1]. Sabiston and Gregg disproved that theory, however, when they showed that asystole causes an abrupt fall in total coronary resistance [2]. The fall in the resistance with arrest was interpreted as removal of the extravascular resistance component which occurs during systole. Repitition of that experiment using microspheres reveals that the extravascular resistance is nonuniformly distributed across the heart wall with a large component in the deep layers and a negligible component at the subepicardium [3].

Pressure development in the ventricular lumen was found to be the primary determinant of the gradient in extravascular resistance [4]. Thus, it was hypothesized that contraction influences coronary resistance by elevating tissue pressure in the heart wall. Attempts at measuring this tissue pressure revealed that during systole there is indeed a gradient of pressure across the ventricular wall with the highest pressure at the subendocardium and near zero pressure at the subepicardium [5–8]. Although the magnitude of the intramyocardial pressure depends on the method used to measure it [6] all of the reports agree that near the subendocardium it is at least equal to ventricular pressure and may exceed it.

The waterfall hypothesis

We proposed that tissue pressure may be reducing coronary flow by the formation of vascular waterfalls much as alveolar pressure affects flow through the lung [9]. We investigated that possibility by first constructing a computer model of a waterfall system for the coronary bed [10]. The waterfall equations describe flow as a discontinuous function of resistance, arterial pressure, venous pressure and tissue pressure. When tissue pressure exceeds arterial pressure the vessel is collapsed and flow is zero. When tissue pressure is less than venous pressure flow is simply proportional to the arterial-venous pressure difference. When tissue pressure is between arterial and venous pressure, however, partial collapse of the vasculature causes flow to be proportional to the arterial pressure-tissue pressure difference. The complicating factor in the heart is that tissue pressure varies both spatially and temporally.

The coronary waterfall model is shown in Figure 1. Ten parallel legs were

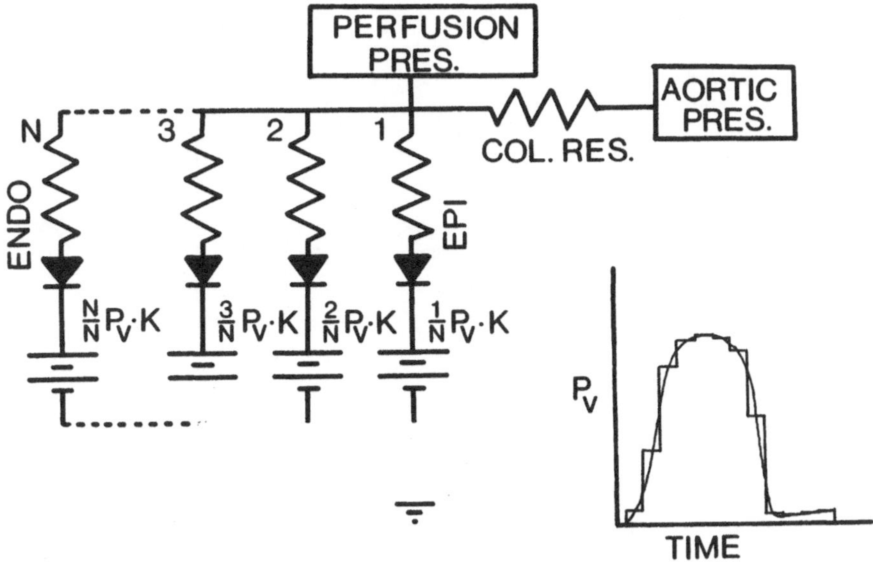

Figure 1. The waterfall model of the coronary circulation. See text for an explanation.

assumed, each representing different depths across the ventricular wall. The waterfall is represented by a resistor, representing the vascular resistance, and a diode with a back-biased battery which represents the collapsed segment. The voltage of the batteries, which correspond to the tissue pressure, was set to be a fixed proportion of ventricular pressure since experimental studies indicate that to be the case in the canine heart. The proportion was highest in the subendocardial leg and fell linearly toward zero for the subepicardial legs. The cardiac cycle was broken into 12 time periods and a typical ventricular pressure was provided. The equations were coded in BASIC and run on a PDP8 minicomputer.

The model predicted that a unique pressure-flow curve should exist for the coronary artery of a beating heart. The curve is is straight above the peak tissue pressure and is convex to the perfusion pressure axis below that peak pressure (see Figure 2). Removal of all tissue pressure as would occur with cardiac arrest, would cause the pressure-flow curve to become straight and to shift upwards. We tested this hypothesis in open chest dogs as shown in Figure 3. A small coronary branch was cannulated and perfused with a positive displacement pump. Intravascular resistance changes in the perfused segment were abolished by maximally dilating it with an adenosine infusion. Flow was measured both before and after cardiac arrest over a wide range of perfusion pressures.

Examination of the pressure-flow data revealed that the predicted behavior was present (see Figure 4). The curve during arrest was straight while that during beating was both straight in the high pressure range and parallel to the arrest curve. At low pressures the beating curve converged toward the arrest curve. The

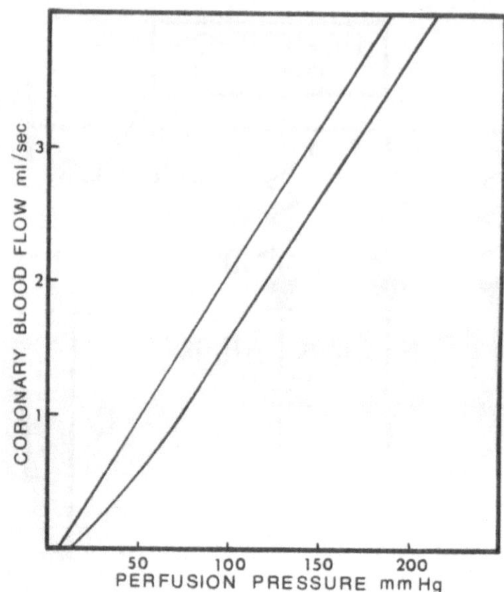

Figure 2. The pressure-flow curve predicted by the model for the coronary circulation during beating (lower curve) and arrest (upper curve).

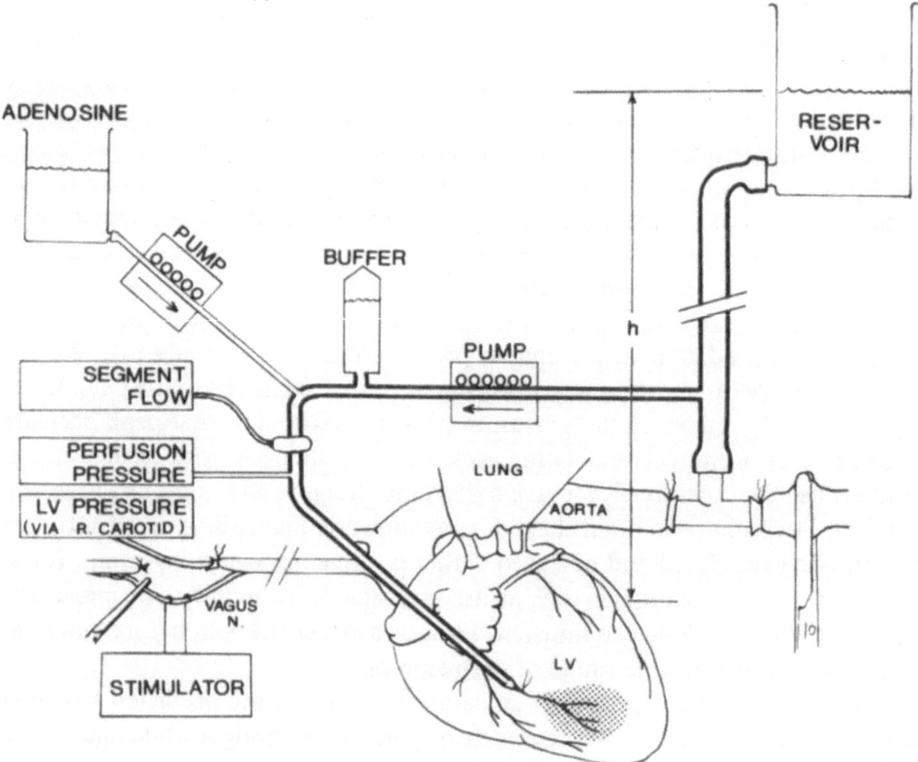

Figure 3. Animal preparation used to test the waterfall model.

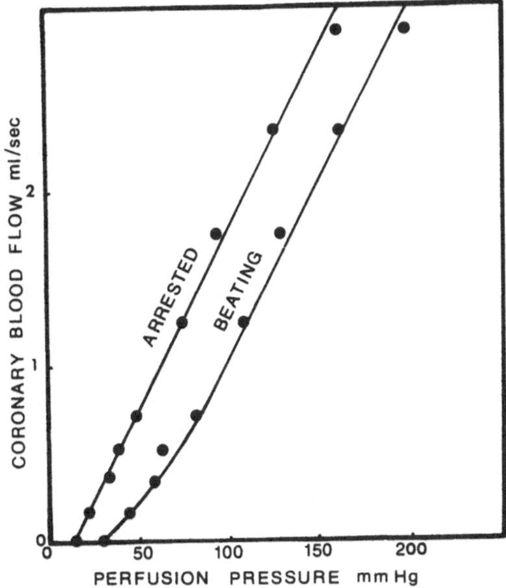

Figure 4. Resulting pressure-flow curve in a maximally dilated canine coronary artery. Note the resembalance to the model's prediction in Figure 2.

model predicted that the transition from linear to curved would occur at a perfusion pressure equal to the peak tissue pressure in the system. That transition was always very near peak ventricular pressure. Thus, we concluded that tissue pressure in the heart probably never exceeds ventricular pressure and that experiments which report such high pressures suffer from a measurement artifact.

We further tested the validity of the model by having the computer collect coronary and ventricular pressure directly from a dog while regional flow was measured by the microsphere method [11]. The coronary artery was maximally dilated to abolish any intravascular influences and a wide variety of hemodynamic conditions were examined. The waterfall model, using peak tissue pressure equal to intraventricular pressure, always gave an accurate prediction of the regional flow to all layers of the heart.

Coronary capacitance

One glaring shortcoming of the simple waterfall model described above was that it was incapable of duplicating the coronary flow profile seen at the coronary ostium. We reasoned that the failure might be due to our omission of capacitance elements in the model. Capacitance results from elasticity in the walls of the blood vessels such that any change in the transmural pressure of a vessel must be met with an appropriate change in its volume. Just as the voltage across capacitor is given by the charge times the capacitance. The transmural pressure in a blood vessel is determined by its volume times its compliance (here refered to as capacitance). A sudden change in the pressure surrounding a vessel will be transmitted to blood within the vessel's lumen. That change will persist until the volume of blood in the lumen can change to bring the system back to equilibrium. Large epicardial coronary arteries see intrathoracic pressure as the surround pressure and thus their volume responds to changes in arterial pressure only. Intramyocardial vessels, on the other hand, are exposed to the high tissue pressure in the myocardium and thus their volume is determined by the difference between intravascular and tissue pressure.

Spaan et al. [12] have published convincing evidence that considerable vascular capacitance resides in the microcirculation and is responding to the fluctuations in tissue pressure. They argue that the capacitance is so large, in fact, that it maintains microvascular pressure above tissue pressure throughout systole which would prevent waterfall formation. This becomes a critical point since the capacitance-only model was incapable of duplicating the coronary pressure flow curves observed in the dog [13]. Could Spaan et al's data be explained by a hybred waterfall and small capacitance model?

We, therefore, modified the the waterfall model to include capacitances as shown in Figure 5. The small vessel capacitance has tissue pressure as the outside pressure. Note that we modeled the capacitance as a single lumped capacitor having both proximal and distal resistance segments. Although, capacitance is probably distributed all along the vascular tree a distributed model would be impossible to test and was, therefore, not attempted. The equations were coded in BASIC and run on a Commodore PET computer. The equations were arranged as a repetitive loop using a 10 ms time slice. The algorithm for the numerical analysis is shown in Figure 6. The pressure at the node, Pn, is determined by the charge on the capacitor, Q, and tissue pressure, Pi. The charge on the capacitor is the running integral of the current onto it, Ic, which is the difference between Iu and Id.

The model predicted that perfusion with a nonpulsitile pressure would give clear transient flow overshoots with the onset of diastole as the capacitance filled. Emptying of the capacitance during systole was obscured by the rising extravascular resistance. Figure 7 indicates that elimination of the waterfall or the capacitance or increasing the magnitude of the capacitance had a profound effect on the coronary flow profile and eliminated the overshoots. We then prepared a dog for constant pressure perfusion of its coronary arteries to see if the actual flow profile fit that predicted by any of the models. Coronary flow for 10 beats was collected by a PDP 12 computer and averaged to yield the coronary flow profile shown in Figure 8. This was done for several heart rates. Note that the overshoot and transient decay was heart rate independent and best approximated the small capacitance waterfall model. Parameter estimation revealed that about 60% of the coronary resistance is proximal to the capacitance site and that C is approx-

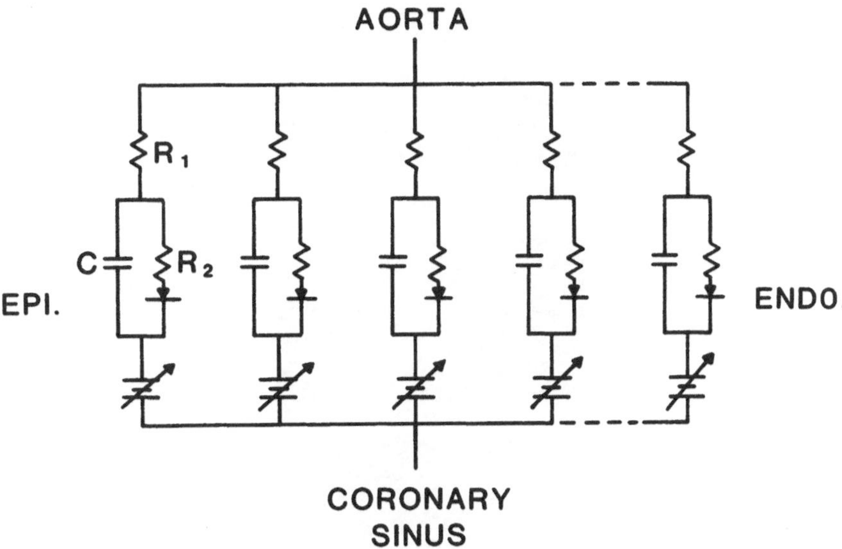

Figure 5. A proposed model of coronary capacitance.

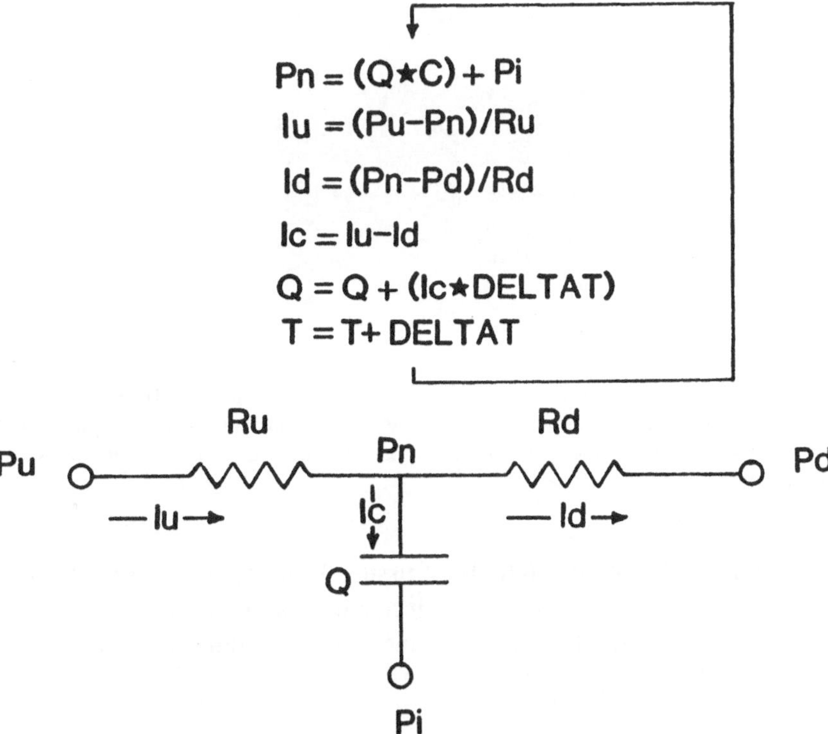

Figure 6. The numerical algorithm used to simulate capacitance behavior in the proposed model. I represents flow, Q is the charge on the capacitor, R is resistance, C is the value of the capacitance, T is time, DELTAT is the time increment, P is pressure, u refers to the upstream segment, d refers to the downstream segment, and Pi refers to the intramyocardial pressure.

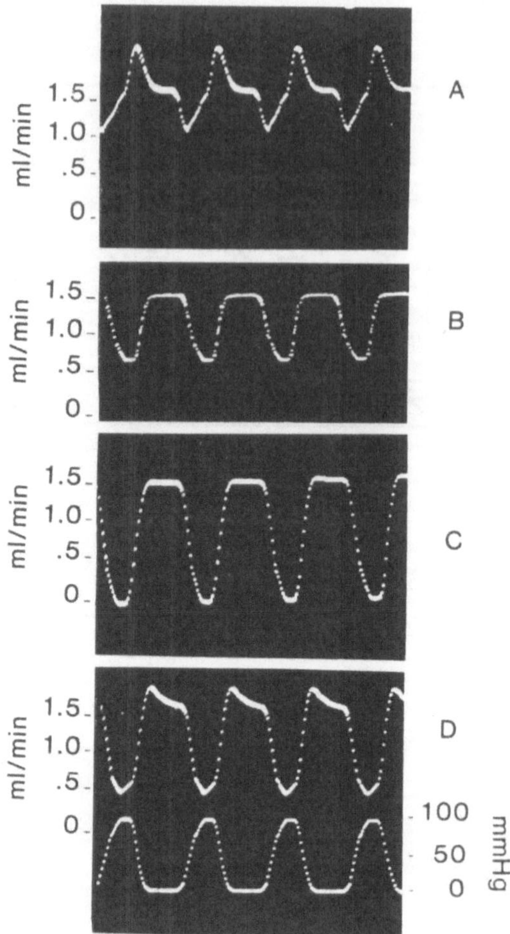

Figure 7. Phasic coronary flow resulting from nonpulsitile perfusion as predicted from 4 versions of the model. A: capacitance only. B: waterfalls only. C: long time constant capacitance plus waterfalls. D: short time constant capacitance plus waterfalls. The bottom trace is the ventricular pressure used for all of the traces.

imately 0.005 to 0.03 ml/mm Hg/100 g of tissue. That value agrees well with that reported by Klocke et al. [14] but is much smaller than that reported by Spaan et al. [12]. We concluded that both capacitance and waterfall effects are present in the coronary system of a beating heart.

The collateral circulation

Let us now turn our attention to the coronary collateral circulation. Collateral

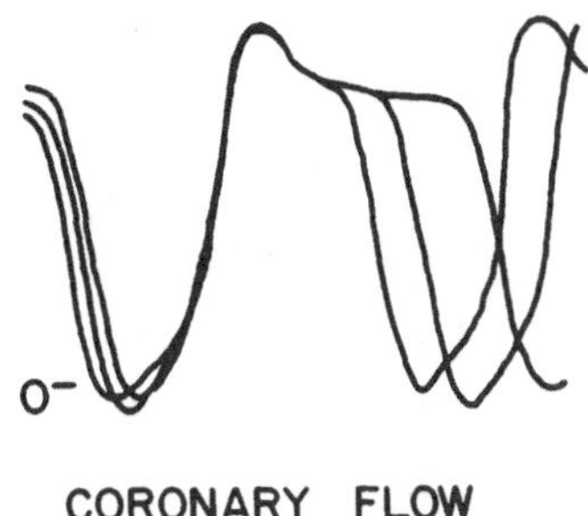

Figure 8. Actual coronary flow resulting from nonpulsitile pressure perfusion of a dog's coronary artery. The three traces represent 3 different heart rates. Note that the overshoot and decay with the onset of diastole is unaffected by the heart rate. The time constant of the decay ranged between 50 and 100 ms depending on whether the coronary artery had tone or was dilated respectively.

vessels interconnect the branches of the coronary tree such that occlusion of a major branch does not completely abolish flow to the capillaries served by that branch. Collateral flow is the critical determinant of necrosis in acute myocardial infarction [15] and, therefore, becomes a parameter of considerable interest to the clinician as well as the coronary physiologist. One of the earliest attempts to estimate collateral flow was to measure the peripheral coronary pressure [16]. That is, the pressure distal to a coronary occlusion. The higher this pressure, the lower the collateral resistance is likely to be. This method does not yield a flow value, however, only a pressure. Anrep and Hausler [17] discovered that collateral flow could be demonstrated by ligating a coronary branch and opening the distal segment to the atmosphere. Under these conditions arterial blood trickled out of the vessel in a retrograde direction and was thought to represent collateral flow destined for the capillaries of the compromised bed.

It has been argued that the retrograde flow method overestimates the true collateral flow since dropping the pressure in the distal segment enhances the pressure gradient across the collateral bed [18]. Others argue that retrograde flow underestimates collateral flow because not all of the collateral flow appears in the retrograde flowing blood. Some blood may still be flowing antegrade to the capillaries [19]. The first argument alone makes the method theoretically incorrect. If retrograde flow does exactly equal collateral flow in any given measurement, it is only because the first artifact listed above was compensated by the second artifact, a coincidence which could hardly be relied on to routinely occur.

We, therefore, constructed a simple model of the collateral circulation as shown in Figure 9. It readily became apparent that if the collateral resistance was constant, and if retrograde flow accounted for all of the collateral irrigation (no antegrade diversion) then collateral flow could be analyzed by a load line method as is commonly used for transistors in circuit design. In Figure 9, flow through the collateral resistance is plotted against the pressure at node A. Note that a straight

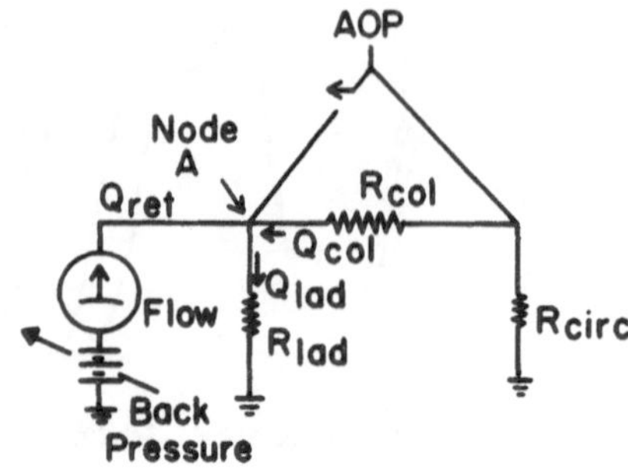

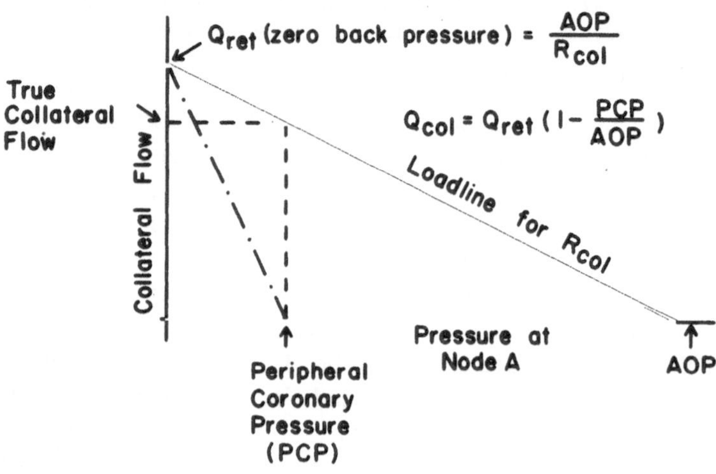

Figure 9. A representation of the coronary collateral circulation and the load line analysis of that circuit. See text for details.

line, the load line, is described which runs from an arterial pressure intercept on the horizontal axis to an intercept on the vertical axis at retrograde flow. The true collateral flow during simple occlusion is determined by the point where peripheral coronary pressure intersects the load line. Thus, if aortic pressure, peripheral coronary pressure and retrograde flow were known, true collateral flow could be calculated as indicated by the equation.

To prove the validity of the model we had to show that the assumptions were correct. If the distal segment were cannulated with a collection system in which back pressure (and thus pressure at node A) could be varied as illustrated in Figure 9, then retrograde flow into that system would be described by the hashed line in Figure 9. At zero back pressure all of the collateral flow will be retrograde into the collection system. At a back pressure equal to peripheral coronary pressure all of the flow would be antegrade into the capillaries and none would enter the collection system. If we could force the antegrade resistance, Rlad, to suddenly become infinite then the retrograde flow-back pressure line would become the load line itself since antegrade flow into the capillaries would be impossible regardless of the pressure.

The simple model derived above was tested in the animal laboratory [20]. Open chest, anesthetized dogs were prepared as shown in Figure 10. A small coronary branch was cannulated and autoperfused from a femoral artery. A branch was provided for retrograde flow collection. Flow was measured with a computerized drop counter at the open end of the tubing. Provision was made to elevate the drop counter so that back pressure to flow could be adjusted. Successive measurements were made at various back pressures so as to describe the pressure-flow curve. The segment was then embolized with 25 μm microspheres until no forward flow could be detected and the retrograde flow measurements were repeated. The microembolization allowed us to cause the antegrade resistance to become infinite and, therefore, charactorize the load line.

A typical result is shown in Figure 11. The squares describe flow before embolization and the +s describe flow after embolization. Two features are apparent. First, retrograde flow at zero back pressure was usually unaffected by embolization. This indicates that retrograde flow at zero back pressure does account for all of the collateral flow. The possibility than no antegrade flow diversion occurs was further ensured by the presence of an apparent critical closure of the distal bed at back pressures below 7.5 mm Hg. This critical closure is revealed by the fact that the pre and post embolization curves were the same at pressures up to 7.5 mm Hg. Another interesting finding was that the post embolization curve always had a pressure axis intercept which was considerably less than aortic pressure. This was interpereted to indicate that the collateral anastomoses originate at a level in the donnor bed where 20% of the arterial pressure has been dissipated. Recent studies by Harrison et al. [21] point out that inability to achieve 100% embolization and, thus, infinite resistance causes the 80% figure to be articfactually low. Ninety percent of aortic pressure is probably a more accurate estimate of the pressure source for the coronary collaterals. In light of the above data we modified our original collateral flow model to incorporate both waterfalls in the distal bed and to a resistance proximal to the origin of the collateral anastomosis. The modified version of the model appears in Figure 12. We propose that collateral flow can be estimated from the equation:

$$\mathrm{Q\,col} = \mathrm{Q\,ret}(1 - (\frac{\mathrm{PCP}}{0.9 * \mathrm{AOP}})),$$

where Q ret is the retrograde flow at 0 back pressure, PCP is peripheral coronary pressure and AOP is aortic pressure.

The post embolization curve consistantly demonstrated curvature away from the pressure axis. This indicates that our first assumption of a linear collateral

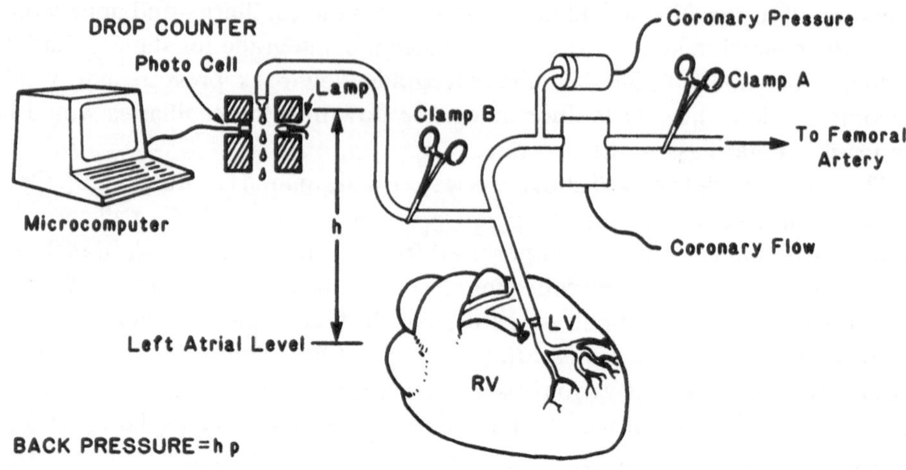

Figure 10. The animal preparation used to test the load line assumptions.

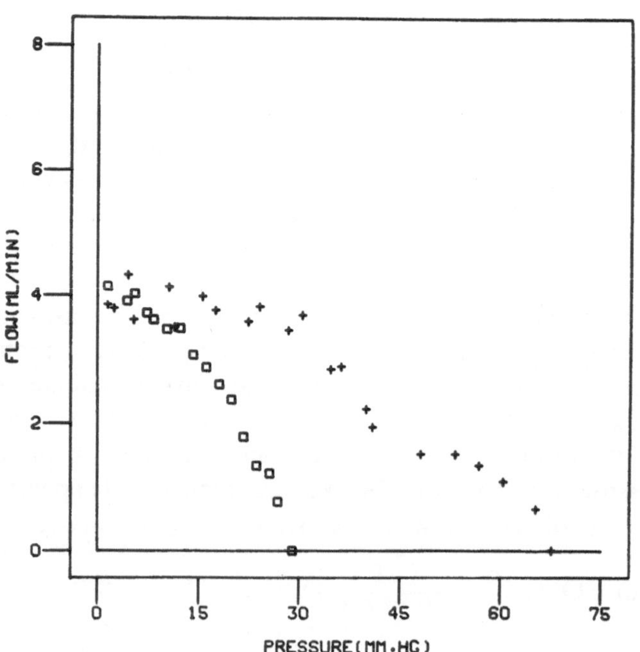

Figure 11. A typical Back pressure-retrograde flow plot from a dogs coronary artery. The boxes depict flow before microembolization of the distal segment and the +s represent flows after embolization.

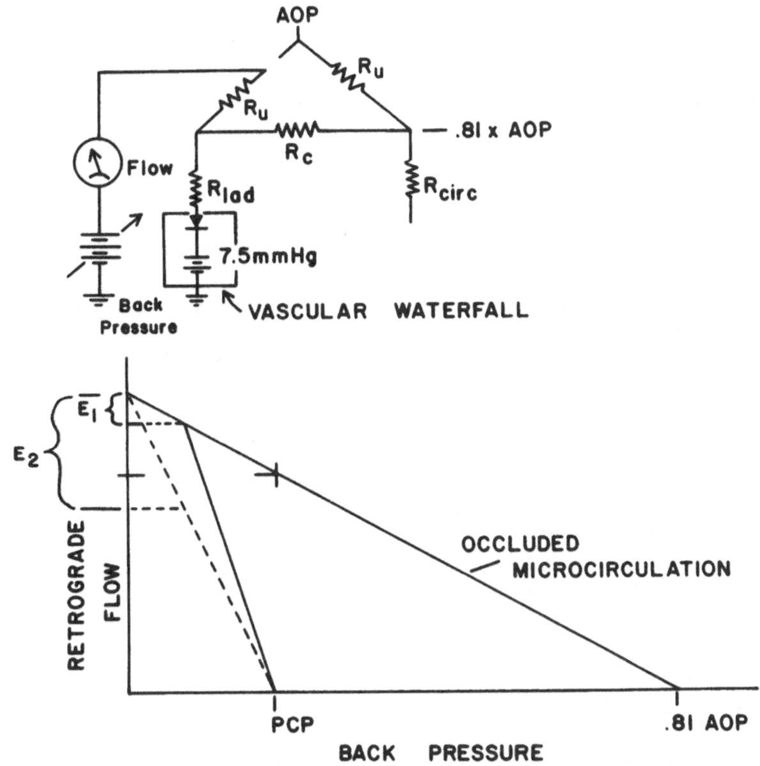

Figure 12. A refined version of the load line model including waterfalls in the distal circulation and resistances proximal to the origin of the collateral anastomosis.

resistance was not entirely met. We assumed that this curvature was the result of pressure dependent distention of the collateral segment. A computer model demonstrated that such pressure dependence could, indeed, duplicate the animal data. Foreman et al. [22] suggest that this curvature may represent waterfall formation in the collateral vasculature. Although this theory is attractive and could also explain the observation, the source of the collapsing forces which could account for the waterfall behavior are difficult to envision.

In conclusion, we have derived models for three aspects of the coronary circulation. These models were tested by performing specific animal experiments to see if predictions from the model could actually be seen in the animal. Animal experiments inturn led to refinements in the models such that current evidence would indicate that these aspects of the coronary circulation have been accurately represented and the underlying mechanisms revealed.

References

1. Porter WT (1898): The influence of the heart beat on flow of blood through the walls of the heart. Am J Physiol 1: 145–163.
2. Sabiston DC, Gregg DE (1957): Effect of cardiac contraction on coronary blood flow. Circulation 15: 14–20.
3. Russell RE, Chagrasulis RW, Downey JM (1977): Inhibitory effect of cardiac contraction on coronary collateral blood flow. Am J Physiol 233: H541–H546.
4. Downey JM,, Downey HF, Kirk ES (1974): Effects of myocardial strains on coronary blood flow. Circ Res 34: 286–292.
5. Kirk ES, Honig CR (1964): An experimental and theoretical analysis of myocardial tissue pressure. Am J Physiol 207: 361–367.
6. Brandi G, McGregor (1976): Intramural pressure in the left ventricle of the dog. Cardiovasc Res 39: 53–57.
7. Heineman F, Grayson J, Bayless CE (1979): Intramyocardial pressure distribution in the ventricular wall. Fed Proc 38: 1038.
8. Stein PD, Marzilli M, Sabbah HN, Lee T (1980): Systolic and diastolic pressure gradients within the left ventricular wall. Am J Physiol 238: H625–H630.
9. Permutt S, Bromberger-Barnea B, Bane HN (1962): Alveolar pressure, pulmonary venous pressure and vascular waterfall. Med Thorac 19: 239–260.
10. Downey JM, Kirk ES (1974): Inhibition of coronary blood flow by a vascular waterfall mechanism. Circ Res 36: 753–760.
11. Munch DF, Downey JM (1980): Prediction of regional blood flow in dogs. Am J Physiol 239: H308–H315.
12. Spaan JAE, Breuls NPW, Laird JD (1981): Diastolic-systolic flow differences are caused by intramyocardial pump action in anesthetized dog. Circ Res 49: 584–593.
13. Lee J, Chambers DE, Akizuki S, Downey JM (1984): The role of vascular capacitance in the coronary arteries. Circ Res 55: 751–762.
14. Klocke FJ, Mates RE, Canty JM, Ellis AK (1985): Coronary pressure-flow relationships: controversial issues and probable implications. Circ Res 56: 310–323.
15. Reimer KA, Jennings RB (1979): The wavefron phenomenon of myocardial ischemic cell death. II. Transmural progression of necrosis within the framework of ischemic bed size (myocardium at risk) and collateral flow. Lab Invest 40: 633–644.
16. Gregg DE (1974): The natural history of collateral development. Circ Res 35: 335–344.
17. Anrep GV, Hausler H (1928): The coronary circulation. I. The effect of changes of the blood pressure and of the output of the heart. J Physiol (London) 65: 357–373.
18. Eckstein RW (1954): Coronary intra arterial anastomosis in young pigs and mongrel dogs. Circ Res 2: 460–465.
19. Scheel KW (1979): The relationship between collateral, true collateral and retrograde flow with collateral growth. Fed Proc 38: 906.
20. Wyatt D, Lee J, Downey JM (1982): Determination of coronary collateral flow by a load line analysis. Circ Res 50: 663–670.
21. Harrison DG, Christy JP, Willhoite DJ, Gumm DC, Chapman MP (1985): The relationship between aortic pressure and the pressure at the origin of the coronary collaterals. Evidence against significant microvascular anastomosis. Fed Proc 44: 822.
22. Forman R, Eng C, Kirk ES (1982): Action of nitroglycerine on coronary collaterals: conductance or waterfall effect. Circulation 66: II-42.

Discussion

Welkowitz: In reality, the capacitance and the resistance are distributed. Thus, the single time constant is not correct. However, the analytical problem with distributed capacitance and resistance is most difficult to solve. It would be interesting to see if it yields similar results.

My second question relates to the waterfall model. There are other possible models that produce similar curves. For example, a turbulence model can be represented by a non-linear resistance which produces essentially the same curve over the physiologically useful range. Have you looked into this as an alternative?

Downey: Obviously, capacitance is distributed all along the coronary vessel. Since its distribution is unknown at present, there is no way to even start with such a model. It is important to note, however, that a very close approximation of coronary behavior can be achieved by a single capacitance site near the capillary bed (as shown here). The frustration is that it is indistinguishable from a damped capacitance site much further up stream, as Dr Mates has proposed. The same problem exists with phenomenon such as turbulent flow. Nevertheless, the waterfall formation, the simplest of hemodynamic responses, still nicely explains the observations with no discrepancies and, therefore, we have not felt compelled to further complicate the model. The beauty of this model is really its simplicity.

Dinnar: I shall describe tomorrow some phasic flow using a similar approach. I have some objection to the waterfall model, for the following reason. In your assumption, the venous pressure remains zero. Actually, if the intermyocardial presure causes collapse of the arterial side, thus bringing the pressure to the same level of the intermyocardial pressure, it must also happen on the venous side. Thus, the relation must be considered between the two pressures on both sides of the capillary. If you take a zero venous pressure you offset this relationship.

Downey: A fundamental premise of the waterfall model is that collapse will occur as close to the outflow region as is possible and that it will not involve a long segment of the vessel. In essence a jet is formed. That means that arterial collapse site is unlikely and is strongly argued against in the data. By venous pressure equal to zero we refer to that in the coronary sinus, the collecting manifold for all of the coronary veins.

Clark: In your presentation you suggested that much can be learned from pulmonary circulation modeling effort, specifically the resistance waterfall model. I would also like to suggest that models used in the area of pulmonary airway mechanics might also be employed to some benefit here, particularly models of the 'collapsible segment' of the airways. In this simple model of the compliant cylindrical airway, single resistive and capacitive elements are utilized; except that both elements are nonlinear. That is, the longitudinal pressure-flow relationship of the resistor is volume dependent and the transmural pressure-volume relationship of the capacitance is curvilinear. The advantage of the nonlinear characterization is that with a relatively small number of parameter values, one can characterize the more complex phenomena that is observed experimentally without resorting to higher-order, piecewise-linear, resistive-capacitive models.

Downey: The airway collapse is really a special case of the waterfall phenomenon. The alvolar pressure is nearly equal to the intrapulmonary pressure. With a forced expiration enough pressure is dissipated along the airway to cause the intra bronchial pressure to fall below the pleural pressure, enough to cause collapse. The waterfall behavior is evidenced in that a maximal expiration velocity is achieved. Above that flow rate the pressure drop would dictate complete collapse and stopage of flow. Below that flow rate the airway is wide open. Thus, the flow rate is regulated. The same thing happens in waterfall behavior which is also jetting, with no complete collapse. Flow is adjusted to cause the pressure inside the vessel at the outflow region to be just on the verge of collapse and form a jet. In that case, however, the flow is adjusted to cause an appropriate pressure drop across the upstream resistance of the vessel.

Arts: I understand from the experiments of Dr Spaan that the time constants within the coronary circulation are in the order of seconds, whereas in your experiments a much shorter time constant is found. I would explain this discrepancy by considering the coronary circulation to be a distributed continuous cable. You are looking at fast phenomena, then the input impedance of the cable behaves according to your findings, having a short time constant. If you consider very slow phenomena you may come into trouble: you may then look along the cable into the deeper parts of the coronary circulation where slower time constants, close to three seconds, are found.

Downey: The primary difference between my studies and those of Dr Spaan is in the capacitive time constant. That, most likely, is explainable in terms of the distribution of the capacitance but not necessarily in terms of a cable model. All of our studies concentrate on capacitance which can be viewed from the arterial side and many of Dr Spaan's studies examine venous level phenomenon not easily measurable from the arterial side. Whether the venous capacitance, which Spaan's studies demonstrate to be quite large, contributes to an intramyocardial pump mechanism or whether waterfalls are forming is the real question. If a waterfall forms upstream of a large low pressure venous capacitance, then that capacitance will, in fact, be isolated from the arterial side and will not be seen. On the other hand, if pressure in the venous capacitance is high during systole, that prevents waterfall formation and forces flow retrograde. If that is the case, however, then it is difficult to explain why systole distributes flow away from the subendocardium.

24. Distensibility of microvasculature and its consequences on coronary arterial and venous flow

J.A.E. SPAAN, P. BRUINSMA, I. VERGROESEN, J. DANKELMAN and H.G. STASSEN

Abstract

In this chapter some effects of pressure dependent changes in vascular volume on resistance and capacitance in the microcirculation will be analysed. First some additional evidence for a significant intramyocardial compliance will be given. This evidence has been obtained from experiments where both arterial and venous coronary signals were measured. Further it is shown that the intramyocardial compliance is not situated at the very end of the coronary circulation, epicardial veins, but that a significant distal resistance must be present. A compartmental model based on pressure dependency of coronary vessels can describe relations between pressure and flow signals quite well. This model shows that time constants characterizing the changes of microvascular volume and relating quantities are in order of a second. The arterial signals show transients with characteristic time constants that are smaller than the duration of diastole and systole. However, the effect of compliance and changing resistance on coronary arterial flow are counteracting and hence concealing each other. We conclude that arterial signals do not provide sufficient information about the events in the microcirculation and models solely based on these signals can provide misleading results.

Introduction

For a long period of time the distensibility of microvessels, especially of capillaries, has, with exceptions, not been considered to be important for organ flow mechanics. In various studies [1, 2] a theoretical basis was looked for to explain the experimentally observed rigidness of capillaries. However, in a well designed study, Smaje et al. [3] could show that at normal physiological pressures and pressure variations the capillaries in the mesentery of the rat were significantly distensible. The discrepancy with the earlier observations were ascribed to the combination of small sensitivity of the earlier techniques and the nonlinear behavior of the vessel wall mechanics.

From our laboratory [4] a model was presented based on the assumption of a significant intramyocardial compliance. This so-called intramyocardial pump model could describe satisfactorily the relation between pulsatilities in coronary arterial flow and pressure. The value for intramyocardial compliance estimated in that study is close to the value that can be estimated from intramyocardial blood volume and capillary distensibility [3, 5].

The concept of rigid capillaries has lead to models of coronary flow mechanics in which the capillary bed is represented by constant resistances. The interaction between heart contraction and coronary flow was thought to be due to the formation of waterfalls [6–8] at, presumably, the venular side of the coronary microcirculation. The high arterial zero flow pressures found in the coronary circulation were ascribed to a similar mechanism in the arterioles of the coronary bed: the Starling resistor effect. However, the found intramyocardial compliance requires a re-evaluation of the interpretation given to the experimental observations.

In this paper we first will present some additional evidence for a significant intramyocardial compliance. Moreover we will show that the time constants for intramyocardial volume variations are larger than a second, hence longer than the duration of a normal systole or diastole. Next, we will present an alternative model of the coronary flow mechanics based on the Ph.D. thesis work of Arts [9]. Finally, an analysis will be given of the discrepancy thought to exist between experimentally found time constants and the intramyocardial pump model.

Evidence for intramyocardial compliance

It is difficult to study intramyocardial compliance effects from the arterial side of the circulation only. Compression of compliant intramyocardial vessels results in a squeezing force on the blood. The tendency of the squeezing is to expel blood from without the intramyocardial blood vessels into both the epicardial arteries and veins. However, normally the arterial pressure is higher than the squeezing pressure and thus arterial flow remains forward. It is like somebody walking backward on a belt moving forward (Fig. 1). As long as the magnitude of the belt speed exceeds that of the person, it will appear to an observer on the fixed ground but without sight on the belt that the person walks forward. The backward movement of the person on the belt is concealed by the forward movement of the belt. It is only under the circumstance that the magnitude of the backwards speed exceeds that of the belt speed that the backward movement becomes apparent to the fixed world observer.

Under special circumstances the backward arterial flow due to the squeezing of the intramyocardial blood becomes apparent. This is the case by lowering mean

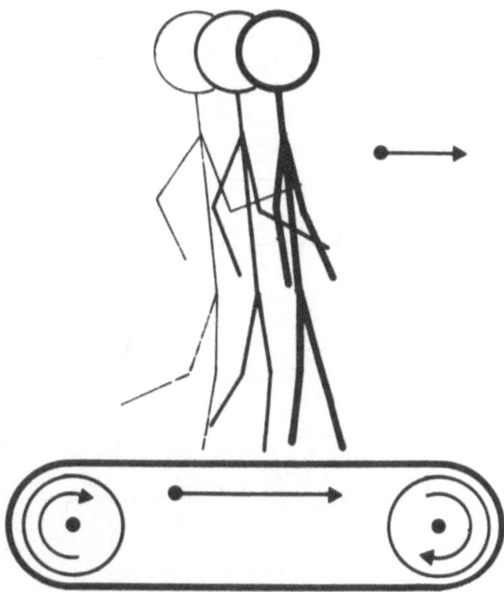

Figure 1. Illustration of the superposition principle. The walker moves forward but walks backward. The observation of the direction of movement depends on the position of the observer: on the fixed world or on the belt. Application of the superposition principle to the coronary circulation makes plausible that backflow and reduced flow may be caused by the same mechanism. With backflow, the 'intramyocardial pump pressure' exceeds the arterial pressure.

arterial pressure and coronary resistance [10], lowering diastolic arterial pressure [11] or increasing the squeezing force on the septum by increasing right ventricular pressure [12]. As with the case of the walker on the belt, the mechanism responsible for backflow must also be active when only reduced arterial flow is seen. Hence, backflow is nothing special. It is a manifestation of the same mechanism that causes reduced systolic flow. This is the attractive side of the intramyocardial pump model [4]. Models, in which the reduced systolic flow is explained on the basis of an increased resistance or on a waterfall have to be extended to explain backflow.

At the venous side of the coronary circulation the squeezing effect results in a driving force for blood directed in the same way as the mainstream. Hence, systolic venous flow is higher in systole than in diastole [5, 13, 14]. Moreover, coronary venous flow continues for a while after cessation of arterial inflow [5, 12, 15, 16] during long diastoles.

Figure 2 depicts the effect of arterial occlusion on great cardiac venous outflow in the beating heart. This experimental result was obtained in the open chest goat with cannulated left main coronary artery and great cardiac vein. Venous flow was drained in a reservoir in which pressure could be controlled. As is clear in the figure, the venous outflow combined with the peripheral pressure decay clearly

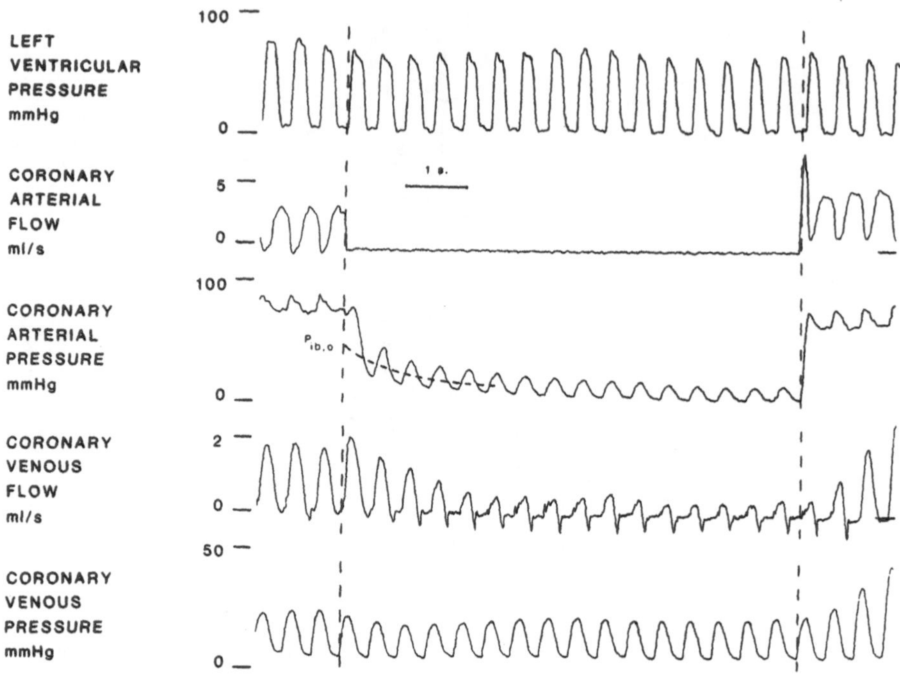

Figure 2. Venous outflow during arterial occlusion. Venous flow was drained into a reservoir where pressure was regulated to keep epicardial venous pressure constant. Coronary venous pressure was measured within a large epicardial vein.

shows the behavior of a wind-kessel. Blood pressure within the compliant intramyocardial blood space decreases when blood is expelled from this space.

In the beating heart, compression and relaxation of the intramyocardial compliance alternate. The relaxation effect on venous outflow becomes very clear in the period after cardiac arrest. This is demonstrated in Fig. 3. In this figure the great cardiac venous flow and left main arterial flow are shown before, during and after cardiac arrest when the coronary bed is dilated with adenosine. Perfusion pressure was maintained during the procedure. The same experimental setup was used as for the experiments described in Fig. 2. In this particular case, the great cardiac venous flow was about half the left main arterial flow. Under the assumption that measured venous flow reflected the complete venous outflow intramyocardial volume variation was calculated.

The diastolic relaxation becomes apparent from the venous outflow signal; the venous outflow is low after the onset of cardiac arrest as a result of the tendency to increase intramyocardial blood volume. In order to characterize the rate at which the volume change occurs the time after cardiac arrest to the moment the volume change was 65% of the change after 4 seconds of arrest was measured. This characteristic time was 0.96 ± 0.06 s (mean $\pm$ sd) for the vasodilated coronary bed and 1.60 ± 0.09 for the coronary bed with active autoregulation. In any case,

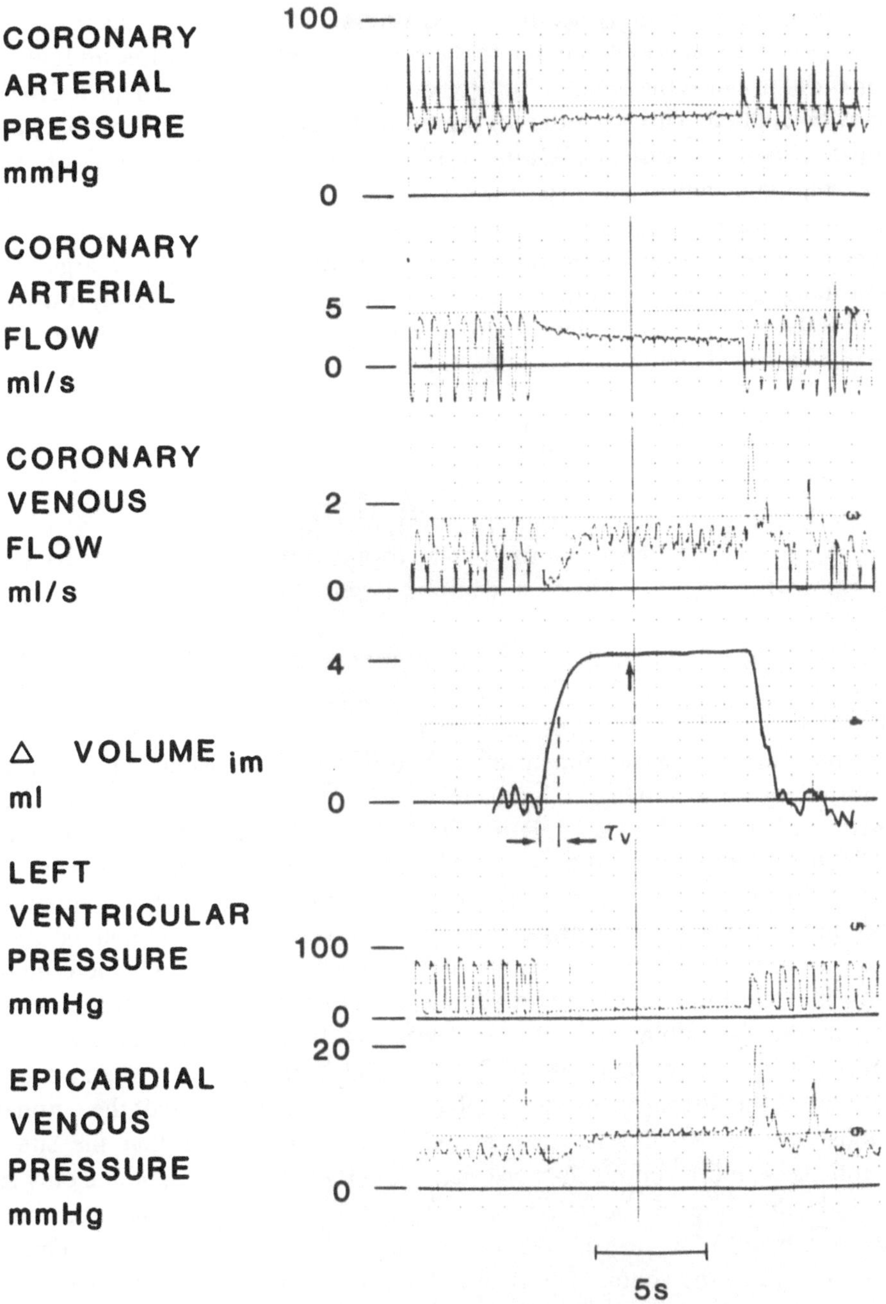

Figure 3. Great cardiac venous flow, CBF, and left main arterial flow (CAF) before, during and after cardiac arrest in the dilated coronary bed. Perfusion pressure (P_{perf}) was maintained. The arrow in the panel of volume change, ΔV_{im} indicates the 4 seconds value of volume change. T_v = time between the onset of diastole and the moment of 67% of the volume change after 4 sec.

the rate at which intramyocardial blood volume, and therefore microvascular pressure change, is slow compared to the normal duration of diastole and systole.

In order to assess the possible location of compliance the model depicted in Fig. 4 may be applied. This is a different representation of the intramyocardial pump model presented before [4]. Because both arterial pressure and venous pressure were kept constant in our experiments the inflow and outflow resistances are parallel with respect to the effect of intramyocardial pressure changes. The capacitance reflects the intramyocardial compliance. The change in charge of the capacitance after the pulsatile voltage has been changed into the steady low value reflects the volume change during cardiac arrest. The characteristic time constant for this electrical circuit can be described as

$$ts = C_{im} * Rs = C_{im} * \frac{R_1 * R_2}{R_1 + R_2}, \tag{1}$$

where Rs = the substitution resistance of R_1 and R_2 in parallel.

With a fixed capacitance and fixed value for the sum $R_1 + R_2$ the time constant is largest when $R_1 = R_2$. The time constant is zero when either R_1 or R_2 equals zero.

In Fig. 5 the relation between time constant and the product $C_{im} * (R_1 + R_2)$ is analyzed. Curves I and II represent the conditions with $R_1 = R_2$ and $R_2 = 0.15 (R_1 + R_2)$ respectively. In theory no data point should be present above curve I, since that curve represents the maximal theoretical time constant at given values of overall resistance. In Fig. 5 also the measured time constants are presented as a function of the product $C_{im} * (R_1 + R_2)$. $(R_1 + R_2)$ was calculated as the ratio between the arterial-venous pressure difference and mean coronary flow prior to cardiac arrest. C_{im} was chosen such that 90% of the autoregulation data points came below curve I. This was the case for $C_{im} = 0.104 \pm 0.012$ ml/mmHg. 100 g. This is close to the value of intramyocardial compliance as could be determined from different studies [5]. With the assumed value of intramyocardial compliance 80% of the data points on autoregulation are between the curves I and II suggesting R_1 is larger than 15% of $R_1 + R_2$. This is only possible when a significant part of the intramyocardial compliance is located upstream of the coronary venous system. Strictly, one can not conclude from Fig. 5 that the site of compliance is more venous than arterial. From the model in Fig. 4 one only can conclude that one of the resistances, R_1 and R_2, is smaller than the other. However from other measurements one may conclude that the compliance is located more to the venous side than to the arterial side of the coronary bed.

One expects the time constant for intramyocardial volume change to depend on the level of autoregulation. A higher arteriolar resistance would result in a larger time constant. Curve III in Fig. 5 represents the theoretical case where inlet resistance, R_1, increases but the outlet resistance, R_2, remains constant. This theoretical result shows that an increase of arteriolar resistance in the autoregul-

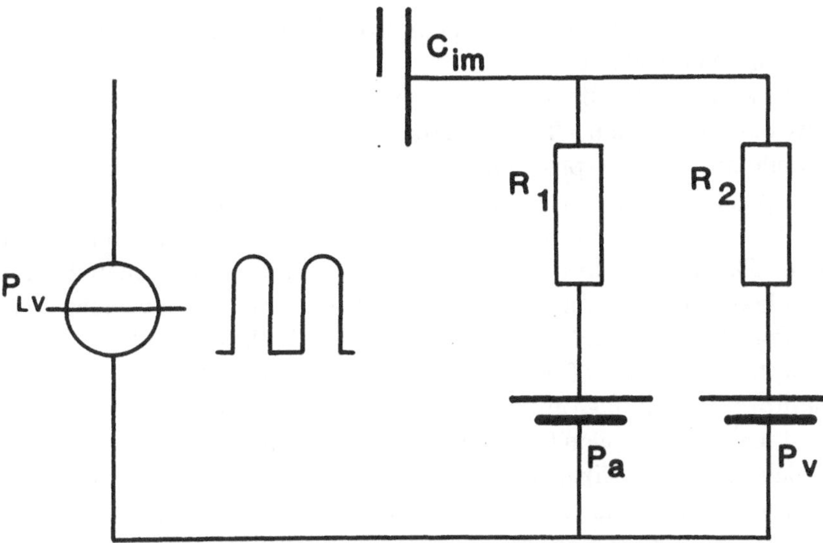

Figure 4. Electrical analog of intramyocardial pump model illucidating the effect of left ventricular pressure changes on the charge of intramyocardial compliance. P_a = arterial perfusion pressure; P_v = the outflow pressure; C_{im} = the intramyocardial compliance; R_1 = the inflow resistance of the coronary system; R_2 = the outflow resistance of the coronary system; P_{lv} = the left ventricular pressure.

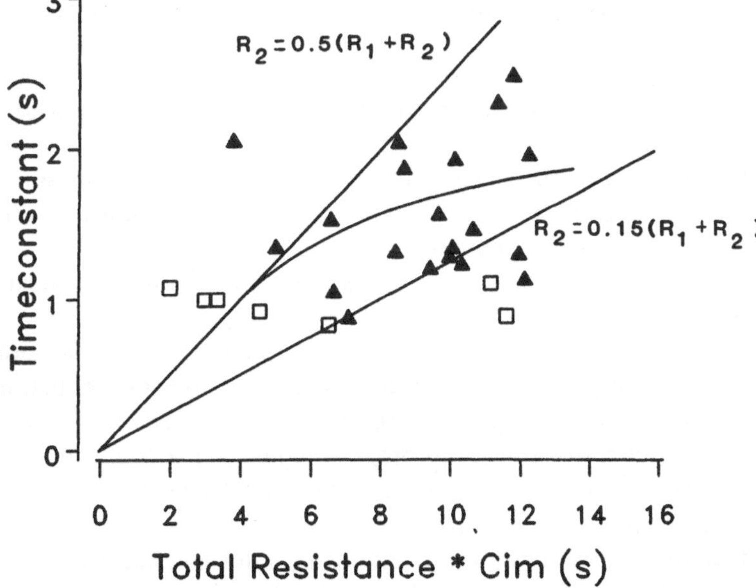

Figure 5. Relation between time constant (= $C_{im} * R_s$) and $C_{im} * (R_1 + R_2)$. Curve I represents the case that R_1 and R_2 are equal. Curve II represents the case for which R_2 is 15% of the total coronary resistance. ▲ and □ measurements in autoregulated bed and vasodilated bed, respectively. For scaling of data points see text. Total coronary resistance is defined as the ratio between arterial-venous pressure difference and mean coronary flow. Curve III represents the effect of autoregulation at a constant R_2 of 24 mm Hg · sec · 100 g/ml and R_1 increasing from 24 to 96 mm Hg · sec · 100 g/ml.

ated coronary bed has a minor influence on the characteristic time for intramyocardial volume change.

We are aware of the limitations of the study reported on above. In the first place we only could drain a fraction of the left main coronary arterial flow. This in itself would not be such a problem, be it not that the partition of coronary venous blood depends on coronary venous pressure. However, our results were not significantly influenced by either the fraction of arterial blood drained (varying between 25% and 75% from animal to animal) and the venous cannula pressure (varying between 0 and 7 mm Hg within each animal). Hence we may conclude that several experimental factors did cause scatter in the data but that our results do show the right order of magnitude for intramyocardial compliance and time constant of microvascular events in the coronary circulation. The second limitation of the model applied to the time constant analysis is that it contained only linear elements. It is unlikely that with the volume changes observed, about 25% of intramyocardial blood volume, that distribution of resistance and compliance would not change during our interventions. The possible consequences of pressure dependent compliance and resistance of the microvasculature will be discussed below.

Model of coronary circulatory mechanics based on the distensibility of the microcirculation

Basically two mechanisms relating to the distensibility of microvessels may influence coronary flow:

1. as a consequence of the balance of blood mass within the intramyocardial space a change of intramyocardial blood volume will result in a difference between arterial and venous flow,
2. a change in the diameters of microvessels will result in a change of microvascular resistance.

Obviously the first mechanism will only play a role during dynamic situations. The second one will play a role in both dynamic and and static situations. The intramyocardial pump model presented earlier [4] concerned only the first mechanism and was only tested for the autoregulated heart. The following model was designed to evaluate quantitatively the possible importance of the distensibility of the vessels in the fully dilated coronary bed.

The left ventricular wall was approximated by a division into eight layers. The circulation in each layer was approximated by three compartments: arteriolar, capillary and venular. Hence the circulation within the left ventricular wall was divided into 24 compartments. The basic assumptions of the model are the relations between vascular transmural pressure and volume of the different compartments. Vascular transmural pressure, or transmural pressure for short, is defined as the difference in fluid pressure between the intravascular and extravascular space. Experimental data on the pressure dependency of the volumes of the different vascular compartments are scarce at the moment. The best one can do is to make an educated guess. We took as a guess that the general relation between volume and pressure found for several different vessels would also apply to the coronary microvessels. This general relation is depicted in Fig. 6 top panel. Essential to this relationship are the final volume at transmural pressure zero, the decreasing compliance at increasing pressure and the possibility to extrude all volume of the vessels when compressed sufficiently.

From a curve like the one in Fig. 6 (top), one can calculate the relation between distensibility, defined as compliance divided by volume, and transmural pressure. As was made plausible in an earlier study [5], the available data on transmural pressure versus distensibility do coincide reasonable well with a compromise curve. Consequently, the pressure volume relations for our compartments where chosen such that for transmural pressures above 10 mm Hg there was reasonable agreement between the pressure-distensibility relation and the compromise curve of Spaan [5]. This agreement is shown in Fig. 7. For the venular compartment this relationship is shown for negative values of transmural pressures as well. This is the only compartment where normally transmural pressures become so low. As a consequence the 24 assumptions for transmural pressure-volume relations are reduced to one assumption for the transmural pressure-distensibility relation and the assumption for volume distribution over the different compartments.

The basic concept of the model is explained in Fig. 6b. The description of the hydrodynamics of each compartment is approximated by a so-called T-network. The resistance of the compartment is split into two equal parts both being pressure dependent. It was assumed that the relation between volume and resistance would change as for Poiseuille flow in tube with constant length and hence

$$R = K1/V^2. \qquad (2)$$

The capacitance, C, reflects the vascular compliance of the compartment and is defined as the slope of the pressure-volume relationship defined in the top panel of Fig. 6. Compliance is pressure dependent because of the slope of the shape of the pressure-volume curve.

In order to arrive at a fully defined model we now have to define for one condition, the reference condition, the distribution of pressure and volume over the different compartments at defined value of arterial, capillary, venous and tissue pressure. These distributions are given in Table 1. It would be beyond the scope of the present paper to present in detail the justifications of the different assumptions. Also the sensitivity of the solutions for these assumptions will not be discussed in detail. However, we may state that from a sensitivity analysis applied to the model that the model solutions are not quite effected by variations of parameter values between 20% and 100%, depending on the parameters involved.

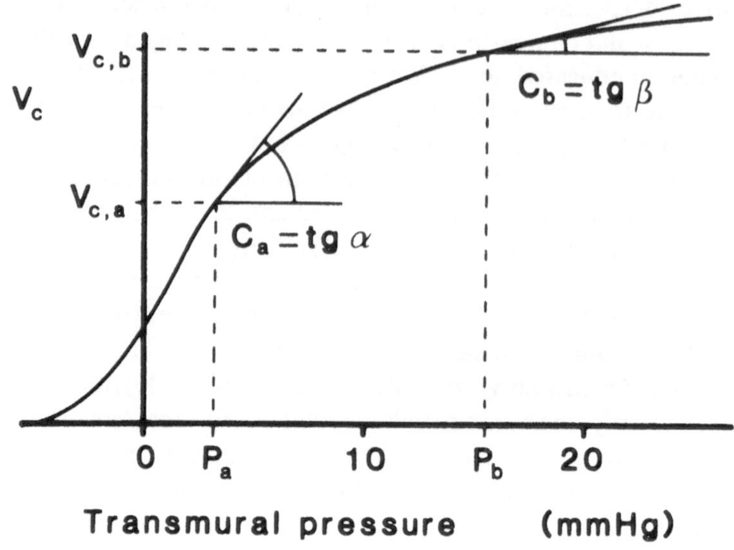

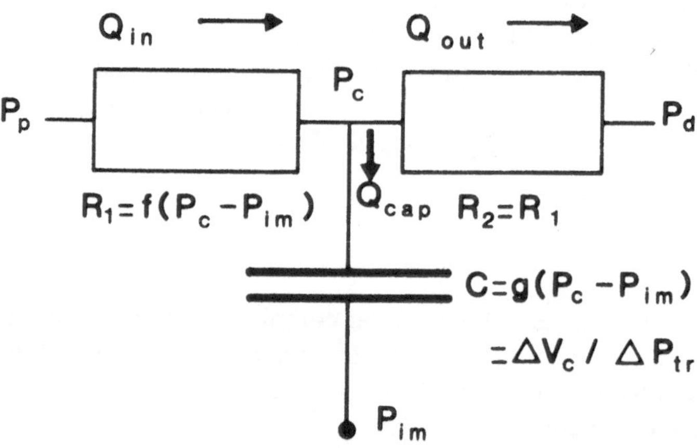

Figure 6. Basic schematic of a compliant vessel compartment. The top panel shows the relation between transmural pressure, P_{tr}, and vascular volume V_c. At each point on the curve the compliance, dV_c/dP_{tr}, equals the tangent at that point. (P_a, $V_{c,a}$) and (P_b, $V_{c,b}$) are two points on the transmural pressure-volume curve resp. Bottom panel gives an electric analogon of a vessel compartment. Resistances and the compliance depend on volume, which in its turn depends on transmural pressure. Q_{in} and Q_{out} are the flow into and out of the compartment resp. For the capacitive flow holds: $Q_{cap} = C\ dP_{tr}/dt$.

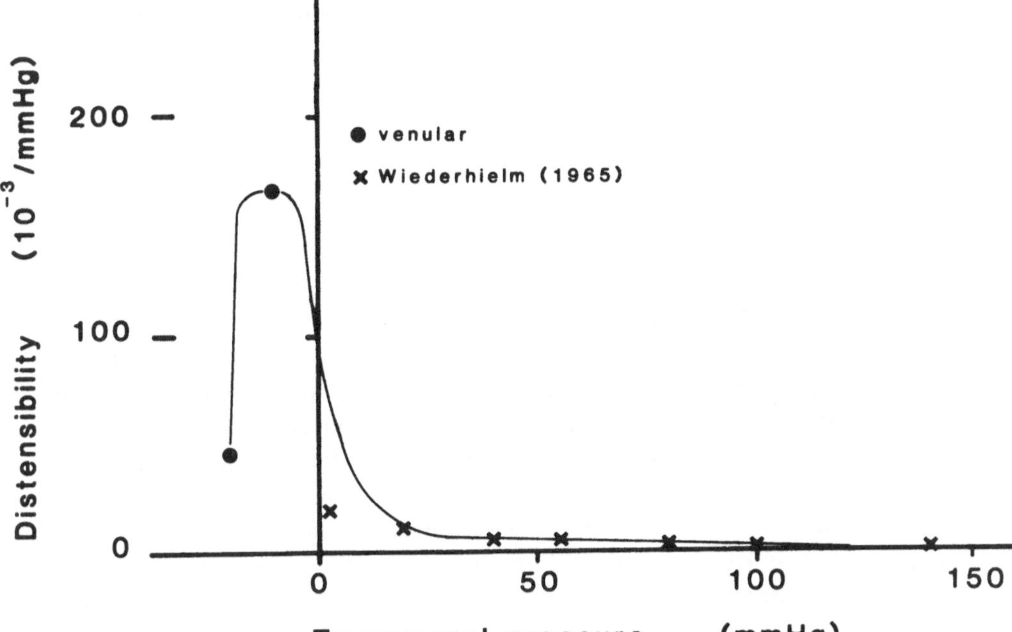

Figure 7. Distensibility as a function of transmural pressure: Above 10 mm Hg there is reasonable agreement between this pressure distensibility relation and the compromise curve of Spaan [5]. The crosses are the data derived from Wiederhielm [17]. The curves for the capillary and arteriolar compartment do incident with the venular curve for P_{tr}>10 mm Hg.

Table 1. Values of the variables in the reference condition.

perfusion pressure	50 mm Hg
arteriolar pressure	35 mm Hg
capillary pressure	15 mm Hg
venular pressure	7.5 mm Hg
venous pressure	5 mm Hg
left ventricular diastolic pressure	0 mm Hg
total coronary blood flow	4 ml/s/100 gr LV
endo/epi ratio of flow	1.56
total arteriolar volume	1.8 ml/100 gr LV
total capillary volume	4.0 ml/100 gr LV
total venular volume	3.6 ml/100 gr LV
endo/epi ratio of volumes	1.14

After having defined the pressure dependency of the compartmental resistances and compliances we have arrived at a set of 24 differential equations that can be solved simultaneously by a 4th order Runge Kutta integration procedure. When knowing the blood pressures and intramyocardial tissue pressures, the arterial and venous flow signals can be calculated as well as the pressure and flow distribution over the different compartments.

Model results

Pressure flow lines for the arrested and beating heart are shown in Fig. 8. In fact, these pressure flow lines were simulated in order to check the compatibility of the present model with the experimental results of Downey and Kirk [6]. These experiments are represented by heavy dots. In order to compensate for the difference in perfused area, the flow data of Downey and Kirk were scaled by a single factor such that the encircled data point coincides with the simulated curve at that very perfusion pressure. We assumed that the heart rate in the particular experiment was 150 beats per minute. The recently published data in the arrested heart presented by Klocke et al. [18] are also depicted. Again, their flow data were scaled such that one data point, encircled, coincides with the theoretical curve.

As to be expected the simulated pressure flow lines are curvilinear as a result of the pressure dependency of resistances in the model. The coincidence between the curvature of the theoretical and experimental curves is fair. We like to note that the parameters in the model were not chosen with the intention of a good fit of these data. There is also fair agreement between theory and experiment for the beating heart. The curvature in our theoretical curve is not due to the progressive formation of systolic waterfalls in different layers of the myocardial wall but to the increased microvascular resistance throughout the complete cycle.

Phasic coronary flow

Phasic coronary arterial flow simulated by the model is represented in Fig. 9. Results are shown for two different constant perfusion pressures, 50 and 100 mm Hg. Results for the whole heart (panels a and d) and for the subendocardium (panels b and e) are given. In the bottom panels, c and f, the calculated resistance variations throughout the cycle are depicted as well. In the figure the transitions to a long diastole are presented too. The thin curves in the upper four panels represent the flow calculated by neglecting the compliance effects. Hence, only the effect of resistance variations due to volume variations were taken into account. Hence, the difference between the bold and thin curves in those panels elicit the intramyocardial compliance effects.

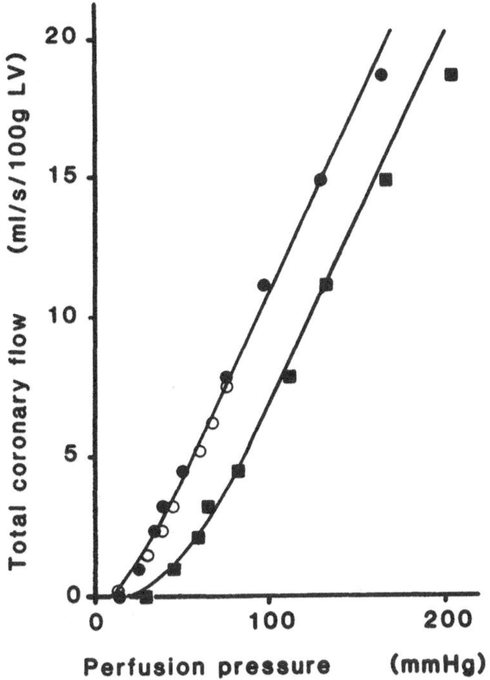

Figure 8. Coronary bloodflow as a function of perfusion pressure in the beating and in the arrested heart. Left and right solid lines represent standard model predictions for the arrested and beating heart (heart rate 150 beats · min⁻¹), respectively. The symbols ● and ■ represent one typical experiment of Downey and Kirk [6] (their Fig. 7) in the arrested and beating heart, respectively. The symbol ○ represents a typical experiment of Klocke et al. [18] (Fig. 1) in the arrested heart only. Flow values are scaled in such a way that the diastolic flows from experiment and calculations coincide at 130 mm Hg [6] and 80 mm Hg [10] perfusion pressure, respectively.

At the higher arterial pressure level the resistance variations occur more rapidly than at the lower pressure level. In fact, at a perfusion pressure of 50 mm Hg, the resistance value hasn't come to a steady state neither at the end of systole nor at the end of diastole. However, the rate of resistance determined flow change is higher at 100 mm Hg and comes to a steady state at the end of the phases in the cardiac cycle. This dependency of rate of resistive flow change on perfusion pressure can easily be understood. Because of the low transmural pressures the resistances but also the compliances of the different compartments are higher. The rate of change of the volume of a compartment, and hence the related quantities, is determined by the product of the resistance and compliance of the compartment.

The pressure dependency of the mechanical events in the model of the coronary circulation, and hence probably in the coronary circulation itself is evident from Fig. 9. At low perfusion pressure the pulsatility of the coronary arterial flow is predominantly due to the intramyocardial pump action, while at higher perfu-

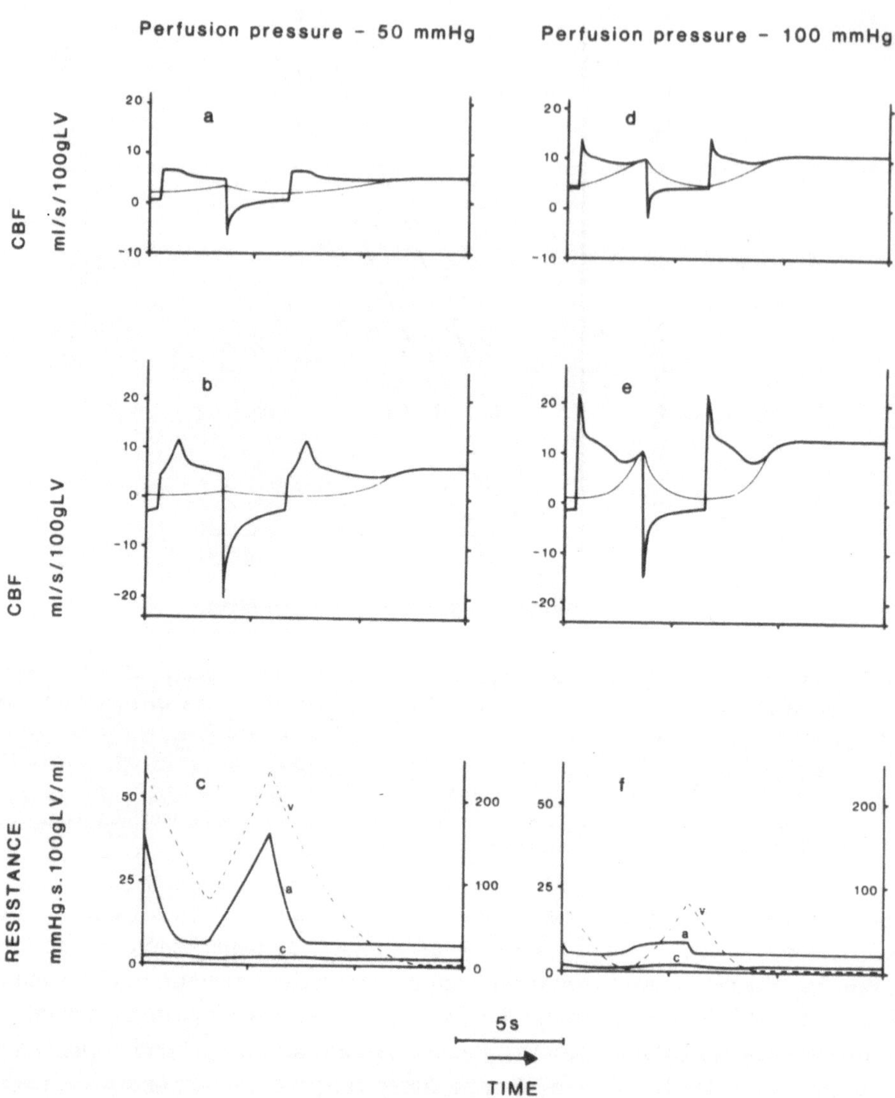

Figure 9. Instantaneous total flow (panels a and d) and subendocardial flow (panels b and c) and resistance variations (panel e and f). Left and right panels depict these variations at a low and high perfusion pressure and are characterized by low and high flow respectively. In the four top panels the total arterial flow variation calculated by the model are presented by the heavy lines and the variations in flow due to resistive effects alone, by the thin lines. At a low level of perfusion pressure the phasic behavior is solely due to intramyocardial pumping, whereas at higher values resistive effects are dominant at end-diastole. Bottom panels show the resistance variations of the arteriolar, a, capillary, c, and venular, v, subendocardial compartment. Scalings for the arterialor and capillary resistance are given at the left hand side. Venular scaling is given at the right hand side.

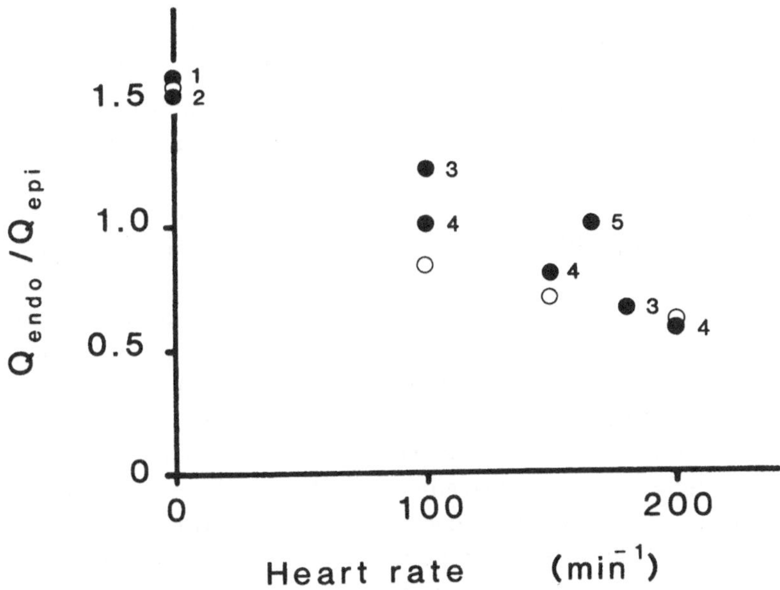

Figure 10. Simulated, ○ and, ●, and experimentally determined transmural distribution of flow as a function of heart rate. In the model, flow through the 8 layers in the reference situation was chosen in such a way that the flow ratio between the two inner layers and the two outer layers was 1.53. Simulations were performed at heart rates, of 0, 100, 150 and 200 beats per minute and perfusion pressure of 100 mm Hg. Experimental results are obtained from [18–22].

sion pressures the resistance change during the cardiac cycle contributes significantly to the pulsatile nature of coronary arterial flow.

Microsphere distribution

As an other test to the validity of the model we simulated the distribution of microspheres over the left ventricular wall at a perfusion pressure of about 100 mm Hg and compared those predictions with data from the literature. The results are shown in Fig. 10. The filled circles are experimental data [19–23]. The open circles are model predictions. Obviously, the value of endo/epi difference in the arrested heart was used as a boundary condition for the model calculations. The model predicts a larger effect of heart rate on the microsphere distribution than experimentally found. However, the difference is not that large.

Discussion of time constants in the coronary circulation

As is clear from measurements on intramyocardial blood volume variations, the characteristic time constants for microcirculation changes are long, in the order of a second. However, analysis of coronary arterial flow and pressure signals suggest much smaller time constants: in the order of 20 ms [18, 24, 25]. The question is: are these observations compatible or not? The answer is obviously yes. The experiments from which the conclusions are deduced were performed correctly. Moreover, since the experiments were all done at the same system the results must be consistent. If we do not see the consistency of the experimental results something is wrong with the theoretical concepts by which we interpret these results.

The model presented above provides a framework for the interpretation of the different results on characteristic time constants. Let us consider the arterial flow signal calculated for the arterial pressure of 100 mm Hg and shown in Fig. 9. The bold lines, representing the model result for the arterial flow measurement, show transient behavior that is compatible with a small characteristic time constant. Seemingly the flow is at steady state in 50 ms. However, the characteristic time of the compliance related flow, the difference between the heavy and thin curves, exhibit a characteristic time which is much longer. Without the intramyocardial compliance effect arterial flow would increase during diastole because of decreasing resistance. Would resistance not vary during the cardiac cycle, the characteristic behavior of intramyocardial compliance would become obvious with a time constant in the order of the duration of diastole. With the combination of both effects, it seems that equilibrium of arterial flow in diastole, and systole is much quicker. Hence, the change in resistance during the cardiac cycle conceals the compliance effects and vice versa. As a result, the small time constant characterizing the behavior of the arterial flow signal can be compatible with a large time constant characterizing the changes of microvascular volume and relating quantities. Hence we must conclude that the arterial signal alone provides not enough information to draw conclusions on events in the microcirculation.

Conclusions

In this paper we have shown from experimental results obtained from a preparation where both arterial and venous coronary flow was measured, that microvascular volume variations within the coronary circulation can be substantial and that the time constants characterizing these variations are in the order of a second. Moreover, we showed that the site of intramyocardial compliance is not in the very end of the circulation, but that a significant distal resistance must exist.

A compartmental model based on the pressure dependency of all micro vessels exhibits several characteristic features of which are also experimentally found in the coronary circulation.

The model study made plausible that small characteristic time constants are compatible with large microcirculatory characteristic time constants. It also was shown that one has to be very prudent to interpret coronary arterial flow and pressure signals by means of models consisting out of elements which are essentially not pressure dependent.

References

1. Fung YC, Zweifach BW, Intaglietta H (1966): Elastic environment of the capillary bed. Circ Res 19: 441–461.
2. Burton AC (1954): Relation of structure to function of the tissues of the wall of blood vessels. Physiol Rev 34: 619–642.
3. Smaje LH, Fraser PS, Clough C (1980): The distensibility of single capillaries and venules in the cat mesentary. Microvasc Res 20: 358–370.
4. Spaan JAE, Breuls NPW, Laird JD (1981): Diastolic-systolic coronary flow differences are caused by intramyocardial pump action in the anesthetized dog. Circ Res 49: 584–593.
5. Spaan JAE (1985): Coronary diastolic pressure-flow relation and zero flow pressure explained on the basis of intramyocardial compliance. Circ Res 56: 293–309.
6. Downey JM, Kirk ES (1975): Inhibition of coronary blood flow by a vascular waterfall mechanism. Circ Res 36: 753–760.
7. Archie JP (1975): Intramyocardial pressure: effect of preload on transmural distribution of systolic coronary blood flow. Am J Cardiol 35: 904–911.
8. Hoffman JIE, Buckberg GD (1976): Transmural variations in myocardial perfusion. Progress in Cardiology 5: 37–89.
9. Arts MGJ (1978): A mathematical model of the dynamics of the left ventricle and the coronary circulation. Ph D Thesis, State University of Limburg, Maastricht, The Netherlands.
10. Spaan JAE, Breuls NPW, Laird JD (1981): Forward coronary flow normally seen in systole is the result of both forward and concealed back flow. Basic Res of Cardiol 76: 582–586.
11. Ellis AK, Klocke FJ (1980): Effects of preload on the transmural distribution of perfusion and pressure-flow relationships in the canine coronary vascular bed. Circ Res 46: 68–77.
12. Chilian WH, Marcus HL (1982): Phasic coronary blood flow velocity in intramural and epicardial coronary arteries. Circ Res 50: 775–782.
13. Porter WT (1898): The influence of the heart-beat on the flow of blood through the walls of the heart. Am J Physiol 1: 145–163.
14. Wiggers CJ (1954): The interplay of coronary vascular resistance and myocardial compression in regulating coronary flow. Circ Res 2: 271–279.
15. Tomonaga G, Tsujioka K, Ogasawara Y, Goto M, Nakai M, Tadaoka S, Kajiya F (1983): Evaluation of phasic blood flow velocity in peripheral coronary vein by laser doppler velocimeter (Abstract). Circulation (Suppl. III): 203.
16. Kajiya F, Tsujioka K, Goto M (1985): Evaluation of phasic blood flow velocity of the great cardiac vein by a laser doppler method. Heart and Vessel 1: 16–23.
17. Wiederhielm CA (1965): Distensibility characteristics of small bloodvessels. Fed Proc 24: 1075–1084.
18. Klocke FJ, Mates RE, Canty jr JM, Ellis AK (1985): Coronary pressure-flow relationships: controversial issues and probable implications. Circ Res 56: 310–323.
19. Wüsten B, Buss DD, Deist H, Schaper W (1977): Dilatory capacity of the coronary circulation and its correlation to the arterial vasculature in the canine left ventricle. Basic Res Cardiol 72: 636–650.
20. Domenech RJ (1978): Regional diastolic coronary blood flow during diastolic ventricular hypertension. Cardiovasc Res 12: 639–645.

21. Domenech RJ, Goich J (1976): Effect of heart rate on regional coronary blood flow. Cardiovasc Res 10: 224–231.
22. Bache RJ, Cobb FR (1977): Effect of maximal coronary vasodilation on transmural myocardial perfusion during tachycardia in the awake dog. Circ Res 41: 648–653.
23. Downey HF, Bashour FA, Boatwright RB, Parker PE, Kechejian SJ (1975): Uniformity of transmural perfusion in anesthetized dogs with maximally dilated coronary circulations. Circ Res 37: 111–117.
24. Dole WP, Alexander GM, Campbell AB, Hixson EL, Bishop VS (1984): Interpretation and physiological significance of diastolic coronary artery pressure-flow relationships in the canine coronary bed. Circ Res 55: 215–226.
25. Lee J, Chambers DE, Akizuki S, Downey JM (1984): The role of vascular capacitance in the coronary arteries. Circ Res 55: 751–762.

Discussion

Mates: You showed a curve in the vasodilated bed, where coronary flow continued to decrease during the long diastole. Our experiments and others do not show this phenomena. Can you explain what the differences are?
Spaan: I am not sure if we really had maximal vasodilation. This is also not very relevant to the point I wanted to make with this figure.
Downey: What appear to be capacitance-related overshoots in flow at the onset of diastole in your model are actually the result of the pressure-dependent resistance. I suggest the validity of the model be tested by presenting it with step changes in coronary arterial pressure during diastole. We get exactly the same time constant for either a step change in perfusion pressure or the onset of diastole. I don't think that will be seen in your model.
Spaan: This has to be tried.
Beyar: A typical waterfall is derived from a segment that has a steep cross sectional area-transmural pressure relationship at low transmural pressures. That phenomenon is actually a collapse or a waterfall. Your model includes this assumption. I fail to see why you resist the waterfall concept when you actually use the basis for it.
Spaan: The model allows for the collapse of vessels. However, systole is just too short for this collapse can occur. There is time needed to squeeze blood out of the microvessels.
Dinnar: Is your capacitance capable of retrograded flow?
Spaan: Yes. This is shown in the results of my paper.

25. Impedance to coronary flow

R.E. MATES, F.J. KLOCKE and J.M. CANTY Jr

Abstract

Impedance to flow in the coronary circulation is time-varying, precluding the use of Fourier transforms of pressure and flow waveforms to determine impedance. Perturbation techniques have been used to determine impedance in long diastoles. Using a hydraulic servovalve, sinusoidal and ramp pressure waveforms were applied to the left circumflex coronary artery of anesthetised, open chest dogs. The resulting flow perturbations were analyzed to determine impedance. A lumped parameter viscoelastic model with pressure dependent parameters was adequate to describe the impedance. At frequencies up to 5 Hz, viscoelastic effects were negligible and a simple resistive-capacitive model was adequate. For slow ramps, this model was used to construct capacitance-free pressure-flow curves which were in good agreement wth those obtained from constant-pressure diastoles. The capacitance affecting coronary inflow appears to be a small fraction of total coronary capacitance.

Introduction

While it has long been recognized that systole impedes coronary inflow, recent observations suggest that even during diastole inflow ceases at arterial pressures which are well above coronary venous pressure [1–4]. Since the vessels comprising the circulation are elastic, phasic flow patterns vary throughout the circulation. Coronary inflow peaks during diastole, while venous outflow reaches a maximum during systole [5, 6].

There is presently no method available to measure phasic flows or pressures throughout the coronary microcirculation. While some attempts have been made to measure epicardial flow using optical techniques [7], flow patterns in the microcirculation probably differ substantially from endocardium to epicardium. Knowledge of the impedance characteristics of the coronary circulation is essential in order to relate flow in the microcirculation to measured inflow and outflow.

The input impedance of other systemic beds has been determined by utilizing Fourier transforms of measured pressure and flow waveforms. This technique requires that the system be stationary, i.e., that the impedance be independent of time. This condition is not met in the coronary circulation, since impedance varies due to compression of embedded vessels during systole.

Sinusoidal perturbations

We have utilized perturbations of coronary arterial pressure to determine input impedance. A servovalve perfusion system was used to control pressure in the cannulated left circumflex coronary artery in anesthetized, open chest dogs [8]. Long diastoles were produced in heart blocked animals by cessation of rapid ventricular pacing. During the long diastole, sinusoidal pressure variations of ± 5–10 mm Hg were superimposed on a constant mean pressure and the resulting flow perturbations were measured. Experiments were conducted in the autoregulating bed and after vasodilation with infusion of adenosine [9].

The modulus and phase of the input impedance were determined over the frequency range 1–10 Hz. The modulus is defined as the ratio of the amplitudes of the pressure and flow oscillations, and the phase as the difference in the phase of the pressure and flow oscillations. This formulation assumes that impedance is constant during the long diastole. In the vasodilated bed, impedance remained constant over the time course of the diastole. In the autoregulating bed, mean flow decreased with time due to the reduced oxygen demand in the non-beating heart. In these experiments, data were analyzed during the first and fifth seconds of diastolic arrest.

The linearity of the system was assessed in two ways. First, pressure and flow waveforms were subjected to Fourier analysis. The amplitudes of higher harmonics were generally less than 10% of that of the fundamental frequency. The impedance was also found to be independent of pressure amplitude for perturbations in the range ± 5–10 mm Hg. Thus, for small perturbations the system is quasi-linear.

Results of the experiments are summarized in Figure 1. For any given mean pressure, the modulus of impedance decreased as frequency was increased. Phase angles were negative (flow led pressure). The modulus of impedance was greater at any mean pressure with smooth muscle tone intact than in the vasodilated bed. The modulus and phase of impedence were found to vary with mean distending pressure. The modulus at a given frequency increased as pressure increased. At low pressures, the phase angle reached a maximum negative value and then returned toward zero. At higher pressures this peak in the phase angle was not observed. The pressure dependence of impedance indicates that, even though the coronary circulation is quasi-linear for small pressure perturbations, nonlinear

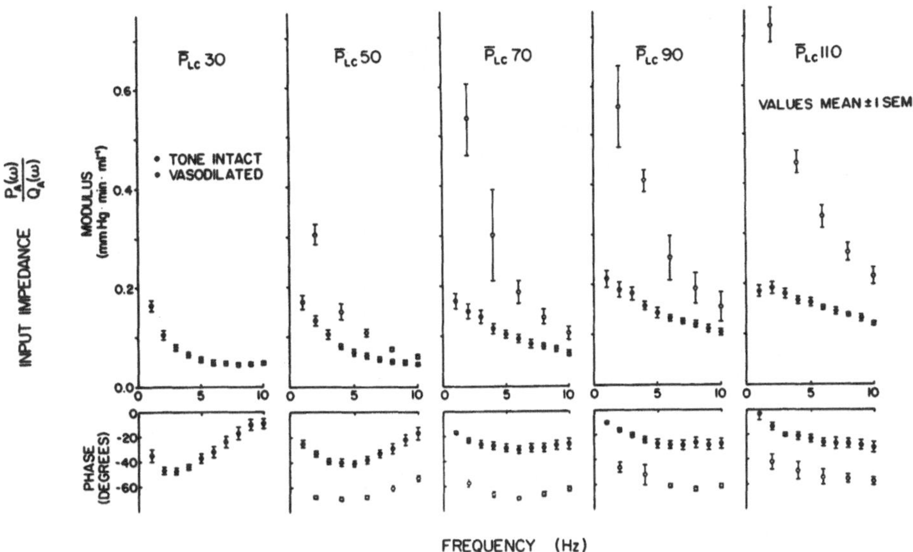

Figure 1. Modulus and phase of input impedance vs. frequency. Each vertical panel shows data at a given mean distending pressure during vasodilation (solid circles) and with tone intact (open circles). Impedance modulus (upper panels) at each distending pressure is lower during vasodilation than with tone intact. Phase angle (lower panel) is greater with tone intact. Reprinted with permission from [8].

effects are important over the range of pressures encountered in normal diastoles.

In order to estimate differences between phasic coronary inflow and flow in the microcirculation, a model describing the dynamics of the circulation is required. Linear lumped parameter models have been used previously in the coronary circulation as well as in other beds because of their mathematical simplicity. Such models represent a crude approximation to the actual circulation and do not describe phenomena associated with wave propagation and reflection. The distance to reflection sites in the coronary circulation is quite short compared to the wavelength of low frequency oscillations of physiological importance. Thus pressure equilibration occurs quite rapidly. In the canine coronary circulation it has been shown that reflections of high frequency waves (>7 Hz) are negligible [10]. Thus, lumped models provide a better approximation to coronary impedance than to the impedance of other systemic beds.

We evaluated a number of lumped parameter models incorporating resistive, capacitive, inductive and viscoelastic elements. An optimization technique was employed to obtain the best least squares fit for a given model to the impedance data [11]. Over the frequency range 1–5 Hz, a parallel combination of a resistance and capacitance provided a good fit to the data. Above 5 Hz, the phase behavior of the impedance data was better fit by replacing the capacitor by a Voigt viscoelastic element as shown in Figure 2. Adding additional elements to the model did not improve the fit.

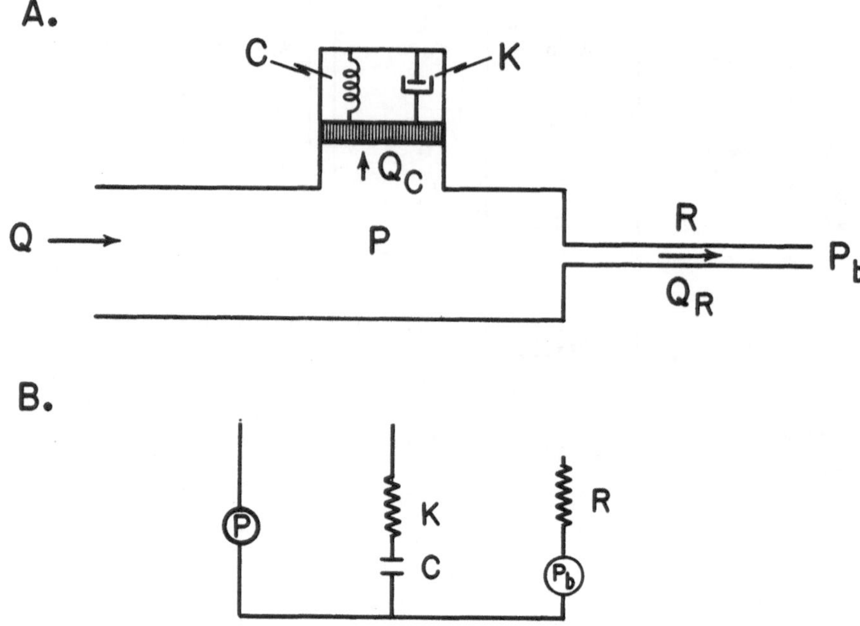

Figure 2. Lumped model of the coronary circulation incorporating a Voigt viscoelastic element (C and K) and a resistor R. Th hydraulic analog of the model is given in (a) and the electrical analog in (b). Q represents inflow, Q_c flow into the viscoelastic element, and Q_R the flow through the resistor. P is the arterial pressure and P_b is the back pressure to flow.

The elastic parameters of the RC viscoelastic model are shown in Figure 3, plotted as a function of pressure. The capacitance decreased with increasing pressure. This is consistent with the observed behavior of excised coronary arteries [12–14]. Other studies of the capacitance of the intact arterial bed have shown variable results. Capacitance measured in beds occluded with 200 micron beads showed a pressure dependence similar to our results [15], while in beds occluded with smaller particles capacitance appeared to be independent of pressure [16, 17]. In the latter studies, the entire arterial bed was at a uniform pressure since there was no through flow. Thus, these studies include a larger than normal contribution from the elasticity of small arterial vessels. If the elasticity of these smaller vessels is not pressure dependent, their contribution may have masked the pressure dependence of the large arteries.

At a given pressure, capacitance in the vasodilated bed was approximately twice as large as with tone intact. This may reflect the effect of smooth muscle tone on the stiffness of individual vessels. In addition, vasodilation will expose more distal vessels to larger pressure fluctuations and may lead to recruitment of additional parallel vessels, both of which would increase the overall capacitance of the arterial bed.

The viscoelastic constant increased with increasing pressure, suggesting that

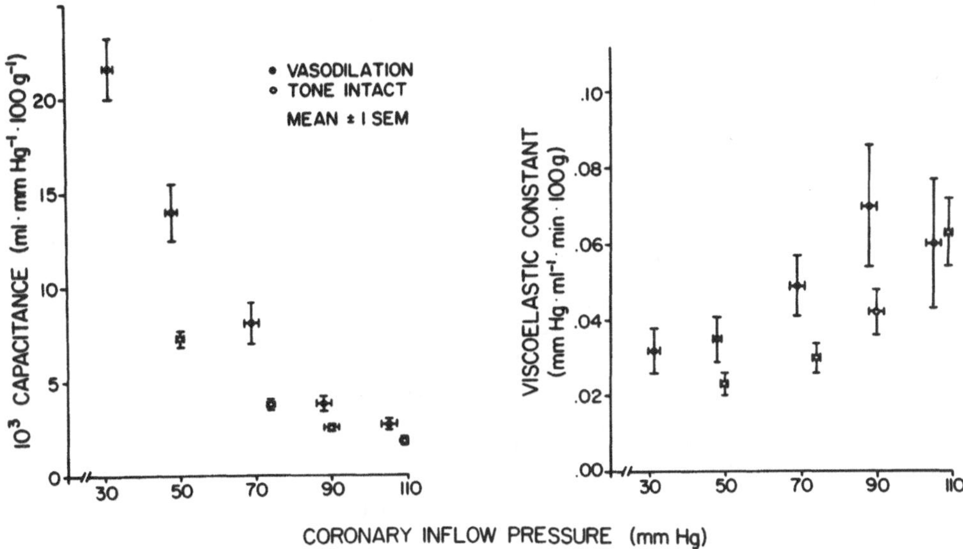

Figure 3. Effects of coronary inflow pressure and vasomotor tone on capacitance (left panel) and viscoelastic constant (right panel) calculated from the RC viscoelasic model. Capacitance decreases as pressure is increased and is larger during vasodilation. The viscoelastic constant increases as pressure is increased and is also larger during vasodilation. Reprinted with permission from [8].

viscoelastic effects are more important as vessels become stiffer. The constant was larger during vasodilation than with vasomotor tone intact. The resistance, which is not shown in the figure, showed a slight decrease with increasing pressure, although the differences were not statistically significant. The resistance at any given pressure was several times higher with tone intact than in the vasodilated bed, as expected.

Ramp perturbations

The use of sinusoidal inlet pressure perturbations provides a method for determining coronary capacitance and hence allows the estimation of resistive, or microcirculatory flow, as a function of inlet pressure. The method requires a substantial amount of data collection and processing. We therefore sought a simpler technique for constructing pressure-flow relationships that are free of capacitive effects.

The success of the simple parallel RC model in fitting the low frequency impedance data suggested the use of ramp waveforms to enable direct construction of capacitance-free pressure flow curves in long diastoles. The method is

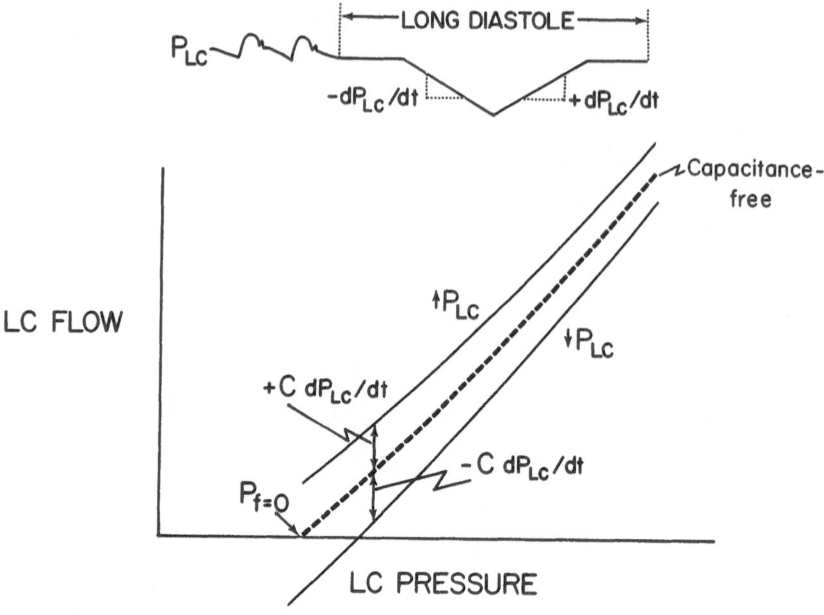

Figure 4. Schematic representation of ramp perturbation. Upper panel shows left circumflex pressure P_{LC} as a function of time. The rates of pressure change dP_{LC}/dt during the down and up ramps are equal and opposite. Lower panel shows left circumflex inflow as a function of pressure. The solid lines are the measured inflow. At any pressure level, the capacitive flows $C\,dP_{LC}$ are equal and opposite during the down and up portions of the ramp. The dotted line is the capacitance-free, or resistive, flow.

shown schematically in Figure 4. The servovalve control system was programmed to decrease pressure at a constant rate with time to a predetermined level, then to increase pressure at the same rate back to the initial level. In the RC model, capacitive flow is given by $Q_c = C\,dP/dt$. Since the values of dP/dt are equal and opposite during the down and up ramps, at any pressure level the capacitive flows will be equal and opposite. The resistive flow at any pressure is then the average of the inflow during the down and up ramps. Since the calculation assumes that impedance does not change during the ramp, the method is applicable only in the vasodilated bed.

Since capacitive flow is the difference between inflow and resistive flow, and dP/dt is known, the capacitance can be determined as a continuous function of pressure from the ramp data. The resistance is simply the slope of the resistive pressure-flow curve. Thus the ramp technique provides not only the capacitance-free pressure-flow relationship, but values of the impedance parameters as well.

A sample record showing ramp pressure and flow as functions of time is given in Figure 5. If the simple RC model were exact, flow should change discontinuously as dP/dt is abruptly changed. In the actual record, a brief flow transient occurs which is probably due to inertial and viscoelastic effects. This transient was not included in the data analysis.

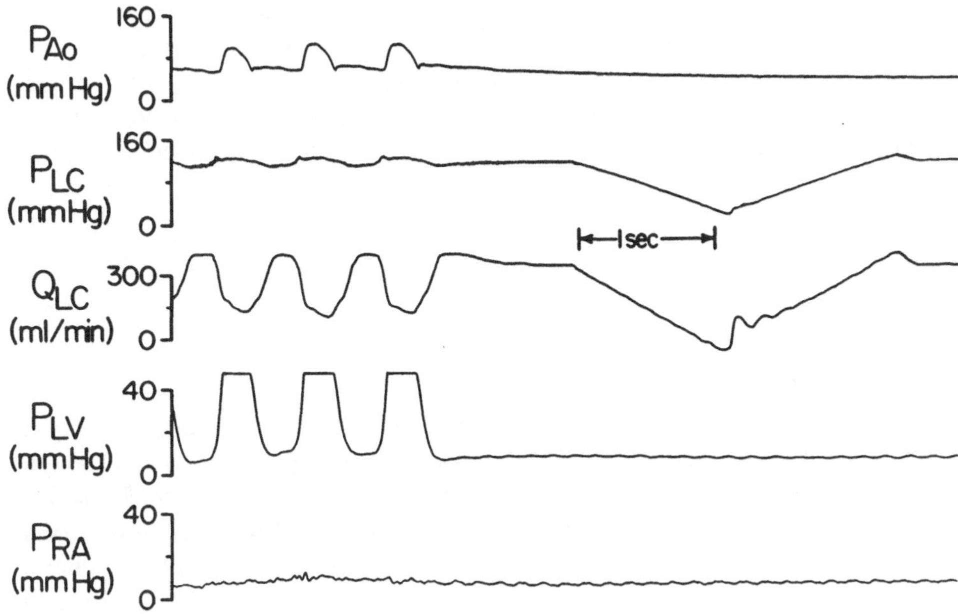

Figure 5. Analog record of a ramp produced during a long diastole. Aortic pressure P_{Ao}, left circumflex pressure P_{LC}, left circumflex flow Q_{LC}, left ventricular pressure P_{LV} (expanded scale) and right atrial pressure P_{RA} are shown as functions of time. Three normal beats are shown, followed by a long diastole. During the diastole, a ramp lasting approximately 2 sec was produced.

Our experience to date with the ramp technique indicates that it provides a quick and accurate method for constructing capacitance free pressure-flow curves during long diastoles [18]. Curves constructed in this manner agree well with those obtained during constant pressure diastoles, in which capacitive effects are absent. In the latter technique, single pressure and flow points are obtained from a series of diastoles in which pressure is maintained constant at different levels. This requires considerably more time than the single ramp, and care must be taken to maintain stable hemodynamics during the series of ramps. In particular, left and right atrial pressures must be held constant to avoid shifts in the pressure-flow curve. Thus the ramp technique greatly simplifies the experimental determination of pressure-flow relationships.

Values of resistance and capacitance calculated from the ramps were in good agreement with those obtained using the sine wave perturbations. The values of capacitance calculated from the ramps at any given pressure showed a modest dependence on the value of dP/dt for the ramp, decreasing as dP/dt increased. This is consistent with the viscoelastic behavior noted in the sine wave perturbations. For values of dP/dt in the range 30–90 mmHg/sec, neither the calculated resistance nor the resistive pressure-flow curve were dependent on dP/dt.

In principle, more rapid ramps can be employed to determine impedance during long diastoles with vasomotor tone intact and during normal cardiac cycles. When dP/dt exceeds 100 mm Hg/sec, viscoelastic effects become appreciable and the RC model no longer adequately describes the system. Analysis of the ramp data on the basis of more complicated models, such as the RC viscoelastic model, is considerably more complex. Because of the pressure dependence of the model parameters, the differential equation describing the system is nonlinear. We are presently investigating the application of nonlinear optimization techniques to this problem.

Discussion

The experiments described above were concerned only with diastolic input impedance. During systole, coronary inflow is drastically reduced even though perfusion pressure is at a maximum. There have been few attempts to characterize systolic impedance to flow. Panerai et al. constructed pressure-flow curves during systole and diastole by varying mean perfusion pressure while the phasic pressure pattern was maintained [19]. Their results showed a systolic increase in both resistance and the back pressure to flow. Distortion of the pressure and flow waveforms required substantial corrections, and capacitive effects were not accounted for.

Spaan et al. have suggested that the reduction in systolic flow is caused by an intramyocardial capacitance coupled to ventricular pressure which discharges during systole and recharges in diastole [20]. This intramyocardial pump provides an explanation for augmented venous outflow during systole. Spaan suggests that the apparent high back pressures to diastolic inflow can be explained on the basis of the intramyocardial capacitance without the need for a vascular waterfall [21]. This point remains controversial [22].

In the vasodilated bed, flows remain constant during long constant-pressure diastoles, indicating negligible charging of the intramyocardial capacitor. The pressure at which inflow ceases is 5–10 mm Hg above right atrial pressure. In the autoregulating bed, reported values of zero-flow pressure are as high as 40–50 mm Hg above right atrial pressure [1]. Here the interpretation is more complicated. Since resistance is changing with time, it is difficult to separate transients due to the charging of a downstream capacitance from those caused by changing resistance. Zero-flow pressures obtained during constant pressure long diastoles in three of four reported studies [2–4] were higher with vasomotor tone intact (18–37 mm Hg) than during vasodilation (11–15 mm Hg) and increased with the level of pre-arrest pressure, which presumably correlates with initial vasomotor tone [22]. These results suggest that charging of a distal capacitance is not sufficient to explain diastolic pressure-flow behavior.

Capacitance estimates made on the basis of the intramyocardial pump model [20] as well as those based on variations in total myocardial blood volume [23–26] and venous outflow [5, 6] are at least an order of magnitude larger than our results [9] and estimates based on inflow occlusion [15–17]. Thus it appears that the capacitance which affects coronary inflow represents a small portion of total coronary capacitance. Nonetheless, it seems clear that capacitance must be accounted for in relating measured inflow to flow in the microcirculation.

The input impedance measurements we have obtained to date have been confined to long diastoles. Systolic-diastolic interactions may alter input impedance, particularly during early diastole. Capacitive flow is the product of capacitance and the rate of change of pressure with time. During diastole, the decline in pressure occurs approximately exponentially, hence the rate of pressure change with time decreases as the diastole proceeds. The value of capacitance, on the other hand, increases as the pressure decreases during diastole. Hence capacitive flow may be appreciable during the entire diastole. There is presently little information available concerning systolic input impedance. The rapid ramp technique described earlier can potentially provide impedance information during the normal cardiac cycle.

Acknowledgment

Supported by grants from the National Heart, Lung and Blood Institute (2-PO1-HLB-15194, 1-KO8-HLB-01168) and American Heart Association with funds contributed by The Western New York Affiliate (83-717).

References

1. Bellamy RF (1978): Diastolic coronary artery pressure-flow relations in the dog. Circ Res 43: 92–101.
2. Klocke FJ, Weinstein IR, Klocke JF, Ellis AK, Kraus DR, Mates RE, Canty JM, Anbar RD, Romanowski RR, Wallmeyer KW, Echt MP (1981): Zero-flow pressures and pressure-flow relationships during single long diastoles in the canine coronary circulation before and during maximum vasodilation: Limited influence of capacitive effects. J Clin Invest 68: 970–980.
3. Dole WP, Bishop VS (1982): Influence of autoregulation and capacitance on diastolic coronary artery pressure-flow relationships in the dog. Circ Res 51: 215–226.
4. Lee J, Chambers DE, Akizuki S, Downey JM (1984): The role of vascular capacitance in the coronary arteries. Circ Res 55: 751–762.
5. Spaan JAE (1981): Intramyocardial compliance studied by venous outflow at arterial occlusion (Abstract). Circulation 66 (Suppl III): 307.
6. Chilian WM, Marcus ML (1984): Coronary venous outflow persists after cessation of coronary arterial inflow. Am J Physiol 247: H984–H990.
7. Tillmans H, Ikeda S, Hansen H, Sarma JSM, Fauvel J-M, Bing RJ (1974): Microcirculation in the ventricle of the dog and turtle. Circ Res 34: 561–569.
8. Canty JM, Mates RE (1982): A programmable pressure control system for coronary flow studies. Am J Physiol 243: H796–H802.
9. Canty JM Jr, Klocke FJ, Mates RE (1985): Pressure and tone dependence of coronary diastolic

input impedance and capacitance. Am J Physiol 248: H700–H711.
10. Arts T, Kruger RTI, van Gerven W, Lambregts JAC, Reneman RS (1979): Propagation velocity and reflection of pressure waves in the canine coronary artery. Am J Physiol 237: H469–H474.
11. Mates RE, Burns T, Canty JM Greenberg R, Neeson J (1983): Modeling diastolic impedance to coronary blood flow. In: Mates RE, Nerem RM, Stein PD (eds) Mechanics of the coronary circulation. American Society of Mechanical Engineers, New York, pp 41–44.
12. Gow BS, Schonfeld D, Patel DJ (1974): The dynamic elastic properties of the canine left circumflex coronary artery. J Biomech 7: 389–395.
13. Patel DJ, Janicki JS (1970): Static elastic properties of the left coronary circumflex artery and the common carotid artery in dogs. Circ Res 27: 149–158.
14. Hayashi K, Igarashi Y, Takamizawa K (1985): Stiffness of human coronary arteries. In: Butler D, Hung TK, Mates RE (eds) 1985 Biomechanics Symposium. ASME, New York, NY.
15. Douglas JE, Greenfield JC Jr (1970): Epicardial coronary artery compliance in the dog. Circ Res 27: 921–929.
16. Gregg DE, Green HD, Wiggers C (1935): Phasic variations in peripheral coronary resistance. Am J Physiol 112: 362–373.
17. Eng C, Kirk ES (1983): The arterial component of the coronary capacitance. In: Mates RE, Nerem RM, Stein PD (eds) Mechanics of the coronary circulation. ASME, New York, NY.
18. Canty JM Jr, Mates RE, Klocke FJ (1983): Rapid determination of capacitance-free pressure-flow relationships during single diastoles (Abstract). Fed Proc 42: 1092.
19. Panerai RB, Chamberlain JH, Sayers BMCA (1979): Characterization of extravascular component of coronary resistance by instantaneous pressure-flow relationships in the dog. Circ Res 45: 378–390.
20. Spaan JAE, Breuls NPW, Laird JD (1981): Diastolic-systolic coronary flow differences are caused by intramyocardial pump action in the anesthetized dog. Circ Res 49: 584–593.
21. Spaan JAE (1985): Coronary diastolic pressure-flow relation and zero flow pressure explained on the basis of intramyocardial compliance. Circ Res 56: 293–309.
22. Klocke FJ, Mates RE, Canty JM Jr, Ellis AE (1985): Coronary pressure-flow rlationships – Controversial issues and probable implications. Circ Res 56: 310–323.
23. Moe GK, Wood EH, Visscher MB (1939): Aortic pressure and the diastolic volume law of energy output in cardiac contraction. Proc Soc Exp Biol Med 40: 460–463.
24. Salisbury PF, Cross CE, Rieben PA (1961): Physiological factors influencing blood volume in isolated dog hearts. Am J Physiol 200: 633–636.
25. Scharf SM, Bromberger-Barnea B (1973): Influence of coronary flow and pressure on cardiac function and coronary vascular volume. Am J Physiol 224: 918–925.
26. Morgenstern C, Holjes U, Arnold G, Lochner W (1973): The influence of coronary pressure and coronary flow on intracoronary blood volume and geometry of the left ventricle. Pflügers Archiv 340: 101–111.

Discussion

Bassingthwaighte: I am delighted by the idea of presenting models as alternative hypotheses tested against each other, rather than making more or less preordained conclusions from a single model.

Downey: Is your viscoelastic model equivalent to our two resistance (RCR) model?

Mates: The transfer functions for the two models are dynamically equivalent. One of the problems with simple lumped parameter models is that they may not be unique. Because of this it is dangerous to assign too much anatomic significance to model elements.

Downey: This may explain a lot of what we see since there may be a finite velocity with which the vessel wall can respond.

Spaan: To what part of the circulation does your resistance refer?

Mates: We considered only one lumped resistance, so it is not possible to specify a precise location. The strong influence of smooth muscle tone suggests that most of the resistance is in arteriolar and pre-capillary vessels.

Bassingthwaighte: You may want to relate your data to those of Vince Rideout who used similar sinusoidal driving functions.

26. Intramyocardial blood volume – implications for analysis of myocardial mechanical characteristics via in vivo imaging of the heart

E.A. HOFFMAN and E.L. RITMAN

Abstract

Volume of intravascular blood within the myocardium can be estimated in the intact, in situ heart using fast CT. The ratio of increased roentgen opacity in the myocardium and in the aortic root was used to estimate the blood volume. In five dogs an average value of 13.4% of myocardium was estimated to be blood and in another nine dogs adenosine infusion into the pulmonary artery increased this value to 22%. A more direct estimate of this value in isolated hearts was obtained by perfusing the coronary circulation with dilute contrast agent. Values obtained ranged from 8% to 14% over a 75 mm Hg to 110 mm Hg perfusion pressure.

Using fast CT the intramyocardial blood volume seems to vary throughout the cardiac cycle. This phasic change is found both by measuring absolute volume of the left ventricular (LV) myocardium and by measuring changes in LV intramyocardial roentgen opacity as a ratio of intra aortic opacity. Using fast CT with lungs held at functional residual capacity, myocardial blood content appears to increase in early systole by about one-seventh the blood volume at end diastole. This transient increase is reversed in mid systole and blood volume is minimum at end systole. The transient increase in myocardial blood volume seems to correspond to the rapid transient decrease in pericardial pressure measured in dogs with a percutaneously introduced catheter in the pericardial space.

Introduction

A portion of the myocardium is made up of intravascular blood. Depending on what fraction of the myocardium is blood, and how easily this blood moves within the intravascular space in response to changes in regional compression, this may have considerable impact on myocardial mechanical properties. The myocardium can be considered basically a two component structure: a tension-resisting container surrounding a compression resisting fluid under pressure. Consequently, the myocardium has many of the anatomic features noted in erectile tissues [1].

The question as to whether this characteristic is of physiologic significance is discussed fairly extensively in the literature [2, 3] but unfortunately is based on observations made primarily in isolated heart or open chested preparations.

The focal point of this discussion is the recent observations of myocardial blood volume indices using the Dynamic Spatial Reconstructor to image the myocardium of the in situ heart, in the never opened thoracic cavity. Findings suggest that, perhaps, the undisturbed intrathoracic milieu imposes mechanical conditions which alter the cardiac cycle dependent variations in coronary blood volume from those observed using opened thorax or isolated heart preparations. These observations require that the accuracy of myocardial blood volume measurements via fast CT be carefully evaluated.

Background

Evidence that myocardium has the anatomic structures needed to function as erectile tissue is documented in various disciplines. At an histological level, many investigators [4, 5] have shown that there is a 1:1 relationship between the capillaries and muscle fibers of the heart of adult animals. While the diameter of the capillaries and/or of the muscle fibers may change with pathological conditions such as hypertrophy, this numerical relationship seems to be constant. The fraction of myocardium that is intravascular space is estimated by such methods to be between 3.5 and 5%. This value would appear to be highly dependent on the conditions under which the myocardium was fixed prior to histological examination, and it does not include vessels larger than capillaries. If a more macroscopic analysis [6] is performed, so that intra arterial and intravenous volumes are included, the fraction of myocardial volume that is blood is thought to be between 11–17% in the isolated heart.

One method for estimating this value in the working heart is to measure wall thickness. Decrease in wall thickness accompanying coronary artery occlusion in the isolated heart is reported [7] to be 10% under control conditions and a 20+% rebound thickening occurs when flow is permitted to reperfuse the now hyperemic myocardium. That the intramyocardial blood content affects myocardial mechanical characteristics was indicated by the observation that wall stiffness decreased with loss of blood pressure in the coronary arteries.

Myocardial blood volume by x-ray contrast enhancement: isolated hearts

We have tried to more directly estimate intramyocardial blood volume by perfusing the left main coronary artery of fresh isolated hearts with saline containing dilute roentgen contrast agent (Figure 1). In four dogs hearts, using perfusion pressures between 75 and 110 mmHg, we measured the increase in roentgen

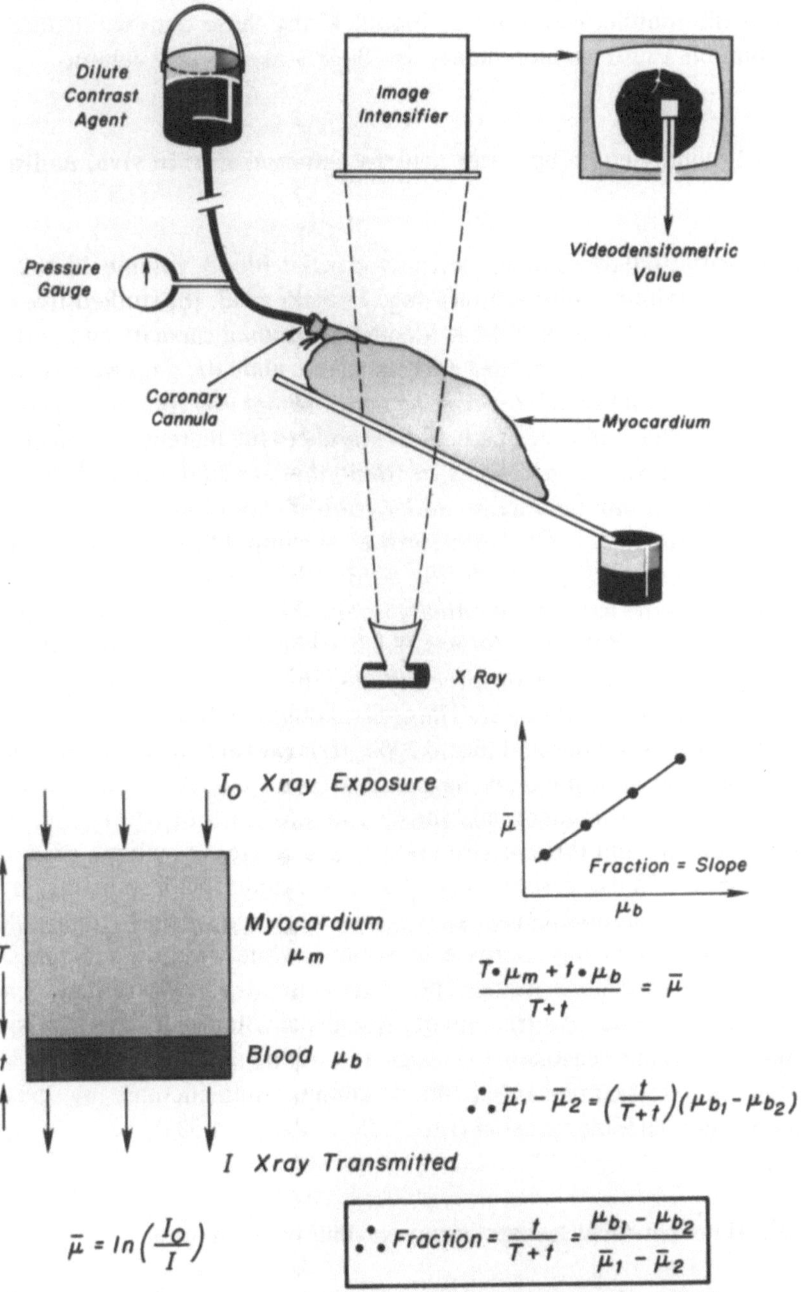

Figure 1. Schematic of in vitro estimation of intramyocardial blood volume. As shown in the top panel, an isolated left ventricle is cut along the posterior wall and flattened. The decrease in x-ray transmission is measured with each increase in concentration of contrast agent in the perfusion fluid. Upto 1:3 diluted contrast agent was used. As shown in the equations of the bottom panel, the percent of myocardium that is blood is derived from the slope of the line through the data points.

opacity of the myocardium as a fraction of the increase in opacity that should have occurred if the muscle were entirely blood. Using these data we deduced that blood volume in these isolated hearts was 8–14% myocardial volume.

Myocardial blood volume by x-ray contrast enhancement: in vivo, undisturbed thorax

We have also tried to estimate intramyocardial blood volume in the intact anesthetized (sodium pentobarbital) dog. Iwasaki et al. [8] studied five supine anesthetized dogs with lungs held at functional residual capacity and performed an aortic root injection of roentgen contrast agent while the dogs were scanned in the DSR [9]. The fraction of blood in the myocardium was computed as the ratio of increased roentgen opacity of the heart muscle to the increase in opacity of the aorta (Figure 2). From these studies we found that at end diastole blood volume was $13.4 \pm 0.3\%$ of muscle volume under control conditions.

In a similar study (J. Stray-Gundersen et al., unpublished) four anestetized dogs were scanned in the DSR during aortic root injection during continuous infusion of adenosine into the pulmonary artery. The average fraction of myocardium that was deduced to be blood was 22.5% (range 21–24%). Two of these dogs were subsequently exercised for three months, the other two were not, and they were restudied three months later. The control dogs had blood volumes of 21 and 22% and the exercised dogs had 16 and 20%. If, however, the myocardial volume for each dog was multiplied by its percent blood content, the control dogs changed from an intramyocardial blood volume of 21.8 to 22.7 cc and 29.0 to 27.2 cc respectively and the exercised dogs changed from a volume of 22.2 cc to 21.0 cc and 35.2 to 35.4 cc respectively. Hence no change in absolute intramyocardial blood volume was noted in any of the dogs. This is consistent with histological findings that the myocytes increase in volume while the number and size of capillaries does not change much. The image data also indicate that adenosine increases blood volume, as a fraction of myocardial volume, from ~14% to 22%. That these values are reasonable is suggested by the study of Crystal et al. [10] who found that intra myocardial blood volume could increase by 75% over control during adenosine infusion (i.e., $1.75 \times 14\% = 24.5\%$).

Cardiac cycle dependent changes in myocardial blood volume

Clearly a vasodilator can result in a considerably increased intramyocardial blood content (Figure 3). Whether this is mediated primarily by distension (relaxation of smooth muscle) of the smaller vessels and/or to what extent this is caused by recruitment of non-patent capillaries remains to be demonstrated. The extent to which perfusion pressure alone (i.e, aortic pressure – right atrial pressure) can

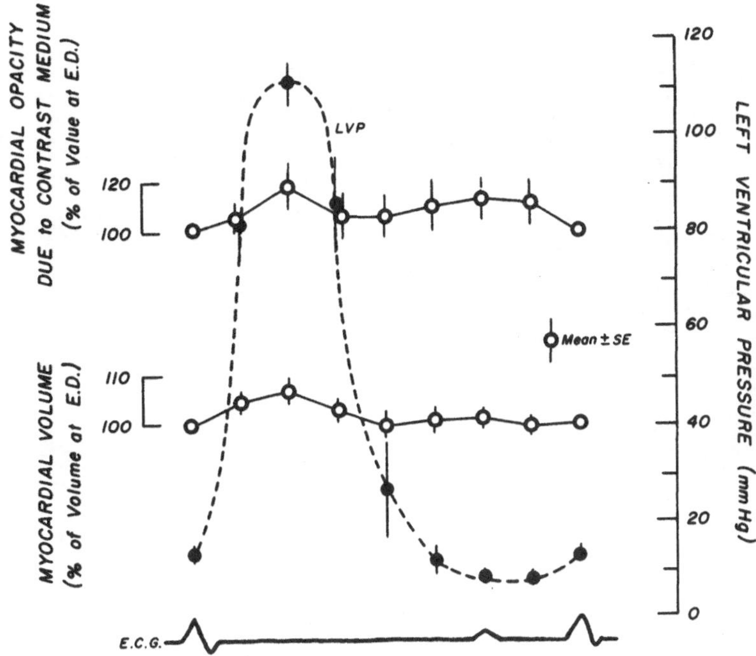

Figure 2. Cyclic variation of left ventricular myocardial volume and roentgen opacity measured by DSR in anesthetized intact dogs. These data are average of eleven dogs under pentobarbital anesthesia.

contribute is also not known. These are difficult questions to address in the intact, never invaded animal because coronary perfusion pressure is generally accompanied by the increased transmural pressure needed to generate the increased aortic pressure. Increased transmural pressure presumably compresses the intramyocardial vasculature, especially in the subendocardial layers [11]. In the intact animal that has never had the chest opened, however, there may be other localized transient pressure gradients that have a significant effect on the amount of blood within the myocardium. Thus, Iwasaki and colleagues found that the roentgen opacity of the myocardium increased during early systole by up to one-seventh relative to the roentgen opacity at end diastole [12]. This translates to at least 1 cc/gm/sec which is comparable to the blood flow through the myocardium. This change should be reflected in the myocardial volume, as indeed it is observed to do. Iwasaki reported this observation in dogs [8] and more recently Whiting et al. [13] reported this in an human subject studied in an Imatron fast CT scanner. While this observation may be incorrectly interpreted, and certainly seems to be at odds with the observations in isolated hearts and instrumented in situ hearts with the pericardium opened, it is possible that the heart, in the never opened chest, does behave differently due to its rather tight mechanical coupling

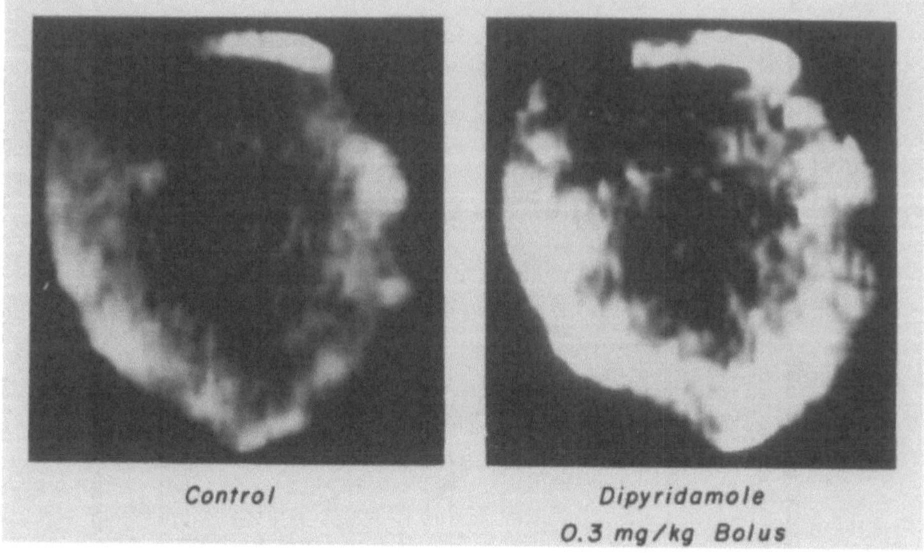

Figure 3. A single 3.6 mm thick, cross section of the in situ heart of an anesthetized dog before and during dipyridamole. The increase in brightness indicates the increased roentgen opacity of the myocardium due to increased blood content of the myocardium. Blood was opacified by a 2 ml/kg injection of the nonionic contrast agent Iohexol injected into the aortic root. Dog under morphine and pentobarbital anesthesia.

to the lung via the intact pericardium.

Many years ago Avasthey et al. [14] showed (Figure 4) that a rapid negative pressure transient, in early isovolumetric systole, occurred in the intact pericardial space. The timing of this negative pressure transient corresponds closely to the timing of the deduced transient increase in blood volume of the myocardium. This negative pressure pulse is almost certainly due to the stiffness of the surrounding lung which may prevent the ventricles from reducing volume unless there is a reciprocal increase of the size of the atria and, to a limited extent, an increase in volume of the myocardium [15, 16]. If in addition the endocardial muscle contracts before the epicardial muscle, there may, indeed, be a tendency to distend the myocardium by the transiently frustrated pulling of the not yet contracting subepicardial myocardium away from the relatively unyielding lungs.

Effect of total heart volume on myocardial blood volume

It has previously been shown [15–17] that the total volume of the heart (contents of the pericardial sac) at end systole remains within 5% of the value at end diastole (Figure 5). We have demonstrated [15] that throughout the cardiac cycle, the epicardial apex of dogs remains fixed while the A-V valve region moves in a

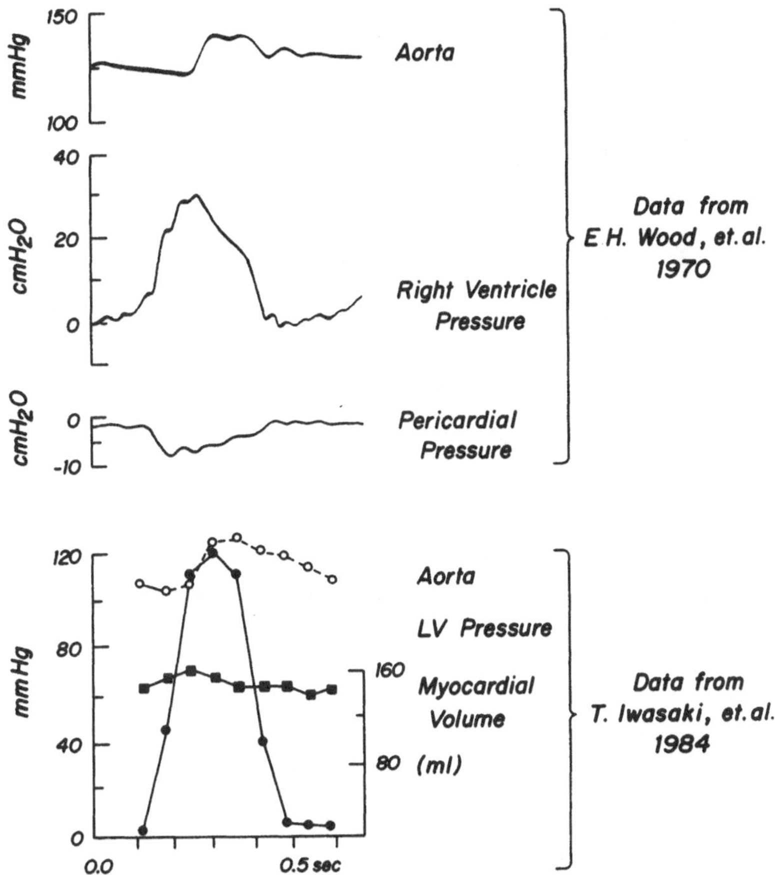

Figure 4. Data from two sources. Upper panel show temporal relationship of intrapericardial pressure relative to the cardiac cycle of an anesthetized dog with intact, never invaded thorax. The lower panel are data from a different dog obtained with the DSR. Note how the transient increase in myocardial volume matches the transient decrease in pericardial pressure. (Lower panel reproduced with permission from [8].)

piston-like motion such that volume reciprocity between atria and ventricles may largely explain this observed 'law of constant heart volume'. (A fixed epicardial apex throughout the cardiac cycle can frequently be observed in normal humans via echocardiography.) As shown in Figure 6, we are able to subtract the total 'chamber volume' (intrapericardial x-ray contrast enhanced blood excluding coronary blood volume) from the total heart volume to obtain a measure of total 'myocardial volume'. These measurements include the intrapericardial portions of the ascending aorta and pulmonary trunk. Preliminary findings [16] suggest that when the total heart volume is reduced (4 dogs) by lung inflation to 15 cm H_2O P_{AWY}, end diastolic total myocardial volume is reduced by a mean of 10%.

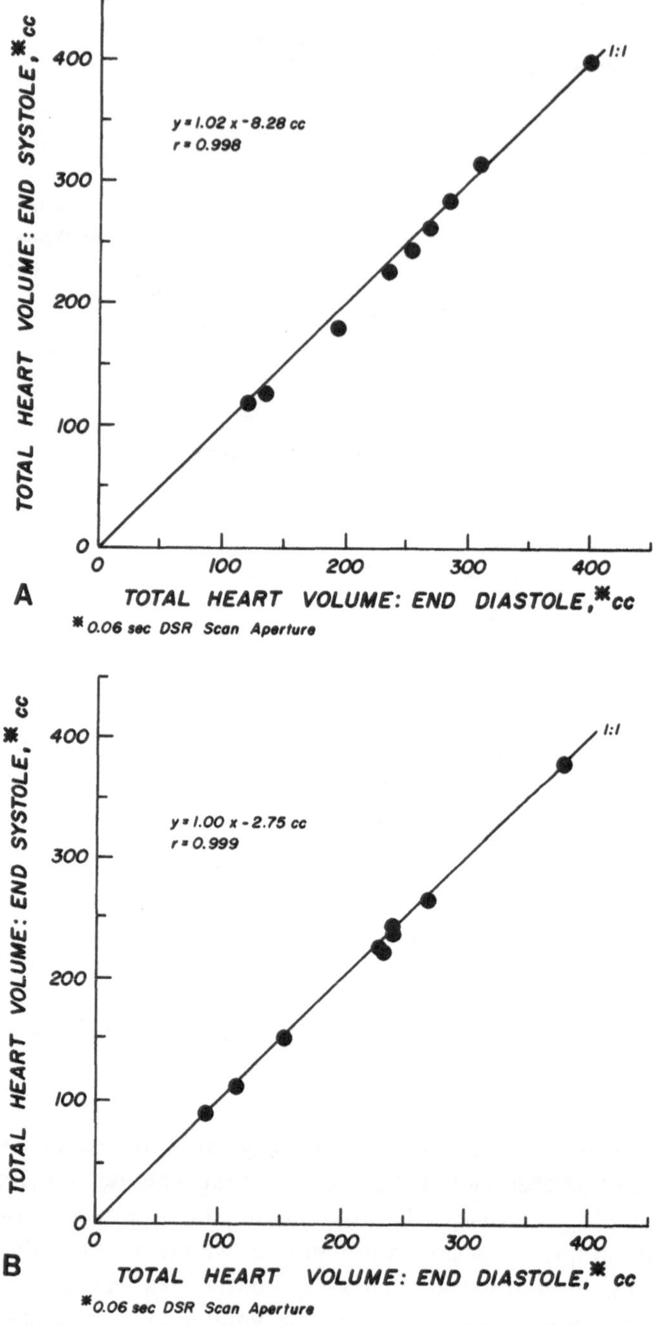

Figure 5. Heart volume (within the pericardial sack) does not change significantly between systole and diastole with the lungs held at either 0 or 15 cm H_2O P_{AWY} (panel A and B, respectively). DSR scan aperture 0.06 second duration. (Reproduced with permission from [15].)

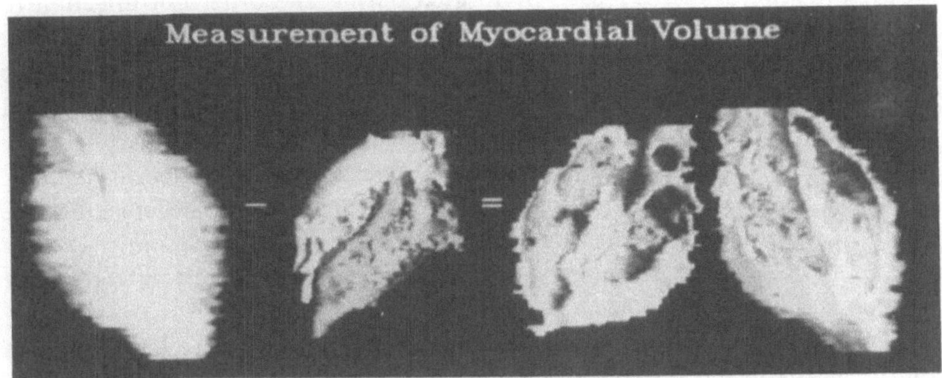

Figure 6. Total myocardial volume is calculated by subtracting the total chamber volume from the total heart volume measurements both at end diastole and end systole. Since cardiac muscle volume presumably remains constant between diastole and systole, a change in myocardial volume should reflect a change in intramyocardial blood volume. (Reproduced with permission from [20[.)

Under conditions of reduced total heart volume and reduced total myocardial volume, we find that at end systole (minimal LV volume) total myocardial volume is greater (12.75%) than the value at end diastole and approximates the end diastolic total myocardial volume found with lungs held at 0 cm H_2O P_{AWY}. Further study is required to clarify the alterations in cardiac geometry which contribute to this difference in our measurement of 'total myocardial volume'. We hypothesize that, if the cardiac muscle is essentially incompressible, then this volume change represents a change in myocardial blood volume.

Atrial compliance also appears to play a role in the maintenance of a constant heart volume [18]. This is suggested by our observation in hearts with atrial fibrillation that, with the lungs held at 0 cm H_2O P_{AWY}, total heart volume is significantly smaller at end systole compared with the end diastolic volume. This is consistent with the observation [15] that atrial/ventricular volume reciprocity is an important factor in the maintenance of a constant heart volume. Atrial function could play an additionally important role in the maintenance of a constant total heart volume through an effect on myocardial blood volume. Atrial contraction could 'pull' on the ventricular muscle and affect the intramural pressures of the ventricular myocardium. Bellamy [19] has observed that in dogs and pigs with complete heart block atrial systole causes an increase in intramyocardial pressure associated with a decrease in coronary arterial flow and an increase in coronary venous flow (thus a reduction in myocardial blood volume).

Conclusion

These data suggest that intramyocardial blood volume can be estimated in the in situ heart using a fast CT scan performed during an aortic root injection of roentgen contrast agent, and the changes in myocardial blood volume may be assessed by the differences in myocardial volume. Applications of the blood contrast enhancement method suggest that almost a doubling of coronary blood volume can be caused by a vasodilator and that in the control state, coronary blood volume increases transiently by about one-seventh during early systole.

Cardiac cycle dependent alterations in myocardial blood volume may be altered by a number of intra- and extra-cardiac parameters within the never opened thorax. These parameters include atrial fibrillation, diastolic total heart volume and lung compliance.

These alterations in coronary blood volume may well have considerable impact on the mechanical properties of the myocardium. Furthermore, the role of the myocardial blood volume alterations in maintaining a constant heart volume may well have an effect on cardiac mechanical efficiency, assuming that it is more efficient to only move blood rather than moving extra-cardiac structures such as the lungs in the process of moving blood.

Acknowledgment

The authors thank Drs J. Stray-Gundersen and J.H. Mitchell for allowing us to use some of their unpublished data in this paper. The figures were prepared by Steven Orwoll and James Hanson. This work was supported in part by NIH grant HL-04664, HL-32300 and RR-02540. Dr E.A. Hoffman is partly funded by a John G. Searle Award.

References

1. Wainwright SA (1970): Design in hydraulic organisms. Naturwissenschaften 57: 321–326.
2. Ahn J, Apstein CS, Hood WB (1977): Erectile properties of the left ventricle: direct effect of coronary artery perfusion pressure on diastolic wall stiffness and thickness (Abstract). Clin Res 25: 201A.
3. Vogel WM, Apstein CS, Briggs LL, Gaasch WH, Ahn J (1982): Acute alterations in left ventricular diastolic chamber stiffness. Role of the 'erectile' effect effect of coronary arterial pressure and flow in normal and damaged hearts. Circ Res 51: 465–478.
4. Rakusan K, Wachtlova M, Poupa O (1969): An attempt to determine indirectly the vascularity of the heart muscle by measuring the tissue concentration of haemoglobin in normal and anaemic rats. Physiol Bohemoslov 18: 1–5.
5. Eliasen P, Amtorp O, Tondevold E, Haunso S (1982): Regional blood flow, microvascular blood content and tissue haematocrit in canine myocardium. Cardiovasc Res 16: 593–598.
6. Morgenstern C, Holjes U, Arnold G, Lochner W (1973): The influence of coronary pressure and coronary flow on intracoronary blood volume and geometry of the left ventricle. Pflungers Archiv 340: 101–111.
7. Gaasch WH, Bing OHL, Franklin A, Rhodes O, Bernard SA, Weintraub RM (1980): The influence of acute alterations in coronary blood flow on left ventricular diastolic compliance and

wall thickness. Eur J Cardiol 7(Suppl): 147–161.

8. Iwasaka T, Sinak LJ, Hoffman EA, Robb RA, Harris LD, Bahn RC, Ritman EL (1984): Mass of left ventricular myocardium estimated with the dynamic spatial reconstructor. Am J (Heart Circ) Physiol 15: H138–H142.
9. Ritman EL, Robb RA, Harris LD (1985): Imaging physiological functions: experience with the dynamic spatial reconstructor. Praeger, Philadelphia, PA, p. 302.
10. Crystal GJ, Downey HF, Bashour FA (1981): Small vessel and total coronary blood volume during intracoronary adenosine. Am J (Heart Circ) Physiol 10: H194–H201.
11. Feigl EO (1983): Coronary physiology. Physiol Review 63: 1–205.
12. Iwasaki T, Ritman EL (1984): Intramyocardial blood volume dynamics in the cardiac cycle (Abstract). Fed Proc 43: 422.
13. Whiting J, Bateman T, Pfaff M, Eisenberg H, Forrester J (1985): Semi-automated method for quantitating LV mass and chamber volume from Cine-CT scans. Circulation 72 (Part II): III–181.
14. Avasthey P, Coulam CM, Wood EH (1970): Position-dependent regional differences in pericardial pressures. J Appl Physiol 28: 622–629.
15. Hoffman EA, Ritman EL (1985): Invariant total heart volume in the intact thorax. Am J (Heart Circ) Physiol 249: H883–H890.
16. Hoffman EA, Ritman EL (1987): Heart-lung interaction: effect on regional lung air content and total heart volume. Ann Biomed Eng 15: Nos. 324 (in press).
17. Hamilton WF, Rompf JH (1932): Movement of the base of the ventricle and the relative constancy of the cardiac volume. Am J Physiol 102: 559–565.
18. Hoffman EA, Ritman EL (1986): Law of constant heart volume disrupted by atrial fibrillation (Abstract). Fed Proc 45: 776.
19. Bellamy RF (1981): Effect of atrial systole on canine and porcine coronary blood flow. Circ Res 49: 701–710.
20. Hoffman EA, Heffernan PB (1986): Investigation of the intrathoracic determinants of cardiac geometry aided by an improved interactive approach to the manipulation of surfaces. Proc NCGA III: 151–161.

Discussion

Downey: One of the things that became obvious from the capacitance model when you use aortic pressure as the perfusion source is that during the onset of systole the capacitance is filling due to the rising aortic pressure and emptying due to the rising intramyocardial pressure. The opposite happens at the onset of diastole (we often use a no-pulsatile perfusion pressure to overcome this problem). Which effect predominates is hard to say and, therefore, it may be difficult to correlate intravascular volume and resistance in this preparation.

Marcus: There are some studies by Wolfgang Schaffer that demonstrate that the endocardial blood volume is substantially larger than in the epicardial layers. Can you see this gradient in your DSR?

Ritman: Yes, during an aortogram we do see a gradient in transmural radio opacity which we interpret to be due to the subendocardium having more blood volume per unit volume of myocardium than does the subepicardium.

Spaan: You have very small, and larger, vessels in the myocardium. Do you see a change in distribution of blood related to the vessel size? Have you tried a mass balance to check how much should the arterial flow differ if one seventh of the blood volume will change during one cycle?

Ritman: No, we rarely resolve vessels within the myocardium, and no, we have not done mass balance analysis.

27. Effect of wall forces on coronary flow

M.B. STEVENS, A.C. HILL, H. MORI, W. HUSSEINI and
J.I.E. HOFFMAN

Abstract

When coronary vessels are maximally dilated, flow through them is linearly related to coronary arterial perfusing pressure over the physiological range. The flows are also affected by the left ventricular systolic pressure. At a mean coronary perfusion pressure of 12 kPa (90 mm Hg), an increase in left ventricular systolic pressure fromm 14 to 19.1 kPa (105 to 143 mm Hg) decreases maximal subendocardial blood flow by 30% and at a mean coronary perfusing pressure of 8 kPa (60 mm Hg) similar increase in left ventricular systolic pressure decreases maximal subendocardial flow by 50%. Subepicardial flows were not affected by changes in left ventricular systolic pressure. These findings are important in practice, as illustrated by the effects of right ventricular systolic hypertension on right ventricular myocardial ischemia. Furthermore, because subendocardial blood flow is entirely diastolic, the mechanism by which a raised systolic wall force impairs diastolic flow must involve an interaction between systole and diastole and may be related to intramyocardial vascular resistances and compliances.

Introduction

Any good model of the coronary circulation must fit existing pathophysiologic data, that is, the input-output relations that are known to occur in experiments should be reproducible by the model. Once a model fits existing data well, a stringent test of it would be its ability to predict what would happen experimentally for types of experiments that have not yet been done. Thus there is continued need for perturbations that reveal new experimental data. In the discussion to follow we will present data on the effects of changes of wall stress on regional myocardial flow and flow reserve, effects not hitherto described in detail.

To introduce this subject, conside the measurement of coronary flow reserve which is the difference between resting and maximal coronary flow at a given coronary perfusing pressure. In dogs, this measurement is best made after cannulating the left main coronary artery so that coronary perfusion pressure can be varied independently of aortic pressure. As a result the coronary perfusing pressure can be changed while aortic pressure and heart rate – two major determinants of myocardial work, oxygen demand and blood flow – do not change. Under normal circumstances, changes of coronary perfusing pressure between 6.67 and 16 kPa (50 and 120 mm Hg) are accompanied by only small changes of coronary flow. The relative constancy of coronary flow at constant myocardial oxygen demand is termed autoregulation. It is achieved by a fall in coronary vascular resistance when perfusing pressure falls and a rise in resistance when perfusing pressure rises. The mechanisms by which this adjustment takes place are imperfectly understood. If in the same dog the coronary vessels are maximally dilated by an agent like adenosine or chromonar, then coronary flow is increased at all perfusing pressures, and the resultant pressure flow relationship is very steep and reasonably linear within the physiological pressure range. The difference between the autoregulated and maximally dilated flows at any perfusing pressure is the coronary flow reserve at that pressure [1]. Two aspects of coronary flow reserve are particularly important. First, there are differences of coronary flow reserve in different layers of the left ventricular wall, with the flow reserve being less in the subendocardium than the subepicardium at any pressure [2, 3]. Secondly, the flow reserve as measured by injecting a pharmacologic vasodilator is not necessarily available to the heart during ischemia because ischemia is not a maximal vasodilator stimulus [4–7].

There are two major problems to consider when measuring coronary flow reserve in humans. One is that because the flow reserve is very sensitive to coronary perfusing pressure, the normal variation is large. In fact, most clinical reports that deal with coronary flow reserve do not mention the perfusing pressures at which the flow reserve was measured. The second problem is that measurement of coronary flow reserve as performed in animals cannot be done in humans because it is not feasible to separate coronary and aortic pressures in human. As a result, to vary perfusing pressure the aortic pressure must be changed, and the dependance of maximal flow on aortic pressure, and thus on left ventricular wall stress, has not been systematically examined. We do know that a high aortic pressure increases resting (regulated) coronary flow because it increases myocardial work. What we do not know is what happens to flow reserve at the same pressure.

To study this, we performed two series of experiments. In one, the Gregg cannula preparation was used, coronary vessels were dilated maximally with chromonar, and regional flows were measured with radioactive microspheres at coronary perfusing pressures of 12, 8 and 6 kPa (90, 60 and 45 mm Hg) while there was a normal mean aortic pressure of 12.8–14.0 kPa (96–105 mm Hg) and then again after elevating mean aortic pressure to 16.8–19.1 kPa (126–143 mm Hg). In the second series of experiments, no cannula was used and coronary and aortic pressures were raised or lowered together during autoregulation and then after maximal coronary vasodilatation.

The first series of studies showed that at normal mean aortic pressures lowering coronary perfusing pressure prduced a steep decrease in flow and decreased flow in all layers of the myocardium. The inner:outer flow ratio (the ratio of flow per gram in the subendocardial and subepicardial layers of the wall of the left ventricle) decreased as perfusion pressure was lowered. When the measurements were repeated at the higher aortic pressure, subepicardial flows were essentially unchanged but all the subendocardial flows were reduced, as were the inner:outer flow ratios at all coronary perfusing pressures (Figure 1).

In the second series of experiments, raising both pressures during normal regulation increased flow slightly in all layers, but did so more in the inner layer as has been described before [8, 9]. During maximal vasodilatation, flows rose markedly by similar amounts in both layers, so that flow reserve at the higher pressures was substantially higher than it was at the lower pressures; the increase was a little greater for the subepicardial than for the subendocardial layer. Comparison of the two sets of experimental data showed that the flow reserve was less at the higher pressures when aortic and coronary pressures rose together than when coronary pressure was increased while aortic pressure remained constant. In other words, the change of coronary flow reserve as pressures changed was less steep when both pressures rose together than they were dissociated.

Discussion

When aortic pressure is elevated acutely, there is an increase of end-diastolic volume (Starling's law) and an increase in end-systolic volume (Frank's law). The raised aortic pressure stimulates baroreceptors and causes cardiac slowing. There may be an increase in contractility. If heart rate is kept constant, as was done in our studies, then the net effect of these changes is to decrease ejection fraction, increase left ventricular diastolic pressure, and increase both diastolic and systolic wall stresses.

The decrease in subendocardial flow for given coronary perfusing pressures when aortic pressure was raised in series I is of interest. The large increase in systolic wall stress is a likely major factor in this change, but a direct mechanism of action is unlikely because little myocardial flow occurs in systole. Therefore either the decrease in subendocardial flow is due to the raised diastolic pressure and wall stress or else it is due to some effect that an increased systolic wall stress has on flow in the subsequent diastole. That an increased left ventricular diastolic pressure decreases subendocardial blood flow has been described many times, both in beating hearts [8, 10–12] and when the heart is fibrillating [13–15].

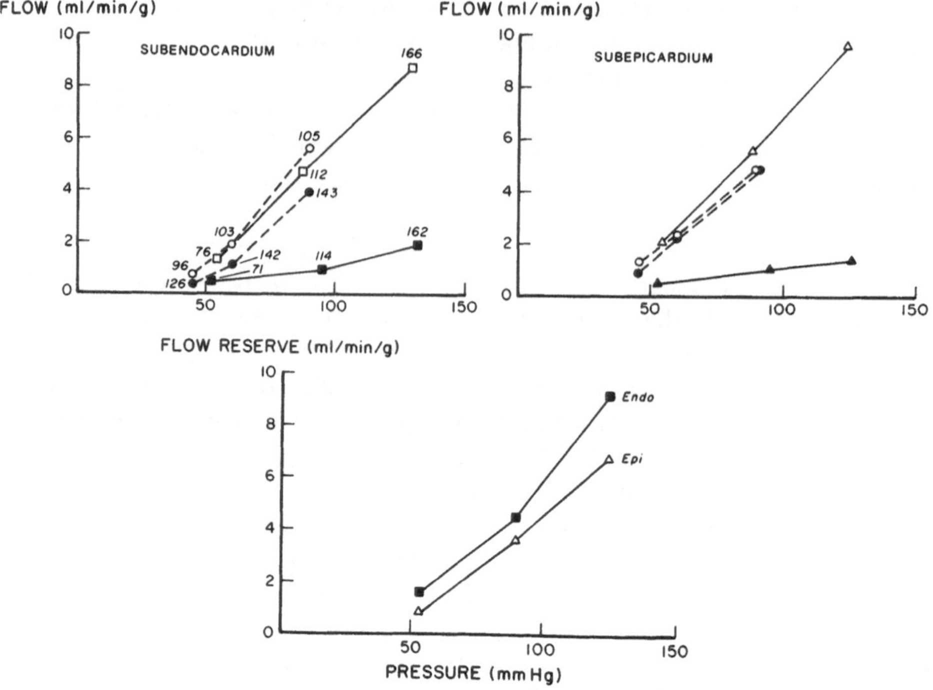

Figure 1. Upper panels: flow versus mean coronary perfusing pressure. Numbers opposite data points in left panel indicate left ventricular systolic pressure at which the measurements were made. These pressures are the same for the equivalent data points in the right panel. ○---○ Cannula study, maximally dilated vessels, normal aortic pressure. ●---● Cannula study, maximally dilated vessels, raised aortic pressure. □—□, △—△ No cannula, maximally dilated vessels. ■—■, ▲-▲ No cannula, autoregulating. *Lower panel:* flow reserve versus mean coronary perfusing pressure from non-cannula study.

However, in all these studies end-diastolic pressures of 2.7–6.7 kPa (20–50 mm Hg) with normal or sometimes with very low perfusion pressures had to be used before substantial decreases in subendocardial blood flow were observed. In our experiments the end-diastolic pressures were about 0.9–1.1 kPa (7–8 mm Hg) in the control state and rose to only 1.3–1.6 kPa (10–12 mm Hg) at the higher aortic pressures; these small changes seem unlikely to be able to cause the marked decreases in subendocardial flow that we observed. Therefore we are left with having to consider whether an increase in systolic wall stress can explain the decreased subendocardial flow.

Previously we have hypothesized that during systole the higher systolic intramyocardial pressure in the subendocardium causes more blood to move out of the subendocardial vessels than out of the subepicardial vessels in systole [16]. Consequently at the beginning of the next diastole the subendocardial vessels are narrower and have a higher resistance to reflow than have the subepicardial vessels. This would lead to a distribution of time constants across the wall that

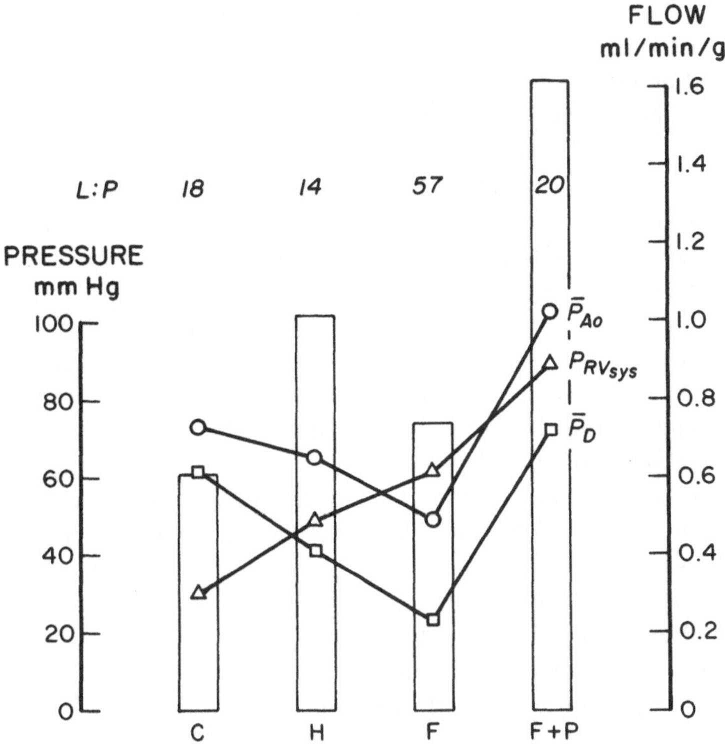

Figure 2. Effects of pulmonary arterial banding on mean aortic pressure ($\bar{P}Ao$), right ventricular systolic pressure (P_{RVsys}), mean pressure difference between aortic and right ventricular pressures ($\bar{P}_D$) and right ventricular myocardial blood flow (open rectangles). The lactate:pyruvate ratios (L:P) are placed above each set of measurements. C = control with normal pressures, H = moderate right ventricular systolic hypertension, F = tighter pulmonary band causing severe right ventricular systolic hypertension and right ventricular failure, F + P = elevation of aortic pressure without loosening pulmonary band. Data taken from Vlahakes et al., Circulation, 63: 87–95, 1981.

would favor flow into the subepicardium. It is possible that higher than normal wall stresses in systole exaggerate this effect and thereby reduce subendocardial flow.

An example of the effects of wall stress that has probable clinical importance is based on studies of acute right ventricular hypertension [17]. For many years it has been known that in experimental animals banding the pulmonary artery causes severe right heart failure long before systemic pressures are attained in the right ventricle. Similar findings have been reported soon after massive pulmonary embolism in humans, in whom pulmonary arterial pressures above 5.3 kPa (40 mm Hg) mean or 6.7 kPa (50 mm Hg) systolic are seldom found [18–22]. Vlahakes et al. [17] proved that the right ventricular failure was associated with ischemia of the right ventricular wall and that it could be reversed without relieving the pulmonary arterial obstruction by raising aortic pressure and thereby increasing right ventricular myocardial blood flow. The mechanism underlying these changes is that with the increased afterload the right ventricle dilates and can at first maintain an output by the Frank-Starling mechanisms. As the heart dilates more and the systolic pressures in the right ventricular wall increase further, not only is the gradient of pressure from aorta to right ventricle reduced but the increased wall stress an additional impediment to myocardial blood flow. This can be inferred because the flow in the right ventricular wall decreases at an aortic to intramyocardial pressure gradient that would still allow adequate flow in the normal left ventricular wall. That is, the decrease in pressure gradient is not enough by itself to prevent an adequate flow from occurring. Once a sufficient pressure gradient is provided by increasing aortic pressure, myocardial flows increase and right ventricular function return to normal (Figure 2).

These findings on the effect of wall stress thus produce some new data that can be used for testing existing models of the coronary circulation. As part of the test, the model would have to allow an effect that is maximal on subendocardial flow and absent on subepicardial flow. They also give some directions for pursuing studies of coronary vascular reserve that can be applied to humans, particularly because animal studies with cannulas in the left coronary artery have limited relevance to humans and because the effects of an acute rise in aortic pressure might be exaggerated in ventricles that are already dilated, have an abnormal compliance, or are without the external support provided by the pericardium.

Acknowledgment

This study was supported in part by Program Project Grant 24857 from the United States Public Health Service and grant 85-N18 from the Central Valley and Long Beach Chapters of the California Affiliate of the American Heart Association (Dr Mori).

References

1. Hoffman JIE (1984): Maximal coronary flow and the concept of coronary vascular reserve. Circulation 70: 153–159.
2. Hoffman JIE (1986): A critical review of coronary reserve. Circulation. In press.
3. Hoffman JIE (1986): Transmural myocardial perfusion. Prog Cardiovasc Dis. In press.
4. Gold FL, Bache RJ (1982): Transmural right ventricular blood flow during acute pulmonary artery hypertension in the awake dog: Evidence for subendocardial ischemia during right ventricular failure despite residual vasodilator reserve. Circ Res 51: 196–204.
5. Aversano T, Becker LC (1985): Persistence of coronary vasodilator reserve despite functionally significant flow reduction. Am J Physiol 248: H403–H411.
6. Pantely GA, Bristow JD, Swenson LJ, Ladley HD, Johnson WB, Anselone CG (1985): Incomplete coronary vasodilation during myocardial ischemia in swine. Am J Physiol 249: H638–H647.

7. Grattan MT, Hanley FL, Stevens MB, Hoffman JIE (1986): Transmural coronary flow reserve patterns in dogs. Am J Physiol. In press.
8. Buckberg GD, Fixler DE, Archié JP, Hoffman JIE (1972): Experimental subendocardial ischemia in dogs with normal coronary arteries. Circ Res 30: 67–81.
9. Boatwright RB, Downey HF, Bashour FA, Crystal GJ (1980): Transmural variation in autoregulation of coronary blood flow in hyperperfused canine myocardium. Circ Res 47: 599–609.
10. Domenech RJ (1978): Regional diatolic coronary blood flow during diastolic ventricular hypertension. Cardiovasc Res 12: 639–645.
11. Kjekshus JK (1973): Mechanism for flow distribution in normal and ischemic myocardium during increased ventricular preload in the dog. Circ Res 33: 489–499.
12. Dunn RB, Griggs DM Jr (1983): Ventricular filling pressure as a determinant of coronary blood flow during ischemia. Am J Physiol 244: H429–H436.
13. Cutarelli R, Levy MN (1963): Intraventricular pressure and the distribution of coronary blood flow. Circ Res 12: 322–327.
14. Hottenrott C, Buckberg G (1974): Studies of the effects of ventricular fibrillation on the adequacy of regional myocardial flow. II. Effects of ventricular distension. J Thorac Cardiovasc Surg 68: 626–633.
15. Downey J (1976): Compression of the coronary arteries by the fibrillating canine heart. Circ Res 39: 53–57.
16. Hoffman JIE, Baer RW, Hanley FL, Messina LM, Grattan MT (1985): Regulation of transmural myocardial blood flow. J Biomech Eng 107: 2–9.
17. Vlahakes GJ, Turley K, Hoffman JIE (1981): The pathophysiology of failure in acute right ventricular hypertension. Hemodynamic correlations. Circulation 63: 87–95.
18. Dalen JE, Banas JS Jr, Brooks HL, Evans GL, Paraskos JA, Dexter L (1969): Resolution rate of acute pulmonary embolism in man. New Engl J Med 280: 1194–1199.
19. Miller GAB, Sutton GC (1970): Acute massive pulmonary embolism. Clinical and haemodynamic findings in 23 patients studied by cardiac catheterisation and pulmonary arteriography. Br Heart J 32: 518–523.
20. McIntyre KM, Sasahara AA (1971): The hemodynamic response to pulmonary embolism in patients without prior cardiopulmonary disease. Am J Cardiol 28: 288–294.
21. Stanek V, Riedel M, Widimsky J (1978): Hemodynamic monitoring in acute pulmonary embolism. Bull Eur Physiopath Resp 14: 561–572.
22. Mangano DT (1980): Immediate hemodynamic and pulmonary changes following pulmonary thromboembolism. Anesthesiology 52: 173–175.

Discussion

Marcus: Do you think that the effect of right ventricular pressure on perfusion may be related to adrenergic vasoconstriction and that this may be different from what you see in the left ventricle?
Hoffman: Sure. This is another possible difference, but I don't know if it is enough to explain the findings.
Bassingthwaighte: Could you comment on the loading of the myocardium with water as you increase the intervascular intercapillary pressure. This is very evident in isolated perfused hearts. You quickly flood them with water when you raise the perfusion pressure in the rabbit even up to 100 mm Hg. Do you think that these hearts get loaded with water and that there is an increased edema even prior to the metabolic imbalance?
Hoffman: This is very unlikely.
Gallagher: There are at least two studies that suggest that right ventricular flow is not autoregulated. Could this be a factor in your studies?
Hoffman: To my mind, there have been no good studies of this in a preparation which has been shown to have left coronary autoregulation.
Sonnenblick: I wonder how much of the effects of the pressure may be due to the prolongation of diastole into the systole and spoiling some of the easy recoils that take place due to prolongation of contraction. In other words, is there a heart rate effect that you would see and will it be manifest also as pressure in the rate of relaxation?
Hoffman: This is a possible cause that we are now investigating.

28. Experimental validation studies related to clinical applications of cine computed tomography

M.L. MARCUS, J.A. RUMBERGER, S.J. REITER, A.J. FEIRING, D.J. SKORTON, S.M. COLLINS and W. STANFORD

Abstract

Cine computed tomography is a relatively new research/diagnostic technique that allows for high speed (50 millisecond) images of the heart following injection of intravenous contrast media. Recent validation studies in dogs have demonstrated that global and regional left and right ventricular geometry and function can be accurately assessed with cine computed tomography. For example, left ventricular mass can be measured with an accuracy of ± 3–4 g, right ventricular stroke volumes ± 2–3 ml and aortic regurgitant volume ± 1–3 ml. Also, vein bypass patency can be defined with about 90% accuracy. Two approaches to estimating changes in myocardial blood flow are actively under investigation. Studies in animals indicate that changes in bypass graft flow reserve can be accurately measured with cine computed tomography. Furthermore, preliminary animal studies suggest that changes in left ventricular perfusion can also be defined with this technology. Thus, cine computed tomography promises to become an important research technique and a valuable clinical approach to the diagnostic evaluation of patients with cardiac disease.

Introduction

Projection cardiac imaging techniques such as contrast ventriculography, planar radionuclide ventriculograms, and digital subtraction angiographic techniques are beset by many limitations. These include limited ability to define the anatomy of the left ventricular wall, relatively crude ability to analyze regional ventricular function, difficulties in precise quantitative analysis of volume and mass of cardiac chambers and problems with separation of superimposed cardiac structures. The improved spatial resolution of tomographic imaging techniques allows one to overcome these deficiencies.

At present there are five cardiac imaging techniques that provide tomographic pictures of the heart: single photon emission computed tomography, positron emission tomography, two-dimensional echocardiography, nuclear magnetic resonance, and cine computed tomography. The resolution of current single photon emission tomograpohic and positron image tomographic systems is in the range of 5–15 mm. Two-dimensional echocardiographic images of the heart can only be obtained in a few cross-sectional planes because of a limited acoustic window in many patients with coronary disease. Moreover, it is difficult to maintain anatomic registration of these images. Cine computed tomography and nuclear magnetic resonance provide high spatial resolution (0.5–2 mm) tomographic images that allow superb definition of cardiac structure and almost an unlimited number of registered tomographic images. At present only with CT is possible to obtain high temporal resolution (50 msec/frame) tomographic images of the heart with superb anatomic detail. Cine computed tomography, positron emission tomography and nuclear magnetic resonance may permit measurements of intravascular blood volume and myocardial perfusion. In this regard preliminary studies with cine computed tomography and positron emission tomography are particularly encouraging.

This review will briefly summarize our recent validation studies related to cine computed tomography.

Methods and protocols

The cine computed tomographic unit utilized in our studies is manufactured by Imatron® [C-100]. Magnetic deflection and focusing of an electron beam results in the rapid activation one of four semicircular tungsten targets that surround the object being scanned and produce dual level tomographic scans in 50 msec (17 frames/sec because there is an 8 msec interscan delay). As many as 80 scans in rapid sequence can be taken during a single contrast injection. Multislice tomographic images can also be obtained yielding as many as eight tomographic sections through the myocardium from base to apex in 224 msec. Tomographic scan thicknesses are approximately 0.8 cm with an average interscan distance of 0.2 cm.

The cine computed tomographic device operates in two modes. One mode, referred to as the 'flow mode', employs electrocardiographic triggering at a designated time during each cardiac cycle. During each scan acquisition two contiguous 8 mm thick tomographic scans are obtained. As many as 40 serial triggered stop action scans can be obtained at two contiguous scanning levels. Additional levels can also be scanned with up to 8 tomographic levels scanned at various times during the cardiac cycle. Subsequent data analysis of contrast wash in and wash out within computer generated cardiac regions of interest can be made. In the 'cine mode' dual or multislice tomographic sections can be obtained throughout an entire cardiac cycle at up to 17 frames per second. This allows for recording of contraction sequences during individual cardiac cycles.

During scan acquisition a non-ionic contrast medium, Iohexol, is infused intravenously with a computer controlled power injector. A typical scan sequence requires between 0.3 and 0.6 ml of contrast/kg body weight. The rate and volume of contrast injection must be adjusted to maximize opacification of the structure being imaged. In general,, flow studies employ rapid bolus injections (1–4 sec) of contrast media whereas cine mode studies require 10–20 sec contrast infusion to insure that both righ and left ventricular cardiac chambers are opacified during scan acquisition.

The cine computed tomograms are analyzed off-line. Time density curves from specific regions of interest can be generated to provide the raw data needed to calculate vein bypass flow rates or assessments of regional myocardial perfusion. The endocardial and epicardial borders of the cardiac chambers are defined with an operator interactive computer assisted program [1]. Cardiac chamber volumes and left ventricular mass are calculated utilizing a modified Simpson's rule.

Results

Left ventricular mass

In closed chest dogs, end-diastolic cine computed tomographic images obtained following intravenous contrast infusion have been analyzed to assess left ventricular mass [1]. With this approach, left ventricular mass can be measured with a high degree of accuracy and precision (Figure 1). Also, inter-observer variability for analysis of the images yielded a high degree of concordance (Figure 2). Furthermore, repeated measurements of left ventricular mass in the same animal, studied under varying hemodynamic conditions, demonstrated that the measurements of left ventricular mass were remarkably similar (Figure 3).

Left and right ventricular stroke volumes

Comparisons between left ventricular stroke volume measured with cine CT versus left ventricular stroke volume determined with either a chronically implanted electromagnetic ascending aortic flow probe or multiple measurements of thermodilution cardiac output (divided by heart rate) have shown that absolute left ventricular stroke volume can be measured to within 2–3 ml with cine computed tomography [2]. Similar results were obtained comparing right ventricular stroke volume measurements with cine computed tomography versus thermodilution cardiac output divided by heart rate [2]. Also, during 10–15 sec of suspended respiration, in anesthetized dogs the difference between right and left ventricular stroke volume was less than 2 ml [2, 3].

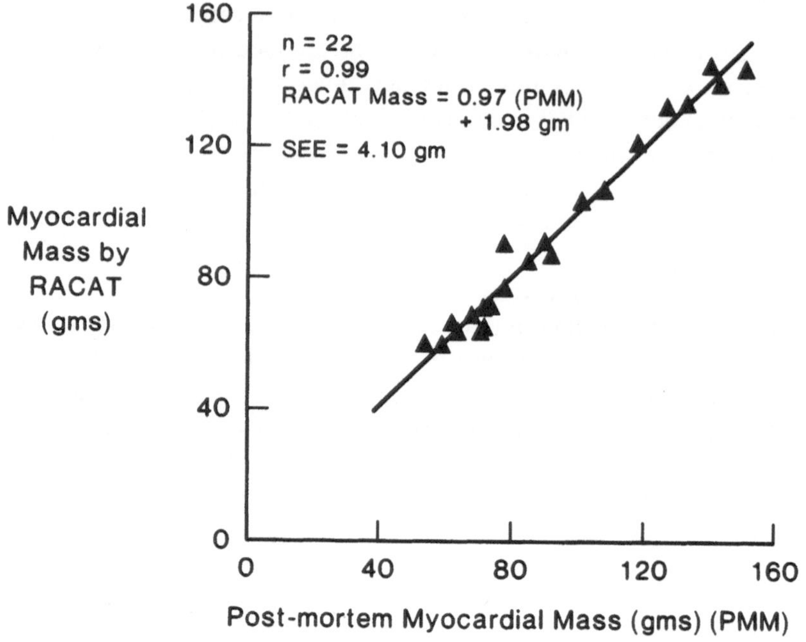

Figure 1. Relationship between RACAT (Rapid Acquisition Computer Axial Tomography) or cine computed tomography and postmortem left ventricular mass in dogs. The regression equation slope (0.97) and y intercept (1.98%) are not significantly different from 1.0 and 0.0, respectively. Standard error of the estimate is 4.1g. This figure is reprinted with permission from the American Heart Association, Inc. [1].

Aortic regurgitant volume

Because left and right ventricular stroke volumes are nearly identical under control conditions, in the setting of aortic regurgitation, the difference between left and right ventricular stroke volumes reflects the volume of aortic regurgitation. To test this hypothesis directly, aortic regurgitation was produced with a basket catheter in dogs. Aortic regurgitant volume was measured with a chronically implanted electromagnetic flow probe on the proximal aorta and compared with measurements of regurgitant volume obtained with cine computed tomography [3]. These studies demonstrated that with cine computed tomography the absolute volume of aortic regurgitation over a broad range could be assessed to within 2–3 ml/cardiac cycle.

Regional left ventricular function

Studies of segmental endocardial contraction of the left ventricle in dogs and

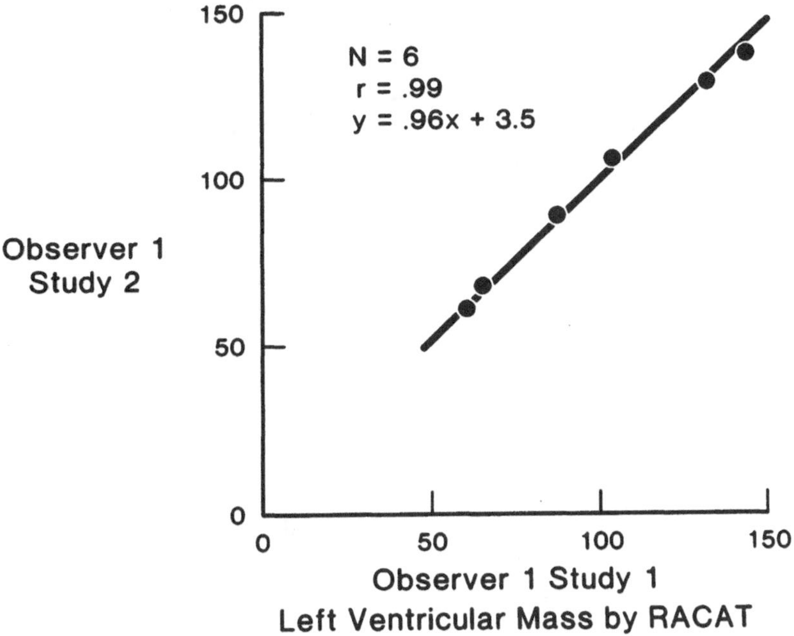

Figure 2. Intraobserver variability in determinations of left ventricular mass from six representative dogs with masses ranging from 50 to 150 g. This figure is reprinted with permission from the American Heart Association, Inc. [1].

normal patients with cine computed tomography employing either an endocardial or epicardial centroid have demonstrated considerable homogeneity of contraction [4]. In contrast, circumferential left ventricular wall thickness measurements in normal subjects with cine computed tomography have been strikingly heterogeneous [5]. It is likely that the marked heterogeneity of left ventricular wall thickening observed with cine computed tomography occurs because of the complex nature of three-dimensional cardiac contraction resulting in technical difficulties when any tomographic imaging technique is employed to analyze wall thickening. Cine computed tomographic images are obtained at a fixed point in space throughout the cardiac cycle. However, because of apex to base accordion-like motion, torsion and rotation the left ventricular chamber moves through the scan plane of a given computed tomographic slice during a single cardiac cycle. Consequently, the left ventricular wall images obtained at end-systole and end-diastole are not of the same segment of the left ventricle. In our opinion this contributes substantially to the heterogeneity of left ventricular wall thickening observed with cine computed tomography. This problem is not seen when segmental area contraction of the left ventricle is analyzed. The problem related to the evaluation of wall thickening may be resolved in the future by either true volume imaging which would require a major hardware modification or three-

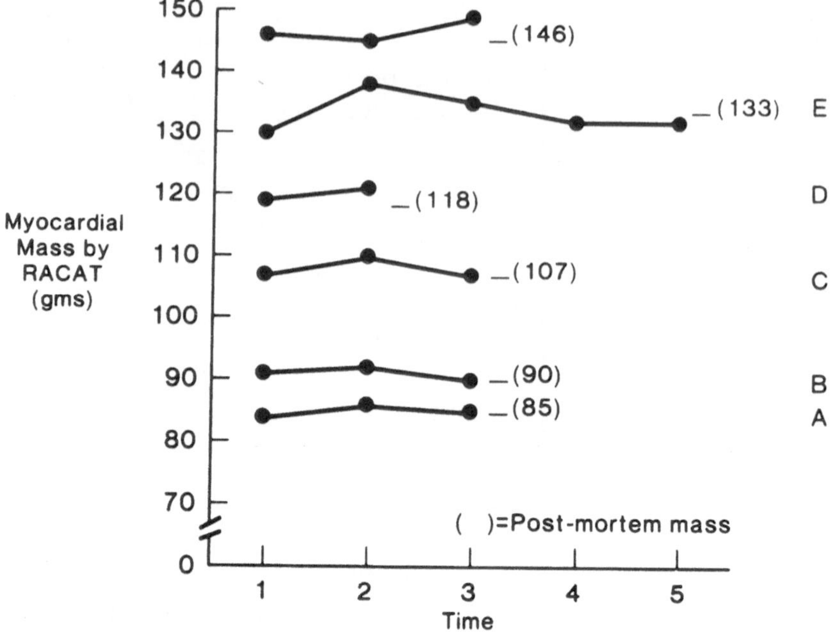

Figure 3. Reproducibility of scans and determinations of left ventricular mass in each of six animals. Each dog was rescanned between two to six times. The second point on each line (A to E) represents animals that were scanned at a 40° angle clockwise to the usual short-axis orientation. This figure reprinted with permission from the American Heart Association, Inc. [1].

dimensional reconstruction and retrospective computation of computed tomographic slices that can account for the complexities of left ventricular translational motion.

Vein bypass grafts

Several clinical studies indicate that the patency of vein bypass grafts and internal mammary artery implants can be measured with about 90% accuracy with cine computed tomography [6]. In addition, preliminary attempts to define absolute graft flow rates and graft flow reserve with cine computed tomography are encouraging [6, 7]. In dogs, changes in bypass graft flow velocity measured with an implanted Doppler probe correlate highly ($r = 0.85$) with changes in graft flow measured with cine computed tomography.

Left ventricular perfusion

Changes in left ventricular perfusion measured with labelled microspheres in dogs have been compared to data obtained with cine computed tomography. Although the reported correlations are in the range of r = 0.7–0.9 [8, 9], the standard error of the estimates is substantial and cine computed tomography significantly underestimates changes in perfusion. Spatially heterogeneous imaging artifacts are likely the cause of the significant standard errors. Attempts to substantially reduce or properly account for these artifacts through hardware and software modifications are currently under evaluation.

Conclusions

The primary conclusions that can be made from the data presented are as follows:
1. experimental studies in dogs indicate that with cine computed tomography global and regional left and right ventricular function, left ventricular mass and aortic regurgitant volume can be measured precisely;
2. vein bypass patency and bypass flow reserve can be measured accurately with cine computed tomography; and
3. at present, the ability of cine computed tomography to measure changes in left ventricular perfusion is limited.

Although the animal validation studies are encouraging, it is of great importance to extend these investigations to the clinical arena. Furthermore, it will be important to employ this powerful research modality to pursue important physiological and pathophysiological questions.

Many research questions which were heretofore difficult to pursue, particularly in humans, can now be investigated with cine computed tomography. For example, the rates of progression and regression of left ventricular hypertrophy in various pathological states can now be examined and the factors responsible for modulating the progression and regression of ventricular hypertrophy can be elucidated. Also, the three-dimensional motion of various cardiac structures such as the ventricular septum can be examined in great detail. Lastly, as the ability of cine computed tomography to measure the transmural distribution of myocardial perfusion improves, it may finally be possible to study transmural myocardial perfusion in humans. Such studies will almost certainly improve our understanding of the regulation of the coronary circulation in humans in normal and pathological states.

Acknowledgment

The original studies reviewed in this chapter were supported by the following grants: Ischemic SCOR (HL 32295), Clinician Scientist Awards to John A. Rumberger and Andrew J. Feiring, a National Institutes of Health Career Development Award (KO4 HL 01290) to David J. Skorton, and support from Imatron, Inc.

References

1. Feiring AJ, Rumberger JA, Skorton DJ, Collins SM, Higgins CB, Lipton MJ, Ell S, Marcus ML (1985): Determination of left ventricular mass in the dog with rapid acquisition cardiac CT scanning. Circulation 72: 1355.
2. Reiter SJ, Rumberger JA, Feiring AJ, Ell SR, Stanford W, Marcus ML (1985): Precise determination of left and right ventricular stroke volume with cine computed tomography. Circulation 72: II-719.
3. Reiter SJ, Rumberger JA, Feiring AJ, Stanford W, Marcus ML (1986): Measurement of aortic regurgitation with cine CT. J Am Coll Cardiol 7(2): 155A.
4. Rumberger JA, Feiring AJ, Skorton DJ, Collins SM, Ell SR, Higgins CB, Lipton MJ, Marcus ML (1984): Spatial uniformity of endocardial wall motion as demonstrated by rapid acquisition computed tomography. Circulation 70: II-169.
5. Feiring AJ, Rumberger JA, Collins SM, Skorton DJ, Noel MP, Reiter SJ, Stanford W, Marcus ML (1986): Regional ventricular function with cine CT. J Am Coll Cardiol 7(2): 44A.
6. Bateman TM, Whiting JS, Forrester JS, Aronson AL, Schauer MS, Gray RJ, Matloff JM, Berman DS, Swan HJC (1986): Noninvasive evaluation of aorto-coronary bypass grafts using cine-CT. J Am Coll Cardiol 7(2): 154A.
7. Rumberger JA, Feiring AJ, Hiratzka LE, Reiter SJ, Stanford W, Marcus ML (1986): Determination of changes in coronary bypass graft flow rate using cine-CT. J Am Coll Cardiol 7(2): 155A.
8. Rumberger JA, Feiring AJ, Lipton MJ, Higgins CB, Marcus ML (1985): Measurement of myocardial perfusion by ultrafast CT. J Am Coll Cardiol 5(2): 500.
9. Ferguson JL, Chomka E, Wolfkiel C, Law WR, Brundage B (1985): Meaurement of regional myocardial perfusion by computed tomographic assessment of contrast medium washout. Fed Proc 44(3): 821.

Discussion

Dinnar: Have you noticed any changes in diameter, or tapering, of coronay bypass grafts with time?
Marcus: It has been known for a long time that coronary bypass grafts are larger in the early post-operative period than at a later time. Whenever they ask us to perform a cine CT study in a patient who is one week post-operative, it is always an easy study because the vein grafts are very large at this point in time. Other groups have done serial studies in these patients and there is significant narrowing of the grafts with time.
Dinnar: In estimating graft flow reserve, what do you intend to use as a basis for prognostic evaluation?
Marcus: It would be helpful if we knew the flow reserve in the graft in the early post-operative period and use this as a basis for future prognostic evaluation. If, for example, we knew that two weeks after operation the bypass graft could deliver five times basal flow to the area it was perfusing at a given perfusion pressure and that two years down the road it could only increase flow to that region by only about 1.5 fold, this would indicate a tremendous deterioration. I think that serial studies of flow reserve in patients with coronary bypass grafts or implanted internal mammary arteries performed with cine CT will turn out to be very helpful.
Spaan: How can you distinguish between the reserve limitation of the microcirculation and the reserve of the bypass graft conduit by itself?
Marcus: With the cine CT evaluation of vein bypass graft flow reserve we cannot distinguish between the microcirculation and the conduit. However, if we study a patient and the bypass grafts are fine, that is to say that flow reserve is excellent, it does not make any difference. If flow reserve in one of the grafts is seriously decreased, we would have to do angiogram to determine if this was due to distal downstream disease or to a stenosis someplace in the bypass graft.
Sideman: Do you take advantage of the dynamics of your CT?
Marcus: With our present CT instrument we can obtain 17 frames/cardiac cycle. That could provide substantial dynamic information about cardiac function. At the present time, we have focused our analysis primarily on end-systolic and end-diastolic images. In the future with more automated analysis of the tomographic data, it will be possible to obtaine detailed studies of three-dimensional systolic and diastolic function of the entire ventricle throughout the cardiac cycle at relatively frequent intervals.
Lab: What is the relationship between bypass graft flow and regional function? Does regional function vary as the graft is stenosed with time?
Marcus: I would expect it to behave like a coronary stenosis. That is to say, a moderate graft stenosis will impair exercise ventricular function and a severe stenosis might impair resting ventricular function. I imagine that this could eventually be demonstrated with cine CT.

Dysfunction of the diseased ventricle: mechanical and metabolic aspects

29. Regional ventricular function in myocardial ischemia

J.K.-J. LI

Abstract

The time dependence of ischemia and reperfusion and the mechanism of ischemia precipitated pulsus alternans are not clear. In addition, the assessment and improvement of regional ventricular function need to be established. To investigate these, experiments were performed on open-chest anesthetized dogs. Central and peripheral arterial pressures, aortic flow, electrocardiogram and endocardial segment lengths in normal and ischemic zones were measured during 15 minutes of coronary artery ligation and during reperfusion. Results show different time courses of occlusion and reperfusion. Pressure-segment length loops are useful representations of regional ventricular function during control, digitalis, coronary artery ligation and propranolol, and parallel force-length relations in the isovolumic contraction and relaxation phases. The constant end-diastolic lengths in strong and weak beats indicate that the alternating contractile state is the responsible mechanism for the occurrence of pulsus alternans.

Introduction

Myocardial ischemia is produced as a result of a decreased oxygen supply to tissues of the myocardium. It is associated with a reduction in coronary arterial blood flow. The branching characteristics of the coronary arterial tree suggests that ischemia is predominantly regional. Failure in global ventricular function however, often results from such prolonged initial regional abnormalities. Regional dysfunction of the myocardium is frequently masked in the assessment of ventricular pump performance.

In assessing regional ventricular function, investigators have tackled the problem from a geometric perspective. Longitudinally, occlusion of a coronary artery produces three zones: the normal, the border ischemic and the central ischemic [1, 2]. Transversely, ischemia affects differentially the subepicardial and the subendocardial layers of the myocardium [3]. Transmural wall thickness changes have also been observed [4, 5]. The complexity of the structure and function of the myocardium is apparent, although it is often modelled globally as a thin-walled or thick-walled, sphere or ellipsoid.

This paper approaches myocardial ischemia from a broad perspective. It examines the time dependence of ischemia and reperfusion, the mechanism of ischemia precipitated pulsus alternans and the assessment and improvement of regional ventricular function during ischemia.

Methods

Healthy mongrel dogs of either sex with body weights of 20–24 kg were used for the experiments. In each, the dog was anesthetized with intravenous Nembutal (25 mg/kg). Electrocardiogram was established and continuously monitored. Respiration was maintained with a positive pressure respirator (Harvard Apparatus) after tracheal intubation. Chest was open via a left thoracotomy at the fifth intercostal space. The heart was supported in a pericardium cradle for ease of instrumentation. Left ventricular pressure was measured through the apex with a catheter-tip transducer (Millar PC-350). Aortic pressure was measured by another catheter-tip transducer introduced through the left femoral artery. In some dogs, the right femoral pressure was also recorded with a catheter (30 cm; 2 mm i.d.)-manometer (P23 ID) system. An electromagnetic probe was cuffed around the isolated section of the ascending aorta to measure flow. The signal was obtained by a flowmeter (Biotronex BL-610) and lowpass filtered at 50 Hz. Pairs of ultrasonic dimension gages (LZT, 5 MHz) were placed through stub wounds in the endocardial layers to measure segmental contraction along the circumferential direction of the short axis. Transit time detection allows distance to be quantified by the Schuessler Dimensioning System.

Left anterior descending coronary artery was isolated distal to the first major branching. Segment lengths were measured in the normal and in the central ischemic zones. Regional myocardial ischemia was imposed for 15 min and reperfused for an equal period. Ventricular and arterial hemodynamic parameters were collected at 5, 10 and 15 min during occlusion and after reperfusion. Regional ventricular function was assessed by segmental shortening and end-systolic and end-diastolic pressure-length relations. Pressure-length loops were also constructed. To assess the usefulness and limitations of pressure-length loops in characterizing the intrinsic properties of the myocardium, the following experiments were performed: digitalis bolus infusion (1 μg/kg), brief occlusion (10 sec) of the descending thoracic aorta and propranolol (1 mg/kg) infusion. To examine force-length and pressure-length relationship, isometric tension gages were sutured to the deep layers adjacent to segment lengths measurements.

Dogs which exhibited pulsus alternans after induction of coronary artery

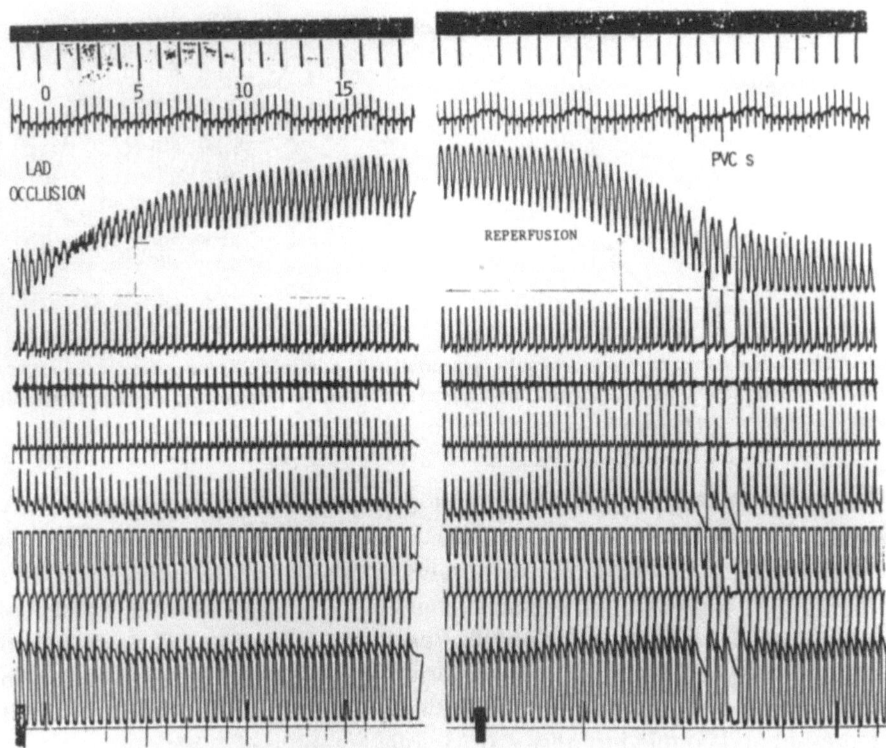

Figure 1. Simultaneously measured hemodynamic parameters at the onset of occlusion of the left anterior descending coronary artery (left) and during reperfusion (right) after 15 minutes of occlusion. Time marks in seconds. Tracings from top: Electrocardiogram (ECG), ischemic zone segment length (LI), ascending aortic flow (AOQ), flow acceleration (dQ/dt), femoral arterial pressure derivative (FA dp/dt), femoral pressure (FAP), left ventricular end-diastolic pressure (LVEDP), first derivative of left ventricular pressure (LV dp/dt), aortic pressure (AOP) and left ventricular pressure (LVP).

occlusion were grouped to determine the responsible mechanism, i.e. the Frank-Starling mechanism or the alternating contractile state theory.

Results

Figure 1 shows simultaneously measured hemodynamic parameters during control, coronary occlusion and reperfusion. It is clear that segment length in the ischemic region is the most sensitive parameter at the onset of ischemia. Global measurements of pressures and flow are much less sensitive. Left ventricular end diastolic pressure (LVEDP) increased, indicating the utilization of the Frank-Starling mechanism. Negative dp/dt_{max} is sharply reduced. Preload compensation and slowed ventricular relaxation are apparent. Ischemic segment length increased, both end-systolic and end-diastolic, more rapidly during the first 5 sec,

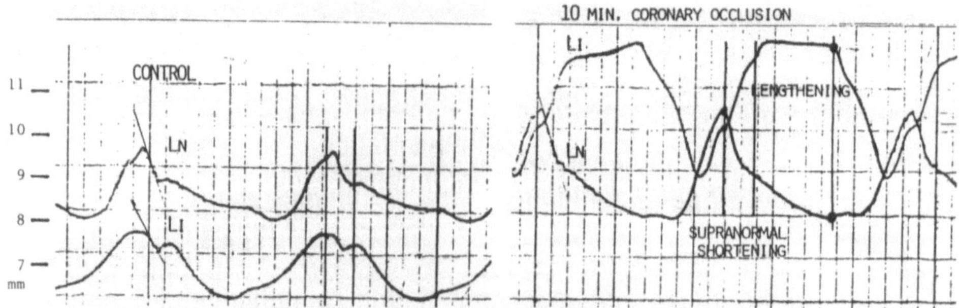

Figure 2. Endocardial muscle segment lengths measured in the normal (LN) and ischemic (LI zones at control (left) and after 10 minutes of coronary artery occlusion. Isovolumic and ejection phases are identified by heavy vertical lines.

gradually thereafter. Peripheral femoral arterial pressure decreased slightly, following ventricular and aortic pressures. Femoral negative dp/dt however, did not follow −LV dp/dt since the aortic valve is closed and the arterial system is decoupled from the ventricle. Segment length morphology following reperfusion differed from that following the onset of occlusion. Negative LV dp/dt did not return to control as rapidly after reperfusion as it decreased during occlusion. LVEDP returned to about control level. Premature ventricular contraction beats were present and coupled to post-extrasystolic potentiated beats.

Figure 2 shows the normal zone (L_N) and ischemic zone (L_I) segment lengths measured during control and at 10 min post occlusion. The hyperactivity i.e. supranormal shortening in the normal segment and the passive lengthening in the ischemic segment during the isovolumic phase are evident. Notice also the akinetic motion of the ischemic segment during the ejection phase. The time courses of indices of diastolic compliance (EDL/EDP) and regional contractility (ESP/ESL are shown in Fig. 3.

Pressure-length loops constructed for control and various interventions are shown in Fig. 4. Loop area increased during digitalis ($p<.001$) and descending thoracic aorta occlusion ($p<.01$). In the former it is accompanied by an increased shortening and in the latter by a decreased shortening. Coronary ligation produced negative loop area (clockwise) with a negative shortening (lengthening). Propranolol reduced loop area, with a concurrent reduction in shortening. The P-L loop is shifted to the right with a reduction in ESP/ESL ratio, opposite to that observed for digitalis.

In coronary occlusion induced pulsus alternans (Fig. 5), the R-R intervals and end-diastolic lengths are constant, while end-systolic lengths alternates between strong and weak beats.

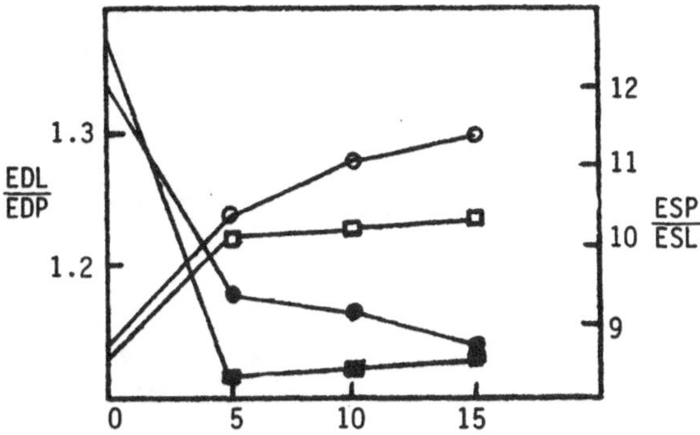

Figure 3. Regional contractility (ESP/ESL; circles; mm Hg/mm squares) and diastolic compliance (EDL/EDP; mm/mm Hg; circles) indices plotted as a function of time. Closed symbols: occlusion. Open symbols: reperfusion. Time in min.

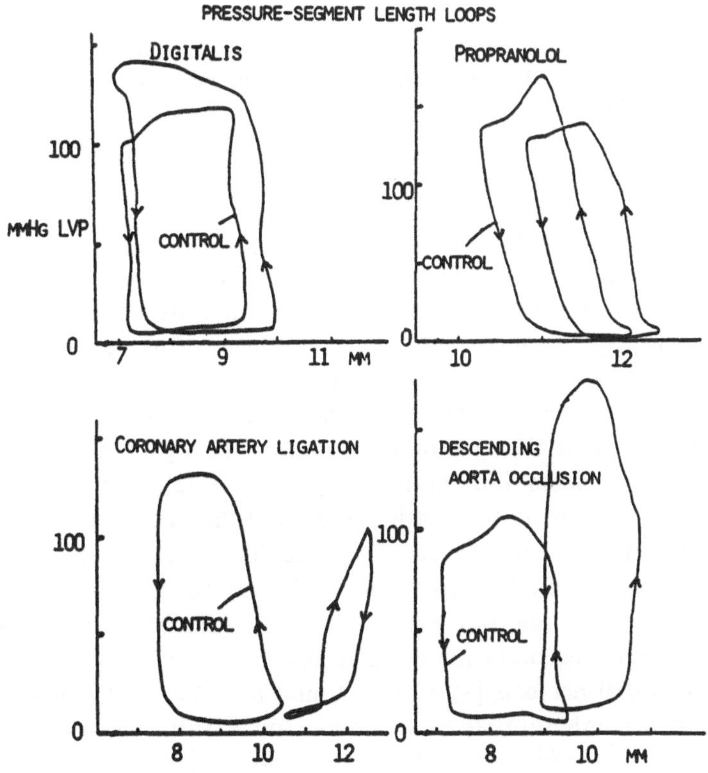

Figure 4. Left ventricular pressure-length loops. Interventions are compared to control.

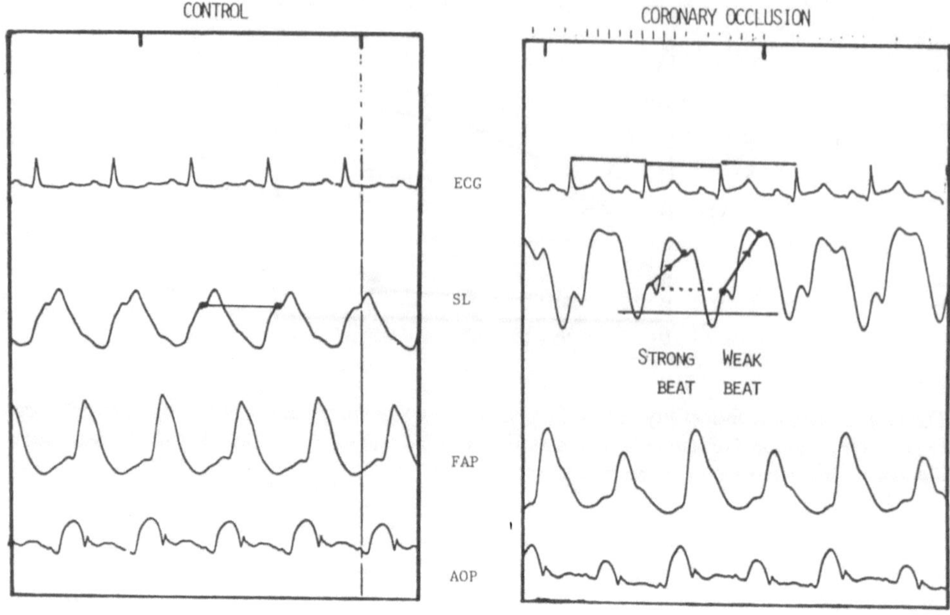

Figure 5. **Illustrating coronary artery occlusion induced pulsus alternans (right). End-diastolic lengths are constant (dotted line)., while end-systolic lengths alternate between strong and weak beats. Acronyms as identified in Fig. 1.**

Discussion

Regional ventricular response to acute occlusion of a coronary artery is characterized by paradoxical systolic bulging in the ischemic zone, as first observed half a century ago [6]. Differential mechanical responses of myocardial layers and zones defined by ischemia have been documented by studies of segment muscle contraction, wall thickness and blood flow measurements in these regions. These studies reported segmental lengthening, thinning of the myocardium and reduced myocardial oxygen consumption in the ischemic zone, reduced shortening, wall thickness and blood flow in the border zone, and the utilization of the Frank-Starling mechanism [7, 8] and increased systolic shortening and wall thickness in the normal zone. Such initial changes however, do not persist. Some investigators reported depressed systolic function and diastolic dilatation can persist progressively with repeated occlusion without histochemical or ultrastructural evidence of myocardial necrosis [9]. Others found that repeated ischemia caused cumulative histochemic injuries to the myocardium [10]. It is found here that although diastolic compliance has returned close to control, regional contractility remained somewhat depressed after15 minutes of reperfusion. The time courses of mechanical alteration during ischemia and reperfusion differ. It is not yet clear how the time course of hemodynamic parameters during reperfusion is correlated to the length of occlusion or the number of repeated occlusions. There are however, evidences that there is delayed metabolic resynthesis at the cellular level after even a brief period of reversible ischemia [11, 12].

Pressure-volume loop is also termed the 'work-loop', because it represents the external mechanical work generated during ventricular ejection. The similarity of pressure-length loop and pressure-volume loop has been recognized by several investigators. Thus, segment work was used and taken to represent mechanical performance of the local myocardium [13, 14]. It is shown here that the P-L loop is sensitive to regional changes in inotropic states, e.g. during digitalis and propranolol administration. Even in the case of coronary occlusion, the passive lengthening is reflected in the negative segment loop area. However, during descending thoracic aorta occlusion, afterload was greatly increased, the ventricle attemps to compensate by developing a higher pressure and increasing the end-diastolic length by the Starling mechanism. The effective shortening was nevertheless reduced, in a similar fashion seen in the force-length relation in cardiac muscle mechanics [15]. In this case,changes in segment work did not parallel changes in muscle shortening.

It must be cautioned however, that pressure length relation does not exact force-length relation. According to Laplace's law [16], pressure is linearly related to tension if the wall thickness to radius ratio stay constant. For the mammalian heart, pressure is only linearly proportional to force during the isovolumic contraction and relaxation phases (Fig. 6).

Two major mechanisms have been postulated to be responsible for the occurrence of pulsus alternans: the familiar Frank-Starling mechanism and the alternating contractile state theory. It is not uncommon to observe coronary artery occlusion precipitated pulsus alternans. It may exist in the normal, border or ischemic zones. The frequency is the highest in the ischemic zone, however. The constant end-diastolic lengths (Fig. 5) between strong and weak beats effectively eliminated the Frank-Starling mechanism as responsible. If alternating contractile state is the responsible mechanism and since ischemic segment length does not contract, the ischemic zone must still contain active contractile units which do not contribute to the overall shortening process, but resist lengthening. Consequently, a decreased end-systolic length is observed in the strong beat (Fig. 5), although no active shortening is present. Pulsus alternans is therefore a depressed ventricular regional phenomenon [17]

To improve the impaired ventricular function during myocardial ischemia, two general approaches have been taken: pharmacological intervention and mechanical assistance. The common aims are to unload the heart, to improve perfusion and myocardial oxygen supply/demand ratio. Some investigators have reported infarct size reduction with beta-blocker propranolol [18]. Others, however, do not attest to this finding [19] and suggest that beta-blocker may delay but not prevent ischemic cell death i.e. ischemia can be limited with propranolol only if

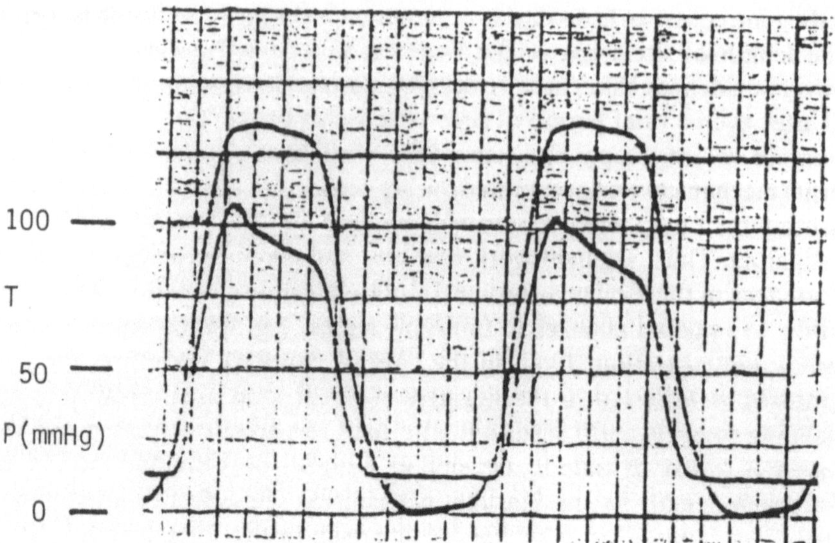

Figure 6. Simultaneously measured left ventricular chamber pressure and endocardial tension (arbitrary units). Notice the responses parallel each other only during isovolumic (contraction and relaxation) phases. The two differ markedly during the ejection phase.

occlusion is followed by *reperfusion* [20]. Mechanical assistance of the failing heart with intra-aortic balloon pump is common, particularly if ischemia is recurrent. It reduces systolic extra-vascular compression by reducing afterload. It also increases coronary perfusion through diastolic augmentation. Its beneficial effects, however, depend critically on proper timing of balloon inflation and deflation [21, 22]. Often there is a compromise to be made between increasing coronary perfusion and afterload reduction. This latter indicates the importance of incorporating analysis of the heart-arterial system interaction in the assessment and improvement of regional ventricular function during ischemia.

References

1. Theroux P, Ross J Jr, Franklin D, Covell JW, Bloor CM, Sasayama S (1977): Regional myocardial function and dimensions early and late after myocardial infarction in the unanesthetized dog. Circ Res 40: 158–165.
2. Yoran C, Sonnenblick EH, Kirk ES (1982): Contractile reserve and left ventricular function in regional myocardial ischemia in the dog. Circulation 66: 121.
3. Weintraub WS, Hattori S, Agarwal JB, Bodenheimer MM, Banka VS, Helfant RH (1981): Relationship between myocardial blood flow and contraction by myocardial layer in the canine left ventricle during ischemia. Circ Res 48: 430–438.
4. Sasayama S, Gallagher KP, Kemper WS, Franklin D, Ross J Jr (1981): Regional left ventricular wall thickness early and late after coronary occlusion in the conscious dog. Am J Physiol 240: H293–299.

5. Gallagher KP, Matsuzaki M, Koziol JA, Kemper WS, Ross J Jr (1984): Regional myocardial perfusion and wall thickening during ischemia in conscious dogs. Am J Psysiol 247: H727–738.
6. Tennant R, Wiggers CJ (1935): Effect of coronary occlusion on myocardial contraction. Am J Physiol 112: 351–361.
7. Braunwald E, Ross J Jr, Sonnenblick EH, (1976): Mechanisms of contractions of the normal and failing heart. Little Brown, Boston.
8. Lew WY, Ban-Hayashi E (1985): Mechanisms of improving regional and global ventricular function by preload alterations during acute ischemia in the canine left ventricle. Circulation 72: 1125–1134.
9. Nicklas JM, Becker LC, Bulkley BH (1985): Effects of repeated brief coronary occlusion on regional left ventricular function and dimension in dogs. Am J Cardiol 56: 473–478.
10. Geft IL, Fishbein MC, Ninomlya K, Hashida J, Chaux E, Yano J et al. (1982): Intermittent brief periods of ischemia have a cumulative effect and may cause myocardial necrosis. Circulation 66: 1150–1153.
11. Reimer KA, Hill ML, Jennings RB (1981): Prolonged depletion of ATP and of the adenine nucleotide pool due to delayed resynthesis of adenine nucleotides following reversible myocardial ischemia injury in dogs. J Mol Cell Cardiol 13: 229–239.
12. De Boer WWV, Ingwall JS, Kloner RA, Braunwald E (1980): Prolonged derangements of canine myocardial purine metabolism after a brief coronary artery occlusion not associated with anatomic evidence of necrosis. Proc Natl Acad Sci (USA) 77: 5471–5475.
13. Hood WB, Covelli VH, Abelman WH, Norman JC (1969): Persistence of contractile behavior in acutely ischemic myocardium. Cardiovasc Res 3: 249–255.
14. Tyberg JV, Forrester JS, Wyatt HL, Goldner SJ, Parmley WW, Swan HJC (1974): An analysis of segment ischemic dysfunction utilizing the pressure-length loop. Circulation 49: 748–754.
15. Brutsaert DL, Paulus WJ (1977): Loading performance of the heart as muscle and pump. Cardiovasc Res 11: 1–16.
16. Li JK-J (1986): Comparative cardiac mechanics: Laplace's law. J Theor Biol 118: 339–343.
17. Li JK-J (1982): Ventricular alternans: relative unimportance of the Starling mechanism. IRCS J Med Sci 10: 19.
18. Rasmussen MM, Reimer KA, Kloner RA, Jennings RB (1977): Infarct size reduction by propanolol before and after coronary ligation in dogs. Circulation 56: 794–798.
19. Peter T, Heng MK, Singh BN, Amber P, Nisbet H, Elliot R, Norris RM (1978): Failure of high doses of propranolol to reduce experimental myocardial ischemic damage. Circulation 57: 534–540.
20. Lange R, Nieminen MS, Kloner RA (1984): Failure of pindolol and metoprolol to reduce the size of non-reperfused infarcts in dogs using area at risk techniques. Cardiovasc Res 18: 37–43.
21. Li JK-J, Welkowitz W, Zelano J, Molony DA, Kostis JB, Mackenzie JW (1983): Effects of balloon inflation and deflation rates on global and regional ventricular performance. Progr Artif Organs 137–140.
22. Welkowitz W, Li JK-J (1984): Modelling and optimization of assisted circulation. IEEE Trans Biomed Eng BME-31: 899–902.

Discussion

Lab: You have said that the pressure-length loop is not identical to the force-length loop. Surely, the comparison is not a true one since you have to simulate a small section of isometric contraction before ejection. So, if you did the simulations carefully, you will be able to produce a force-length loop in a papillary muscle to look the same as a pressure-volume loop.
Li: I have measured the tension simultaneously with the pressure, but only in the isovolumic phase can one see the parallel relationship.
Sideman: What are the physical implications of the medication? Does it affect vasodilation or more oxygen extraction?
Wiess: Propranolol primarily reduces myocardial oxygen demand, though less in the ischemic zone. There it may help to redistribute oxygen supply and demand more efficatiously and potentially improve the efficiency of oxygen consumption there.
Beyar: I believe that when you give an adenergic drug you cause the shortening to increase, but, paradoxicaly, the end-diastolic length increases. This leads you to think that this is more of a preload effect than a contractility effect.
Li: Yes. The data actually indicates this phenomenon. However, propranolol is a β-adrenergic blocker. It decreases myocardial contractility and the pressure-length loop is shifted to the right.

30. Simulation of the mechanics of an infarcted left ventricle

M. PERL and A. HOROWITZ

Abstract

An immediate infarction occurring in a canine left ventricle at the beginning of the ejection phase is simulated, employing a recently developed comprehensive finite element model. The analysis assumes an instantaneous loss of contractility in the infarcted region, whereas the passive mechanical properties of the tissue are yet unaltered. The results indicate a progressive deterioration of the cardiac performance, as well as considerable geometrical changes in the kinematics of the whole ventricle, with increasing infarct size. Due to the reduction in the stroke volume, the simulation predicts a degradation of up to 33% in the ejection fraction for an infarct consisting of 43% of the myocardium volume. Furthermore, moderate bulging of the infarcted region is noticed as well as a decrease of the apex to base twist angle. At the border zone between the infarcted and the intact tissue high stress gradients develop while the stresses within the infarcted zone are considerably lower, as compared to the intact state.

Introduction

Various pathological conditions of the heart may often have direct expression in terms of its mechanical behavior. A pathology that may have a significant mechanical effect is ischemic heart disease, including the acute condition of infarction of the myocardium. The initial manifestation of an ischemic state is in the deterioration of contractility of the affected tissue, furthermore, histological changes may induce a considerable alteration of the passive mechanical properties of the myocardium.

The extension of mechanical models to the simulation of such pathological conditions is a direct option, once the models have been formulated and assessed for the normal state. Swan et al. [1] have employed a lumped two compartmental model in which they examined the effect of infarcts of various sizes on the left ventricle (LV) stroke volume and pressure-volume relations. Janz and Waldron [2], Yettram et al. [3] and Bogen et al. [4, 5] have implemented various finite element (FE) models in which they introduced infarcts of several sizes and material properties. Janz and Waldron [2] have simulated a stiffened apical aneurism using a two-dimensional axi-symmetric model. Yettram et al. [3] implemented a three-dimensional model in order to examine the effect of infarcts at various locations in LV walls of either increased or decreased stiffness, relatively to the intact tissue. Bogen et al. [4, 5], using a spherical membranous model, have simulated regions of reduced contractility in conjunction with altered inotropic conditions of the LV, in addition to various sizes of infarcts. All these models do not allow to account for the loss of contractility separately from the changes in the passive mechanical properties of the ischemic or infarcted tissue, since no active contraction of the LV can be simulated by them.

In the present work, the effects of infarcts of various sizes on the deformation, stress pattern and mechanical performance of the LV during the ejection phase are considered. Following a short description of the mechanical model and the simulation procedure, results regarding several infarcts are presented and discussed. Finally, prospects for future applications of the present model to pathological states involving changes in the mechanics of the LV are suggested.

The mechanical model

A comprehensive three dimensional model for the simulation of the LV mechanics has been recently suggested by Perl et al. [6, 7]. This model, which is based on the finite element method, is the sole one, simultaneously accounting for all the main parameters affecting the LV kinematics: the real irregular in vivo measured 3-D geometry of the ventricle, the anistropy of its walls, the large deformation it undergoes during the cardiac cycle, the material nonlinearity of the myocardium and the mechanical activation of the heart muscle. Unlike most existing models, the present model describes the entire cardiac cycle in a continuous manner, incorporating the active forces developing in the myocardial fibers, which play an important role throughout most of the cycle. Due to these particular characteristics, this model is notably suitable for simulating partial or total loss of contractility of any given portion of the ventricle as well as of regional changes in the myocardium passive properties. The main features of this model are hereafter presented, a more detailed description being given in [6, 7].

The LV geometry

The 3-D reconstruction of the LV is based on data provided by Ritman et al. [8], obtained by computerized tomography. This data is reduced into a finite element grid, consisting of two layers of 3-D isoparametric elements, arranged into eight stacks vertically, each consisting of 24 elements (Fig. 1). The total number of degrees of freedom in the resulting mesh is 1391.

The anisotropy of the LV wall

The direction-varying anisotropy of the LV induced by its fibrous structure [9, 10] is modelled by superimposing a system of truss elements upon the 3-D elements mesh. These are grouped into 5 layers each with a different fiber orientation, which approximately describes the direction of the myocardial fibers at the corresponding wall [10]. The truss elements have two roles:

a. To increase the stiffness of the wall in the fiber direction, relative to the direction normal to the fibers. The fibers are ascribed the same form of exponential stress-strain relation attributed to the whole muscle strip [11],

$$\sigma = \frac{c}{k}\,[\exp(k\varepsilon) - 1], \tag{1}$$

but with different values of the experimental constants c and k.

b. To define the direction of the active forces which develop within the fibers, and thus coincide with the truss directions.

The geometric nonlinearity

The large deformation analysis required by the significant changes of shape that the LV undergoes during the cardiac cycle is performed by an incremental approach, applying relatively small loading steps and assuming that the resulting displacements are small enough to consider the problem as geometrically linear. The geometry of the structure is adjusted at each step by an updated Lagrangian scheme.

The material nonlinearity

In the absence of quantitative data for the multi-axial mechanical properties of the muscle, the values of the uniaxial experimental constants (c and k) in (1) [11] are adopted for the description of the material behavior of the 3-D finite elements. The exponential material law is implemented in the model in a piecewise linear manner. This approach necessitates defining a single parameter for each element in order to characterize the stress state and consequently to ascribe the appropriate instantaneous Young modulus to this element. As the axial stress

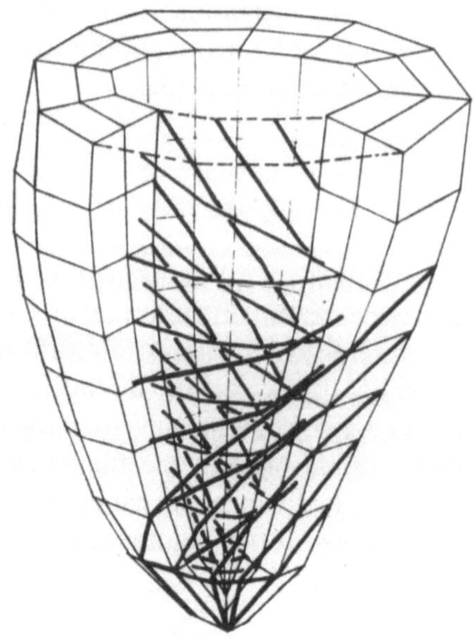

Figure 1. Breakdown of the LV into finite elements. The LV wall consists of two layers of three-dimensional elements, combined with five layers of truss elements.

serves for this purpose for the truss element, for the 3-D element Von Mise's effective stress is used. Since the myocardium, as most of the other soft tissues, is nearly incompressible, Poisson's ratio is chosen to be 0.45.

The active forces

The active forces developing within the myocardial fibers are evidently the dominant factor affecting the deformation and the stress level in the LV during the systole. As for the diastole, the common approach treats the ventricle as a strictly passive material expanded by the rising cavity pressure. However, if the myocardium is ascribed the experimentally measured passive mechanical properties [11], the given increase in the cavity pressure is too small, at least in the early filling phase, to produce the measured change in the cavity volume. This discrepancy may be accounted for in the present model by the release of fiber strains induced by the active forces. The active forces are applied through the truss elements, and their magnitude is determined so as to be proportional to the truss element cross sections.

With the absence of quantitative information regarding the activation function, it is taken as the independent variable of the simulation. Its value is chosen so that the numerically simulated pressure-volume loop coincides with in vivo measured one. Thus, the ventricular volume is maintained constant durig the isovolumic stages by counteracting the contraction effects of the active forces with the expansion effect of the internal pressure. Similarily, the ventricular contraction in the ejection phase is induced by overcoming the rising cavity pressure by increasing the active forces, while the ventricular expansion in the filling phase is produced by the combined effect of the cavity pressure rise and of the release of active strains.

The boundary conditions

The quantitative information required to express actual constraints imposed on the LV by the other parts of the heart and the adjacent organs in terms of kinematic boundary conditions is still unavailable. Nevertheless, such boundary conditions are necessary in order to prevent rigid body displacements and rotations. The appropriate conditions satisfying these requirements while causing only minimal and local distortion of the deformation field chosen here are clamping two adjacent nodal points on the LV base and prevention of the vertical movement of all the nodal points on the LV base.

The normal pressure applied by the blood volume contained in the LV is assumed to be uniform at any given instant and its time variance is based on experimental measurements acquired simultaneously with the ventricle geometry.

The simulation procedure

In a previous paper by the authors [7] an entire cardiac cycle based on in vivo measured time sequential, canine heart data was simulated. Within the present work it is intended to simulate the first stage of an infarct, commonly termed [4] as an immediate infarction, occuring at the beginning of the ejection phase. The immediate infarction is characterized by an instantaneous total loss of contractility of a certain region of the myocardium, while the passive mechnical properties of the tissue are yet unaltered. Therefore, the simulation consists of two parts:

a. simulation of the intact canine heart, as from the QRS through the systolic isovolumic stage;
b. instantaneous introduction of an infarct, and simulation of the ejection phase, until the end systolic pressure is reached.

Simulation of the systolic isovolumic phase

The onset of the electrical activation (QRS) is chosen to be the starting point of the simulation since at this state the LV is almost stress and strain free, i.e. no active strain prevails in the fibers and only a small intramural pressure exists. The simulation proceeds by applying an increment of intraventricular pressure as well as a tentative increment of active forces on the initial given 3-D geometry at QRS. The FE analysis is performed, yielding the deformed configuration of the LV due to the above applied loads. The new cavity volume is compared to the experimentally measured one. If the numerical value deviates from the experimental finding by more than 1%, the present step is repeated with adjusted incremental active forces until it converges. Once the above requirement is fulfilled, the geometry of the LV and the stresses are updated. Then the effective stress in each element is calculated and an appropriate Young modulus is assigned to it. The process is repeated until the systolic isovolumic stage is terminated. Prior to simulating the ejection phase of the infarcted heart the same phase is simulated for the intact heart. This is done in order to evaluate the active forces during this phase that will serve in part as input for the infarcted case.

Simulation of the ejection phase

Once the systolic isovolumic phase is completed the ventricle is instantaneously infarcted by completely deactivating a certain portion of the myocardium, simulating an immediate infarct. Furthermore, the ejection phase is simulated employing the intraventricular pressure increments and the active forces (only for the non damaged part of the ventricle), previously evaluated for the intact case. This procedure enables a direct assessment of the ventricular functional changes resulting from this particular pathology.

Results

In order to examine the effect of the infarct size on the mechanics of the LV, the simulation of the ejection phase was repeated three times, for infarcts comprising 16.6%, 27.1% and 42.7% of the LV wall volume. The infarcts cover a zone which extends longitudinally from the basal region of the LV to its apical one, not including the base and apex themselves, and circumferentially, the infarcts occupy about 60°, 120° and 240° of the ventricle (see Figs 2–4).

For each of the three cases, the results are presented in terms of the deformations of the LV, the stresses which develop in its walls and the ejection fraction it produces. Subsequently, these parameters are compared with the corresponding ones for the intact case.

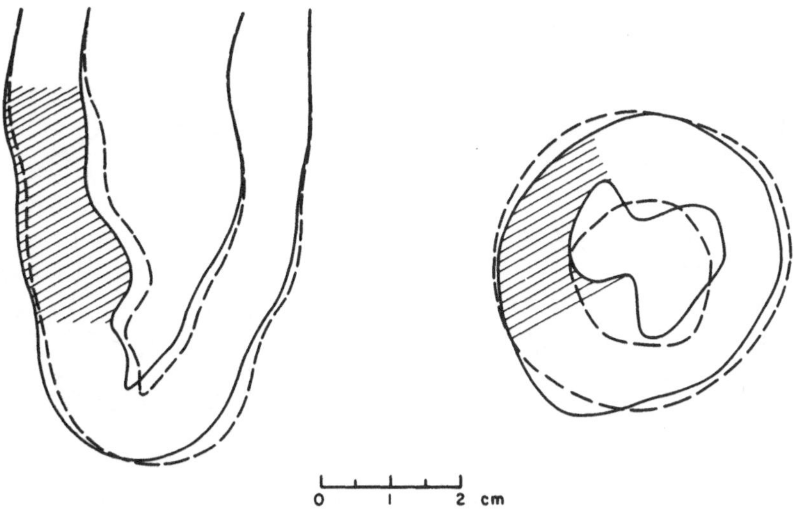

Figure 2. Comparison of transverse and longitudinal contours of an intact LV (broken curves) versus those of an infarcted one. Small infarct.

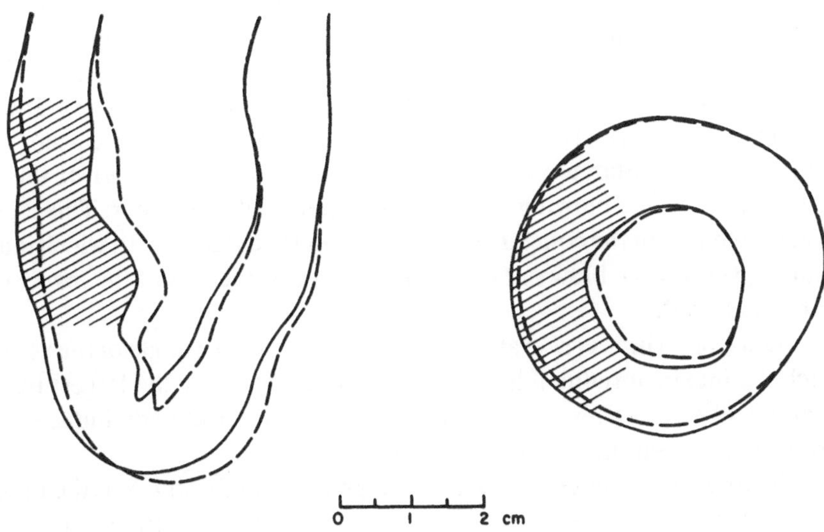

Figure 3. Comparison of transverse and longitudinal contours of an intact LV versus those of an infarcted one (medium infarct).

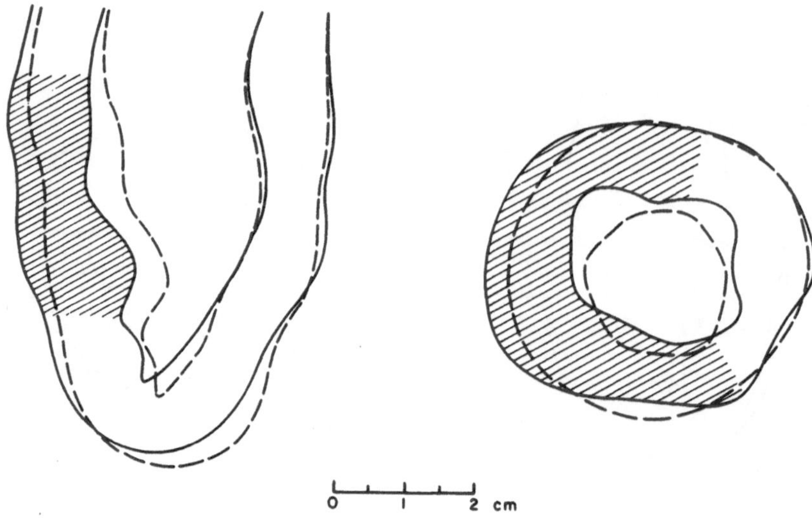

Figure 4. Comparison of transverse and longitudinal contours of an intact LV versus those of an infarcted one (large infarct).

Effect of infarction on LV deformations

The global deformation of the infarcted LV is compared to that of the intact one by referring to the transverse and longitudinal contours of the ventricle. A small infarct results in a local indentation of the wall, with almost no alteration of the overall dimensions and global shape of the LV (Fig. 2). A medium sized infarct induces a smaller overall contraction of the whole ventricle, almost without altering the pattern of the transverse and longitudinal contours (Fig. 3). The large infarct significantly affects the contraction mode of the ventricle, causing larger bulging out of the infarcted regions (Fig. 4). However, in neither of the three cases does an extreme blowing out of the infarcted wall area occur. This seems to be in agreement with the conclusions of Bogen and McMahon [12], which indicate that aneurysms do not blow out unless the passive properties of the myocardium have been altered.

Occurence of an infarct also affects the apex to base twist angle of the ventricle. Though the maximal reduction in the twist angle caused by the largest infarct is only about 10%, the presence of even a smaller infarct already induces a considerable decrease in the twist angle (Fig. 5)

The distribution of the fiber strains through the wall thickness in the infarcted region is by far different from that in the intact parts of the ventricle. In the intact wall, the midwall fibers undergo the highest shortening, while the endocardial and epicardial fibers shorten to a lesser and closely similar extent. In the infarcted portion, where no contraction prevails, the fiber strain distribution progressively

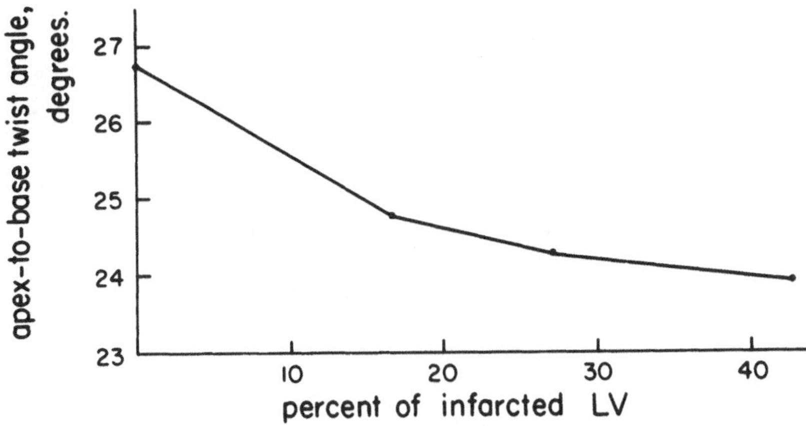

Figure 5. The variation in the apex-to-base twist angle as a function of infarct size.

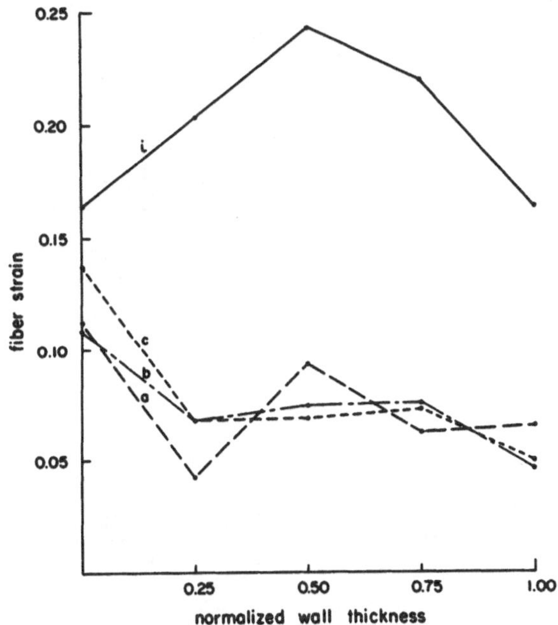

Figure 6. Fiber strain as a function of LV wall thickness for an intact LV (i), and for three cases of a small (a), medium (b) and large (c) infarct.

changes with the infarct size, showing the largest strains in the endocardial fibers and decreasing towards the epicardium (Fig. 6). This distribution is typical to a thick walled vessel acted upon by an internal pressure, and is expected to appear once the active forces are detracted.

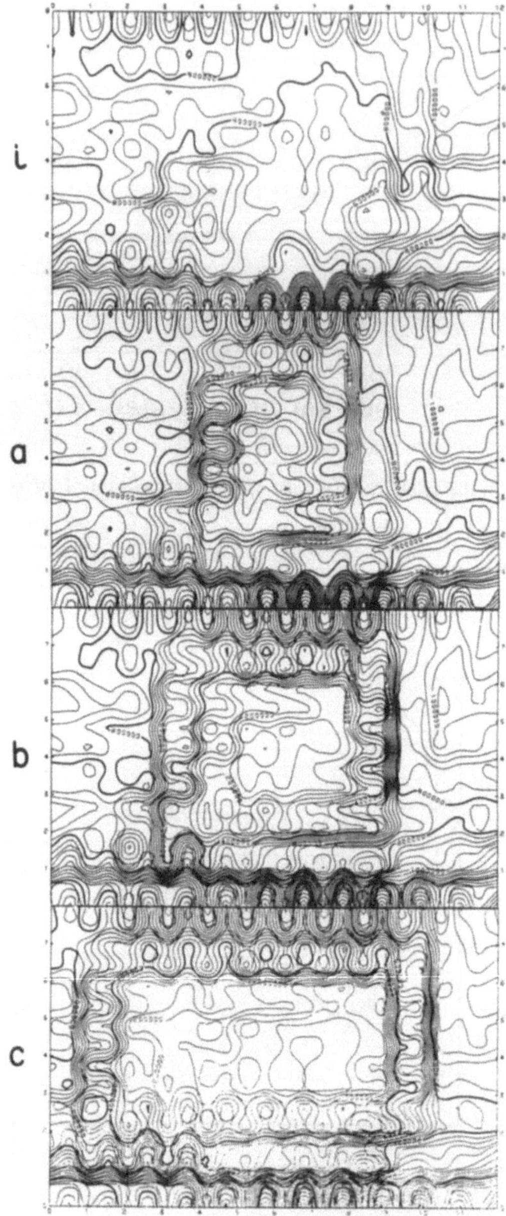

Figure 7. Effective stresses on the midwall surface for an intact LV (i) and for three cases of a small (a), medium (b), and large (c) infarcts.

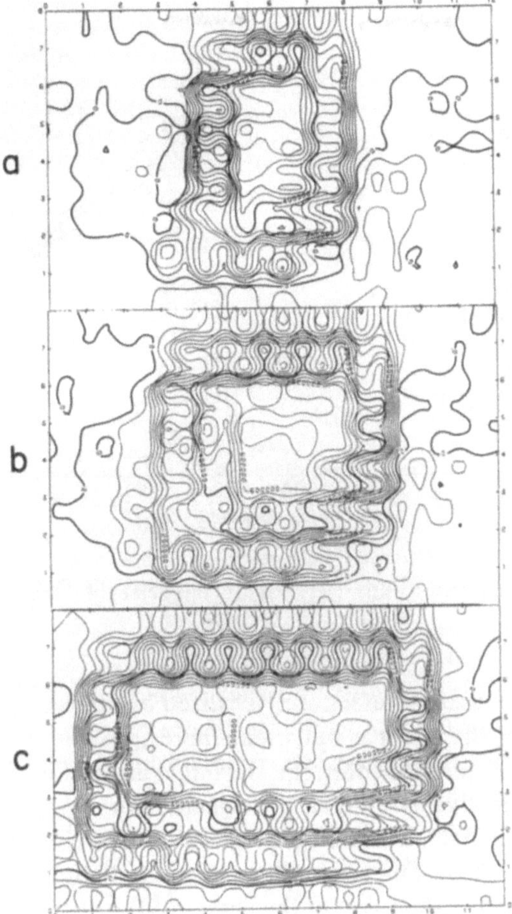

Figure 8. Stress maps resulting from the detraction of the effective stresses on the midwall of the three infarction cases considered from the corresponding one in the intact state.

Effect of infarction on LV wall stresses

The stress distribution in the LV wall is considered here in terms of the Von Mise's effective stress, which is related to the cartesian stress tensor components by

$$\sigma_{eff} = \left\{ \frac{1}{2} \left[(\sigma_{xx} - \sigma_{yy})^2 + (\sigma_{yy} - \sigma_{zz})^2 + (\sigma_{zz} - \sigma_{xx})^2 \right] + 3\,\tau_{xy}^2 + 3\,\tau_{yz}^2 + 3\,\tau_{zx}^2 \right\}^{1/2} \tag{2}$$

and which gives a general notion of the stress state. For purposes of comparison

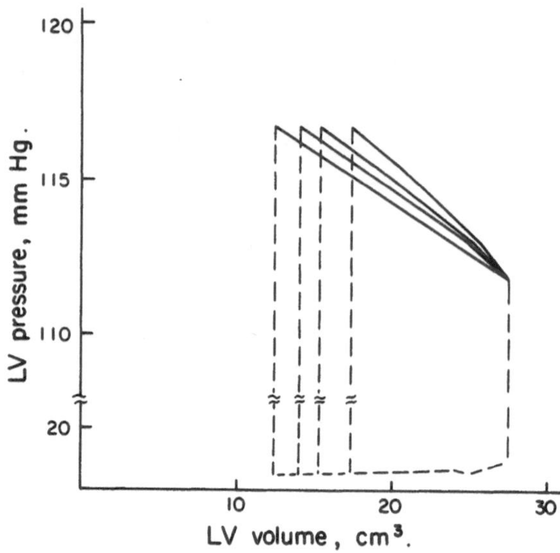

Figure 9. Pressure-volume loops of an intact LV and of three cases of a small (a), medium (b) and large (c) infarct.

with the intact LV, these stresses are visualized by maps of isostress lines for the midwall surfaces of the intact as well as the three infarcted states (Fig. 7). In order to accentuate the differences between the intact and the infarcted ventricles, the corresponding effective stresses are detracted for each of the three infarcts considered, and similarly visualized on isotress maps (Fig. 8). The results show that for all the three cases, there are sharp stress gradients at the boundaries of the infarcted region, while the stress at the center of this region is significantly lower that the one in the surrounding tissue. This may be caused by the disappearance of compressive stresses which would have been exerted by the presently nonexistent active forces. Except for the boundaries, the stress distribution in the infarcted region seems to be relatively even, slightly decreasing towards the center. The stress pattern in the intact parts of the LV wall does not appear to be considerably affected by the introduction of the infarct, except for increased stresses in the apical and basal strips adjacent to it.

Effect of infarct on LV ejection fraction

The introduction of infarcts results in progressively lower end systolic volumes, for increased infarct sizes (Fig. 9). As a result the ejection fraction (EF) is linearly decreasing as the infarct size increases (Fig. 10). Similar relations were reported by Swan et al. [1] and by Bogen et al. [4]. The amount of decrease in EF relative to the intact state is somewhat lower than the relative size of the infarct.

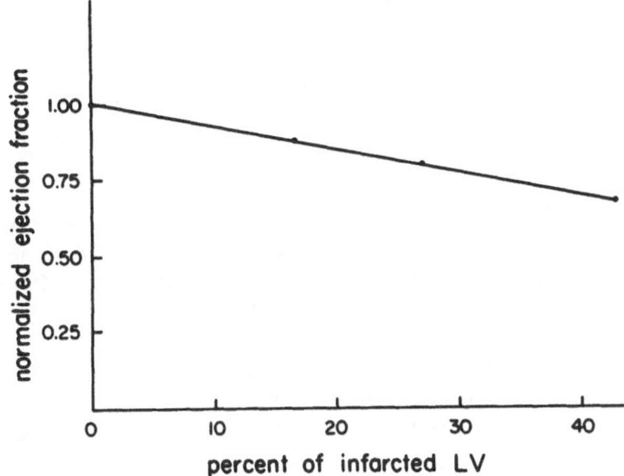

Figure 10. The ejection fraction of the LV as a function of infarct size.

Concluding remarks

Using a recently developed comprehensive model for the mechanics of the LV, immediate infarcts of various sizes have been simulated. The model predicts various geometrical and functional changes in the ventricle that occur due to the total loss of contractility of the infarcted region, which are found to be in good agreement with physiological observations.

Due to the model's distinct feature, that enables the treatment of contractility separately from the passive mechanical properties of the myocardium, various additional pathologies involving mechanical alterations of the ventricle, may be simulated in the future. The first category consists of pathologies in which contractility is partially or entirely lost such as in ischemic disease. The second category involves states in which the passive mechanical properties of the tissue are altered as in fibrosis or scarification that is part of the degenerative processes following infarction. Any pathology belonging to one or both categories can be readily simulated using the present model.

References

1. Swan HJC, Forrester GD, Chaterjee K, Parmley WW, Mirsky I (1972): A conceptual model of myocardial infarction and cardiogenic shock. In: Mirsky I, Ghista DN, Sandler H (eds) Cardiac mechanics, pp. 359–377. J. Wiley and Sons, New York.
2. Janz RF, Waldron RJ (1978): Predicted effect of chronic apical aneuryms on the passive stiffness of the human left ventricle. Circ Res 42: 255–263.
3. Yettram AL, Vinson CA, Gibson DG (1979): Influence of the distribution of stiffness in the

human left ventricular myocardium on shape changes in diastole. Med Biol Eng Comp 17: 553–562.

4. Bogen DK, Rabinowitz SA, Needleman A, McMahon TA, Abelman WH (1980): An analysis of the mechanical disadvantage of myocardial infarction in the canine left ventricle. Circ Res 47: 728–741.
5. Bogen DK, Needleman A, McMahon TA (1984): An analysis of myocardial infarction. The effect of regional changes in contractility. Circ Res 55: 805–815.
6. Perl M, Horowitz A, Sideman S (1986): Comprehensive model for the simulation of left ventricle mechanics. Part 1: Model description and simulation procedure. Med Biol Eng Comp 24: 145–149.
7. Horowitz A, Perl M, Sideman S, Ritman EL (1986): Comprehensive model for the simulation of left ventricle mechanics. Part 2: Implementation and results analysis. Med Biol Eng Comp 24: 150–156.
8. Ritman EL, Kinsey JH, Robb RA, Gilbert BK, Harris LD, Wood EH (1980): Three dimensional imaging of heart, lung and circulation. Science 210: 273–280.
9. Greenbaum RA, Ho SV, Gibson DG, Becker A, Anderson RH (1981): Left ventricular fiber architecture in man. Br Heart J, 45: 248–263.
10. Streeter DD, Hanna WT (1973): Engineering mechanics for successive states in canine left ventricular myocardium. Circ Res, 33: 656–664.
11. Pao YC, Nagendra GK, Padiyar R, Ritman EL (1980): Derivation of myocardial fiber stiffness equation based on theory of laminated composites. J Biomech Engng, 102: 252–257.
12. Bogen DK, McMahon TA (1979): Do cardiac aneurysms blow out? Biophys J, 27: 301–316.

Discussion

Marcus: It is known that if you infarct only half of the thickness of the left ventricular wall, from the endocardium to the mid-wall, you get a transmural mechanical effect. I believe that Jim Weiss at Hopkins has shown that. Also, many investigators have shown that if you produce an infarction in the anterior wall, you get hyperfunction in the posterior wall. I wonder if you tried anything like that in your model simulations.

Perl: No, we have not reached this point as yet.

Arts: You simulated a transmural ischemia. However, most of the ischemias are subendocardial. One of your conclusions was about the decrease of twisting. But in subendocardial infarction twisting will increase, and contraction will decrease. This is the clinical situation.

Perl: That is a good test for the model and I thank you for the advice.

Baan: How do you have the fibers mechanically interact with each other? This is especially important, in the case of infarct particularly, from layer to layer.

Perl: The fibers are not allowed to move separately. They are connected to the nodal points of the 3-D elements.

31. Nonischemic dysfunction at the lateral margins of ischemic myocardium

K.P. GALLAGHER, R.A. GERREN, A.J. BUDA and W.R. DUNHAM

Abstract

To determine the lateral extent of dysfunction in nonischemic myocardium adjacent to ischemic muscle, we measured systolic wall thickening during circumflex coronary occlusion in two groups of anesthetized, open-chest dogs. In one group (n = 12), wall thickening was measured with sonomicrometers arrayed on both sides of the perfusion boundary (PB) between ischemic and nonischemic myocardium. The location of the PB and the distances of the sonomicrometers from the PB were determined from full circumference maps of myocardial blood flow (microspheres) distribution constructed from multiple, small tissue samples. Sigmoid curves were fitted to the data to model changes in wall thickening as a continuous function of distance from the PB. Using this approach, the average extent of dysfunction (defined as wall thickening less than control condition values) was approximately 4–5 mm (or 15–18 degrees) of endocardial circumference. In the second group (n = 18), cross-sectional two-dimensional echocardiograms were obtained to measure regional function. Wall thickening was measured at 22.5 degree intervals around cross-sections of the left ventricle and myocardial blood flow distribution in the corresponding 16 sectors was measured with microspheres or autoradiography. Circumferential maps of wall thickening and blood flow distribution during circumflex coronary occlusion were constructed. By superimposing the maps, the difference between the size of the hypofunctional zone (174 ± 4 degrees) and ischemic zone (125 ± 26 degrees) was estimated. Consistent with the results obtained with sonomicrometry, the extent of nonischemic dysfunction averaged approximately 25 degrees (or 8–9 mm of endocardial circumference) at each lateral border of the ischemic area. We conclude that a 'functional border zone' (defined as nonischemic muscle exhibiting abnormal function) exists adjacent to acutely ischemic myocardium. Because its lateral extent is relatively limited, however, it is possible to estimate the size of the ischemic zone with reasonable accuracy using functional measurements alone.

Introduction

Potential preservation of 'border zone' myocardium at the lateral margins of an ischemic area has received considerable attention. Recent studies, however, have demonstrated that the lateral borders of an infarcted area are sharply delineated [1–9] and are unlikely to be substantially altered with different interventions [2]. Several lines of evidence suggest that the damaged myocardium is surrounded by a zone of normally perfused but functionally impaired muscle [10–20]. This type of border zone, defined in terms of contractile performance rather than perfusion, may begin at the relatively abrupt perfusion boundary between ischemic and nonischemic muscle and extend laterally into myocardium with normal blood flow. The circumferential distribution of impaired wall motion has been reported to overestimate infarct size by most investigators, but the amount of overestimation varies considerably [17, 21–27].

Given the existence of a functional border zone, its dimensions and the potential for altering them are important issues for the correct interpretation of most methods used clinically and experimentally to measure regional myocardial function. Therefore, the objective of the studies reviewed in this article was characterization of the functional border zone in order to answer the following question: Does mechanical dysfunction extent beyond the boundary between ischemic and nonischemic myocardium into normally perfused muscle, and if so, how far does it extend and how severe is the dysfunction? The microsphere technique was used to precisely delineate the ischemic-nonischemic interface and the distribution of functional changes across the perfusion boundary was measured with sonomicrometers [28] or two-dimensional echocardiography [29].

Materials and methods

Two separate but related studies were performed in open-chest, anesthetized dogs. In one of the studies, halothane (end-tidal concentration 0.5–0.7%) anesthesia was used and sonomicrometers were implanted to measure regional wall thickening [28]. In the second study, pentobarbital (30 mg/kg) anesthesia was used and regional function was measured as wall thickening with two-dimensional echocardiography [29].

Experimental preparation in sonomicrometer studies

After performing a left thoracotomy, a Millar high fidelity micromanometer was passed into the left ventricle via the carotid artery and aorta for measurement of left ventricular pressure. Tygon catheters were placed in the left ventricle (via the apex to verify calibration of the Millar micromanometer in mm Hg), left atrium (for injection of microspheres), and femoral and carotid arteries to obtain two simultaneous reference arterial samples for calculation of myocardial blood flow. Around the proximal circumflex artery, a screw clamp occluder was positioned to produce total coronary occlusion.

Regional myocardial function was measured in 12 dogs with sonomicrometers arrayed to measure wall thickness [30, 31]. One crystal of each wall thickness pair was inserted tangentially to the subendocardium and the other crystal was attached to the epicardium over the position of the inner crystal. The epicardial crystal was attached to a dacron patch, enabling us to sew it to the epicardium with shallow sutures after locating the position of least distance between the two crystals while monitoring the signals with an oscilloscope [31]. Data were not used if the crystals were improperly aligned or if the inner crystal was not contained within the inner third of the myocardium [32].

Regional myocardial blood flow was measured with tracer labelled microspheres (15 μm diameter, New England Nuclear) using the reference withdrawal method [33]. Two or three injections of microspheres were made in each experiment, utilizing one of six available isotopes (Ce-141, Sn-113, Cr-51, Ru-103, Nb-95, Sc-46) for each flow determination. Approximately 1–2 million microspheres were injected into the left atrium for measuring blood flows. Arterial reference samples were obtained simultaneously from the femoral and carotid arteries at a constant rate with a Harvard withdrawal pump. The withdrawals were started before injecting the microspheres and they were completed 2 minutes later. The microspheres were thoroughly mixed before injection to ensure that adequate mixing would be achieved.

Blood flow measurements were made during control conditions and five to ten minutes after abruptly occluding the circumflex artery, while continuously recording hemodynamic and dimensional data on strip chart and FM tape recorders. We waited for at least five minutes after coronary occlusion to make certain that steady conditions were achieved before injecting microspheres or obtaining dimensional data for analysis. Longer periods of ischemia were not evaluated in this experimental series.

At the end of the experiments, the dogs were euthanized with intravenous KCl. The heart was removed and placed in formalin to make it easier to section. The sonomicrometers were left in the heart to allow careful assessment of their position and alignment within the myocardial wall. Full thickness sections were obtained around the circumference of left ventricular rings as shown in Figure 1. In the vicinity of the perfusion boundary, the sections (designated A through N in Figure 1) were approximately 3 mm wide, similar to the approach for delineating perfusion boundaries described by Murdock et al. [9]. Each transmural section was divided into three pieces of approximately equal thickness from the endocardial to epicardial surfaces. The location of each piece of tissue and the positions of the sonomicrometers were recorded. Then the tissue samples were weighed and placed in counting vials for assay of radioactivity in a Tracor (Model 1185)

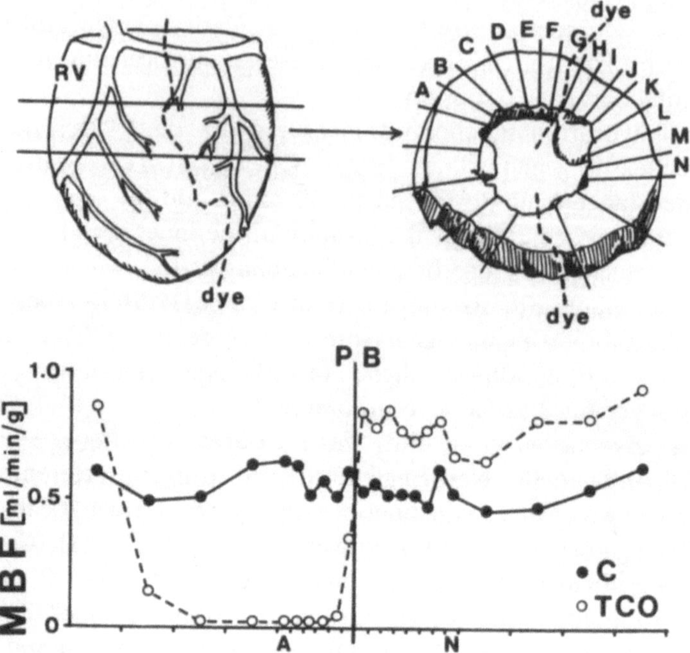

Figure 1. Schematic depiction of the manner in which transverse slices of the left ventricle were sectioned. In the upper left is shown the left ventricle alone with one transverse ring indicated. In the upper right is shown the technique for sectioning the transverse slice. Small samples (Samples A through N) were obtained in the vicinity of the perfusion boundary and larger samples were obtained remote from the perfusion boundary. In the lower portion of the figure is shown an actual circumferential 'map' of myocardial blood flow (MBF) from one of the experiments in this study. For the sake of clarity, only subendocardial blood flow is presented in the graph. Control (C) condition blood flow is depicted with solid symbols; blood flow during coronary occlusion (TCO) is shown with open symbols. A sharp demarcation between ischemic and nonischemic areas is evident, with only one sample demonstrating an intermediate flow value.

γ-scintillation counter. The output of the gamma counter was recorded on a floppy disk for subsequent calculation of myocardial blood flows using standard techniques [33].

Myocardial blood flow 'maps' around the circumference of the left ventricle were generated in which the position of the dimension measurements could be located. The perfusion boundary was identified by the position of the flow gradient in the circumferential blood flow map (Figure 1). Because the samples delineating the perfusion boundary were quite small, we could successfully localize the boundary in most of the experiments. When a sharp boundary was not evident, however, the data from such experiments were not used. The locations of the wall thickening measurements were superimposed on the perfusion maps and the distance from each measurement to the perfusion boundary was determined.

The main parameter of systolic function we concentrated on was the extent of wall thickening, defined as the difference between end-diastolic and end-systolic wall thickness. End-diastole was identified as the point corresponding to the onset of the positive dP/dt signal and end-systole was defined as the point 20 msec prior to peak negative dP/dt [34]. The dimensional and hemodynamic data were analyzed from recordings made at 100 mm/s or were analyzed by digitizing the recorded data from analog tape with a DEC Micro PDP 11 computer system. Ten to 20 cardiac cycles were averaged at each condition, using the beats occurring during the microsphere injection.

Experimental preparation in echocardiographic studies

Eighteen dogs were studied as part of this experimental series. Although pentobarbital anesthesia was used, the preparation was similar to the sonomicrometer studies described above. A left thoracotomy was performed to allow placement of left atrial and arterial catheters. The circumflex artery was exposed by dissection and a hydraulic occluder was placed around it to produce coronary occlusion. Thereafter, the left thoracotomy was partially closed and the dog was turned over. A small right thoracotomy was performed to allow placement of the two-dimensional echocardiographic transducer over the right ventricle. This approach minimized distortion of the left ventricle by the echocardiographic transducer and maximized image quality of the echocardiograms [29].

The two-dimensional echocardiograms were obtained with a Diasonics 3400R scanner and 2.25 MHz transducer. Full cross-section (short axis) views were obtained at the level of the mid-posterior papillary muscle. After this location was identified, the transducer position was fixed with clamps to make certain the same cross-section of the left ventricle was visualized throughout the study.

Echocardiograms were obtained during control conditions and 60 minutes after circumflex coronary occlusion. In seven of the 18 dogs, standard tracer labeled (15 μm diameter, New England Nuclear) microspheres were injected to measure myocardial blood flow before and after coronary occlusion. The same procedures for using the microspheres were followed as those described for the sonomicrometer study. In 13 dogs (of which five overlapped with the standard microsphere studies), microspheres labeled with technetium-99m (20 μm diameter, 3 M Co.) were injected for subsequent autoradiographic analysis to define the location of the perfusion boundary [35].

After completing the measurements at 60 minutes following coronary occlusion, the dogs were euthanized with intravenous KCl. The hearts were removed and placed in formalin to facilitate sectioning (for studies in which microspheres were used) or were immediately sliced into cross-sections (5 mm thick) and placed in X-ray cassettes to perform autoradiography. The slices were exposed for 18 hours on 8×10 inch sheets of high speed X-ray film and developed.

Normally perfused tissue was obvious as the area with high radiographic density. The ischemic area was characterized by much lower or no radiographic density. Tracings of the slices (made on clear plastic sheets) were superimposed on the autoradiograms to identify the boundaries between ischemic and nonischemic myocardium. For comparison with echocardiograms, the midpapillary slices were used. In the five animals in which standard microspheres were injected, as well as technetium microspheres, the midpapillary slices were sectioned (as described previously) for determination of blood flows. Excellent correspondence between the perfusion boundaries delineated with the two techniques was observed.

Results

Group 1: systolic wall thickening, measured with sonomicrometry, across the perfusion boundary

After abrupt circumflex coronary occlusion, heart rate increased from 107 ± 15 (mean ± SD) beats/min to 111 ± 18 beats/min ($p<0.03$). Peak systolic pressure in the left ventricle decreased significantly from 114 ± 10 mm Hg to 96 ± 11 mm Hg ($p<0.01$) and end-diastolic pressure increased from 8.2 ± 1.5 mm Hg to 13.3 ± 2.8 mm Hg ($p<0.01$). In the cross-sections of left ventricle containing dimension gauges, the size of the ischemic area averaged 42 ± 6% of total cross-sectional area, or 149 ± 21 degrees of circumference.

Wall thickness and blood flow data were evaluated in four locations:

1. the central ischemic area,
2. the ischemic border zone,
3. the nonischemic border zone, and
4. central nonischemic or control area.

The average distances from the perfusion boundary in these four categories were 13 ± 3 mm (central ischemic area), 5 ± 3 mm (ischemic border zone), 4 ± 2 mm (nonischemic border zone), and 15 ± 4 mm (nonischemic area).

During control conditions, myocardial blood flow was similar in the four locations defined to analyze wall motion. As shown in Figure 2, blood flow was markedly reduced in the ischemic area and ischemic border zone during circumflex coronary occlusion. There were no significant differences between blood flow values in these two locations. In the nonischemic area, there were no significant differences between blood flow in the nonischemic border zone (immediately adjacent to the perfusion boundary) and the central nonischemic area (Figure 2). The relative abruptness of the perfusion boundary is demonstrated in Figure 3, which shows the circumferential perfusion map (subendocardial and subepicardial blood flow) after coronary occlusion in one of the experiments from this study.

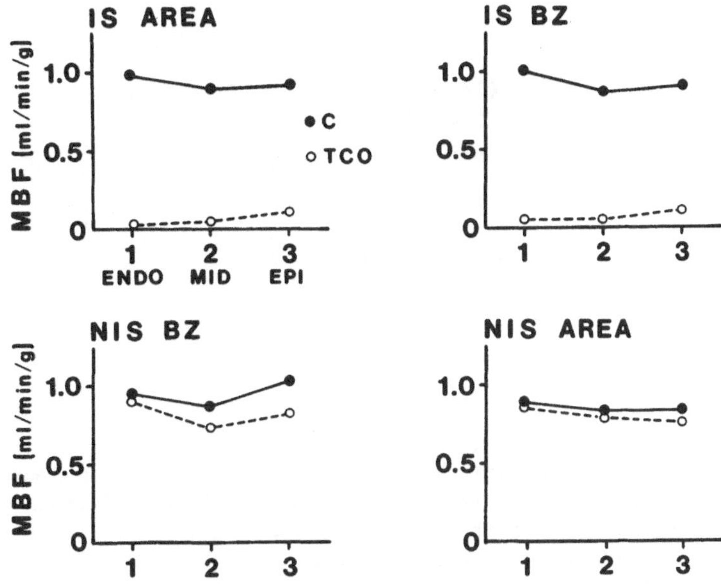

Figure 2. Average myocardial blood flow data in four locations where regional wall thickening was measured. Blood flow is shown in three layers across the myocardial wall: Subendocardium (1), midmyocardium (2), and (3) subepicardium. Blood flow during control (C) conditions is shown with solid symbols and blood flow during total coronary occlusion (TCO) is presented with open symbols. Blood flow was similar in all four locations before occlusion. After coronary occlusion, blood flow was drastically reduced in the two ischemic locations but there was no significant change in the non-ischemic area. Blood flow in the central ischemic area (IS AREA) was not significantly different from flow in the ischemic border zone (IS BZ). Likewise, blood flow in the nonischemic border zone (NIS BZ) was not significantly different from flow in the central nonischemic area (NIS AREA).

Examples of wall thickness waveforms are presented in Figure 4. During control conditions, wall thickening was not significantly different among the four location categories, averaging 3.00 ± 0.61 mm (n = 9) in the ischemic area, 2.84 ± 0.83 mm (n = 10) in the ischemic border zone, 2.72 ± 0.80 mm (n = 12) in the nonischemic border zone, and 2.56 ± 0.57 mm (n = 12) in the central non-ischemic area. After coronary occlusion, thickening was replaced by systolic thinning in the ischemic area. The wall thickness gauges in the ischemic border zone also exhibited paradoxical motion (Figures 3 and 4) that was not significantly different from that in the central ischemic area.

As demonstrated in Figure 5, ischemic and nonischemic border zone wall thickening were markedly different. These gauges were separated by approximately 1 cm, on the average, yet a striking disparity in the extent of wall motion was evident (Figure 4). Systolic thinning averaged -0.24 ± 0.40 mm in the ischemic border zone gauges whereas nonischemic border zone wall thickening was well maintained at 2.44 ± 0.79 mm. This constituted a small (10%) but significant reduction from control condition values. In the nonischemic area,

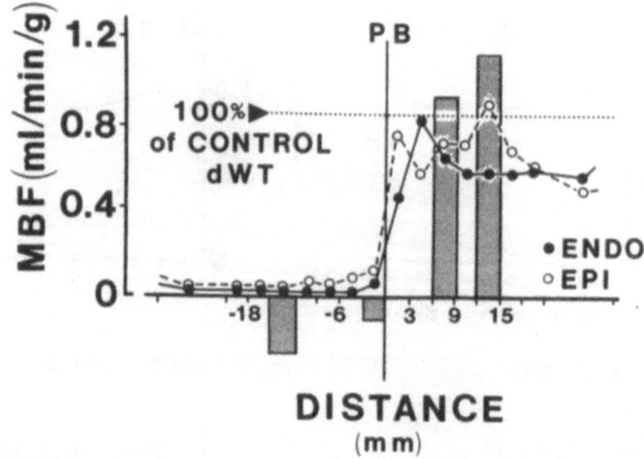

Figure 3. Example of a blood flow map in the vicinity of the perfusion boundary from one experiment in which wall thickening was measured with sonomicrometers. The locations of the sonomicrometers are shown with the stippled bars. The height of the bars indicates the percentage of control condition thickening evident after the circumflex artery was occluded. The relative abruptness of the perfusion boundary as delineated with this microsphere technique (modified from that described by Murdock et al. [9]) is evident and there is a striking difference between the extent of wall thickening on each side of the perfusion boundary (PB). The distance measurements are referenced to the position of the perfusion boundary which was designated as zero. Abbreviations: ENDO, subendocardial; EPI, subepicardial; MBF, myocardial blood flow.

approximately 1.5 cm from the perfusion boundary, wall thickening increased by 27% to 3.24 ± 0.72 mm ($p<0.01$).

In addition to the categorical analysis (Figure 5), wall thickening data were evaluated as a continuous function of distance from the perfusion boundary in order to determine the distribution of wall thickening impairment across the ischemic-nonischemic interface. By using sonomicrometers to monitor wall thickness, we obtained high resolution, discrete regional measurements of transmural function at different locations relative to the perfusion boundary. Sonomicrometers have the disadvantage, however, of allowing limited functional sampling in each experiment. By applying sigmoid curve fits to the data, we attempted to minimize the sampling problem as much as possible.

To mathematically model the distribution of wall thickening change across the ischemic-nonischemic interface we assumed that the nonischemic tissue had a wall thickening asymptote, N, and that the ischemic tissue had a wall thickening asymptote, I. A mathematical function with these asymptotes and that changes monotonically between them is a form of the Normal Distribution Function [36] shown below:

$$y = I + \frac{N - I}{(2\pi\sigma^2)^{1/2}} \int_{\infty}^{x} \exp\left[-(a-\mu)^2/2\sigma^2\right] da.$$

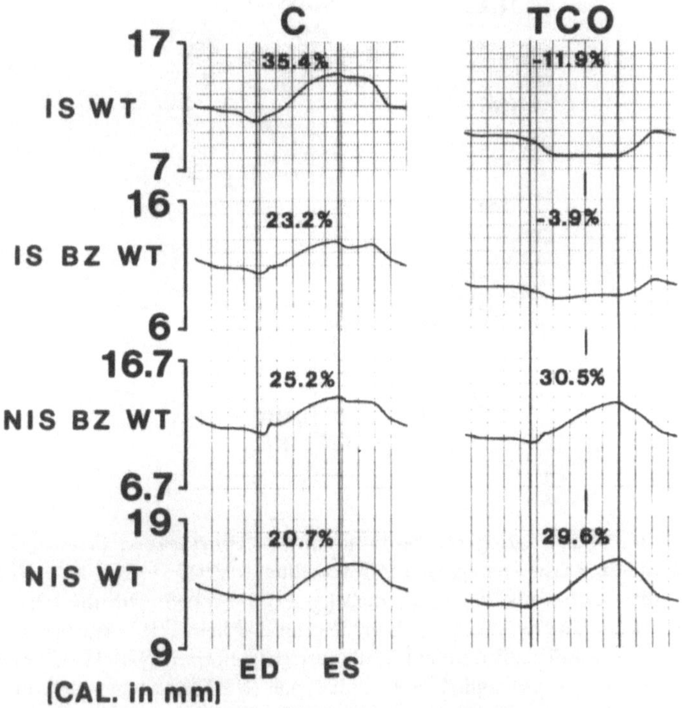

Figure 4. Examples of recorded analog tracings from the same experiment shown in Figure 3. Wall thickness (WT) waveforms are presented during control (C) conditions on the left and during total coronary occlusion (TCO) on the right. The solid lines indicate end-diastole (ED) and end-systole (ES). Percentage wall thickening (averaged over ten consecutive cycles during the microsphere injections) are superimposed on the tracings. The ischemic (IS) and ischemic border zone (IS BZ) wall thicknesses were characterized by systolic thinning after coronary occlusion. Although separated from the ischemic border zone wall thickness by only 8 mm (see Figure 3), nonischemic border zone (NIS BZ) wall thickening increased post-occlusion. Nonischemic (NIS) or control wall thickening, however, increased more substantially after coronary occlusion consistent with its location at a greater distance from the perfusion boundary.

The value μ is equal to the position on the x-axis of the midpoint of the change between the asymptotes and σ is a value (analogous to the standard deviation) that discribes how rapidly the change is made. A change in x from $\mu - 2\sigma$ to $\mu + 2\sigma$ means that the function y changes over 95% of its range (N to I). A low value of σ implies that the transition between asymptotes occurs over a short distance; a high value of σ indicates that the transition between abnormal and normal wall thickening occurs over a broader distance. Computerized nonlinear minimization techniques [37–39] were used to fit the modeling function to the data from each dog and to the pooled data from all of the dogs.

Regional function is plotted on the y-axis as a decimal fraction or percentage of control condition wall thickening in Figures 6 and 7. The position of each data

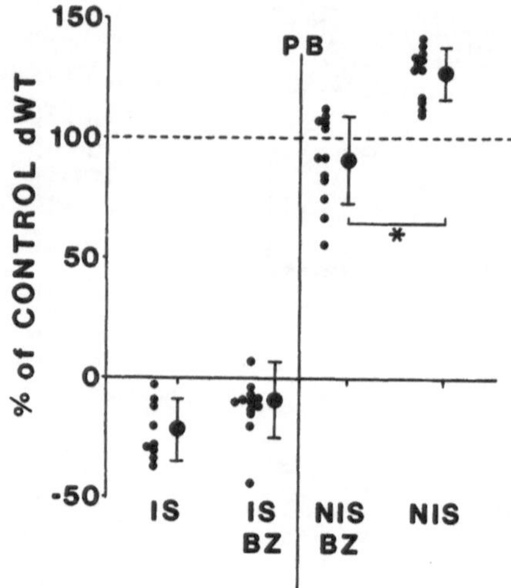

Figure 5. Wall thickening data during coronary occlusion from all of the sonomicrometry experiments. The data were normalized as percentages of control condition wall thickening (dWT). Individual data are shown with the small symbols; average data (± SD) are shown with the large symbols and standard deviation bars. The relative changes in the central ischemic (IS) area and ischemic border zone (IS BZ) were not significantly different. Both were characterized by dyskinesia or wall thinning after coronary occlusion. In the nonischemic border zone (NIS BZ) a small (10%) but significant reduction in wall thickening was observed. The relative change in the NIS BZ was significantly different than the change in central nonischemic (NIS) wall thickening which increased significantly after coronary occlusion.

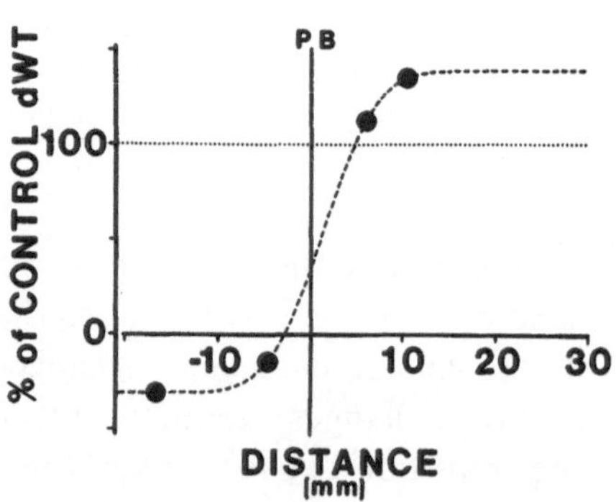

Figure 6. Individual example of a sigmoid curve fit (to wall thickening data from the same experiment shown in Figures 3 and 4). Wall thickening (on the y-axis) is expressed as a percentage of control condition values. Distance on the x-axis is in mm of endocardial circumference, with the position of the perfusion boundary designated as zero. The lateral extent of nonischemic dysfunction (defined as wall thickening less than 100%) was approximately 5 mm or 18 degrees.

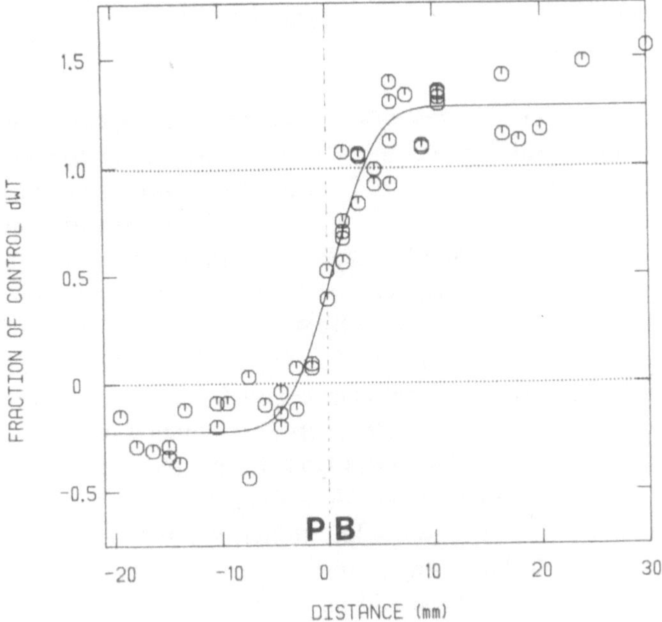

Figure 7. Composite graph of wall thickening data from all 12 of the sonomicrometry experiments relative to the position fo the perfusion boundary. The x and y-axes (with wall thickening expressed as a decimal fraction of control values) are arranged in the same manner as Figure 6. The solid line represents the composite sigmoid fit. Although from different experiments, the data points are distributed closely around the composite fit. A continuum of dysfunction is evident, demonstrating that reduced contractile performance extends beyond the boundary of the ischemic area but the average extent of dysfunction (defined as wall thickening less than 100%) was restricted to approximately 4 mm or 15 degrees.

point relative to the x-axis corresponds to the distance of the measurement from the perfusion boundary, designated as zero, with positive numbers indicating nonischemic myocardium and negative numbers indicating ischemic myocardium. In Figure 6, an individual example of a sigmoid surve fit is presented from the same experiment shown in Figures 3 and 4. The solid line represents the sigmoid curve for the data set. The composite data set and composite sigmoid curve fit (dashed line) are shown in Figure 7. A continuum of functional change was apparent extending across the perfusion boundary. Nonischemic dysfunction, defined as wall thickening less than the control value, extended only 4–5 mm (measured in mm of endocardial circumference) beyond the perfusion boundary. The entire transition zone from dyskinetic to normal wall thickening was restricted to approximately 10 mm.

Group 2: two-dimensional echocardiographic evaluation of wall thickening across the perfusion boundary

In this experimental group, hemodynamic changes after circumflex coronary occlusion were not significant due to the different anesthetic that was employed (pentobarbital). Heart rate was 141 ± 25 beats/min before occlusion and 137 ± 34 beats/min after occlusion. Likewise, mean arterial blood pressure was not altered (100 ± 17 mm Hg to 107 ± 21 mm Hg, NS). Sustantial effects of coronary occlusion on left ventricular end-diastolic area were documented, however, which increased significantly from 12.4 ± 3.0 cm^2 to 15.4 ± 4.2 cm^2 ($p<0.01$). Area ejection fraction decreased from 49 ± 9% to 29 ± 7% ($p<0.01$). Despite large changes in ejection fraction and regional wall thickening secondary to circumflex occlusion, the cross-section of the left ventricle remained symmetrical. The ratio of anterior-posterior diameter to septal-lateral diameter was 1.04 ± 0.08 at baseline and did not change (1.03 ± 0.06) after occlusion.

Circumferential maps of regional left ventricular function were derived by measuring systolic wall thickening at intervals of 22.5 degrees around a cross-section of the left ventricle at the mid-papillary muscle level. End-diastolic and end-systolic frames were selected for analysis using a minicomputer based video digitizing system. An observer traced the endocardial and epicardial borders from the video display for three consecutive beats using the largest cavity area as the end-diastolic frame and smallest cavity as the end-systolic frame. Percent wall thickening was calculated with a radial contraction model and fixed diastolic center of mass for 16 sectors over the full circumference of the cross-section [40].

Myocardial blood flow distribution was also measured in the 16 sectors of the left ventricular cross-section imaged with two-dimensional echocardiography. In this manner, maps of blood flow distribution and wall thickening were produced from the same cross-section of the heart before and during circumflex coronary occlusion. By combining the information from the two types of 'maps', it was possible to calculate the amount of lateral nonischemic dysfunction as the difference between the circumferential extent of ischemia (defined as blood flow reduced to less than 50% of control levels) and the circumferential extent of dysfunction (defined as wall thickening less than the mean control condition value minus two standard deviations).

An example of a blood flow and a function map from one of the experiments is presented in Figure 8. The distribution of subendocardial and subepicardial blood flow during occlusion demonstrates, again, that an abrupt perfusion boundary was produced by circumflex coronary occlusion, similar to the observations made in the other group of experiments (Figure 3). The circumferential distribution of wall thickening was characterized by intense dysfunction in the center of the ischemic area and normal wall thickening in the nonischemic area less than two 22.5° sectors from the perfusion boundary (lower graph, Figure 8). The extent of nonischemic dysfunction (or functional border zone), using the definitions de-

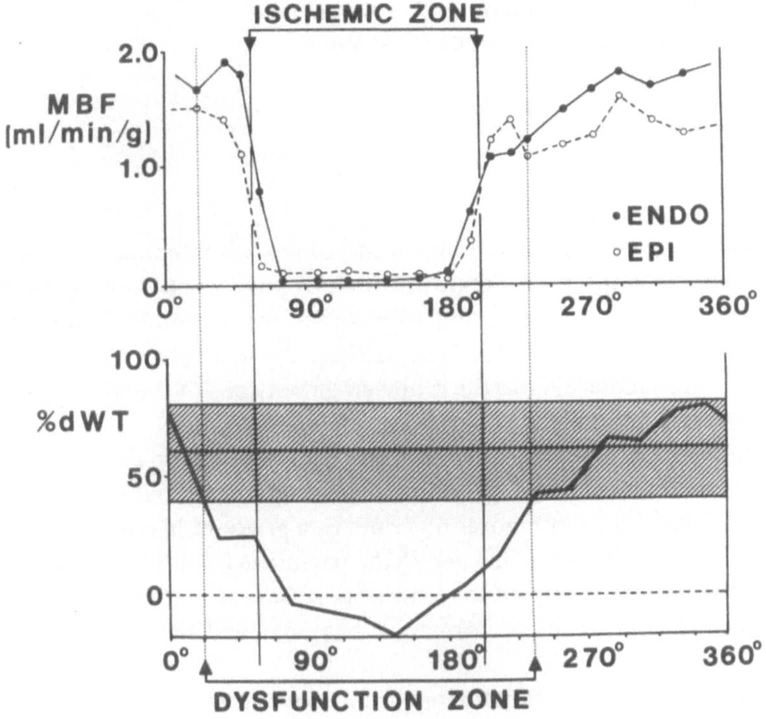

Figure 8. Examples of a circumferential perfusion and circumferential function map from one of the experiments in which two-dimensional echocardiography was used. In the upper graph, subendocardial (ENDO) and subepicardial (EPI) blood flow 60 minutes after circumflex coronary occlusion are plotted relative to position around a full circumference cross-section of the left ventricle. In the lower graph, the corresponding functional data are plotted in terms of percentage wall thickening. The heavy line represents the distribution of wall thickening after coronary occlusion; the cross-hatched area represents mean wall thickening ± 2 standard deviations during control conditions. The size of the ischemic zone is indicated with the solid vertical lines, which represent the perfusion boundaries. The dysfunctional zone, indicated with the dotted lines, is larger than the ischemic area by approximately 30 degrees at each lateral margin. The areas between the solid and dotted lines represent the 'functional border zone'.

scribed above, was approximately 30 degrees at each lateral border.

In all of the experiments, the dysfunctional zone detected by two dimensional echocardiography extended over 174 ± 4 degrees (48% of cross-sectional circumference). The ischemic zone was significantly smaller, encompassing 125 ± 26 degrees (35% of circumference), which means that a functional border zone existed averaging 49 ± 34 degrees. This corresponded to dysfunction in 8–9 mm or 25 degrees of nonischemic myocardium (measured at the endocardium) at either lateral border, a result that agrees well with results based on the sonomicrometric measurements (Figure 7). The reduction in wall thickening in myocardium that constituted the functional border zone (Figure 8) averaged 56%, although no significant reduction in myocardial blood flow was evident in the muscle where those measurements were made.

Discussion

The goal of the studies reviewed here [28, 29] was to determine the distribution of functional change across the lateral margins of acutely ischemic myocardium. In so doing, we attempted to define the extent and severity of dysfunction in normally perfused muscle adjacent to ischemic myocardium. Several previous studies have demonstrated that nonischemic dysfunction exists lateral to an ischemic or infarcted area, but the reported dimensions of the 'functional border zone' varied considerably.

Our findings, obtained with two different modalities for measuring regional myocardial function, support the existence of a significant but narrow functional border zone. As shown in Figures 6, 7, and 8, a gradient in contractile performance was present adjacent to and across the perfusion boundary. Although not as abrupt as the interface defined in terms of perfusion, the transition from abnormal to normal contractile performance was achieved over a relatively small distance.

The lateral extent of the functional border zone, measured with sonomicrometers, was approximately 4–5 mm or 15–18 degrees of endocardial circumference at one lateral margin. In the experiments using two-dimensional echocardiography, the corresponding values were 8 mm or approximately 25 degrees of circumference. Given the differences between echocardiography and sonomicrometry in terms of resolution (and the associated difference in how 'dysfunction' was defined), we consider the disparity between the echocardiographic and sonomicrometric results remarkably small. The complementary results strengthen our confidence in the conclusions on the dimensions of the functional border zone and also suggest that the results may be useful clinically. Because marked dysfunction was restricted to only a few mm immediately adjacent to the perfusion boundary (Figures 7 and 8), the circumferential extent of *severe* dysfunction corresponded closely to the size of the ischemic area. Consequently, if severe dysfunction is used to define the boundaries of an acutely infarcted zone, our findings indicate that ischemic area size can be estimated with reasonable accuracy using imaging techniques based on functional measurements.

Although earlier studies reported that dysfunction extended beyond an infarcted area into surrounding (normally perfused) myocardium, only recent investigations included quantitative data on the relationship between position of the perfusion boundary and the location of functional measurements. For example, Homans et al. [24] used two-dimensional echocardiography and subendocardial segment lengths to measure regional function in anesthetized, open-chest dogs. Contractile performance was evaluated as endocardial wall motion in eight

(45 degree) sectors around the circumference of the left ventricle and as segment shortening, measured with sonomicrometers, close to the perfusion boundary. Like us, they concluded that dysfunction extended beyond the ischemic area but that the degree of nonischemic dysfunction was relatively mild and that the extent of severe dysfunction was comparable to the size of the ischemic zone. An average of 10 mm from the perfusion boundary (delineated with post-mortem dye injections), wall motion was reduced only 24% from control. Simultaneously measured segment shortening, less than 9 mm from the boundary, decreased 19% after coronary occlusion, a relatively small difference compared with our own results. There are several differences between the study of Homans et al. [24] and ours, reviewed here, but the results complement one another and the conclusions are the same.

Sakai et al. [27] measured epicardial segment shortening parallel to the perfusion boundary (delineated with dye injection) in open-chest, anesthetized pigs. They observed that dysfunction extended approximately 15 mm into nonischemic myocardium at the epicardium. The relationship could be described with a exponential equation which documented that proximity to the perfusion boundary was associated with significantly greater reductions in systolic shortening. By 9 mm from the perfusion boundary, however, shortening was 75% of that evident during control conditions. Reductions in function greater than 50% were apparent only within 5 mm of the ischemic-nonischemic interface, in close agreement with our findings. In a recent preliminary report, Prinzen et al. [41] made similar observations on the distribution of epicardial functional changes after coronary occlusion.

The experimental results of Homans et al. [24], Sakai et al. [27], and Prinzen et al. [41] support our conclusion that nonischemic dysfunction is limited to a short distance. Theoretical proposals by Bogen et al. [42, 43] also support this conclusion and may provide a means of rigorously explaining the mechanism of lateral nonischemic dysfunction. They calculated the degree of stress amplification at the interface between infarcted and noninfarcted myocardium based on modeling of the left ventricle as a sphere composed of isotropic material. Stress amplification was highest at the interface between infarcted and noninfarcted myocardium, then recovered logarithmically to control levels over approximately 45 degrees of circumference in the presence of an acute, extensible infarct. The lateral extent of stress amplification decreased with elevated infarct stiffness but was relatively unaffected by infarct size over the range 15–41% of the left ventricle. Given that stress amplification can be equated with restriction of normal motion, the distribution of stress amplification may describe (approximately) the distribution of dysfunction. Although this has yet to be verified, the predictions of Bogen et al. [42, 43] correspond closely to the observations we and others [24, 27, 41] have made on the lateral extent and severity of nonischemic dysfunction. The predictions are even closer if the assumptions made by Bogen et al. [24] on the relativeness stiffness of an acute infarct prove to be in error. We suggest this may be the case, given the reports by Hess et al. [44] and Edwards et al. [45] that acutely ischemic myocardium is much stiffer than what Bogen et al. [42, 43] assumed. This would mean the lateral extent of stress amplification was restricted to a narrower zone (approximately 30–35 degrees of circumference) that is more in line with our results. Although we think stress amplification may explain the mechanism of nonischemic dysfunction, it remains a theoretical possibility only until additional experiments are performed to rigorously test this hypothesis.

The term 'tethering' has been used in the context of nonischemic dysfunction, as well. Tethering implies some sort of mechanical constraint or 'resistive loading' of motion in normally perfused muscle. As such it is intuitively appealing but no definition of tethering exists as yet. We have used the term ourselves but must acknowledge that it is a concept with limited usefulness until it can be defined rigorously. Because stess amplification can be defined and because its distribution appears to resemble that of regional dysfunction near the perfusion boundary, we think stress amplification should be considered the most likely mechanism of nonischemic dysfunction at the lateral margins of ischemic or infarcted myocardium.

Methodologic considerations

Several earlier studies, using myocardial blood flow distribution [1, 5, 9], NADH fluorescence [4], histology [2, 7] or metabolic indices [3, 6] to focus on the size of the junction between ischemic and nonischemic tissue demonstrated that it is a relatively narrow zone, characterized by quite limited overlap of perfusion beds. Recently, Murdock et al. [9] analyzed the distribution of myocardial blood flow (measured with microspheres) during acute coronary occlusion. Using postmortem angiograms as a guide to identifying occluded and nonoccluded regions, serial 3 mm tissue samples were obtained to define the ischemic-nonischemic interface. Overlapping perfusion zones, which resulted from an admixture of ischemic and nonischemic tissue in these samples, were limited to one sample width (3 mm). Thus, the junction between ischemic and nonischemic tissue appeared to be a relatively abrupt interface which was resolveable to approximately 3 mm, using myocardial blood flow 'maps' [9].

Our observations were quite similar in that one 3 mm tissue sample was usually characterized by a level of blood flow intermediate between that in the ischemic and nonischemic areas (Figures 1, 3, and 8). Using the microsphere technique, as described here [28, 29] or by Murdock et al. [9], means that a potential error of 1–2 mm (4–8 degrees) at the endocardium exists in the position of the perfusion boundary as we defined it. The actual perfusion boundary is not a straight line, rather it is irregular, with considerable interdigitation of ischemic and nonischemic muscle [2, 7]. The tissue samples with intermediate blood flow probably represent the muscle with mixed perfusion, where two vascular beds meet and interdigitate [9]. Because we assigned such tissue samples to the ischemic area, we may have overestimated the size of the ischemic zone and underestimated the lateral extent of the functional border zone by 1–2 mm. This approach, however, allowed us to characterize regional contractile performance adjacent to the perfusion boundary with greater confidence that the tissue was perfused at normal levels and was not contaminated by the presence of ischemic muscle. The extent of lateral nonischemic dysfunction remains less than 10 mm even with the addition of 2 mm to adjust for the potential error.

Conclusions

The studies reviewed in this article demonstrated that a functional border zone exists. It may constitute an important feature in the overall impact on the left ventricle of acute regional ischemia. Although statistically significant, the lateral extent and severity of the functional border are limited during acute ischemia and several questions remain to be addressed. The results obtained thus far apply only to myocardium in the basal half of the left ventricle. Whether comparable results would be obtained in the apical left ventricle (rendered ischemic by occlusion of the left anterior descending rather than circumflex artery) remains to be determined. Likewise, the effects of altered loading conditions, changes in contractility, and replacement of infarcted muscle with scar tissue will require additional investigation.

Acknowledgment

We thank Thomas B. McClanahan, Diane Pace, Lisa Krause, and Russell A. Grinage for technical assistance in the performance of these experiments. We also thank Tarry Goble for word processing of the manuscript. This study was supported in part by NIH grants RO1 HL32043 and RO1 HL29716. K.P. Gallagher is recipient of NIH Research Career Development Award KO4 HLO4120.

References

1. Marcus ML, Kerber RE, Ehrhardt J, Abboud FM (1975): Three dimensional geometry of acutely ischemic myocardium. Circulation 52: 254–263.
2. Hirzel HO, Sonnenblick EH, Kirk ES (1977): Absence of a lateral border zone of intermediate creatine phosphokinase depletion surrounding a central infarct 24 hours after acute coronary occlusion in the dog. Circ Res 41: 673–683.
3. Hearse DJ, Opie LH, Katseff IE, Lubbe WF, VanderWerff TJ, Peisach M, Boulle G (1977): Characterization of the 'Border Zone' in acute regional ischemia in the dog. Am J Cardiol 40: 716–726.

4. Harken AH, Barlow CH, Harden WR III, Chance B (1978): Two and three dimensional display of myocardial ischemic 'border zone' in dogs. Am J Cardiol 42: 954–959.
5. Schaper W (1979): Residual perfusion of acutely ischemic heart muscle. In: Schaper W (ed) pathophysiology of myocardial perfusion. Elsevier/North Holland Biomedical Press, Amsterdam, pp. 345–378.
6. Yellon DM, Hearse DJ, Crome R, Grannell J, Wyse RKG (1981): Characterization of the lateral interface between normal and ischemic tissue in the canine heart during evolving myocardial infarction. Am J Cardiol 47: 1233–1249.
7. Factor SM, Okun EM, Monase T, Kirk ES (1982): The microcirculation of the human heart: End-capillary loops with discrete perfusion fields. Circulation 66: 1241–1248.
8. Liedtke AJ, Nellis SH, Whitesell LF (1982): Effects of regional ischemia on metabolic function in adjacent aerobic myocardium. J Mol Cell Cardiol 14: 195–205.
9. Murdock RH Jr, Harlan DM, Morris JJ III, Pryor WW Jr, Cobb FR 1983): Transitional blood flow zones between ischemic and nonischemic myocardium in the awake dog. Analysis based on distribution of the intramural vasculature. Circ Res 52: 451–459.
10. Kerber RE, Marcus ML, Ehrhardt J, Wilson R, Abboud FM (1975): Correlation between echocardiographically demonstrated segmental dyskinesis and regional myocardial perfusion. Circulation 52: 1097–1104.
11. Kerber RE, Marcus ML, Wilson R, Ehrhardt J, Abboud FM (1976): Effects of acute coronary occlusion on the motion and perfusion of the normal and ischemic interventricular septum: An experimental echocardiographic study. Circulation 54: 928–935.
12. Wyatt HL, Forrester JS, daLuz PL, Diamond GA, Chagrasulis R, Swan JJC (1976): Functional abnormalities in nonoccluded regions of myocardium after experimental coronary occlusion. Am J Cardiol 37: 366–372.
13. Ross J Jr, Franklin D (1976): Analysis of regional myocardial function, dimensions, and wall thickness in characterization of myocardial ischemia and infarction. Circulation 53: 188–192.
14. Meltzer RS, Woythaler JN, Buda AJ, Griffith JC, Harrison WD, Martin RP, Harrison DC, Popp RL (1979): Two-dimensional echocardiographic quantification of infarct size alteration by pharmacologic agents. Am J Cardiol 44: 257–262.
15. Lieberman AN, Weiss JL, Jugdutt BI, Becker LC, Bulkley BH, Garrison JG, Hutchins GM, Kallman CA, Weisfeldt ML (1981): Two-dimensional echocardiography and infarct size. Relationship of regional wall motion and thickening to the extent of myocardial infarction in the dog. Circulation 63: 739–746.
16. Likoff M, Reichek N, St. John Sutton M, Macoviak J, Harken A (1982): Epicardial mapping of segmental myocardial function. An echocardiographic method applicable to man. Circulation 66: 1050–1058.
17. Nieminen M, Parisi AF, O'Boyle JE, Folland ED, Khuri S, Kloner RA (1982): Serial evaluation of myocardial thickening and thinning in acute experimental infarction: Identification and quantification using two-dimensional echocardiography. Circulation 66: 174–180.
18. Cox DA, Vatner SF (1982): Myocardial function in areas of heterogeneous perfusion after coronary artery occlusion in conscious dogs. Circulation 66: 1154–1158.
19. Blumenthal DS, Becker LC, Bulkley BH, Hutchins GM, Weisfeldt ML, Weiss JL (1983) Impaired function of salvaged myocardium. Two-dimensional echocardiographic quantification of regional wall thickening in the open chest dog. Circulation 67: 225–233.
20. Guth BD, White FC, Gallagher KP, Bloor CM (1984): Decreased wall thickening in myocardium adjacent to ischemic zones in conscious swine during brief coronary artery occlusion. Am Heart J 107: 458–464.
21. Wyatt HL, Meerbaum S, Heng MK, Rit J, Gueret P, Corday E (1981): Experimental evaluation of the extent of myocardial dyssynergy and infarct size by two-dimensional echocardiography. Circulation 63: 607–614.
22. Pandian NG, Koyanagi S, Skorton DJ, Collins SM, Eastham CL, Kieso RA, Marcus ML, Kerber

RE (1983): Relations between 2-dimensional echocardiographic wall thickening abnormalities, myocardial infarct size and coronary risk area in normal and hypertrophied myocardium. Am J Cardiol 52: 1318–1325.

23. Lima JAC, Becker LC, Melin JA, Lima S, Kallman CH, Weisfeldt ML, Weiss JL (1985): Impaired thickening of non-ischemic myocardium during acute regional ischemia in the dog. Circulation 71: 1048–1059.
24. Homans DC, Asinger R, Elsperger KJ, Erlien D, Sublett E, Mikell F, Bache RJ (1985): Regional function and perfusion at the lateral border of ischemic myocardium. Circulation 71: 1038–1047.
25. Force T, Kemper AJ, Cohen C, Parisi AF (1985): Early loss of postextrasystolic potentiation in acutely ischemic myocardium: evaluation by contrast two-dimensional echocardiography. Circulation 71: 602–609.
26. Gibbons EF, Hogan RD, Franklin TD, Nolting M, Weyman AE (1985): The natural history of regional dysfunction in a canine preparation of chronic infarction. Circulation 71: 394–402.
27. Sakai K, Watanabe K, Millard RW (1985): Defining the mechanical border zone: A study in the pig heart. Am J Physiol 249 (Heart Circ Physiol 18): H88–H94.
28. Gallagher KP, Gerren RA, Stirling MC, Choy M, Dysko RC, McManimon SP, Dunham WR (1986): The distribution of functional impairment across the lateral border of acutely ischemic myoardium. Circ Res 58: 570–583.
29. Buda AJ, Gallagher KP, Zotz RJ, Turla M, Pace D, Krause L (1986): Characterization of the functional border zone around regionally ischemic myocardium using circumferential regional flow-function maps. J Am Col Cardiol 8: 150–158.
30. Bugge-Asperheim B, Leraand S, Kiil F (1969): Local dimensional changes of the myocardium measured by ultrasonic technique. Scand J Clin Lab Invest 24: 361–371.
31. Sasayama S, Franklin D, Ross J Jr, Kemper WS, McKown D (1976): Dynamic changes in left ventricular wall thickness and their use in analyzing cardiac function in the conscious dog. Am J Cardiol 38: 870–879.
32. Gallagher KP, Osakada G, Matsuzaki M, Miller MM, Kemper WS, Ross J Jr (1985): Nonuniformity of inner and outer systolic wall thickening in conscious dogs. Am J Physiol 249 (Heart Circ Physiol 18): H241–H248.
33. Heymann MA, Payne BD, Hoffman JIE, Rudolph AM (1977): Blood flow measurements with radionuclide-labeled particles. Prog Cardiovasc Dis 20: 55–79.
34. Theroux P, Franklin D, Ross J Jr, Kemper WS (1974): Regional myocardial function during acute coronary artery occlusion and its modification by pharmacologic agents in the dog. Circ Res 35: 896–908.
35. De Boer LWV, Strauss HW, Kloner RA, Rude RE, Davis RF, Maroko PR, Braunwald E (1980): Autoradiographic method for measuring the ischemic myocardium at risk. Effects of verapamil on infarct size after experimental coronary occlusion. Proc Natl Acad Sci 77: 6119–6123.
36. Morrison DF (1967): Multivariate statistical analysis. McGraw-Hill, New York, p. 133–148.
37. Dunham WR, Wu CT, Polichar RM, Sands RH, Harding LJ (1977): Added precision in 57Fe Mossbauer Spectroscopy. Nucl Inst Meth 145: 537–553.
38. Dunham WR, Fee JA, Harding LJ, Grande HJ (1980): Application of fast Fourier transforms to EPR spectra of free radicals in solution. J Mag Res 40: 351–359.
39. Hagen WR, Hearshen DO, Harding LJ, Dunham WR (1985): Quantitative numerical analysis of g strain in the EPR of distributed systems; its importance for multicenter metalloproteins. J Magn Reson 61: 233–244.
40. Buda AJ, Delp EJ, Meyer CR, Jenkins JM, Smith DN, Bookstein FL, Pitt B (1983): Automatic computer processing of digital two-dimensional echocardiograms. Am J Cardiol 52: 384–389.
41. Prinzen FW, Prinzen TT, Arts T, Reneman RS (1985): Gradients in epicardial shortening and transmural blood flow from ischemic towards normal left ventricular myocardium (Abstract). J Moll Cell Cardiol 17 (Suppl 3): 225.
42. Bogen DK, Rabinowitz SA, Needleman A, McMahon TA, Abelmann WH 1980): An analysis of

the mechanical disadvantage of myocardial infarction in the canine left ventricle. Circ Res 47: 728–741.

43. Bogen DK, Needleman A, McMahon TA (1984): An analysis of myocardial infarction. The effect of regional changes in contractility. Circ Res 55: 805–815.
44. Hess OM, Osakada G, Lavelle JF, Gallagher KP, Kemper WS, Ross J Jr (1983): Diastolic myocardial wall stiffness during partial and complete coronary occlusion in the conscious dog. Circ Res 52: 387–400.
45. Edwards CH II, Rankin JS, McHale PA, Ling D, Anderson RW (1981): Effects of ischemia on left ventricular regional function in the conscious dog. Am J Physiol 240 (Heart Circ Physiol 9): H413–H420.

Discussion

Li: Does wall thickening parallel muscle segment shortening even though they are orthogonal to each other?
Gallagher: Two answers. Under normal conditions if you measure a deep (subendocardial) segment length and wall thickness with sonomicrometers in adjacent locations, you will find that changes in one parallel changes in the other. If they are both in the middle of an ischemic area, they will act in the same manner but provide mirror images. However, trying to apply segment shortening to the question of what happens at the border zone is a potential problem. Because the zone of nonischemic dysfunction is relatively narrow, if you use a standard segment length you have a good chance of missing it.
Li: Did you observe muscle shortening at the ischemic border zone boundary?
Gallagher: This is a tricky question, particularly in light of Cox and Vatner's study from 1982 (Circulation 66: 1154–1158, 1982) suggesting that segment length shortening is entirely dominated by ischemic muscle if the segment spans both ischemic and nonischemic muscle. Our view is that segment shortening in that situation represents an integral of normally functioning and dysfunctional muscle, i.e. it is not governed solely by the ischemic muscle. Consequently we would predict that substantial, albeit somewhat reduced, shortening should be evident in nonischemic muscle adjacent to the perfusion boundary when conventional segment lengths are used.
Marcus: Did you use data from gauges implanted in myocardium with mixed sources of perfusion? This might represent a problem because you can not be sure how much normal and how much ischemic tissue is in the muscle subtended by the sonomicrometers.
Gallagher: We tried to be as rigorous as we could. If we could not define the perfusion boundary within the limits stated, we discarded the data. We proceeded on the assumption that the flow boundary is a perpendicular line between the epicardium and endocardium. In fact it is actually somewhat irregular. The manner in which we sectioned the heart meant that we observed a very poorly defined perfusion boundary if the true boundary was particularly irregular or oblique. In this case, the crystals would cross muscle with normal flow and abnormal flow. For the time being we have kept data derived from those sonomicrometers out of the analysis. We hope to be able to deal with irregular flow boundaries in the future.
Sideman: We have a combination of low perfusion, low mechanical stress, less oxygen demand in the border of the ischemic region. How would the electrical activation be affected?
Bassingthwaighte: My question is almost related. Did you examine the zone-thickness with respect for fiber direction? The reason for my question is that in the injured area you have depolarization and dysfunction, and the time length constant may be longer in the direction of the fiber than perpendicular to it. You then may see a longer border zone along the fibers than across the fibers.

Gallagher: We did the wall thickening studies because it gave us a relatively discrete measurement. We tried to categorize what happens in cylinders 3 mm in diameter parallel to the perfusion boundary. The other reason for wall thickening studies is to avoid the fiber orientation problem completely so we do not have to worry how it affects our measurement. It is thus difficult to draw solid conclusions from wall thickening data as to what happens in the direction of the fibers, whether in terms of depolarization of velocity of conduction.

Sonnenblick: You may be going at a fine question with a sledge hammer. You are trying to look at fine edges and anticipated a wide border but you showed that there was a narrow border. But what you found may have been due to artifacts from anatomical irregularities. The fine precision that you postulate is impossible, given the method you use to measure wall thickness. The dilemma is that you want to find details about a fine edge, but you use something that by its very nature had a width that does not let you to define the area that you want to look at.

Gallagher: From where we stood, this was the best technique to attack the problem. We actually expected that the functional border zone would be larger than what we found. We still think it is worthy of study in more detail, using these methods.

Arts: I would like to relate to data I got from our laboratory, from Dr Frits Prinzen. We plotted blood flow in the inner myocardial layers, across the border zone area. We also measured segment length shortening at the epicardium and superimposed these data onto the 'map' of blood flow data. Percent shortening was low in the central ischemic area and was normal in the central nonischemic area. Of course, it is not ideal, but is is the best we could do. These are the raw data. The functional border zone, in the data of Kim Gallagher is quite steep. If you take the average of our curves then you see on average a wider border of functional impairment in nonischemic muscle. The distance between each point on the slide is about 4 mm so the length of the zone of nonischemic dysfunction is about 8–10 mm.

Gallagher: Using the average data from all the dogs we had, assuming that the distribution of functional changes are the same at both lateral border created by circumflex occlusion, we constructed this figure which describes the extent of the ischemic area and extent of dysfunction in a cross-section of the left ventricle. The functional border zone is about 4 millimeters wide when measured at the endocardium but about 8–9 millimeters measured at the epicardium because of the difference in endocardial and epicardial circumferences. The measurements of Prinzen were made at the epicardium and we are in pretty close agreement. Because my measurements were at the endocardium and Prinzen's at the epicardium, the larger epicardial than endocardial circumference explains the apparent difference.

32. Assisted circulation as a tool for the study of cardiac models and cardiac performance

W. WELKOWITZ, J.K.-J. LI and J. ZELANO

Abstract

The intraaortic balloon pump (IABP) is a cardiac assist device used for pre- and postoperative support of patients undergoing cardiac surgery. The device exerts its hemodynamic effects by synchronously removing a fixed volume of blood from an aortic compartment out of phase with the natural heart. Balloon inflation during diastole increases systemic and coronary perfusion pressures. Balloon deflation triggered just prior to isovolumetric systole causes a reduction of myocardial afterload leading to increased cardiac output. These hemodynamic parameters may be altered by varying the phasing of the device relative to the cardiac cycle which changes the mechanical interaction between IABP and the cardiovascular system. This allows one to perturb the operating state of the heart and provides a means of studying cardiac function under a variety of pathological conditions.

A number of experiments were performed on anesthetized open chest infarcted dogs. Device phasing was varied by changing the timing of inflation and deflation. Helium and nitrogen were interchanged as balloon shuttle gases to alter inflation/deflation rates. Simultaneous recordings of aortic and left ventricular pressures, coronary (QC) and aortic (SV) flows, ECG, and muscle segment lengths in both normal and ischemic border zones were taken. Changes in tension-time index (TTI), endocardial viability ratio (EVR), hemodynamic power output (Wlv) and aortic input resistance (Rin) were computed from these parameters. The percentage change from control was computed for QC and SV. Pressure-length loops for the ventricular normal zone were plotted for several timing conditions.

Results indicate that greater enhancements in hemodynamic parameters occur for rapid balloon inflation/deflation rates. SV, QC, and Wlv displayed definite maxima as a function of inflation and deflation timing. Rin showed a distinct minimum as a function of deflation timing. Strong correlation was observed between changes in QC and EVR while TTI became larger as Rin was increased for different timing conditions. Enhanced Wlv was apparent as EVR increased, indicating augmented power output as a function of increased myocardial oxygen supply/demand ratio. The intrinsic contractility of the ventricular normal zone was determined from the end systolic pressure-length relationship obtained for different timing conditions.

The results indicate the viability of IABP as a probe of physiological function. The ability of IABP to alter cardiac performance provides a useful tool for the study of myocardial function.

Introduction

In general we would like to describe the structure and function (anatomy and physiology) of the heart in both normal and abnormal states and in greater and greater detail. In order to arrive at this description, it has been found useful to perturb the heart (for example by the use of drugs) to obtain quantitative information concerning the physiological performance. Pharmacological agents have been frequently used to alter the physiological determinants of myocardial oxygen demand. These include vasodilators, beta blockers, and diuretics. Similarly, positive inotropic agents have been used to reduce cardiac volume. While pharmacological agents permit the study of cardiac physiology under much variation, it has now been found useful in animal studies to artificially induce ischemic and infarcted regions into the myocardium (by blocking some coronary arteries) in order to study the responses of both the ischemic tissue and the remaining normal tissue. In addition to pharmacolgical and surgical interventions being used to study the performance of the heart under widely varying conditions, it has been shown [1] that mechanical interaction in the form of mechanical cardiac assistance (or more specifically, intraaortic balloon pumping) when coupled with surgical intervention can radically alter the cardiac state.

The intraaortic balloon pump is a counterpulsation device which removes blood from an intravascular region synchronized with the cardiac cycle. The balloon is inflated during diastole and deflated during systole. The deflation causes a rapid decrease in aortic pressure thus the left ventricle ejects blood against a lesser load, improving ventricular performance. The inflation during diastole causes a rise in aortic pressure which results in increased coronary artery perfusion pressure and flow [2]. It is important to note that the intraaortic balloon cannot produce forward flow in the aorta as does a bypass pump. The entire cardiac output must pass through the left ventricle. The effectiveness of the device comes about by altering hemodynamic parameters and improving ventricular performance by decreasing afterload and oxygen consumption and by increasing coronary flow, cardiac output and myocardial energetics.

Some of the effects of balloon pumping can be analyzed in terms of the endocardial viability ratio [3, 4], the ratio of diastolic pressure time index to tension time index. The tension time index is a measure of myocardial oxygen demand and is the time integral of aortic pressure during systole. The diastolic pressure time index is a measure of the myocardial oxygen supply and is the time integral of the aortic pressure minus the left ventricular pressure over diastole. Balloon pumping increases the difference between aortic and ventricular pressure during diastole and also reduces systolic pressure. Thus it is a technique to decrease oxygen demand and increase oxygen supply. Additionally, the resultant systolic unloading produces improved cardiac performance at reduced myocardial energy requirements.

Besides its effects on the oxygen supply and demand, balloon pumping produces direct hemodynamic effects (particularly in ischemic animals). These include increased cardiac output, reduced end diastole pressure, reduced systolic pressure, and reduced end diastolic volume. Thus, the balloon pump is clearly a tool that can be used to study the heart under varying metabolic conditions as well as varying hemodynamic (or mechanical) conditions.

Description of the balloon pump as an experimental tool

It has been suggested above that the balloon pump could be a tool to study the heart under various conditions of oxygen supply and demand and of hemodynamic state. In order to be of great use in this regard, it must be possible to vary the control parameters over a reasonably wide range in order to assess the sensitivity of cardiac characteristics to such changes of control variables. The following material describes the balloon pump as such a tool and discusses the technique for varying the controls by modifying the rate of rise and fall of the balloon inflation and deflation and by altering the time of inflation and time of deflation.

The hardware used was a Datascope Model 80 System modified to permit timing control from an MC68000 microprocessor. The physiological input signals used to control the timing were the R-wave of the electrocardiogram, the second heart sound (S_2), and the atrial P-wave. The systolic time interval was calculated from the R-wave and the second heart sound on a beat to beat basis. The second heart sound and the computed systolic time interval were used to control and vary balloon inflation time. The P-wave and the calculated P-R interval were used to control and vary deflation time. The hemodynamic parameters that were measured were the coronary blood flow, the aortic blood flow, the aortic pressure, and the left ventricular pressure. Segmental muscle shortening was monitored in the normal and ischemic border zones of the myocardium.

Two series of timing experiments were performed. In the first, the deflation time was held constant while the inflation time was varied by fixed amounts in the period prior to the second heart sound. In the second, inflation time was held constant and deflation time was varied from isovolumic systole into late systole. A series of experiments was also performed varying inflation and deflation rates by using two different driving gases of different densities, nitrogen (N_2) and helium (He). Since the changes in the dependent variables were almost always greater in the He experiments as compared to the N_2 experiments, He was used in all timing variation experiments.

Experimental procedures

The experiments that demonstrate the capability of the balloon pump as a device to produce variations in hemodynamic state were performed on anesthetized dogs on a positive pressure respirator. Myocardial ischemia was induced by occluding the left anterior descending coronary artery just distal to the first major branching. For pumping, a single chambered pediatric intraaortic balloon was placed in the descending aorta 2–4 cm below the aortic arch. Balloon counterpulsation was initiated one hour after occlusion using a Datascope Model 80 System with modified pressure and vacuum modules to minimize balloon inflation and deflation time. Ten dogs were tested in the inflation-deflation rate studies. Ten more dogs were studied in the timing experiments. One hour after occlusion, control data was taken for eight to ten heartbeats and then the balloon pump was activated for ten to fifteen heartbeats. Pumping was terminated for at least fifty beats to allow the cardiovascular system to return to its control state. For data evaluation each assisted data set was paired with the immediately preceding control data set. For the assisted set the second and third heart cycles following the control set were analyzed and averaged. In all cases the effects of balloon pumping were expressed as percent changes between the assisted and unassisted hemodynamic measures.

Experimental results

Varying inflation and deflation rates

The first set of experiments demonstrated the possibility of parameter variation using different inflation and deflation rates. Fig. 1 shows the pressure tracings during inflation of the balloon with aortic occlusion using a non-traumatic clamp. The oscilloscope was triggered simultaneously with the pressure solenoid. For He the rise time was 45 msec and for N_2 it was 100 msec. The delay times after triggering are also different for the two gases, however this was compensated for in the experiments so that initiation of inflation and deflation occured at the same time. Typical hemodynamic measurements taken during the experiments are shown in Fig. 2. Tables 1 and 2 show the different effects of the varying rise and fall rates on a number of hemodynamic parameters. The timing settings were for normal inflation-normal deflation, early inflation-normal deflation, and normal

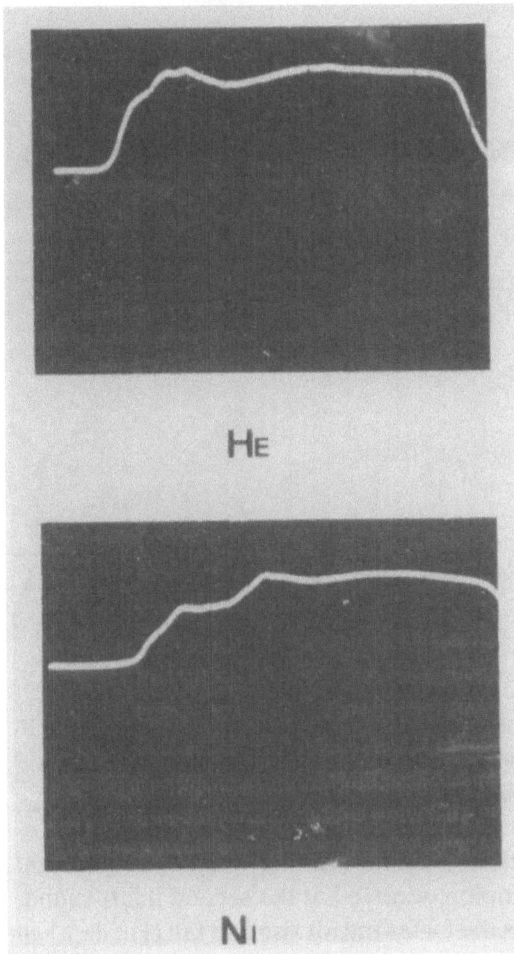

Figure 1. Balloon rise times measured in vivo.

Table 1. Hemodynamic results of intra-aortic balloon pumping using He or N_2 as the driving gas; percent changes from control during IABP.

		QC	SV	EDP	VPP	LN	LB
He	NI-ND	31.0	32.3	10.93	−3.8	6.5	8.7
N_2	NI-ND	12.0	18.0	17.1	−1.0	2.57	1.8
He	EI-ND	37.0	45.0	9.7	−6.3	8.5	9.6
N_2	EI-ND	16.0	25.0	12.6	−4.0	3.89	2.1
He	NI-LD	26.0	21.0	12.0	7.5	2.6	5.0
N_2	NI-LD	7.0	−1.3	14.9	3.0	−6.25	−12.7

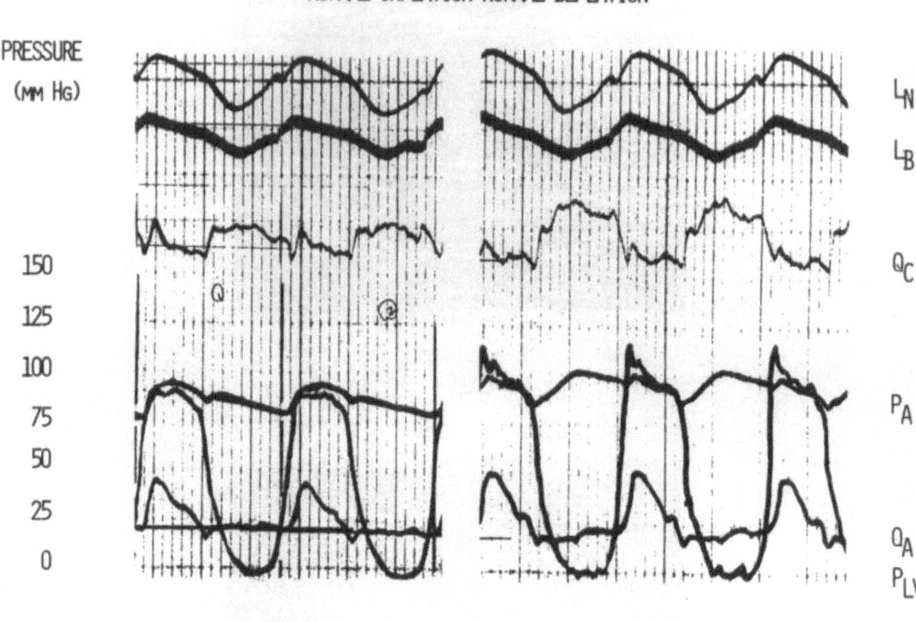

Figure 2. Typical experimental data.

inflation-late deflation. Normal inflation was chosen so that the rise in aortic pressure due to pumping occurred at the second heart sound.

In almost all cases the faster rate of rise and fall (He data) appeared to produce greater changes than the slower rates. The hemodynamic changes were most marked for coronary blood flow and stroke volume. The results in Table 2 for aortic input resistance (afterload) and for left ventricular hemodynamic power output were calculated for the case of normal inflation-normal deflation. Clearly with helium, sizeable afterload reduction and reasonable power output reduction were obtainable.

Varying inflation times

While varying inflation and deflation rates is one way of obtaining varying hemodynamic parameters, it is clearly a limited method since obtaining a wide variation in these rates requires the use of different pumping gases, a cumbersome procedure. An alternate method that can be used for wider control is to vary the timing of inflation and deflation from the approximately normal inflation at

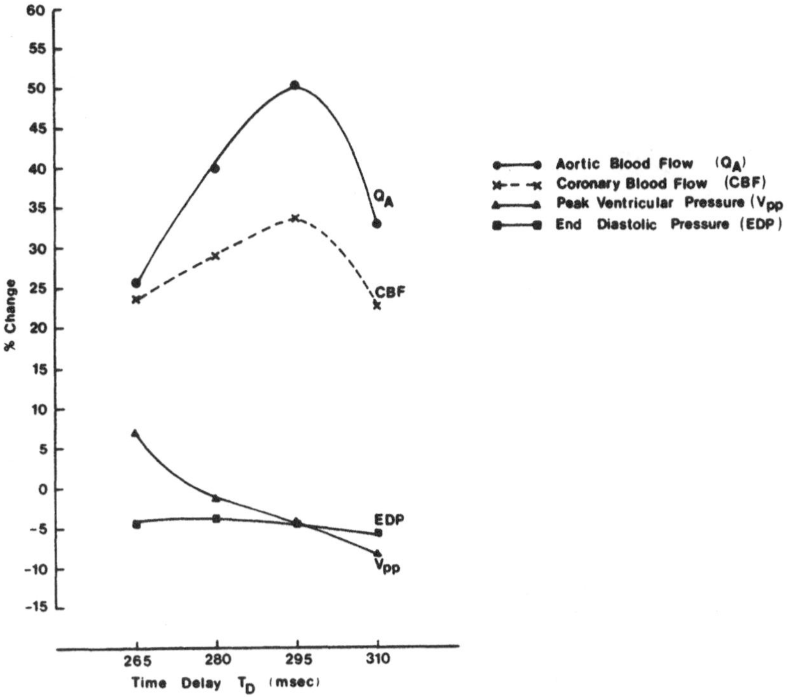

Figure 3. Percentage change from control of hemodynamic parameters vs time delay of balloon inflation (T_D) following the R-wave.

the dichrotic notch and deflation at the R-wave. The first set of such data was taken with balloon deflation time kept constant at the end of isovolumic systole. The initial run was done for inflation at S_2, while in subsequent runs inflation was started earlier in increments of 15 msec. Fig. 3 shows the changes obtainable in hemodynamic variables as a function of this timing variation, while Fig. 4 shows the changes in average term ventricular power and in aortic input resistance. For a somewhat different fixed deflation time, Fig. 5 shows the variation in tension time index (oxygen demand) and, in endocardial viability ratio (ratio of oxygen

Table 2. Percent changes during assistance in Zin and Wlv as a function of balloon driving gases, He and N_2.

Harmonic	N_2		He	
	Zin	Wlv	Zin	Wlv
O(DC)	−9.6	9.16	−31.7	13.9
1	−12.8	2.10	−45.7	11.5

Normal deflation was chosen so that balloon collapse was initiated at the R-wave. Early inflation was initiated 30 msec before S_2. Late deflation started 30 msec after the R-wave.

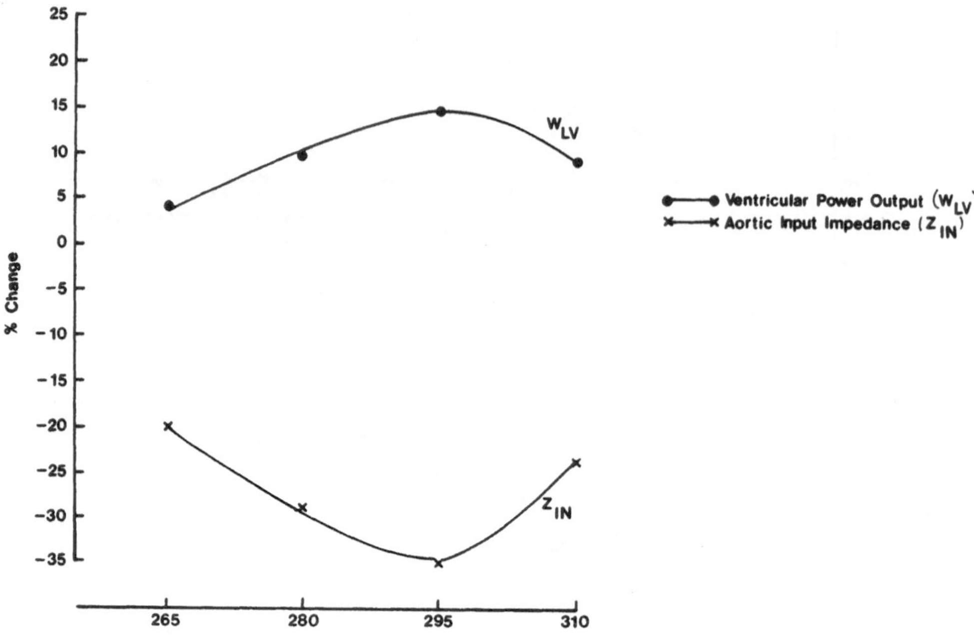

Figure 4. Percentage change from control of average ventricular power output (DC) and aortic input impedance (DC) vs time delay of balloon inflation (T_D).

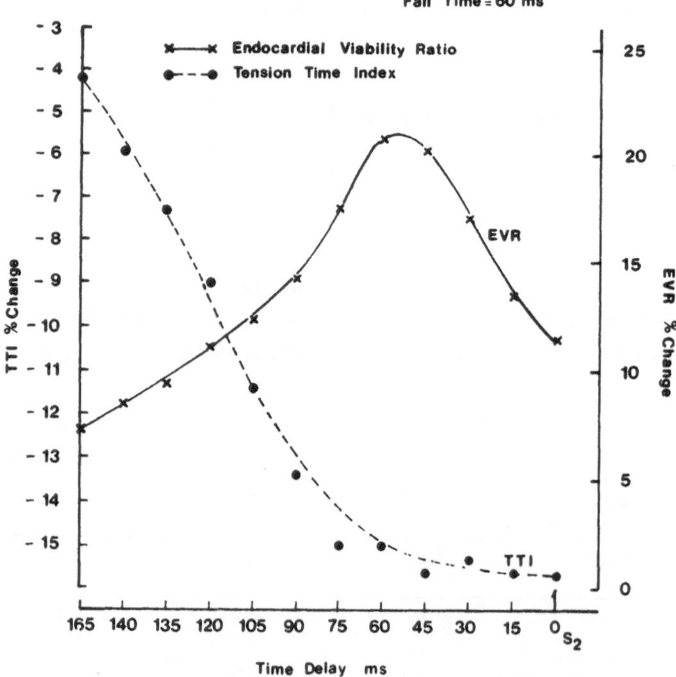

Figure 5. Percentage change from control of tension time index (TTI) and endocardial viability ratio (EVR) vs delay of balloon inflation preceding the second heart sound (S_2).

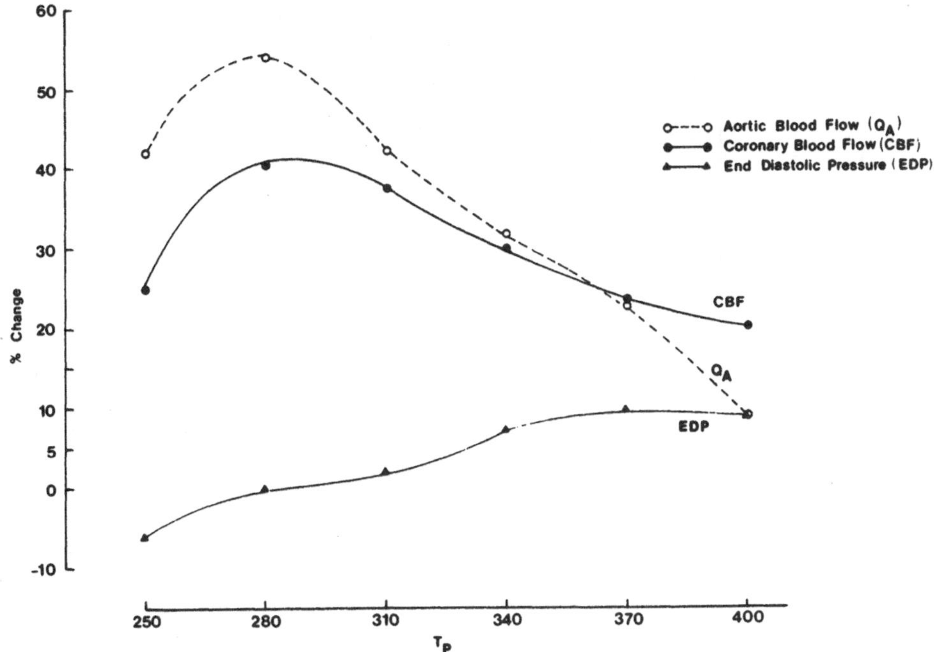

Figure 6. Percentage change from control of hemodynamic parameters vs primary interval (T_p) late deflation mode.

supply to oxygen demand) as a function of varying inflation time. It is apparent from Figures 3, 4, and 5 that induced ischemia plus counterpulsation is a reasonable tool for modifying hemodynamic parameters, controlling ventricular pressure, reducing afterload, and varying oxygen supply and demand.

Varying deflation times

The next set of data taken looked at variations in balloon deflation timing. In this set of data, inflation was held constant at the second heart sound and deflation, which was initially at the end of isovolumic systole, was delayed in 30 msec increments. In a manner comparable to the variable inflation time data, Fig. 6 shows the changes in hemodynamic variables as a function of the deflation timing variation, Fig. 7 shows the changes in average term ventricular power and in aortic input resistance, and Fig. 8 shows the variation in tension time index and endocardial viability ratio. It is again apparent that the procedure outlined provides a tool for modifying the physiology of the heart.

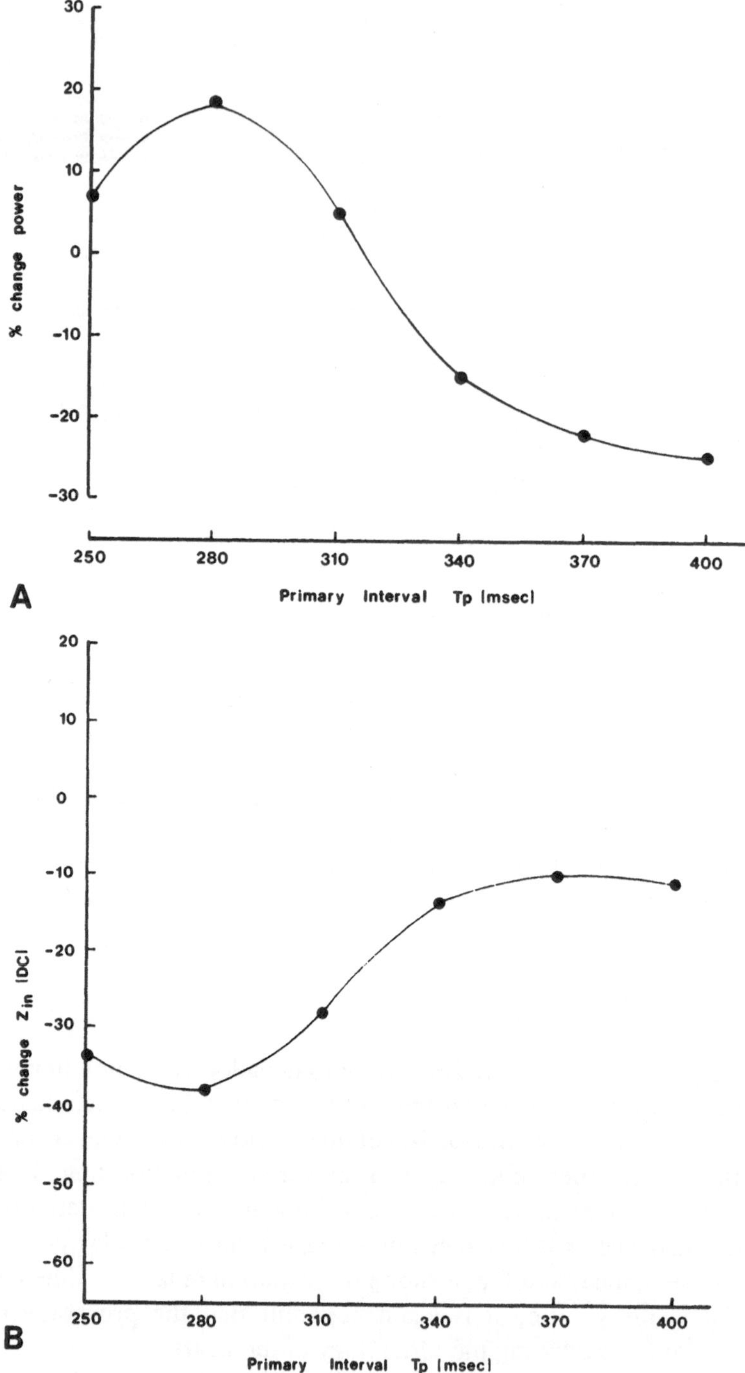

Figure 7. A: percentage change of average ventricular power output (DC) vs primary interval (T_p). B: percentage change of aortic input impedance Z_{in} (DC) vs primary interval (T_p).

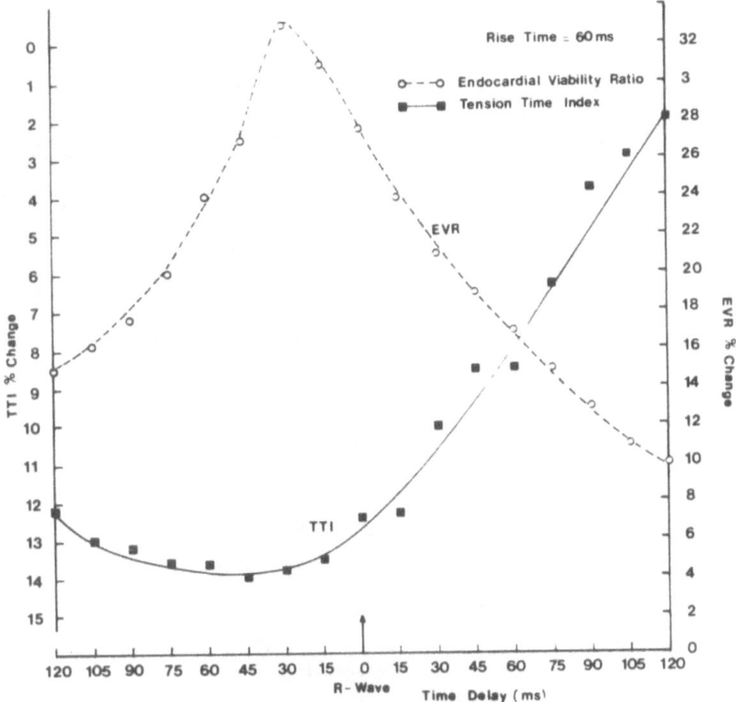

Figure 8. Percentage change from control of tension time index (TTI) and endocardial viability ratio (EVR) vs time delay of balloon deflation.

Relating physiological variables

Thus far, it has been demonstrated that either inflation or deflation timing variations lead to appreciable changes in measurable physiological variables. However, the usefulness of this procedure as a test tool depends upon the ability to interpret the data in terms of the interactions among the physiological and metabolic (or metabolically related) variables. Fig. 9 is one demonstration of this capability. In this case, using variable deflation timing data, the reduction in tension time index is plotted against the reduction in aortic input resistance. The results clearly show the reduction in myocardial oxygen consumption that occurs when there is a measurable reduction in afterload. In Fig. 10 the change in endocardial viability ratio (DPTI/TTI) is plotted against the change in coronary blood flow when inflation timing was varied. As expected, an increase in coronary blood flow produces an increase in oxygen supply and a resultant increase in endocardial viability ratio. Any concomittant decrease in oxygen consumption due to the balloon pumping would even further increase the endocardial viability ratio. Finally, in Fig. 11, the change in the average term ventricular power is

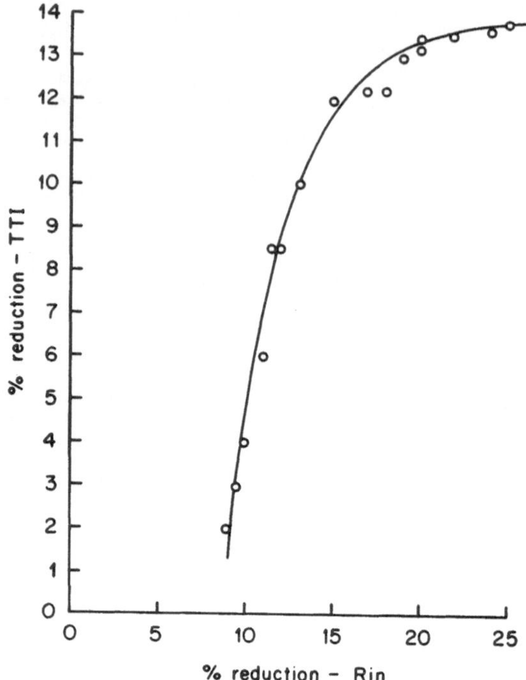

Figure 9. Reduction in tension time index (TTI) vs reduction in aortic input resistance.

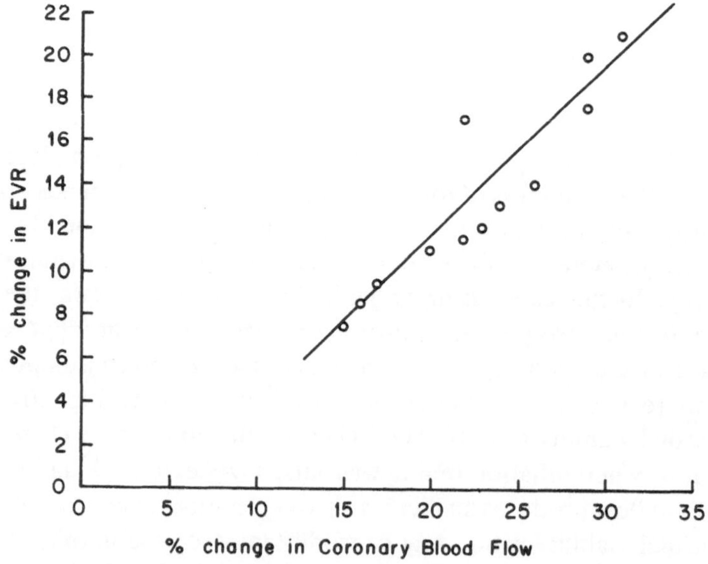

Figure 10. Increase in endocardial viability ratio (EVR) vs increase in coronary blood flow.

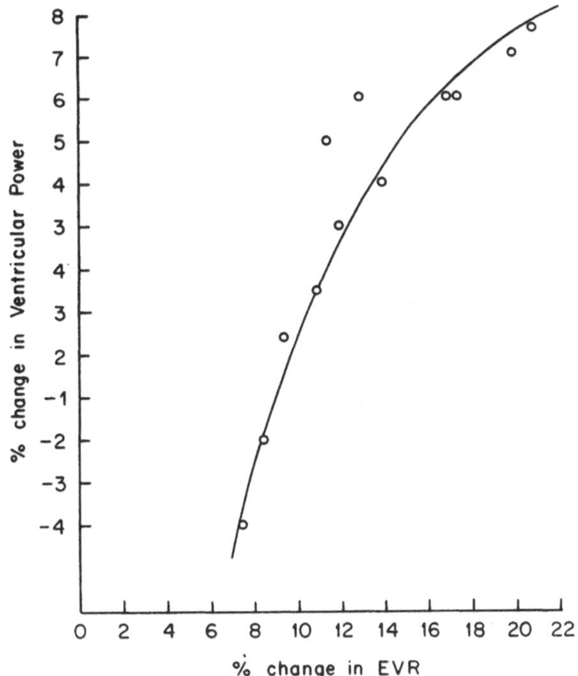

Figure 11. Changes in average ventricular power output (WLV) vs changes in endocardial viability ratio (EVR).

plotted against the change in endocardial viability ratio. These results show that as the ratio of oxygen supply to demand is improved, the average work that the damaged left ventricle can perform is increased.

Conclusions

The extensive measurements and the derived interelationships among variables presented, appear to clearly demonstrate the utility of surgically induced ischemia coupled with mechanical circulatory assistance as a tool for studying the physiology of the heart. With simple timing controls and a small number of hemodynamic measurements, it was possible to carry out this study for a reasonable range of variables and to permit the calculations of sensitivity information as a function of some metabolically related characteristics.

One question that arises is whether this technique can be used to validate different ventricular models and to differentiate between models on the basis of sensitivity to the induced perturbations. Clearly such ventricle models can be incorporated into systems which include balloon pump models for appropriate computer analysis. Welkowitz et al. [5] described such a system that includes a

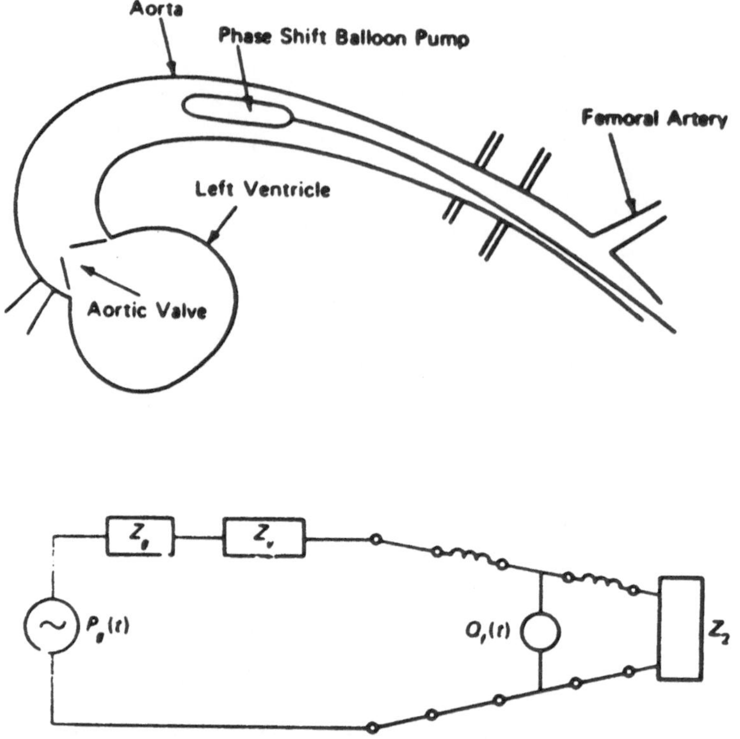

Figure 12. A left ventricle model coupled to balloon pump and systemic circulation models.

source pressure-source impedance ventricle model and derived the appropriate equations for exercising the model. A network representation of this system is shown in Fig. 12.

Another question that should be explored is whether this procedure has any advantages over pharmacological studies. Clearly there are no chemical side effects. On the other hand, the combination of surgically induced ischemia and balloon pumping is certainly a major insult to the cardiovascular system. Possibly the information obtained with this procedure can be complementary to that obtained through drug studies.

A final important consideration is whether this approach could be used to measure intrinsic contractility. At the same time that hemodynamic measurements were made, segmental muscle shortening was monitored by inserting pairs of piezoelectric ultrasonic dimension gauges in the normal and the ischemic border zones of the myocardium. Some of the changes obtainable with these measurements were shown in Table 1. It has been pointed out [6] that a plot of end systolic pressure vs. end-systolic volume for different loading conditions yields a linear relationship that is independent of preload and afterload. The slope of this line is the maximum elastance of the left ventricle. If the heart is given inotropic

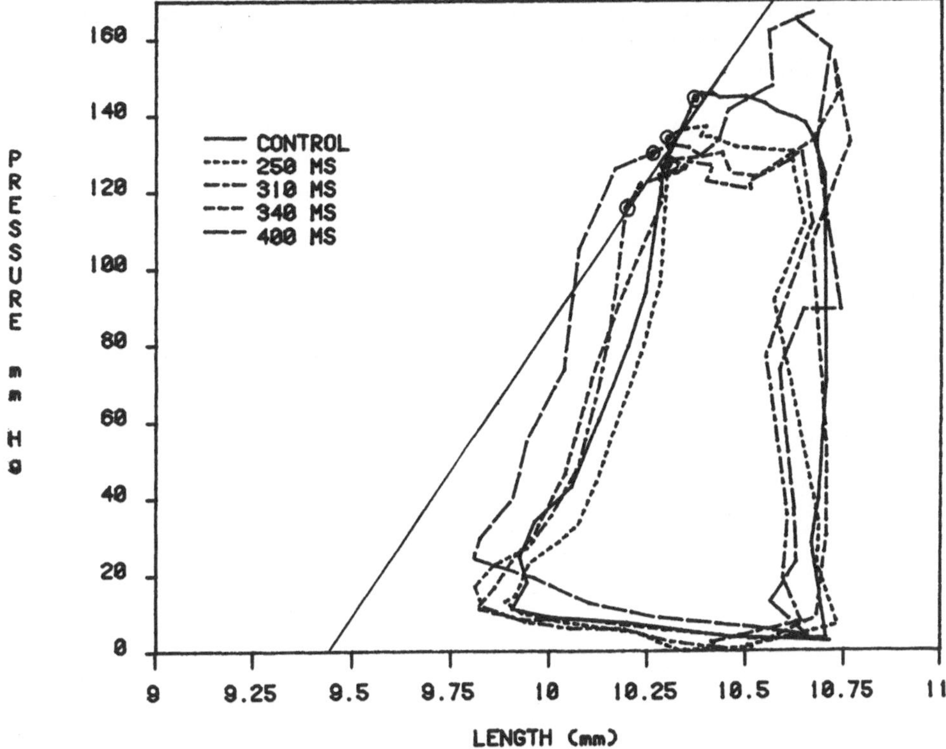

Figure 13. Pressure-length diagrams in the normal zone vs primary interval (T_p), late deflation.

agents, the slope of this line changes. Thus it is a measure of cardiac contractility. Using the segmental length data from the normal myocardial region while deflation timing is varied, it is possible to plot pressure-segment length curves. The variation in timing produces variations in loading. This leads to the set of pressure-length curves shown in Fig. 13 and permits one to draw an experimentally derived maximum elastance curve as shown in the figure. The slope of this line is a measure of intrinsic contractility of the myocardium.

References

1. Welkowitz W (1983): Cardiac control mechanisms in adaptation to the left ventricular assist device. Adv Cardiovasc Phys 5: 102.
2. Clauss RH, Birtwell WC, Albertal G, Lunzer S, Taylor WJ, Fosberg AM, Harken DE (1961): Assisted circulation. I. The arterial counterpulsator. J Thorac Cardiovasc Surg 41: 447.
3. Buckberg GD, Fixler DE, Archie JP (1972): Experimental subendocardial ischemia in dogs with normal coronary arteries. Circ Res 30: 67.
4. Phillips PA, Marty AT, Mirjamoto AM (1975): A clinical method for detecting subendocaridal ischemia after cardiopulmonary bypass. J Thorac Cardiovasc Surg 69: 30.

5. Welkowitz W (1977): Engineering hemodynamics: application to cardiac assist devices. Lexington books, D.C. Heath, Lexington, Mass.
6. Sagawa K (1978): The ventricular pressure-volume diagram revisited. Circ Res 43: C77.

Discussion

Spaan: How was the flow measured? Would it not be wise to measure oxygen consumption?
Welkowitz: The flow was measured with an electromagnetic flowmeter placed around the left main coronary artery. It would definitely be better to measure oxygen consumption rather than to infer it from the calculated tension time index.

33. Modulation of coronary autoregulatory responses

J.M. CANTY Jr and F.J. KLOCKE

Abstract

A number of studies of the coronary circulation in anesthetized animals have established the general features of the autoregulatory relationship between mean coronary pressure and flow and have documented vulnerability of the subendocardium to ischemia as coronary pressure is reduced. Although reductions in subendocardial flow and inner-outer flow ratio have been interpreted to indicate maximal vasodilation of the subendocardial vascular bed, recent studies have confirmed that reductions in resting subendocardial perfusion can occur in the face of vasodilator reserve recruitable by infusion of pharmacologic agents. These findings suggest that factors other than local metabolic mechanisms importantly modulate or potentially limit coronary autoregulatory responses. Interactions among regional myocardial performance, metabolic demand and flow remain incompletely characterized. In addition, although various extrinsic factors influencing coronary flow have been studied at normal coronary artery pressures, their potential influence on coronary autoregulation and subendocardial flow at reduced coronary pressures has been difficult to define. This article reviews limitations of intrinsic coronary autoregulatory responses, modulation of these responses by extrinsic factors, and possible chronic adaptations to reduced coronary artery pressure.

Introduction

Previous studies have demonstrated that coronary blood flow is autoregulated during acute changes in coronary perfusion pressure as metabolic demand and contractile function remain constant[1, 2]. In contrast to the strong autoregulation of flow which has been characteristic of skeletal muscle and kidney, coronary flow is less perfectly controlled within the autoregulatory pressure range, which has usually been considered to be between 70 and 140 mm Hg [3].

The characteristics of coronary autoregulation are complicated by significant transmural variations. These are the result of increased subendocardial metabolic demand and a greater importance of time-averaged compressive effects generated on the subendocardial vascular bed during cardiac contraction [4]. Studies by Rouleau et al. have demonstrated that subendocardial flow begins to fall at a critical diastolic pressure-time index:systolic pressure-time index (DPTI:SPTI) ratio [5]. Their results established that subendocardial vasodilator reserve is exhausted before subepicardial vasodilator reserve in a preparation in which compressive effects on subendocardial vasodilator reserve are relatively great due to high resting heart rates. Similar reductions in subendocardial flow with progressive reductions in coronary pressure distal to a stenosis have been reported by Guyton et al. [6]. Below a coronary pressure of 70 mm Hg, subendocardial flow began to fall, while epicardial flow remained constant to coronary pressures of 40 mm Hg. The possibility of vasodilator reserve at a time when subendocardial flow was reduced was not examined in either study.

The consequence of a reduction in subendocardial blood flow is a concomitant reduction in regional myocardial function as measured by subendocardial circumferential systolic shortening or systolic wall thickening. Downey demonstrated a close correlation between myocardial function measured by an isometric force gauge and mean coronary flow in an anesthetized preparation in which autoregulation was present [7]. Gallagher et al. related systolic wall thickening obtained by sonomicrometry and regional subendocardial flow in anesthetized animals [8]. Moderate reductions in mean coronary pressure to 55 mm Hg reduced subendocardial flow significantly and resulted in ~50% reductions in wall thickening. Weintraub et al. found significant reductions in both subendocardial flow and subendocardial segment shortening at diastolic coronary pressures below 50 mm Hg [9]. Studies by Vatner [10] and Gallagher et al. [11] in conscious animals also documented a close correlation between subendocardial flow and function. The relationship between coronary pressure and subendocardial function during autoregulation in individual animals has not been studied systematically in anesthetized or awake animals.

Although severe reductions in regional subendocardial function are associated with metabolic evidence of myocardial ischemia [12, 13], it is currently not clear whether mild reductions in subendocardial flow and function may represent a new balance between myocardial supply and demand when inflow is limited. Such a mechanism would suggest that local mechanisms are capable of regulating regional myocardial function in response to reductions in coronary inflow which are not severe. Such a phenomenon was originally suggested by Gregg in the late 1950's [14]. The 'Gregg Phenomenon' was studied in numerous laboratories with various preparations and has recently been reviewed by Feigl [15]. The general finding was that an increase in coronary flow from low values to those present during spontaneous autoregulation was associated with an increase in myocardial oxygen consumption of 10–20%. The mechanism of this response remains unclear.

Limitations of intrinsic autoregulatory responses

The generally held concept of coronary autoregulation has been that metabolic stimuli are the predominant factor underlying coronary flow regulation [1, 2, 15]. Although their importance has been difficult to demonstrate and/or quantitate, neural and/or myogenic influences have also been thought possibly to play a role. When autoregulatory mechanisms fail to maintain flow constant, the reduction in flow has usually been interpreted to indicate that some portion of the distal vascular bed is maximally vasodilated (since oxygen extraction is near maximal under resting conditions). However, until recently, transmural vasodilator reserve at a time when coronary flow is reduced during spontaneous autoregulation had not been examined.

Four laboratories have now reported that reductions in subendocardial flow occur regularly in anesthetized animals during spontaneous autoregulation at a time when vasodilator reserve recruitable by intracoronary infusion of adenosine is present. Canty and Klocke studied coronary autoregulation in anesthetized dogs which were paced at a heart rate of 60 bpm after producing AV block [16]. Coronary artery pressure was reduced from 90 mm Hg to 35 mm Hg resulting in a reduction in subendocardial flow of ~40% to a mean value of 0.35 $ml \cdot min^{-1} \cdot g^{-1}$. Despite a substantial reduction in the autoregulated flow value, subendocardial flow was able to increase to 1.1 $ml \cdot min^{-1} \cdot g^{-1}$ during intracoronary infusion of adenosine while heart rate, systemic pressure and coronary artery pressure remained constant. When coronary pressure was reduced to 25 mm Hg, subendocardial flow fell further and subendocardial vasodilator reserve was no longer demonstrable but epicardial reserve was still present. These data established that reductions in resting coronary flow do not necessarily indicate that the distal vascular bed is maximally vasodilated. They also indicated that, despite a low resting heart rate (and correspondingly reduced time-averaged compressive effects), subendocardial vasodilator reserve was exhausted before subepicardial vasodilator reserve but at lower pressures than previously reported in anesthetized animals, i.e., between 25–35 mm Hg.

Similar findings have been reported by Aversano and Becker in an anesthetized preparation in which heart rate and compressive effects were substantially greater [17]. They found that subendocardial flow was regularly reduced at a time when adenosine-recruitable reserve was present. They provided limited measurements of subendocardial function using sonomicrometry and showed an improvement in segment shortening after vasodilation when the reduced coronary pressure was held constant. The overall extent of improvement in subendocardial flow was greater than that in myocardial function. Pantely et al. observed a similar phenomenon in swine using a hydraulic occluder to reduce pressure in the left anterior descending artery [18]. Although adenosine-recruitable vasodilator reserve was always observed at a time when coronary flow and regional function (as determined by wall thickening) were reduced, there was, in contrast to the results of Aversano, no significant improvement in regional function during infusion of adenosine. It is difficult to reconcile the difference in functional response. One possibility is that regional wall thickening is a less sensitive index of myocardial ischemia than segment shortening. In addition, neither study reported control values of myocardial function after the period in which coronary pressure, subendocardial flow and myocardial function were reduced. Many laboratories have reported that brief periods of myocardial ischemia result in prolonged periods of regional myocardial dysfunction or 'stunned myocardium' [19]. Preliminary studies in conscious animals from our laboratory document that this phenomenon occurs regularly when regional function is reduced more than 25% below control levels. It therefore seems necessary to compare functional responses before and after vasodilation, allowing a prolonged period for regional myocardial function to return to baseline levels. This, however, is difficult to accomplish in anesthetized preparations.

Grattan et al. [20] have utilized a canine preparation in which the left main coronary artery rather than one of its branches is cannulated (thereby obviating possible effects of collateral flow at low pressures in the cannulated bed). Radioactive microsphere flow measurements documented that pharmacological vasodilation increases flow in all transmural layers at low coronary artery pressures. The authors concluded that exhaustion of flow reserve is not the mechanism by which subendocardial ischemia occurs in this preparation.

Each of the above studies is in agreement that reductions in subendocardial flow during spontaneous autoregulation occur regularly in the anesthetized animal at a time when adenosine-recruitable vasodilator reserve persists. The significance of recruitable vasodilator reserve in a model employing a fixed coronary stenosis is complicated by effects on distal coronary pressure following vasodilation. The increased pressure drop across the stenosis during vasodilation has, under many circumstances, been demonstrated to result in a transmural steal due to a reduction in post-stenotic coronary pressure [21]. The effects of less intense vasodilatory stimuli, which may potentially result in preferential subendocardial vasodilation (i.e., submaximal adenosine, α-adrenergic blockade or calcium channel blockers), remain to be elucidated.

Grover and Weiss have recently demonstrated that a reduced level of regional myocardial metabolism is able to increase in response to stress despite a significant reduction in resting coronary flow [22]. They measured subendocardial oxygen consumption using a micro-Fick technique. Coronary flow was restricted to 50% of baseline in a group of animals paced at their control rate and in a group of animals subsequently paced 50% above the control rate. Subendocardial oxygen consumption was reduced after partial occlusion but increased during pacing despite the same level of coronary stenosis. These results indicate that although coronary flow and oxygen consumption were reduced distal to the stenosis, metabolic reserve resulting in an increase in oxygen consumption could be recruited. Thus, a reduction in resting flow was accompanied by metabolic evidence of reduced oxygen utilization, with the latter then being able to increase during the additional stress of atrial pacing. The detailed metabolic responses to milder levels of subendocardial functional impairment remain to be elucidated.

Three additional studies have documented reductions in regional perfusion at a time when adenosine-recruitable reserve is present. Gorman and Sparks observed a progressive flow impairment after three hours of regional myocardial ischemia obtained by holding coronary pressure constant at 50 mm Hg during atrial pacing at 180 bpm [23]. Despite a reduction in flow and lactate production indicating subendocardial ischemia, intracoronary adenosine infusion resulted in improved subendocardial flow. Gold and Bache demonstrated reductions in right ventricular subendocardial flow during acute right ventricular pressure overload in sedated dogs at a time when vasodilator reserve could be demonstrated during intravenous infusion of adenosine [24]. In 1980, our laboratories reported reductions in regional flow in the face of adenosine-recruitable vasodilator reserve in an animal model simulating a coronary artery 'muscle bridge' [25].

In summary, there is substantial evidence to suggest that intrinsic autoregulatory flow responses during coronary pressure reduction may be limited in the sense that coronary vasodilation is not always maximal. Extrinsic vascular factors may be responsible for this limitation. Alternatively, it may relate to the intrinsic autoregulatory stimuli available at any given level of metabolic demand.

Modulation of coronary autoregulatory responses

Factors modulating intrinsic autoregulatory flow responses have only recently begun to be clarified and are important with regard to the issues outlined above. If flow regulation is less precise under certain circumstances and reductions in regional flow occur at a time when vasodilator reserve exists, reductions in regional myocardial metabolism and function may represent an important adaptive response. Preliminary studies by Dole et al. [26] have examined the influence of coronary venous oxygen content in determining the steady-state gain [27] of the autoregulatory response at normal coronary pressures. When coronary venous oxygen saturation increased following a reduction in heart rate, the gain of the autoregulatory response was near zero, indicating large changes in coronary blood flow with changes in coronary artery pressure. Increasing heart rate resulted in a reduction in coronary venous oxygen content and an improvement in steady-state flow regulation, manifest by an increase in autoregulatory gain to approximately 0.5. These data suggest that the intrinsic level of myocardial oxygen demand may importantly modulate autoregulatory flow responses. They also support the hypothesis that flow regulation at basal levels of myocardial oxygen consumption may be less precise than during states characterized by elevated metabolic demand. The importance of this regulation on a transmural basis and the functional and metabolic consequences of a reduced autoregulatory response have not been examined.

The importance of arterial oxygen supply on coronary autoregulation also remains unclear. Weisfeldt reported that increasing arterial PO_2 improved the characteristics of flow regulation in terms of maintaining flow constant [28]. Although coronary venous PO_2 was not measured, it seems likely that it was increased during hyperoxia. The results seem at odds with those outlined above suggesting that coronary venous PO_2 is an important determinant of the adequacy of flow regulation [26]. Previous studies [15, 29] have suggested that oxygen is a coronary vasoconstrictor and are supported by recent in vitro experiments on excised vascular rings [30]. Vasoconstrictor effects, however, are difficult to separate from appropriate metabolic constriction due to the increased oxygen supply without determining the adequacy of subendocardial oxygen delivery or the characteristics of steady-state autoregulation. Surjadhana et al. studied the effects of polycythemia on coronary autoregulation by examining the relation between DPTI and SPTI [31]. Their results showed that despite an increased oxygen carrying capacity, polycythemia resulted in vulnerability of the subendocardium to ischemia at a higher diastolic pressure-time index, indicating an important effect of viscosity on transmural vasodilator reserve. Direct effects of arterial oxygen content on autoregulation have been difficult to separate from effects on resting coronary flow and vascular resistance due to changes in viscosity when hemoglobin is manipulated.

Studies of extrinsic vascular factors affecting coronary vasomotor tone have generally been conducted at resting levels of coronary pressure. Since most pharmacologic agents have been infused systemically, it has been difficult to separate direct effects of the agents on coronary vasomotor tone from reflex effects on coronary vascular resistance secondary to changes in systemic hemodynamics. Interventions which do not affect resting coronary blood flow may alter flow regulation at reduced coronary pressure during spontaneous autoregulation. This is due to the fact that relatively small changes in coronary vascular resistance become proportionately more important when the vascular bed becomes progressively vasodilated as coronary pressure is reduced.

Mohrman and Feigl demonstrated the ability of sympathetic vasoconstriction to modulate coronary flow during intracoronary norepinephrine infusion and carotid sinus hypotension [32]. Their studies established the importance of α-adrenergic tone competing with intrinsic metabolic vasodilation to produce reductions in coronary flow while maintaining oxygen delivery by increased oxygen extraction. Buffington and Feigl studied the transmural distribution of flow during sympathetic activation at reduced coronary pressure [33]. Their results demonstrated significant α-adrenergic constriction despite metabolic evidence of myocardial ischemia during norepinephrine infusion, with the α-constriction overriden during severe ischemia. Heusch and Deussen have suggested that adrenergic constriction distal to a coronary artery stenosis is unmasked at reduced coronary pressures and mediated by a postjunctional α_2-receptor mechanism [34]. The consequences of adrenegeric constrictor tone on regional function at reduced coronary pressure have not been examined.

Recent studies by Khayyal et al. have shown that intracoronary vasopressin can reduce resting coronary flow and regional contractile performance while the coronary artery is perfused at a normal coronary pressure [35]. Importantly, their study also demonstrated that the functional consequences of vasopressin infusion could be reversed by simultaneous infusion of adenosine. Despite significant reductions in resting coronary blood flow and regional contractile performance at the spontaneous coronary pressure, coronary blood flow was autoregulated as coronary pressure was reduced. They interpreted their results to indicate that coronary autoregulation may be modulated by extrinsic vasoconstriction which limits coronary flow. The fact that autoregulation was maintained at a time when functionally significant reductions in resting coronary flow were produced argues against a dominant metabolic control mechanism. An alternative possibility would be that a myogenic mechanism is responsible for pressure-induced autoregulation. The effects of coronary vasodilators outlined earlier may also be compatible with this concept [16–18].

Chronic adaptations to reduced coronary pressure

Chronic adaptations to reductions in coronary flow and coronary pressure may be more complex than adjustments to acute reductions in coronary pressure. Measurements of myocardial perfusion in man employing inert gas techniques which adequately assess heterogeneous perfusion have shown reductions in resting myocardial flow distal to severe coronary stenoses, as compared to normal areas at similar levels of myocardial oxygen demand [36, 37]. Similar conclusions have been reported in studies measuring regional coronary flow using wash-out of radioactive xenon [38]. Resting myocardial flow has also been shown to be reduced in collateral-dependent myocardium distal to total anterior descending artery occlusions [39]. The mechanisms responsible for these chronic reductions in resting coronary flow remain unclear. They generally occur in the absence of clinically detectible myocardial ischemia and do not appear to be the result of myocardial scarring. Chen et al. [40] have suggested that myocardial hypertrophy in the area of the perfused segment could play a role. It is currently uncertain whether vasodilator reserve exists in these areas of reduced perfusion, although a recent preliminary report has shown that some patients may have significant full-thickness vasodilator reserve as measured in response to radiographic contrast administration [41]. These findings suggest that states of reduced perfusion at coronary pressures encountered chronically distal to severe stenoses may represent limitations and/or modulation of autoregulatory flow adjustments having similarities to those which have been demonstrated in response to acute pressure reduction.

The functional performance of myocardium distal to high-grade coronary artery stenoses may be depressed on a chronic basis. St. John Sutton and colleagues measured fractional wall thickening and rates of systolic and diastolic thickening and thinning in patients with significant disease of the left main or anterior descending coronary artery [42]. Although only the rate of diastolic relaxation distinguished patients with >90% stenosis from those with lesser degrees of stenosis, all three parameters were depressed in coronary patients without prior myocardial infarction when compared to normal controls. Studies by Tillisch et al. have documented improvement in wall motion following revascularization by coronary artery bypass surgery in myocardial regions having reduced resting blood flow and increased glucose uptake as assessed by positron emission tomography [43]. These studies support the possibility that chronic reductions in regional function represent an adaptation to chronically reduced coronary pressure and flow and are not always the result of myocardial necrosis.

Metabolic and biochemical responses to chronic pressure and flow reductions may be more involved than those present during acute reductions in pressure and flow. Recent studies by Schwaiger et al. have demonstrated this to be the case in myocardium salvaged by reperfusion [44]. Regional myocardial metabolism in viable myocardium was shifted from the utilization of free fatty acids to the aerobic metabolism of glucose as measured by positron emission tomography. The functional consequences of such changes in metabolism and substrate utilization remain unclear but the end result may be a more efficient oxygen utilization. Other adaptations could include alterations in myosin ATPase which have been demonstrated to occur in myocardial hypertrophy and during changes in thyroid hormone level [45]. Alternatively, changes in sympathetic responsiveness which have been demonstrated following acute myocardial ischemia [46] and in viable myocardium following myocardial infarction [47] may play a role in the adaptive response to chronic reductions in regional coronary pressure and flow.

Our knowledge of chronically reduced states of myocardial perfusion remains hampered by the lack of an appropriate animal model. Most investigators have characterized coronary dynamics in a collateral-dependent zone produced by an ameroid occluder [48] or multiple brief coronary artery occlusions [49]. Differences in resting myocardial function have not been observed before or after total coronary occlusion in either model. When either model is employed in the canine circulation, collaterals develop rapidly and result in vasodilator reserve in the collateral-dependent zone which is only modestly reduced from that present in the normal zone. Other laboratories have attempted to use animal models in which the development of collateral vessels is less complete than the dog. Studies using ameroid occluders in pigs have resulted in a high incidence of sudden death at the time of occlusion and an extremely high frequency of nontransmural myocardial infarction [50]. Thus, at one extreme in the dog, collateral vessel development is so great that it is sometimes difficult to demonstrate relative myocardial ischemia during stress and at the other, in the pig, it is so poor that myocardial infarction nearly always develops. The state of the collateral bed in man likely lies between the two extremes under most circumstances [51].

Our laboratory has recently undertaken studies in a modified ameroid preparation in the hope of obtaining a more suitable animal model for studying functional adaptations to chronically reduced pressure [52]. At the time of initial instrumentation, the usual ameroid occluder is implanted on the proximal circumflex artery. In addition, visible epicardial connections between the circumflex and other arterial beds are ligated. The latter procedure is intended to limit collateral flow into the circumflex artery during and following ameroid occlusion. Distal circumflex pressure, aortic pressure and left ventricular pressure are measured chronically. In addition, regional subendocardial function is monitored using wall thickness crystals implanted in the circumflex and anterior descending beds. In initial studies, serial measurements have been made before and after ameroid occlusion in the conscious state in seven animals. Resting circumflex wall thickness became depressed relative to that in the anterior descending bed as a resting aortic-circumflex gradient began to develop. Circumflex function reached a nadir near the time of total ameroid occlusion, falling to 68 ± 7 (SEM) percent of that in the anterior descending bed at the time of total occlusion. Circumflex function then gradually returned toward normal over 1–4 weeks. These findings are taken to indicate that collateral-dependent myocardial function can be reduced at rest when collateral flow is limited.

Conclusion

Knowledge of factors which control coronary autoregulatory responses remains limited. Previous studies of coronary autoregulation have been conducted in anesthetized animals. Substantial reductions in subendocardial flow have recently been observed in the face of pharmacologic vasodilator reserve, challenging the widely held notion that reduced resting flow implies the presence of maximal regional coronary vasodilation. The functional and metabolic significance of these responses are unclear. The presence of a chronic state of reduced regional flow and function in patients with ischemic heart disease remains controversial, with further understanding of chronic adaptations to reduced coronary pressure and flow needed.

Acknowledgement

This study was supported by grants from the National Heart, Lung and Blood Institute (2-PO1-HLB-15194, 1-KO8-HLB-01168) and the American Heart Association with funds contributed from the WNY Affiliate (83-717).

References

1. Berne RM (1964): Regulation of coronary blood flow. Physiol Rev 44: 1–29.
2. Rubio R, Berne RM (1975): Regulation of coronary blood flow. Prog Cardiovasc Dis 18: 105–122.
3. Mosher P, Ross J Jr, McFate PA, Shaw RF (1964): Control of coronary blood flow by an autoregulatory mechanism. Circ Res 14: 250–259.
4. Hoffman JIE (1978): Determinants and prediction of transmural myocardial perfusion. Circulation 58: 381–391.
5. Rouleau J, Boerboom LE, Surjadhana A, Hoffman JIE (1979): The role of autoregulation and tissue diastolic pressures in the transmural distribution of left ventricular blood flow in anesthetized dogs. Circ Res 45: 804–815.
6. Guyton RA, McClenathan JH, Newman GE, Michaelis LL (1977): Significance of subendocardial ST segment elevation caused by coronary stenosis in the dog. Am J Cardiol 40: 373–380.
7. Downey JM (1976): Myocardial contractile force as a function of coronary blood flow. Am J Physiol 230: 1–6.
8. Gallagher KP, Kumada T, Koziol JA, McKown MD, Kemper WS, Ross J Jr (1980): Significance of regional wall thickening abnormalities relative to transmural myocardial perfusion in anesthetized dogs. Circulation 62: 1266–1274.
9. Weintraub WS, Hattori S, Agarwal JB, Bodenheimer MM, Banka VS, Helfant RH (1981): The relationship between myocardial blood flow and contraction by myocardial layer in the canine left ventricle during ischemia. Circ Res 48: 430–438.
10. Vatner SF (1980): Correlation between acute reductions in myocardial blood flow and function in conscious dogs. Circ Res 47: 201–207.
11. Gallagher KP, Matsuzaki M, Koziol JA, Kemper WS, Ross J Jr (1984): Regional myocardial perfusion and wall thickening during ischemia in conscious dogs. Am J Physiol 247 (Heart Circ. Physiol. 16): H727–H738.
12. Griggs DM Jr, Tchokoev VV, Chen CC (1972): Transmural differences in ventricular tissue substrate levels, due to coronary constriction. Am J Physiol 222: 705–709.
13. Dunn RB, Griggs DM Jr (1975): Transmural gradients in ventricular tissue metabolites produced by stopping coronary blood flow in the dog. Circ Res 37: 438–445.
14. Gregg DE (1985): Regulation of the collateral and coronary circulation of the heart: possible utilization of deep coronary venous drainage circuits in the normal heart. III. The coronary circulation. In: McMichael J (ed) Circulation. Blackwell, Oxford, pp. 163–186. (Proc. Harvey Tercentenary Congr.).
15. Feigl EO (1983): Coronary physiology. Physiol Rev 63: 1–205.
16. Canty JM, Klocke FJ Jr (1985): Reduced regional myocardial perfusion in the presence of pharmacologic vasodilator reserve. Circulation 71: 370–377.
17. Aversano T, Becker LC (1985): Persistence of coronary vasodilator reserve despite functionally significant flow reduction. Am J Physiol 248 (Heart Circ. Physiol. 17): H403–H411.
18. Pantley GA, Bristow JD, Swenson LJ, Ladley HD, Johnson WB, Anselone CG (1985): Incomplete coronary vasodilation during myocardial ischemia in swine. Am J Physiol 248 (Heart Circ. Physiol. 18): H638–H647.
19. Heyndrickx GR, Baig H, Nellins P, Leusen I, Fishbein MC, Vatner SF (1978): Depression of regional blood flow and wall thickening after brief coronary occlusions. Am J Physiol 234 (Heart Circ. Physiol. 3): H653–H659.
20. Grattan MT, Hanley FL, Stevens MB, Hoffman JIE (1986): Transmural coronary flow reserve patterns in dogs. Am J Physiol 250 (Heart Circ. Physiol. 19): H276–H283.
21. Gallagher KP, Folts JD, Shebuski RJ, Rankin JHG, Rowe GG (1980): Subepicardial vasodilator reserve in the presence of critical coronary stenosis in dogs. Am J Cardiol 46: 67–72.
22. Grover GJ, Weiss HR (1985): Effect of pacing on oxygen supply-to-consumption ratio in ischemic myocardium. Am J Cardiol 46: 67–72.

23. Gorman MW, Sparks HV Jr (1982): Progressive vasoconstriction during relative ischemia in canine myocardium. Circ Res 51: 411–420.
24. Gold FL, Bache RJ (1982): Transmural right ventricular blood flow during acute pulmonary artery hypertension in the sedated dog. Circ Res 51: 196–204.
25. Krawczyk JA, Dashkoff N, Mays A, Klocke FJ (1980): Reduced coronary flow in a canine model of 'muscle bridge' with inflow occlusion extending into diastole; possible role of downstream vascular closure. Trans Assoc Am Physicians 93: 100–109.
26. Dole WP, Nuno DW, Johannsen UJ (1984): Dependence of coronary autoregulation on myocardial oxygenation. Circulation 70 (suppl. II): 230.
27. Norris CP, Barnes GE, Smith EE, Granger HJ (1979): Autoregulation of superior mesenteric flow in fasted and fed dogs. Am J Physiol 237 (Heart Circ. Physiol. 6): H174–H177.
28. Weisfeldt ML, Shock NW (1970): Effect of perfusion pressure on coronary flow and oxygen usage of nonworking heart. Am J Physiol 218: 95–101.
29. Sobol BJ, Wanlass SA, Joseph EB, Azarshahy I (1962): Alteration of coronary blood flow in the dog by inhalation of 100 percent oxygen. Circ Res 11: 797–802.
30. Rubanyi G, Paul RJ (1985): Two distinct effects of oxygen on vascular tone in isolated porcine coronary arteries. Circ Res 56: 1–10.
31. Surjadhana A, Rouleau J, Boerboom L, Hoffman JIE (1978): Myocardial blood flow and its distribution in anesthetized polycythemic dogs. Circ Res 43: 619–631.
32. Mohrman DE, Feigl EO (1978): Competition between sympathetic vasoconstriction and metabolic vasodilation in the canine coronary circulation. Circ Res 42: 79–80.
33. Buffington CW, Feigl EO (1983): Effect of coronary artery pressure on transmural distribution of adrenergic coronary vasoconstriction in the dog. Circ Res 53: 613–621.
34. Heusch G, Deussen A (1983): The effects of cardiac sympathetic nerve stimulation on perfusion of stenotic coronary arteries in the dog. Circ Res 53: 8–15.
35. Khayyal MA, Eng C, Franzen D, Braell JA, Kirk ES (1985): Effects of vasopressin on the coronary circulation: reserve and regulation during ischemia. Am J Physiol (Heart Circ. Physiol. 17): H516–H522.
36. Klocke FJ, Bunnell IL, Greene DG, Wittenberg SM, Visco JP (1974): Average coronary blood flow per unit weight of left ventricle in patients with and without coronary artery disease. Circulation 50: 547–559.
37. Klocke FJ, Bunnell IL, Greene DG, Arani DT, Roberts DC, Nakazawa HK, Mates RE, Orlick AE, Visco JP, Wittenberg SM (1977): Myocardial blood flow determined with helium desaturation and great cardiac vein/coronary sinus sampling in patients with left anterior descending or circumflex artery stenosis. Herz 2: 11–15.
38. Cannon PJ, Schmidt DH, Weiss MB, Fowler DL, Sciacca RR, Ellis K, Casarella WJ (1975): The relationships between regional myocardial perfusion at rest and arteriographic lesions in patients with coronary atherosclerosis. J Clin Invest 56: 1442–1454.
39. Arani DT, Greene DG, Bunnell IL, Smith GL, Klocke FJ (1984): Reductions in coronary blood flow under resting conditions in collateral-dependent myocardium of paients with complete occlusion of the left anterior descending coronary artery. J Amer Coll Cardiol 3: 668–674.
40. Chen PH, Nichols AB, Weiss MB, Sciacca RR, Watter PD, Cannon PJ (1982): Left ventricular myocardial blood flow in multivessel coronary artery disease. Circulation 66: 537–547.
41. Hodgson J.McB, Most AS, Williams DO, Gewirtz H (1985): Coronary flow reserve not abolished in humans with coronary stenosis and reduced basal flow. Circulation 72 (suppl. III): 387.
42. St. John Sutton MG, Frye RL, Smith HC, Chesebro JH, Ritman EL (1978): Relation between left coronary artery stenosis and regional left ventricular function. Circ 58: 491–497.
43. Tillisch J, Brunken RB, Marshall R, Schwaiger M, Mandelkern M, Phelps M, Schelbert H (1986): Reversibility of cardiac wall-motion abnormalities predicted by position tomography. New Eng J Med 314: 884–888.
44. Schwaiger M, Schelbert HR, Ellison D, Hansen H, Yeatman L, Vinten-Johansen J, Selin C,

Barrio J, Phelps ME (1985): Sustained regional abnormalities in cardiac metabolism after transient ischemia in the chronic dog model. J Amer Coll Cardiol 6: 336–347.
45. Scheuer J, Bhan AK (1979): Cardiac contractile proteins: adenosine triphosphatase activity and physiological function. Circ Res 45: 1–12.
46. Ciuffo AA, Ouyang P, Becker LW, Levin L, Weisfeldt ML (1985): Reduction of sympathetic inotropic response after ischemia in dogs: contributor to stunned myocardium. J Clin Invest 75: 1504–1509.
47. Barber MJ, Mueller TM, Davies BG, Gill RM, Zipes DP (1985): Interruption of sympathetic and vagal-mediated afferent responses by transmural myocardial infarction. Circulation 72: 623–631.
48. Hill RC, Kleinman LH, Tiller WH Jr, Chitwood WR Jr, Rembert JC, Wechsler AS (1983): Myocardial blood flow and function during gradual coronary occlusion in awake dogs. Am J Physiol 244 (Heart Circ. Physiol. 13): H60–H67.
49. Yamamoto H, Tomoike H, Shimokawa H, Nabeyama S, Nakamura M (1984): Development of collateral function with repetitive coronary occlusion in a canine model reduces myocardial reactive hyperemia in the absence of significant coronary stenosis. Circ Res 55: 623–632.
50. Bloor CM, White FC, Sanders TM (1984): Effects of exercise on collateral development in myocardial ischemia in pigs. J Appl Physiol: Respirat Environ Exercise Physiol 56: 656–665.
51. Gregg DE (1974): The natural history of coronary collateral development. Circ Res 35: 335–344.
52. Canty JM Jr, Klocke FJ (1987): Reductions in regional myocardial function at rest in conscious dogs with chronically reduced regional coronary artery pressure. J Am Coll Cardiol 9 (Suppl. A): 253A.

Discussion

Beyar: It has been shown in the past that endocardial layers show a greater reduction in flow as a function of coronary pressure. Now you have shown that at the middle of your experiment you have a reduction in wall thickening to 73% of the control level, yet an equal decrease in endocardial and epicardial flows. I would expect the endocardial decrease to be more than the epicardial decrease. Can you explain this?
Klocke: Although we think our wall thickness measurements represent function in the inner half of the wall reasonably well, we have only limited data on subendocardial segment shortening and flow.
Downey: The coronary pressures were not really that low and I am surprised there was that much dysfunction. Is there a possibility that something about this preparation is causing the tissue in that region to 'take it easy' for a while?
Klocke: We agree this is a possibility. We have begun to make observations in a sham-operated animal in which the ameroid constrictor is removed just before closing the chest. In thinking about myocardium which is 'taking it easy', we have suggested the term 'idling' myocardium rather than 'ischemic' or 'stunned' myocardium. The presence of a flow reduction clearly cannot be taken to reflect exhaustion of vasodilator reserve.
Hoffman: I am not sure that your sham operation is going to answer the question. I would rather look at myocardial norepinephrine level and response to nerve stimulation, because the chronic ameroid occlusion might cause more damage to nerves than the acute ameroid placement and removal.
Sonnenblick: Another possible factor is that when the contractile behavior of one portion of the heart is altered chronically, reactive hypertrophy occurs in other areas. You then have a problem affecting the total heart arising out of a segmental change and it can get very interesting.
Klocke: I agree with both comments. We are initially trying to look at pathology to make sure we are not dealing with subendocardial fibrosis, but will need also to consider these points.
Marcus: Do you have flow measurements?
Klocke: We are just beginning to collect these systematically. We take the flow in the circumflex area and relate it to simultaneous flow in the anterior descending area. The ratio on the initial day of study is taken as our control value. Ratios on subsequent studies are evaluated in relation to this control value.

34. Is stunned myocardium energy deficient?

L.C. BECKER

Abstract

Prolonged myocardial dysfunction following a brief period of ischemia has been termed 'stunned myocardium' since no permanent tissue damage can be identified, and function eventually returns to normal. Tissue ATP levels are reduced in stunned myocardium and recover slowly along with function. The delayed restoration of ATP has been attributed to a loss of purine precursors, and energy deficiency has therefore been thought to represent the underlying cause of stunned myocardium. To evaluate the energy deficiency hypothesis further, we produced two models of stunned myocardium:

1. regional stunning in the dog caused by repetitive occlusions of the anterior descending coronary artery for 5 minutes, interrupted by 10 minutes of reperfusion, and
2. global stunning in the buffer perfused rabbit heart caused by 20 minutes of hypothermic total global ischemia.

In both models electron microscopy revealed essentially normal ultrastructure. Despite reduced function at rest, regionally stunned myocardium responded promptly to maximal doses of intravenous epinephrine and maintained augmented function during 60 minutes of continuous infusion, without any evidence of post-stimulation depression. The response to post-extrasystolic potentiation also appeared to be normal. The globally stunned myocardium demonstrated moderately reduced ATP levels, as measured by ^{31}P nuclear magnetic resonance, but despite a doubling of the rate-pressure product during isoproterenol stimulation, tissue ATP levels were maintained constant, indicating an ability of stunned myocardium to increase ATP turnover. Infusions of adenosine induced globally stunned hearts to accelerate repletion of ATP, producing a 50% restoration of ATP levels, but this was not accompanied by an improvement in function. Our results are consistent with normal functional and metabolic reserve in stunned myocardium and do not support the concept that energy deficiency is the basis for post-ischemic myocardial dysfunction.

Introduction

Myocardial dysfunction following brief coronary artery occlusions, persisting long after blood flow has been restored, has been recognized in the experimental laboratory for over 10 years [1–3]. Heyndrickx et al. [3] found that after occlusions of only 5 minutes in the dog, function remained depressed for up to 3 hours despite rapid normalization of the intramyocardial electrogram and blood flow. Kloner et al. [4] reported that after a 15 minute coronary occlusion, systolic shortening remained abnormal at 72 hours but returned to normal by 1 week.

Because function eventually returned to normal and no permanent myocardial injury could be identified, Braunwald and Kloner [5] coined the term 'stunned myocardium' to describe the prolonged but reversible myocardial dysfunction following brief periods of ischemia. Important in the definition of stunned myocardium is that post-ischemic reperfusion is complete. 'Stunned' myocardium refers to dysfunction in the face of normal blood flow, and not merely to acutely or chronically ischemic myocardium.

Interest in 'stunned myocardium' has heightened with the increasing use of thrombolytic therapy and coronary angioplasty to achieve reperfusion in patients with acute myocardial infarction. Despite successful opening of an occluded artery, the return of function may be delayed, obscuring the true benefit of reperfusion [6]. In addition, the presence of stunned myocardium may seriously compromise left ventricular function and lead to heart failure despite a relatively small area of truly irreversible myocardial damage [7].

What is known about the causes of stunned myocardium?

Ultrastructurally, remarkably few abnormalities have been found in dysfunctional stunned myocardium [4, 8–10]. Although major structural changes are absent, the findings, consisting of scattered mitochondrial swelling, glycogen loss, and accumulation of lipid, are consistent with some degree of membrane damage, particularly to the mitochondria [2]. Damage to the myofibrillar proteins is unlikely to be the cause of post-ischemic dysfunction since even prolonged episodes of ischemia do not alter myosin [11], actin [12], or actomyosin [13]. Early impairment in the uptake and release of calcium by sarcoplasmic reticulum has been shown to occur within 15 minutes of ischemia [14, 15] and could contribute to abnormal myocardial function. Longer periods of ischemia, especially with reflow, are associated with an increase in intracellular calcium content and precipitation of calcium in the mitochondria. Although increased cellular calcium may occur in stunned myocytes, gross calcium precipitates are not characteristic.

Most previous attention has focused on impaired energy production as the cause of stunned myocardium. Functional depression following an ischemic episode apears to parallel reduced tissue ATP levels in several regional and global animal models [4, 8, 9, 16, 17]. During ischemia, ATP is degraded to ADP and AMP via myokinase to support energy requiring reactions within the cell. AMP is subsequently converted by 5-nucleotidase to adenosine, which diffuses across the sarcolemmal membrane [18], resulting in a decrease in the total purine pool. Following reperfusion, ATP repletion is markedly delayed [4, 8, 9, 16, 17, 19–21], and recovers with a time course similar to the recovery of function [4]. In short term reperfusion studies, Reibel and Rovetto [17] reported that tissue ATP content and ventricular function were closely correlated in post-ischemic and post-anoxic isolated rat hearts. Vial et al. [20] found that regional ATP and function were both depressed following 45 minutes of coronary artery occlusion in the dog, but that the correlation between function and ATP content in individual animals was poor. Similarly, Vary et al. [22] also found little correlation between post-ischemic mechanical recovery and tissue energy levels in the perfused rat heart.

ATP repletion is thought to be limited in the post-ischemic myocardium by the loss of precursors. Through 'salvage pathways' ATP is regenerated from adenine nucleotides and nucleosides: adenosine is converted to AMP by adenosine kinase and inosine is converted to inosine monophosphate (IMP) via hypoxanthine phosphoribosyl transferase [23]. De novo synthesis is much slower and costlier in terms of energy requirements: IMP is manufactured from the precursor ribose-5-phosphate [24]. Several days are required to fully replace a 50% loss of ATP by this mechanism [16]. Zimmer [24] has measured the rate of de novo synthesis of ATP from labelled glycine to be only 1.3 nmol/g wet weight/hr in perfused hearts and approximately 6 times this rate in situ. In contrast, Reibel and Rovetto [25] found that ATP synthesis through salvage pathways from adenosine was 300 nmol/g/hr in the post- ischemic rat heart, or approximately 200 times the de novo synthesis rate. This amounted to a replacement of 10% of the total ATP pool per hour.

The concept that ATP repletion is limited by loss of critical precursors is supported by several studies in which ATP repletion after reflow has been accelerated by administration of purines, including 5-amino-4-imidazole carboxamide riboside (AICARiboside) [26, 27]; adenosine, alone and in combination with an adenosine deaminase inhibitor (erythro-9-2-hydroxy-3-nonyl) adenine hydrochloride, (EHNA) [25, 27–30] and inosine [31, 32]. Ribose has been a less effective agent for ATP repletion with a much longer time required for ATP normalization [27, 33]. However, Hoffmeister et al. [34] showed that adenosine did not improve post-ischemic function despite a restoration of half of the depleted ATP.

Thus, although there is considerable evidence to support a reduction of high energy phosphate content in stunned myocardium, it is not yet clear that inadequate energy production actually underlies the phenomenon. The steady state tissue levels of ATP represent the net balance between ATP synthesis and utilization, and therefore do not necessarily reflect the rate of ATP production.

The studies described below from my laboratory were designed to provide further evidence for or against energy deficiency as a cause of stunned myocardium.

Experimental preparations

We have used two different experimental models to study stunned myocardium. In collaboration with Drs Lloyd Stahl, Joseph Levine, Thomas Aversano, John Nicklas and Mr Anthony DiPaula, regionally stunned myocardium has been produced in the dog by repetitive 5 minute occlusions of the anterior descending coronary artery [35, 36]. A global model of stunned myocardium has also been created in the isolated buffer perfused rabbit heart in collaboration with Drs Giuseppe Ambrosio, William Jacobus, Harlan Weisman, and Andrew Bergman [37, 38].

In the dog studies, following pentobarbital anesthesia and left thoracotomy, pairs of sonomicrometer crystals are inserted into the anterior and posterior LV walls, at mid-wall depth, 10–15 mm apart, oriented parallel to the minor axis to measure regional left ventricular function. A pneumatic occluder is placed around the proximal anterior descending coronary artery to create 5 min periods of ischemia, separated by 10 min periods of reperfusion. Up to 16 repetitive cycles of ischemia/reperfusion are performed in order to create maximal post-ischemic dysfunction without producing necrosis. Ultrastructurally, most tissue samples taken from the stunned region are entirely normal (Figure 1). Although the first ischemia/reflow cycle typically produces the greatest amount of dysfunction, a cumulative effect on post-ischemic dysfunction is regularly seen with additional ischemic periods (Figure 2). Generally the effect plateaus after the 6th–8th episode, but significant variability is seen in this pattern and also in the amount of myocardial stunning that can be produced. After 12–16 repetitive ischemic episodes, no significant recovery of function is usually seen with reperfusion of up to 2 hours (Figure 2).

In this model, stunned myocardium exhibits an interesting and characteristic shortening pattern: early systolic lengthening is followed by late systolic shortening, which continues into diastole (Figure 3). The shortening curve appears to be shifted to the right, i.e., into diastole. This could represent delayed or prolonged electrical activation [39] or an inability to shorten against a normal systolic load, with passive recoil occurring in diastole.

In the isolated rabbit heart studies, perfusion is carried out at constant pressure (80 mm Hg) within the bore of a superconducting magnet. Non-blood containing perfusate is used, consisting of 117 mM sodium chloride, 6.0 mM potassium chloride, 2.5 mM calcium chloride, 1.0 mM magnesium sulphate, 0.5 mM EDTA, 16.7 mM glucose, and 24 mM sodium bicarbonate, pH 7.4, at 27° C, bubbled with a gas mixture of 95% oxygen and 5% carbon dioxide. To measure function, a latex balloon is inserted into the left ventricle through the left atrium and filled

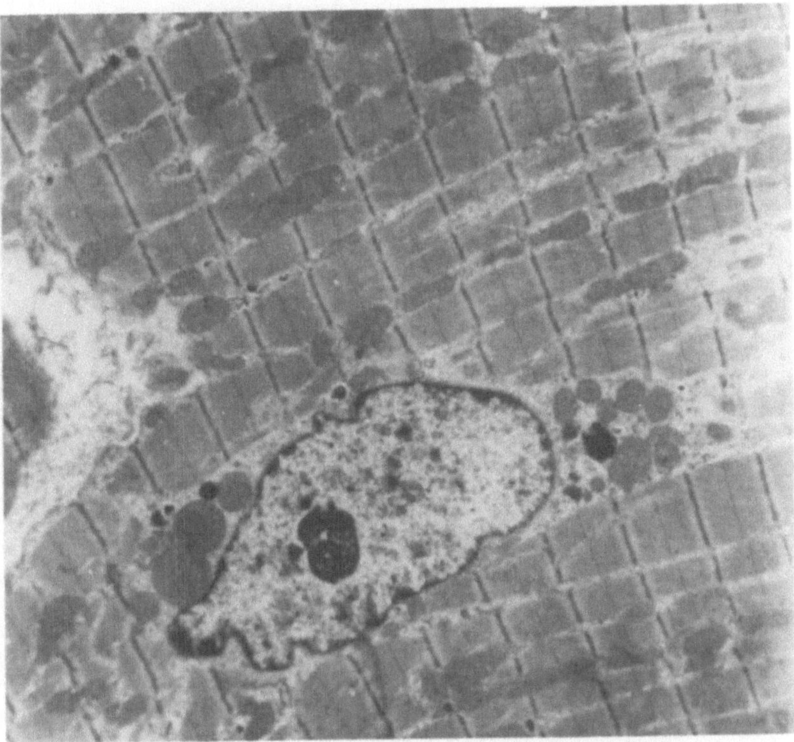

Figure 1. Electron micrograph of myocardium stunned by repetitive 5 minute occlusions in the dog. Ultrastructure is essentially normal, without mitochondrial swelling or calcium precipitates, abnormal fiber architecture or edema.

with saline to produce an end diastolic pressure of 10 mm Hg. 31-Phosphorus nuclear magnetic resonance (NMR) spectra are obtained at 4.2 Tesla every 10 minutes and the amounts of phosphocreatine (PCr), inorganic phosphate (Pi) and ATP are obtained by integrating the areas under the appropriate peaks (Figure 4). Myocardial stunning is created by temporarily cross clamping the perfusion line for 20 minutes. During global ischemia there is cessation of contraction and a gradual fall in myocardial temperature to ambient levels. Function after reperfusion, measured by developed pressure (systolic minus end diastolic), returns on the average to only about 80% of baseline. Myocardial ATP also remains reduced by about 20% while pH and PCr return rapidly to normal (Figure 4). In most hearts, ultrastructural analysis by electron microscopy reveals no abnormalities.

The regional and global models of myocardial stunning we have developed are different but complementary. In the canine regional model, post-ischemic dysfunction is marked and full recovery may require hours to days of reperfusion [3–5]. The global model has only a modest reduction in function, but the potential effects of nerves, circulating hormones and blood products, as well as repeated

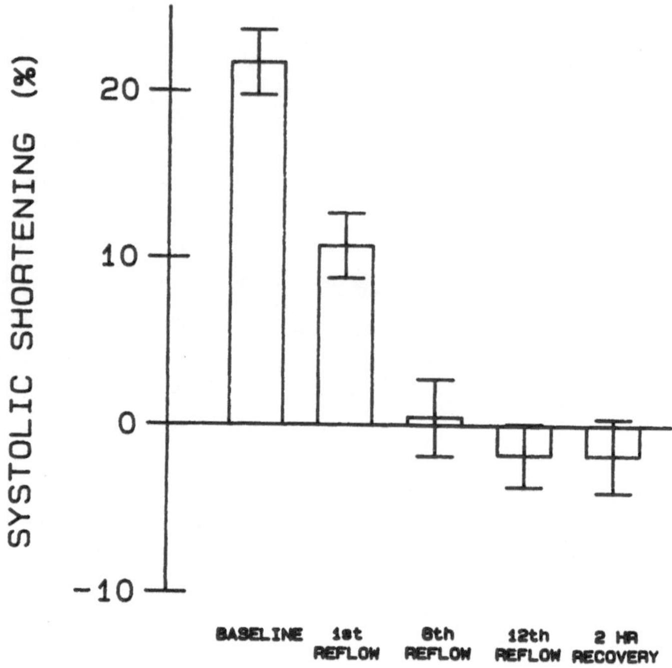

Figure 2. Mean systolic segment shortening measured by sonomicrometry in 9 dogs (18 crystal pairs) after repetitive 5 minute coronary occlusion/10 minute reflow cycles. The greatest decrease in function occurs after the first occlusion/reflow period, but the functional depression is cumulative. No recovery is seen during 2 hours of reperfusion after the 12th ischemic period.

systolic stretching of the ischemic region, are eliminated. Myocardial necrosis is absent in both. The global model has the advantage that high energy phosphate metabolism can be monitored continuously by 31-P NMR, but the extent of long-term functional recovery cannot be determined because of the inherent instability of the isolated buffer-perfused preparation.

Is stunned myocardium energy deficient?

We undertook 3 series of experiments, one in the regional and two in the global stunned model,to explore the ability of stunned myocardium to produce sufficient ATP for normal contraction. We reasoned that if stunned myocardium were energy deficient and unable to supply high energy phosphate rapidly enough to the myofibrils, it should be unable to respond normally to inotropic interventions. Furthermore, if it were unable to generate sufficient energy, a decline in tissue levels of ATP (representing the balance between production and utilization) should occur during inotropic stimulation. Finally, if the stunned myocar-

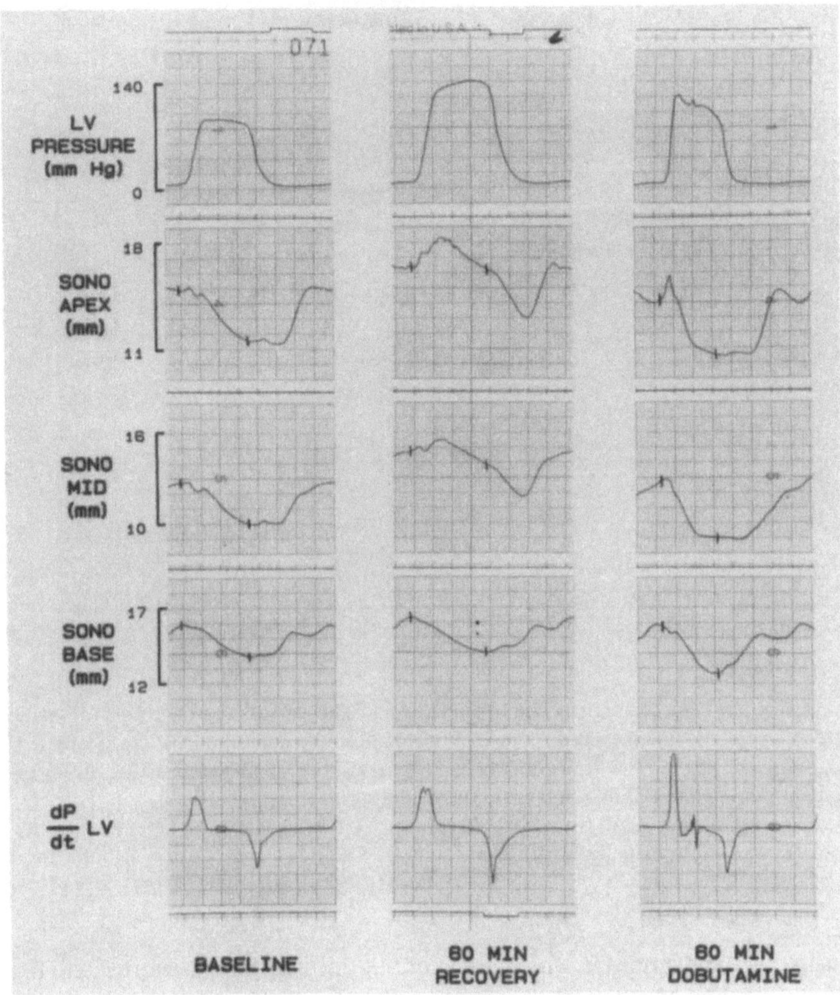

Figure 3. Abnormal shortening pattern characteristic of stunned myocardium is seen in 'apex' and 'mid' sonomicrometer crystal pairs after repetitive occlusions and 60 min recovery period (middle panels). The crystal pair located at the 'base' is outside the ischemic region. The response to intravenous dobutamine is rapid and dramatic with reversal of the 'stunned' shortening pattern.

dium were energy deficient due to loss of precursors, enhancement of the adenine nucleotide pool should result in improved function.

Response of regionally stunned myocardium to inotropic stimulation

In the first series of experiments we found that there was an essentially normal response of stunned myocardium to inotropic stimulation [36]. Figure 3 illustrates

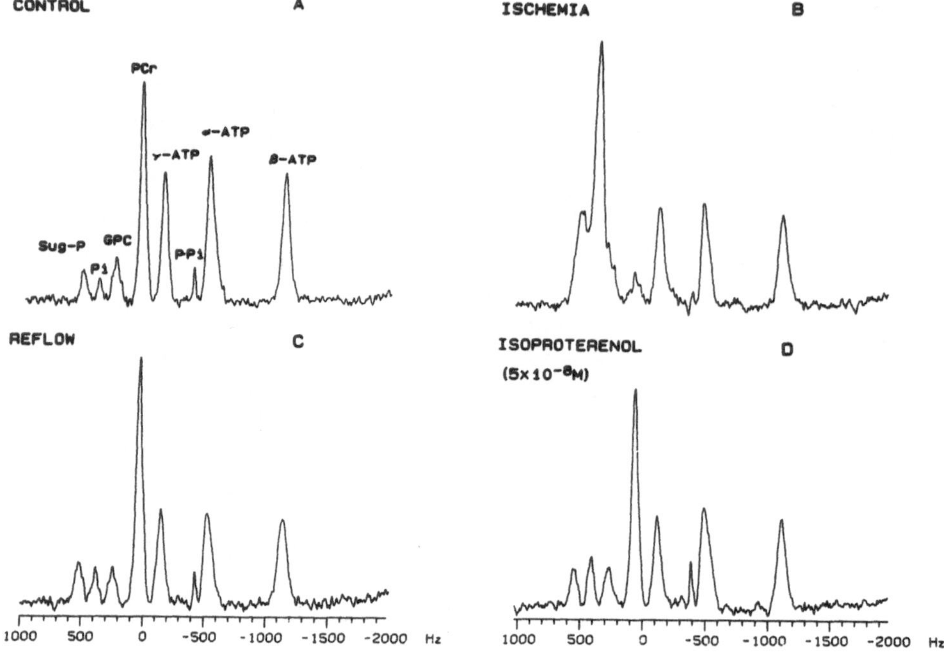

Figure 4. Pooled ^{31}P-NMR spectra from perfused rabbit hearts. The abscissa represents the resonance frequency (relative units). Note the almost complete fall of phosphocreatine and the large increase in inorganic phosphate during the last 10 min of ischemia (Panel B). Both findings normalize during the second 10 min of reflow (Panel C). No changes occurred during isoproterenol stimulation (Panel D). Peaks are labelled as follows: Sug-P = phosphated surgars; Pi = inorganic phosphate; PCr = phosphocreatine; PPi = pyrophosphate (internal standard); α, β, γ-ATP = resonance of each of the three phosphates of the ATP molecule.

the results in one experiment in which intravenous dobutamine was infused in the dog after production of stunned myocardium by the repetitive occlusion technique described above. Despite an increase in left ventricular pressure, systolic segment shortening increased dramatically and the time to minimum segment length decreased so that minimum length occurred at end systole, as defined by peak negative LV dp/dt, instead of in diastole.

The effect of a 60 minute continuous infusion of IV epinephrine was studied in a series of 11 dogs [36]. As a result of myocardial stunning, systolic segment shortening decreased from 21.8% to 4.3% and recovered to only 7.9% after 1 hour of reperfusion. Intravenous epinephrine, titrated to produce a maximal inotropic response, caused segment shortening to increase to 21.6% after 10 minutes and to 24.8% after 1 hour of infusion, despite a 20 mm Hg increase in systolic pressure. The same dose of epinephrine given before ischemia had increased segment shortening to 30.5%. The higher level of shortening achieved with epinephrine before ischemia could reflect an inability of stunned myocardium to mount a normal maximal responce. However, control non-ischemic segments demonstrated the same response pattern: 14.5% shortening at baseline, 22.1% during epinephrine (before ischemia), 12.3% after stunning of the opposite wall, 16.7% after 10minutes and 17.0% after 60 minutes of IV epinephrine. The lesser response to epinephrine after stunning, in both stunned and control segments, was probably due to a gradual increase in systolic pressure during the experiment, so that during epinephrine, systolic pressure averaged 125 mm Hg before stunning and 140 mm Hg afterwards. After discontinuing epinephrine, there was a decline of shortening toward the 'stunned' level but no post-stimilation depression occurred (i.e. no decrease below the pre-epinephrine level).

In six of the dogs, post-extrasystolic potentiation (PESP) was used to elicit the maximal inotropic response from stunned and normal myocardium, independent of β-adrenergic receptors. Using programmed atrial stimulation, the shortest premature stimulus was applied that did not result in atrioventricular block or arrhythmias, followed by a compensatory pause. Before ischemia, PESP increased segment shortening from 21.8 to 31.1%, while after stunning the increase was from 7.9% to 24.8%. As with epinephrine, control segments showed the same response pattern.

Other investigators had demonstrated that stunned myocardium was capable of at least a short term response to catecholamines [40–42]. Our results extended these observations by showing that

1. stunned myocardium could continue to respond maximally during a 60 minute continuous infusion of epinephrine,
2. the response did not depend on β-receptors since it was equally good to PESP, and
3. the maximal response was probably 'normal' since stunned and non-ischemic segments behaved similarly and the response to epinephrine and PESP was equivalent.

Are high energy phosphates maintained in stunned myocardium during inotropic stimulation?

The globally stunned perfused rabbit heart was used for these studies, with measurement of tissue high energy phosphate levels by 31-P NMR. After reperfusion following 20 minutes of total global ischemia at room temperature, developed pressure returned to 77.8% of baseline, while ATP was reduced to 80.9% of baseline (n = 8 hearts). Isoproterenol (5×10^{-8} M for 10 minutes) caused large increases in developed pressure and rate pressure product (to 134.1% and 195.0% of baseline, respectively) (Figure 5). However, there was no decrease in ATP content (80.7% of baseline) (figure 4, 6). PCr content was increased following reperfusion (103% of baseline) and remained constant during isoproterenol stimulation. Control hearts (n = 8) not subjected to ischemia re-

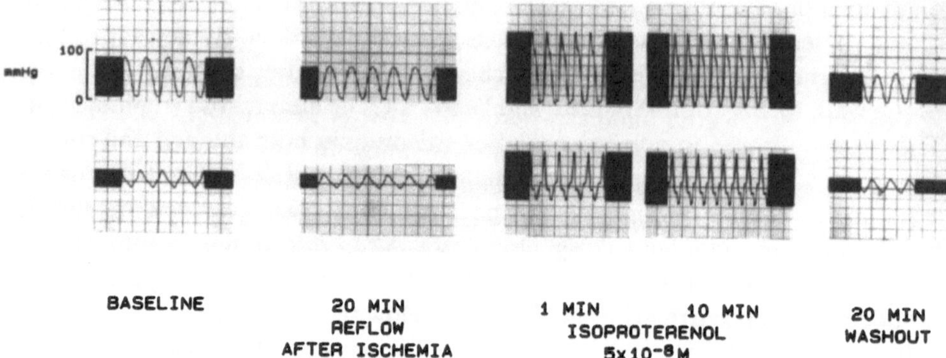

Figure 5. Isoproterenol produced a dramatic and immediate increase in developed left ventricular pressure (top row) and dp/dt (bottom row) in isolated perfused rabbit hearts, as shown in this typical tracing.

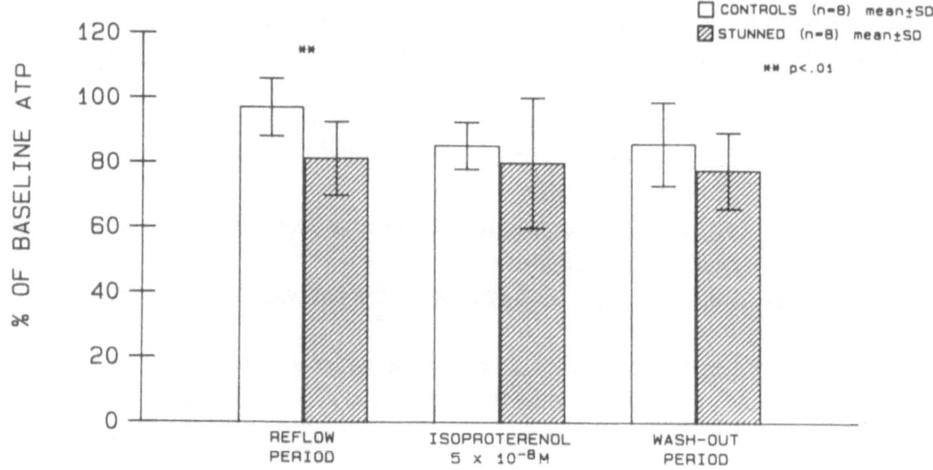

Figure 6. Mean levels of ATP, expressed as a percentage of the baseline value, after stunning (hatched bars) or after a similar period of normal perfusion (open bars) before, during, and after isoproterenol in perfused rabbit hearts. Stunned myocardium is associated with a significant decrease in ATP, but no further decrease is seen during isoproterenol.

sponded similarly to isoproterenol: developed pressure increased to 142% and rate-pressure product to 194% of baseline, while ATP and PCr were maintained. Interestingly, intracellular pH decreased slightly but significantly in both stunned and control hearts during isoproterenol (7.18 to 7.11 and 7.16 to 7.09, respectively). This finding is compatible with a stimulation of anaerobic glycolysis. Neither group of hearts demonstrated functional or metabolic deterioration after discontinuation of the isoproterenol.

Our results appear to rule out a primary deficit of mitochondrial function as the limiting factor for the recovery of ATP and function in stunned myocardium. The myocardial content of PCr was higher than baseline in stunned hearts suggesting that the phosphorylation capability of mitochondria was intact. In addition, the PCr/Pi ratio, an index of the energy supply/demand balance [43], was also increased. The finding of stable tissue ATP levels during isoproterenol stimulation suggests that stunned hearts were able to cope with the large increase in the rate of ATP turnover by proportionally increasing the rate of ADP rephosphorylation.

Does accelerated repletion of ATP improve function in stunned myocardium?

In these experiments in the globally stunned rabbit heart, we investigated whether accelerated repletion of ATP induced by administration of nucleotide precursors would be translated into improved myocardial function [38]. Following production of stunned myocardium by 20 minutes of hypothermic total global ischemia, hearts were perfused with normal perfusate (n = 6 hearts) or perfusate containing 100 μM/l adenosine (n = 6) or 100 μM/l 5-aminoimidazole-4-carboxamide riboside (AICAR) (n = 6) for 2 hours. Tissue levels of ATP, PCr and Pi and intracellular pH were monitored every 10 minutes by ^{31}P NMR.

After stunning, developed pressure was reduced to approximately 84% of baseline, and ATP to about 80% of baseline, while PCr increased above normal to about 120% of the control value. Over an additional 120 minutes of reperfusion with normal buffer, developed pressure, ATP, and PCr all gradually declined to about 70%, 65%, and 95% of baseline, respectively. However,during reperfusion with adenosine, ATP content increased in every heart and, on the average, returned about 50% of the way of baseline; the PCr overshoot was also blunted, perhaps a reflection of increased phosphorylation of ADP. Despite the increased ATP levels, however, there was no improvement at all in developed pressure. Perfusion with AICAR produced no measurable improvement in either ATP content or function. Recent data suggests that ATP repletion proceeds about 10 times more rapidly during intracoronary infusion of adenosine compared to AICAR [27].

Thus, although post-ischemic dysfunction is associated with reduced tissue ATP content, more rapid restoration of ATP induced by infusion of purine precursors does not result in improved function. This suggests that although the two findings occur together, they are not causally related.

Conclusion

Despite the striking temporal relationship between recovery of function and myocardial ATP levels, our results do not support the concept that stunned myocardial is energy deficient. Based on its ability to respond normally to maximal inotropic stimulation in two different animal models, along with evidence for preservation of high energy phosphates in the face of intense inotropic stimulation, stunned myocardium appears to be capable of synthesizing adequate, if not normal, amounts of ATP to support contractile activity.

What, then, is the mechanism of myocardial stunning? More research is clearly needed to answer this question, but perhaps the two most intriguing possibilities involve a disturbance in excitation-contraction coupling. Recent studies have shown depressed action potential parameters and reduced excitability in myocardial tissue after 15 minutes of ischemia [39], consistent with the hypothesis that a primary impairment in excitation may result in defective electro-mechanical coupling. Alternatively, the defect may involve intracellular calcium handling. It has been demonstrated that periods of global ischemia as short as 7.5 minutes are sufficient to produce an impairment in sarcoplasmic reticulum calcium transport [15], characterized by a significant depression and a shift of the calcium sensitivity curve of $Ca^{2+}Mg^{2+}$ ATPase activity. The observation that depression of function in stunned hearts can be partly reversed by interventions which increase intracellular calcium [44] is consistent with this finding and lends support to a disturbance in calcium transport as the basis for stunned myocardium.

Acknowledgment

This study was supported by a Specialized Center for Research in Ischemic Heart Disease, Grant P50 HL 17655 from the National Instituts of Health, Bethesda, MD.

References

1. Weiner JM, Apstein CS, Arthur JH, Pirzada FA, Hood WG Jr (1976): Persistence of myocardial injury following brief periods of coronary occlusion. Cardiovasc Res 10: 678–86.
2. Wood JM, Hanley HG, Entman ML, Hartley CJ, Swain JA, Busch U, Chang C-H, Lewis RM, Morgan WJ, Schwartz A (1979): Biochemical and morphological correlates of acute experimental myocardial ischemia in the dog. IV. Energy mechanisms during very early ischemia. Circ Res 42: 52–61.
3. Heyndrickx GR, Baig H, Nellens P, Leusen I, Fishbein MC, Vatner SF (1978): Depression of regional blood flow and wall thickening after brief coronary occlusions. Am J Physiol 234: H653–59.
4. Kloner RA, DeBoer LWV, Darsee Jr, Ingwall JS, Braunwald E (1981): Recovery from prolonged abnormalities of canine myocardium salvaged from ischemic necrosis by coronary reperfusion. Proc Natl Acad Sci USA 78: 7152–56.
5. Braunwald E, Kloner RA (1982): The stunned myocardium: prolonged, post-ischemic ventricular dysfunction. Circulation 55: 1146–49.
6. Charuzi Y, Beeder C, Marshall LA, Sasaki H, Pack NB, Geft I, Ganz W (1984): Improvement in

regional and global left ventricular function after intracoronary thrombolysis: Assessment with two-dimensional echocardiography. Am J Cardiol 53: 622–5.

7. Nixon JV, Brown CN, Smitherman TC (1982): Identification of transient and persistent segmental wall motion abnormalities in patients with unstable angina by two-dimensional echocardiography. Circulation 65: 1497–1503.
8. Schaper J, Mulch J, Winkler B, Schaper W (1979): Ultrastructural, functional, and biochemical criteria for estimation of reversibility of ischemic injury: A study on the effects of global ischemia, on the isolated dog heart. J Molec Cell Cardiol 11: 521–41.
9. DeBoer LWV, Ingwall JS, Kloner RA, Braunwald E (1980): Prolonged derangements of canine myocardial purine metabolism after a brief coronary artery occlusion not associated with anatomic evidence of necrosis. Proc Natl Acad Sci USA 77: 5471–75.
10. Sharma G, Varley KG, Kim S, Barwinsky J, Cohen M, Dhalla N (1975): ALterations in energy metabolism and ultrastructure upon reperfusion of the ischemic myocardium after coronary occlusion. Am J Cardiol 36: 234–43.
11. Barany M, Gaetjens E, Barany K, Karp E (1964): Comparative studies of rabbit cardiac and skeletal myosins. Arch Biochem Biophys 106: 280–93.
12. Katz AM, Maxwell JB: Actin from heart muscle: Sulfhydryl groups. Circ Res 14: 345–50.
13. Kako K, Bing RJ (1958): Contractility of actomyosin bands prepared from normal and failing human hearts. J Clin Invest 37: 465–70.
14. Schwartz A, Wood JM, Allen JC, Bornet EP, Entman ML, Goldstein MA, Sordahl LA, Suzuki M, Lewis RM (1973): Biochemical and morphological correlates of cardiac ischemia. I. Membrane Systems. Am J Cardiol 36: 46–61.
15. Krause S, Hess ML (1984): Characterization of cardiac sardoplasmic reticulum dysfunction during short-term, normothermic, global ischemia. Circ Res 55: 176–84.
16. Reimer KA, Hill ML, Jennings RB (1981): Prolonged depletion of ATP and the adenine nucleotide pool due to delayed resynthesis of adenine nucleotides following reversible myocardial ischemia injury in dogs. J Mol Cell Cardiol 13: 229–39.
17. Reibel DK, Rovetto MJ (1978): Myocardial ATP synthesis and mechanical function following oxygen deficiency. Am J Physiol 234: H620–24.
18. Fox AC, Reed GE, Meilman H, Silk BS (1979): Release of nucleosides from canine and human hearts as an index of prior ischemia. Am J Cardiol 43: 52–58.
19. Vial C, Font B, Goldschmidt D, Pearlman AS, Delaye J (1978): Regional myocardial energetics during brief periods of coronary occlusion and reperfusion: Comparison with S-T segment changes. Cardiovasc Res 12: 470–76.
20. Vial C, Crozatier B, Goldschmidt D, Font B (1982): Adenine nucleotide content and regional function during ischemia and reperfusion in canine ventricular myocardium. Basic Res Cardiol 77: 645–55.
21. Swain JL, Sabina RL, McHale PA, Greenfield JC Jr, Holmes EW (1982): Prolonged myocardial nucleotide depletion after brief ischemia in the open-chest dog. Am J Physiol 242: H818–26.
22. Vary TC, Angelakos ET, Schaffer SW (1979): Relationship between adenine nucleotide metabolism and irreversible ischemic tissue damage in isolated perfused rat heart. Circ Res 45: 218–25.
23. Namm DH (1973): Myocardial nucleotide synthesis from purine bases and nucleosides. Comparison of the rate of formation of purine nucleotides from various precursors and identification of the enzymatic routes for nucleotide formation in the isolated rat heart. Circ Res 33: 686–95.
24. Zimmer H-G, Trendelenburg C, Kammermeier H, Gerlach E (1973): De novo synthesis of myocardial adenine nucleotides in the rat. Acceleration during recovery from oxygen deficiency. Circ Res 32: 635–42.
25. Reibel DK, Rovetto MJ (1979): Myocardial adenosine salvage rates and restoration of ATP content following ischemia. Am J Physiol 237: H247–52.
26. Swain JL, Hines JJ, Sabina RL, Holmes EW (1982): Accelerated repletion of ATP and GTP pools in post-ischemic canine myocardium using a precursor of purine de novo synthesis. Circ Res 51: 102–5.

27 Mauser M, Hoffmeister HM, Nienaber C, Schaper W (1985): Influence of ribose, adenosine, and 'AICAR' on the rate of myocardial adenosine triphosphate synthesis during reperfusion after coronary artery occlusion in the dog. Circ Res 56: 220–30.

28. Isselhard W, Eitenmuller J, Maurer W, DeVreese A, Reineke H, Czerniak A, Sturz J, Herb H-G (1980): Increase in myocardial adenine nucleotides induced by adenosine: Dosage, mode of application and duration, species differences. J Mol Cell Cardiol 12: 619–34.

29. Foker JE, Einzig S, Want T (1980): Adenosine metabolism and myocardial preservation. Consequences of adenosine catabolism on myocardial high-energy compounds and tissue blood flow. J Thorac Cardiovasc Surg 80: 506–16.

30. Haas GW, DeBoer LWV, O'Keefe DD, Bodenhamer RM, Geffin GA, Drop IJ, Teplick RS, Daggett WM (1984): Reduction of post-ischemic myocardial dysfunction by substrate repletion during reperfusion. Circulation 70 (Suppl I): I-65–74.

31. Duval-Arnold M, Ingwall JS, Menashe P, Fossel ET (1981): Beneficial effects of inosine on cardiac metabolism during and after ischemic cardioplegic arrest-P-31 NMR study. Circulation 64 (Suppl IV): IV:–148 (Abstract).

32. DeWitt DF, Jochim KE, Behrendt DM (1983): Nucleotide degration and functional impairment during cardioplegia: Amelioration by inosine. Circulation 67: 171–78.

33. Zimmer H-G (1983): Normalization of depressed heart function in rats by ribose. Science 220: 81–82.

34. Hoffmeister HM, Mauser M, Schaper W (1984): Failure of post-ischemic ATP repletion by adenosine to improve regional myocardial function. In: Mohl W, Woher E, Gloger D (eds) The coronary sinus. Proceedings of the First International Symposium on Myocardial Protection via the Coronary Sinus. Springer-Verlag, NY, pp. 148–52.

35. Nicklas JM, Becker LC, Bulkley BH (1985): Effects of repeated brief coronary occlusion on regional left ventricular function and dimension in dogs. Am J Cardiol 56: 473–78.

36. Becker LC, Levine JH, DiPaula AF, Guarnieri T, Aversano T (1986): Reversal of dysfunction in post-ischemic stunned myocardium by epinephrine and postextrasystolic potentiation. JACC 7: 580–89.

37. Ambrosio G, Jacobus WJ, Becker LC (1985): Evidence for functional and metabolic reserve in stunned hearts. Clin Res 33: 165A (Abstract).

38. Ambrosio G, Jacobus WE, Becker LC (1985): Effect of the direct purine precursor 'AICAR' on post-ischemic isolated rabbit hearts. Clin Res 33: 738A.

39. Levine JH, Moore EN, Becker LC, deLangen C, Weisman HL, Spear JF (1985): Abnormal action potential characteristics and cell coupling present in post-ischemic 'stunned' myocardium. Circulation 72 Suppl III): III–238 (Abstract).

40. Mercier JC, Lando U, Karmatsuse K, Ninomiya K, Meerbaum S, Fishbein MC, Swan JHC, Ganz W (1982): Divergent effects of inotropic stimulation on the ischemic and severely depressed reperfused myocardium. Circ 66: 397–400.

41. Roan P, Scales F, Saffer S, Buja IM, Willerson JT (1979): functional characterization of left ventricular segmental responses during the initial 24h and 1 wk after experimental canine myocardial infarct. J Clin Invest 64: 1074–88.

42. Ellis SG, Wynne J, Braunwald E, Henschke C, Tamas Sandor D, Kloner RA (1984): Response of reperfusion salvaged, stunned myocardium to inotropic stimulation. Am Heart J 107: 13–19.

43. Chance B, Eleff S, Leigh JS Jr, Sokolow D, Sapega A (1981): Mitochondrial regulation of phosphocreatine/inorganic phosphate ratios in exercising human muscle: a gated ^{31}P NMR study. Proc Natl Acad Sci 78: 6714–18.

44. Ito BR, Tate H, Schaper W (1985): Calcium induced increases in regional contractile function before and after transient coronary occlusion in the dog. Circulation 72 (Suppl III): III–68 (Abstract).

Discussion

Sonnenblick: It is a very beautiful story. The type of left ventricular dysfunction you describe is somewhat similar to the myopathy we have talked about occurring with microvascular spasm or small vessel disease. What happens when you stop the epinephrine? Does it maintain recovery after epinephrine or does it always just go back to how it was before epinephrine? does it ever say 'Thanks Doc' and go on its way normally, or is stunning independent of that inotropic support which nicely corrects it?

Becker: I think the inotropic support only corrects the dysfunction while it is ongoing. In our experience when we stop the epinphrine the function always returns to where it was before the epinephrine. It does not go below it, but it does not demonstrate long-lasting improvement either.

Sonnenblick: You do not produce any extensive damage to the myocardium by supporting it for this time?

Becker: I do not think that we do, based on the lack of post-epinephrine depression of function.

Sonnenblick: It could be useful when you need it.

Beyar: Are there any data regarding the oxygen consumption of the stunned myocardium, independent of the flow or the level of metabolites?

Becker: We have measured oxygen consumption in the perfused rabbit heart and have found that it is reduced after the heart is stunned. However, the rate-pressure product is reduced proportionally even more, so that the oxygen consumption is actually inappropriately high relative to the 'work' being performed. These results are similar to findings by Dr John Nicklas of the University of Michigan in the regionally stunned dog heart.

Beyar: Will this generate a situation where you have a low efficiency of protein synthesis?

Becker: There appears to be oxygen wastage. The oxygen may be going into supporting processes other than contractile function, such as membrane repair.

Bassingthwaighte: Your story suggests that a very large fraction of adenosine infused intravascularly was taken up by endothelial cells. This fits some other data. Our analysis of these data indicate that the endothelial cells with take up some 90%–95% of the infused adenosine and which would not reach the myocyte.

Becker: Do you think that the elevated ATP we measured in these perfused hearts could be in the endothelial cells rather than in the myocytes?

Bassingthwaighte: That is a possibility since ATP is very rapidly formed from adenosine in endothelial cells. One could examine this on isolated cells by NMR or chemistry.

Becker: With NMR we measure the total amount of a substance present and cannot differentiate where it is in the sample.

Bassingthwaighte: Do you think that free radicals may be playing an important

role in causing stunned myocardium?
Becker: Free radicals should not be taken too lightly since administering the free radical scavengers superoxide dismutase and catalase partially prevented stunning in 3 different studies. I agree that free radicals may be important here. We are focusing on very short periods of ischemia, and it may be the reperfusion that occurs after each episode of ischemia that is really injurious.

35. Concentric left ventricular hypertrophy: a simulation study of mechanics related to transmural oxygen demand and perfusion

R. BEYAR and S. SIDEMAN

Abstract

A comprehensive model which incorporates the local instantaneous and global time dependent cardiac mechanics, perfusion and energetics is used to study related parameters in concentric left ventricular hypertrophy (LVH) due to pressure overload. The mechanical aspects are analyzed with special attention to the effect of hypertrophy on E_{max} and on the source resistance of the LV. The local balance between mechanics, oxygen demand and coronary flow are studied and compared to experimental data taken from the published literature. The model presented here represents an attempt to develop a quantitative tool for the study of some phenomena related to LVH.

Introduction

Left ventricular hypertrophy (LVH) due to pressure overload is not a primary disease of the heart but rather an adaptive response to a pressure stimulus. In view of the large prevalence of this problem, major research efforts were carried out attempting to characterize the mechanical and metabolic aspects of this phenomenon. The effect of LVH on the global LV function [1–7] and its relation to fiber properties [1, 5, 8] are well documented. The effect of LVH on the coronary circulation is also well recognized [9–16]. It seems that LVH is accompanied by a decrease in coronary reserve especially at high heart rates [12, 13, 16]. In view of the intensity of the research in this area, an integrated picture of the cardiac behavior due to LVH is highly required.

The present analysis utilizes a recent model of LV mechanics which accounts for LV geometry and structure, fiber properties, electrical activation velocity, the twist of the LV over its long axis, and the typical arterial parameters [17], extended to include the transmural oxygen demand based on a local 'stress-length-area' (SLA) method, which is a modification of the pressure-volume-area

(PVA) approach of Suga et al. [18–19]. Further extension of the model includes coronary hemodynamics and perfusion [20], limited to a simplified algorithm of coronary autoregulation based on the oxygen demand and supply balance [21]. The comprehensive model thus developed can describe the interrelation between transmural and global mechanics, energetics (oxygen demand), and perfusion in the normal heart.

It is the purpose of this presentation to utilize this model for the analysis and description of a relatively symmetric disease of the heart, the pressure overload hypertrophy. It is hoped that this attempt may enhance the understanding of the important parameters effecting the cardiac function and provide a semi-quantitative tool which may help analyze the sequence of events associated with the development of related cardiac diseases.

General description of the simulation model

A brief summary of the assumptions used in the construction of the comprehensive model is given in Table 1. The mechanical model predicts the global LV function as well as the transmural mechanical characteristics as a function of the LV geometry and structure, the fiber properties, the velocity of the transmural

Table 1. A summary of the major assumptions used in the construction of the comprehensive model of LV function.

Mechanical model	Oxygen demand model	Coronary perfusion model
Geometry: spheroidal nested shell. Fan-like fibrous structure. Reference state: unpressurized passive state.	Oxygen demand is proportional to the local sarcomere stress-length area (SLA).	Multilayered. Distributed intramyocardial resistance.
Fiber characteristics: typical active and passive sarcomere stress length relationship. Laws of mechanics: forces are transmitted along fibers; pressure gradient across each layer is calculated based on Laplace's law. Electrical propagation: radial (endo to epicardium). Arterial model: simple windkessel.	SLA is defined as the 'active' area of the stress-length loop drawn by the sarcomere plus the area between this loop and the maximum sarcomere stress length line (Fig. 1).	Distributed arterial, intramyocardial and lumped epicardial compliance. Back pressure is the sum of the local intramural pressure and the microcirculatory critical closing pressure, P_{cr}. Autoregulation occurs locally to account for local oxygen supply demand balance and affects both resistance and P_{cr}.

electrical propagation and the major parameters of the arterial tree. The reference state volume V_o is defined in the passive state at zero transmural LV pressures. LV volumes greater than the reference volume result in extension of the sarcomeres and the thinning of the wall. The sarcomere length at the reference state is assumed to be evenly distributed across the wall, and equals to 1.9 μm, except for the endocardial sarcomeres at V_o which, based on physiological data [22] are taken to be somewhat shorter than 1.9 μm.

The oxygen demand is evaluated by a 'local' analogy [18] to Suga's global PVA approach to predict LV energetics. The sarcomere stress-length area (SLA) (the dashed area in Fig. 1) links the local mechanical and metabolic parameters. When the SLA is normalized by the unstressed sarcomere length, the resulting parameter $SLA_n(y)$ has the units of pressure (energy per unit volume) which relates linearly to the local oxygen demand per beat, $VO_2(y)$, by:

$$VO_2(y)/\text{beat} = K_1\ SLA_n(y) + K_2, \tag{1}$$

where K_1 and K_2 are constants.

The coronary circulation model assumes a distributed 'small vessel' resistance which decreases linearly from the epicardium to the endocardium [20]. The flow across this resistance is proportional to the input pressure minus the local back pressure, $P_{zf}(y, t)$. The latter is assumed to be the sum of the critical closing pressure, $P_{cr}(y)$ (typical of microcirculation), and the 'external' local intramural pressure $P_{im}(y)$. A distributed intramyocardial capacitance $C_{im}(y)$ and a global epicardial arterial capacitance, C_{ep}, are also included in the model. Local autoregulation modifies the microcirculatory resistance and is introduced by utilization autoregulatory function, Twf(y), which equals zero at maximum vasodilation and unity at maximum vasoconstriction. Twf(y) may also be viewed as an approximate expression for local coronary reserve. The autoregulation of the local resistance is adjusted by a balance of oxygen demand and supply. This is achieved by relating to the hemoglobin dissociation curve and assuming that the myocardial tissue extracts oxygen from the blood, until a venous PO_2 of 20 mm Hg is achieved, but the extraction can increase to yield a venous PO_2 not lower than 15 mm Hg.

Application of the simulation model to LV hypertrophy

Geometrical aspects

Concentric hypertrophy is associated with an increase in the end diastolic (ED) wall thickness. If no decomposition of cardiac function has occurred, the LV cavity may be normal, or even smaller than normal, in the hypertrophic case. The geometrical parameters of the ventricle can be introduced into the model via the

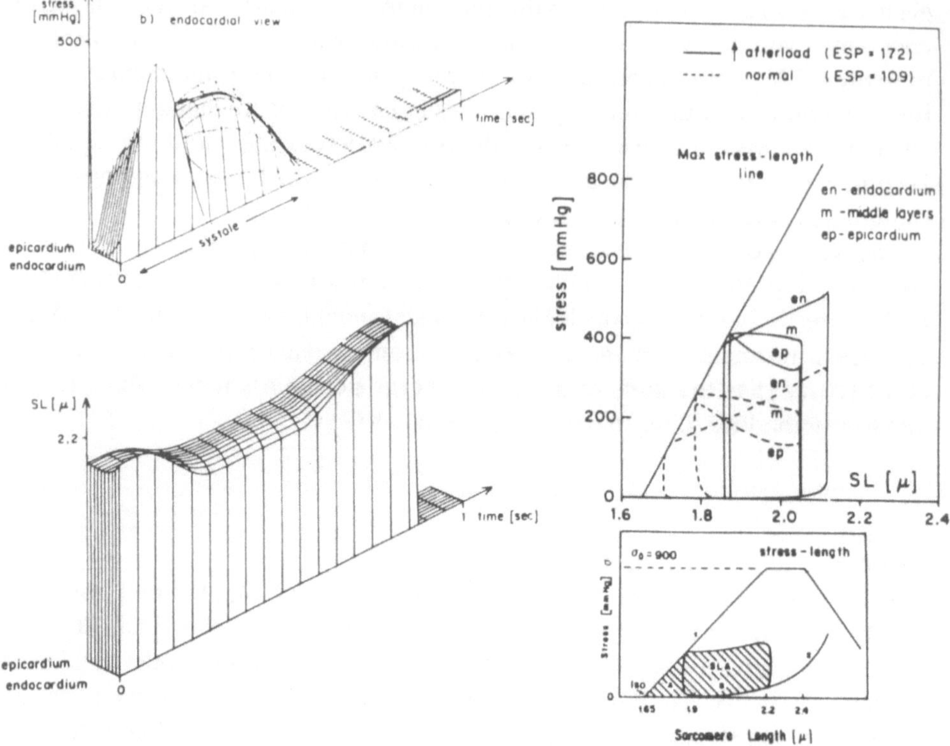

Figure 1. Left: Endocardial view of the 'axial' (along the fibers) sarcomere stress (top) and length (bottom) distribution vs. time (bottom). Right: The sarcomere stress-length loop for the endocardial, middle and epicardial layers for two loads (top). The dashed area (bottom) is the area defined as SLA and used to calculate the local oxygen consumption.

'reference dimensions' which, by definition, are load-independent. However, no conclusive evidence as to the value of the reference volume at compensated LVH is presently known. Thus, LVH can be simulated either by assuming a constant reference semi-minor axis (and thus a constant V_0) and an increased reference wall thickness, h_0, or, alternatively, by relating to a constant reference midwall position, which is associated with a decreased V_0 and b_0 (Fig. 2).

Fiber mechanics

The fiber mechanical properties are usually studied based on their force-length and force-velocity relationship. Experimental studies of the evolution of hypertrophy indicate that at the early LVH stages, the force generated by the fibers is maintained, or even increased, while the maximum velocity of shortening is reduced [1, 5]. This is related to changes in the biochemical properties of the myosin type [23, 24] and is not associated with an impaired function of the myocardium but is rather viewed as an improved economy of force generation [24].

A decrease in myocardial contractility may occur at a later stage of hypertrophy [1, 7, 14] leading to the development of the congestive heart failure associated with hypertrophic cardiomyopathy [25, 26].

Energetic aspects

The simple SLA approach used here for the prediction of transmural oygen demand requires the estimation of the two constants K_1 and K_2. Changes in the value of these parameters with isotrophic changes [27, 28] are being investigated using the PVA approach. However, the possible effect of the changes in the myosin type, or the force velocity relationships, on the constants K_1 and K_2 are neglected here for lack of data concerning the human heart (although some yet unmeasurable changes in the myosin type may affect sarcomeres efficiency and have an effect on K_1 and K_2).

Coronary circulation aspects

Some experimental data [11, 12] indicate that the coronary minimal resistance increases in LVH, although the flow distribution at rest may be normal [16]. Bache et al. [12] have calculated an increase of about 50–60% in the minimum resistance, from 16.5 to 22.6 mm Hg · sec/ml, in LVH as compared with normal dogs. Okeefe et al. [11] showed an 80% increase in the minimum resistance. For lack of a better value it is assumed here that the LVH resistance increased 1.5 times the normal value in coronary circulation. Note that this assumption is the only coronary-related parameter which is taken in this simulation model to be different in the LVH as compared to the normal heart.

Results and discussion

Mechanical aspects

The reference state is used here to define changes in LV geometry during LVH. Two possible simulations of LVH are depicted in Fig. 2. One is based on an increase in the LV wall thickness while the reference cavity volume, V_0, remains unchanged. The other possible geometry relates to a constant midwall dimension at the reference configuration, resulting in a decreased V_0 value. As shown in Fig. 3, the E_{max} line in both cases is shifted to the left, thus allowing the ventricle to

REFERENCE STATE IN LVH

A. Constant V_o

h_o V_o b_o h_o V_o b_o

NORMAL HYPERTROPHY

B. Constant midwall surface

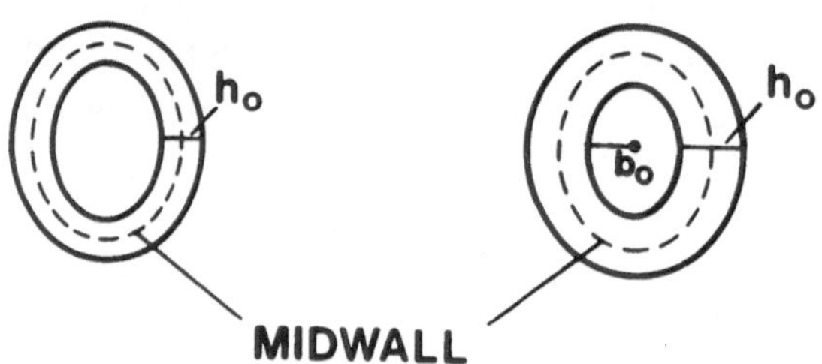

Figure 2. The reference state, defined as the geometry at the passive state for zero transmural pressure. b_o, h_o and V_o are the semiminor axis, wall thickness and cavity volume at the reference state. Two types of possible hypertrophy models are illustrated: (A) increase in h_o with constant V_o, and (B) constant midwall location.

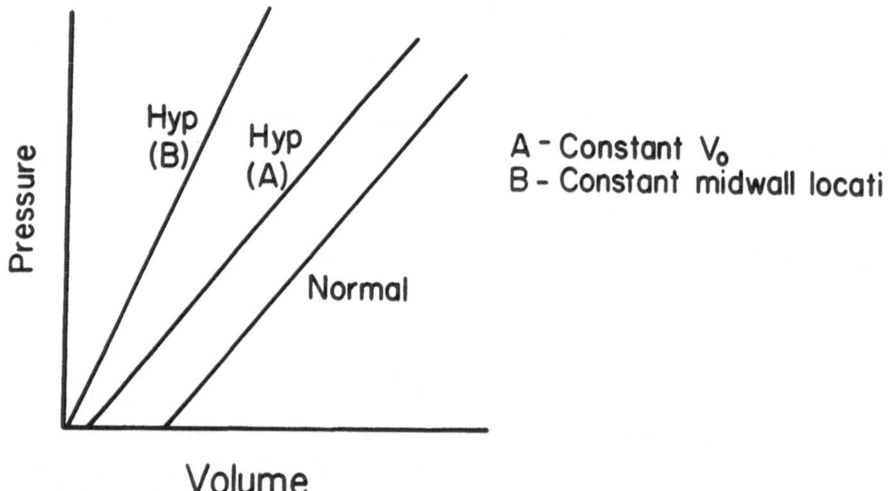

Figure 3. E_{max} line for the normal case compared to hypertrophy simulated by (A) a constant V_o and (B) a constant midwall location.

eject against higher loads. As seen in Table 2, all the contractile parameters are enhanced during LVH simulated by an increased wall thickness (constant V_o). Interestingly, the E_{max} slope does not increase in this case of a constant V_o, but increases in the case of an assumed constant reference midwall thickness.

It is noted that published data [6] indicate that E_{max} increases during hypertrophy. It is also suggested that hypertrophied hearts without decompensation may be smaller than normal comparable hearts. This information indicates that the simulation of the LVH with a constant midwall and a decreased V_o relative to the normal case is the more appropriate model. However, more data are needed before final conclusions can be drawn on this point.

The effect of changes in the force velocity relationship (FVR) can now be studied. As shown before [29], the dynamic FVR (Fig. 4) can be translated to a dynamic LV internal resistance, R_S, by:

$$R_S = \frac{\triangle P(t)}{Q(t)}, \tag{2}$$

where $\triangle P(t)$ is the instantaneous difference between the theoretical isovolumic pressure at that instant and the measured LV pressure, and Q(t) is the simultaneous time dependent aortic flow. As shown in Fig. 4 [29], assuming a fan-like dynamic FVR (wherein the maximum shortening velocity at zero stress develops very fast, and the force acts as a slow time dependent function) yields a linear pressure resistance relationship with a slope α similar to that reported by Shroff et al. [30].

Table 3 represents a simulation of some stages in the evolution of hypertrophy. Chronic hypertension, and compensated hypertrophy leading to normal ejection fraction, does not significantly affect either R_S or the R_s vs P_o slope α. However, a marked increase in both R_S and α is noted if one reduces the maximum unloaded fiber velocity to half its normal value. Interestingly, a decrease in the fiber force

Table 2. The effect of different degrees of LVH at the same LV pressure on different indices of contractility. Hypertrophy is simulated by an increase in wall thickness h_o while V_o (= 57 ml), Ved (= 102 ml) are held constant. End diastolic aortic pressure is kept constant at 70 mm Hg.

	ho [cm]	ho/bo	h_{ed} [cm]	$(h/b)_{ed}$	Vm [ml]	EF %	$(dP/dt)_{max}$ [mm Hg · sec^{-1}]	U_{cf} [sec]$^{-1}$]	E_{max} [mm Hg/ml]
Normal	1.2	0.63	0.99	0.43	44	65	1833	1.33	4.8
LVH	1.6	0.73	1.16	0.50	179	69	1954	1.43	5.0
LVH	1.8	0.84	1.34	0.58	219	73	1947	1.61	4.2

b_o = reference semi-minor axis; V_m = muscle volume, U_{cf} = average circumferential shortening rate (at endocardial level), E_{max} = maximum elastance representing slope of end systolic pressure-volume points.

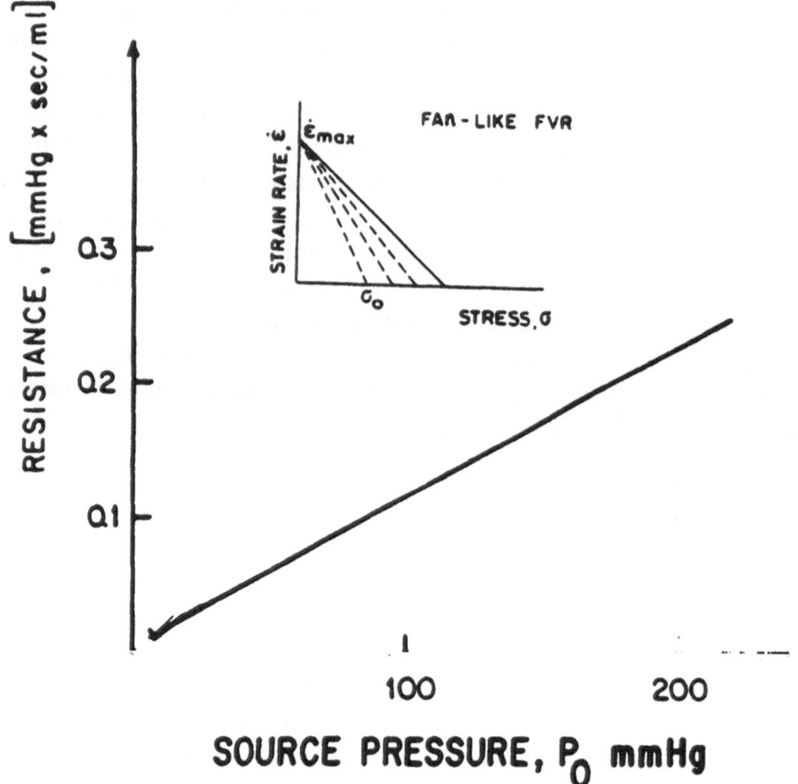

Figure 4. Source resistance vs. source pressure corresponding to the dynamic, fan-like, force-velocity relationship with a constant $\dot{\varepsilon}_{max}$ and a time variable stress.

results in the reversal of R_S and α towards the normal values. Thus, it seems that the R_S reflects the ratio between the fiber force and the unloaded velocity. The high slope generated by a decrease in the $\dot{\varepsilon}_{max}$ value is important for optimal ventricular-arterial impedance matching during hypertension. When the myocardial function deteriorates and the fiber force decreases, this ratio decreases and a normal R_S may be noted. Some evidence supports the theoretical prediction of increased R_S during the early stages of LVH (Shroff, personal communication). However, more experiments are needed to elucidate this point.

Oxygen demand and coronary flow

The effect of LV mechanics during hypertrophy on the transmural oxygen demand and perfusion was studied by a simulation based on experimental data of Bache et al. [12]. LVH was generated by chronic aortic banding and the mechanical as well as perfusion parameters were compared to normal dog values at a variable heart rate.

The following assumptions were used in deriving the model parameters.

a. The LV mass increases as hypertrophy develops.
b. End diastolic (ED) LV volume remains constant throughout.
c. The (average) sarcomere length at ED in both the normal and LVH cases is equal to 2.07 μm. Normal fiber force is assumed.
d. The arterial parameters and the constriction area are derived based on the contraction is assumed to be given by:

$$P = \frac{1}{2} \varrho \, V_{jet}^2, \tag{3}$$

where ϱ = specific gravity and V_{jet} – velocity of the blood jet.

The geometrical, structural (fibers) and arterial system parameters used in the simulation are shown in Table 4. For very rapid heart rates LVH may be associated with ischemia (and decreased contractility). In both cases, rapid heart rates have probable effects on the LV end diastolic volume.

The comparison between the general mechanical parameters of the normal and hypertrophic cases is shown in Table 5. Note the high transtenotic pressure gradients generated in the hypertrophic dogs at HR = 100. Note that a marked decrease in the gradient is observed for HR = 240. However, an isolated increase of the heart rate in the model does not predict a decrease in the gradient, as observed experimentally. Thus, either a decrease in contractility or a decrease in the ED volume, or both, may explain the observed decrease in the peak LV pressure in LVH at HR = 240. In order to explain the decrease in the transtenotic pressure gradient as the HR increases, a decreased ED volume was assumed for

Table 3. The effect of different stages of hypertrophy (LVH) and hypertension (HT) on LV source resistance and other contractility indices. Human parameters are used.

	V_{ed} (ml)	V_m (ml)	Blood pressure (mm Hg)	EF (%)	(dP/dt) (mm Hg · sec−1)	U_{cf} (sec^{-1})	R_S (mm Hg · sec · ml^{-1})	α (sec ml^{-1} × 10^{-3})
1. Normal heart	102	179	122/82	66	2008	1.37	0.60	0.84
2. LVH & HT with normal fiber parameters	102	337	205/114	66	2474	1.30	0.18	0.90
3. As above but with $\dot{\varepsilon}_{max}$ reduced from 3 to 1.5 sec^{-1}	102	337	191/114	65	2774	1.21	0.42	1.50
4. Same as (3) but with decreased contractility (σ_0: 1140→840)	102	337	184/114	54	1841	0.95	0.33	1.05

V_{ed} = end diastolic volume; V_m = LV muscle volume; U_{cf} = average circumferential shortening velocity.

both the normal and the hypertrophic cases and an additional decrease in contractility was assumed for the LVH. This is based on evidence that some subendocardial hypoxia was generated here (to be discussed below).

Table 6 presents the principal parameters of energetics and perfusion used in the simulation. The SLA constants of (1) are based on Suga's [27] experiments ($K_1 = 1.7\,10^{-5}$ ml O_2/mm Hg · gr · beat, $K_2 = 3.0\,10^{-4}$ O_2/gr · beat) and are assumed to be the same in the normal and the hypertrophic hearts. As indicated above, the minimum coronary resistance in LVH is assumed to be 1.5 times the normal resistance.

Table 4. Parameters related to LV mechanics used in the simulation of perfusion in LVH.

LV geometry	Normal heart	Hypertrophic heart
LV muscle volume [ml]	83	127
b_{ed} – ED semiminor axis [cm]	1.8	1.8
h_{ed} – ED wall thickness [cm]	0.9	1.2
b_o – reference seminimor axis [cm]	1.51	1.45
$(h/b)_{ed}$	0.5	0.66
Fiber properties		
Max. stress at optimal sarcomere length – [mm Hg]	1000	1000[a]
ED sarcomere length [μm] average	2.07	2.07
Arterial parameters		
Peripheral resistance [mm Hg · sec/ml]	2	2
Arterial capacitance [ml/mm Hg]	0.6	0.4
Banded aortic orifice [cm^2]	4	0.22

[a] HR = 100 bpm. Value goes to 700 mm Hg at HR = 240 bpm.

Table 5. Comparison of calculated results with experimental hemodynamic data (dogs).

	HR = 100 bpm				HR = 240 bpm			
	Normal		Hypertrophy		Normal		Hypertrophy	
	Exp	Calc.	Exp	Calc.	Exp	Calc.[a]	Exp	Calc.[b]
LV systolic pressure [mm Hg]	126	116	241	238	117	104	163	165
Aortic pressure [mm Hg]	126/79	117/85	109/76	96/83	106/76	104/87	96/67	90/85
Average transtenotic pressure gradient [mm Hg]	–	0.46	–	72	–	2.09	–	35
U_{cf} [sec^{-1}]	–	1.76	–	1.34	–	2.17	–	0.99

U_{cf} = average endocardial circumferential shortening rate
[a] V_{ed} = 34 ml assumed for a normal heart at HR = 240.
[b] b_{ed} = 1.65 cm; V_{ed} = 34 ml; σ_o = 700 mm Hg for LVH.

The autoregulation function Twf(y) [20] is allowed to adjust so that the venous oxygen tension is set at 20 mm Hg. Whenever, if the oxygen demand is not supplied in spite of maximum vasodilation, the venous oxygen tension may go as low as 15 mm Hg, thus reflecting higher oxygen extraction. The hemoglobin concentration in the blood is taken as 12 gr%.

The experimental and simulated transmural flow distribution in the normal heart at two heart rates for an autoregulated and a maximum vasodilated heart are shown in Fig. 5. Note that the flow at HR = 100 bmp is almost equally distributed throughout the wall. Note also that at HR = 240, with maximum autoregulation, the endocardial layers have only a slight coronary reserve and the flow is much higher at the epicardial than endocardial layers. Evidently, the compressive forces acting on the endocardial layers are much more effective at high heart rates than at low heart rates. Note that a decreased preload case (as detailed in Table 5) is only slightly different from a constant preload case.

The comparable plots for the hypertrophic heart are shown in Fig. 6. The experimental studies show close to normal perfusion distribution at HR = 100, but the autoregulated flows are higher than in the normal hearts. However, pacing at HR = 240 bpm causes a transmural decrease in the flow rate at maximum vasodilatation, although the subendocardial decrease in flow is most prominent. Flow in the autoregulated case is increased so as to supply the increased demand in the outer LV wall, but fails to increase in the subendocardial layers.

Table 6. Parameters related to perfusion and energetics.

	Normal heart	Hypertrophic heart
Local oxygen demand by SLA approach	$K_1 = 1.74 \times 10^{-5}$ [ml] O_2/beat · gr · mm Hg] $K_2 = 3 \times 10^{-4}$ [ml O_2/beat · gr]	same as for normal
Coronary perfusion		
	Linear:	
Minimum coronary resistance	R_{min} (o) = 600 [mm Hg · sec/ml]	
	R_{min} (h) = 900 [mm Hg · sec/ml]	$R_{min} = 1.5\, R_{min}$ of normal
Maximum coronary resistance	$5 \times R_{min}$	same as for normal
Autoregulation		
Twf(y) is adjusted so that venous oxygen pressure varies between set 1 and set 2	Set 1 = 15 mm Hg Set 2 = 20 mm Hg	Set 1 = 15 mm Hg Set 1 = 20 mm Hg
Hb concentration	12 gr%	12 gr%
Hb dissociation curve const.:		
P_{50}	26 (mm Hg)	26 (mm Hg)
Cooperation constant	2.3	2.3

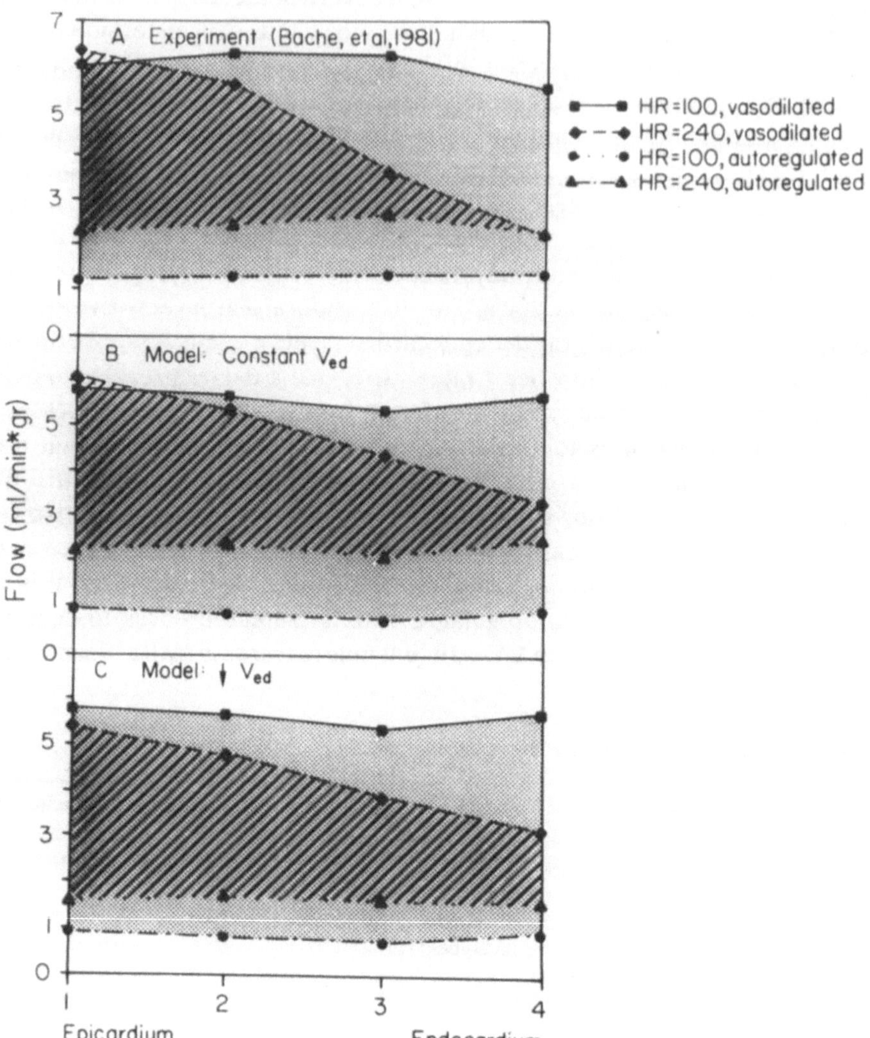

Figure 5. Comparison of experimental and calculated transmural flows in the normal LV. The experimental measurements (A) are compared to model simulation with a constant end diastolic volume V_{ed}, (B), and a decreased V_{ed}, (C).

The calculated results, assuming no change in preload or contractility, shown in Fig. 6b indicate an increase in the maximum vasodilation flow in the subepicardium. This is a result of the highly increased aortic preconstriction pressure which seems to affect mostly the epicardial layers. This is obviously not a real situation and panel 6C was calculated to represent a more realistic simulation which is consistant with experimental data. The autoregulatory function Twf(y) repre-

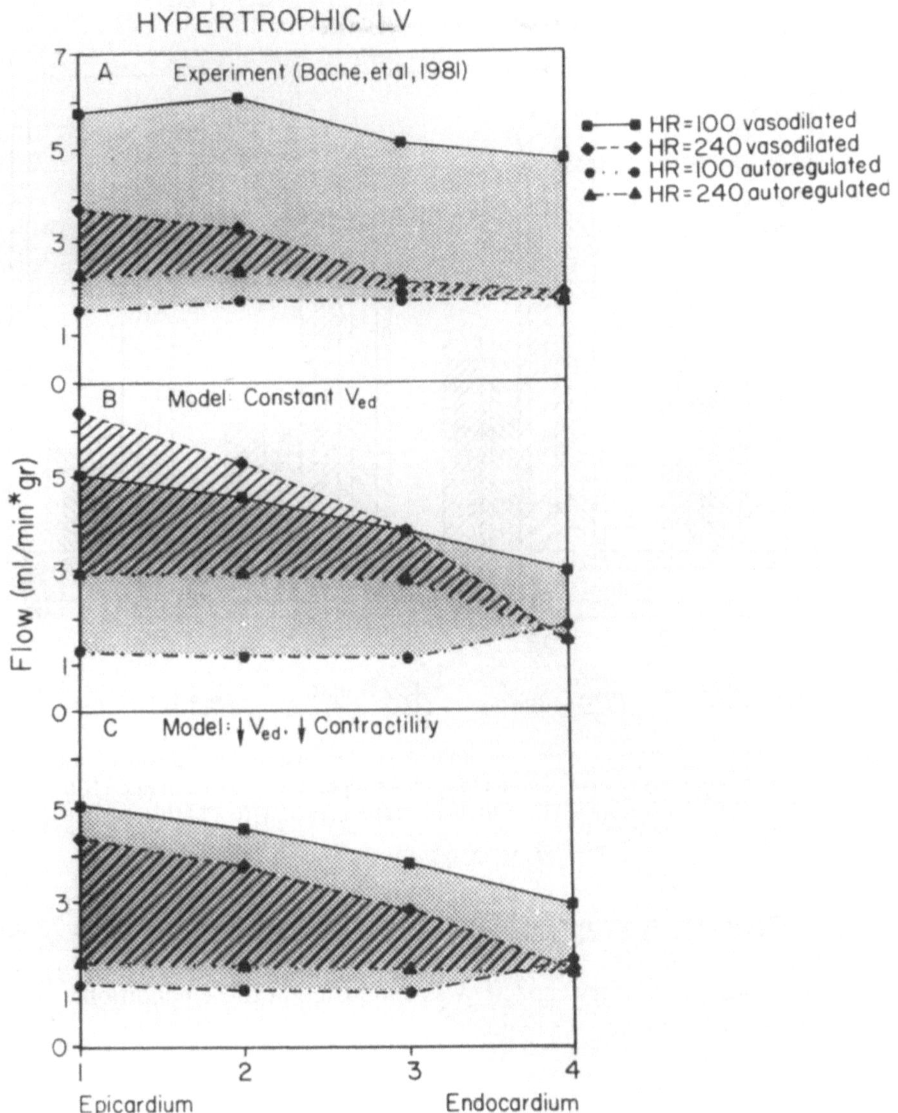

Figure 6. Comparison of experimental and calculated transmural flows in the hypertrophic LV. The model simulation for a constant V_{ed} is compared to a simulation assuming decreased V_{ed} and contractility (see Table 5).

sents the vasodilatory capacity of each layer. Thus, Twf(y) = 0 corresponds to zero vasodilatory capacity and Twf(y) = 1 denotes maximum vasodilatory capacity. A plot of the transmural Twf(y) for the above cases is shown in Fig. 7 for 4 (epicardium to endocardium) layers. Note that the vasodilatory capacity decreases from the epicardium to the endocardium, both for HR = 100 bpm and

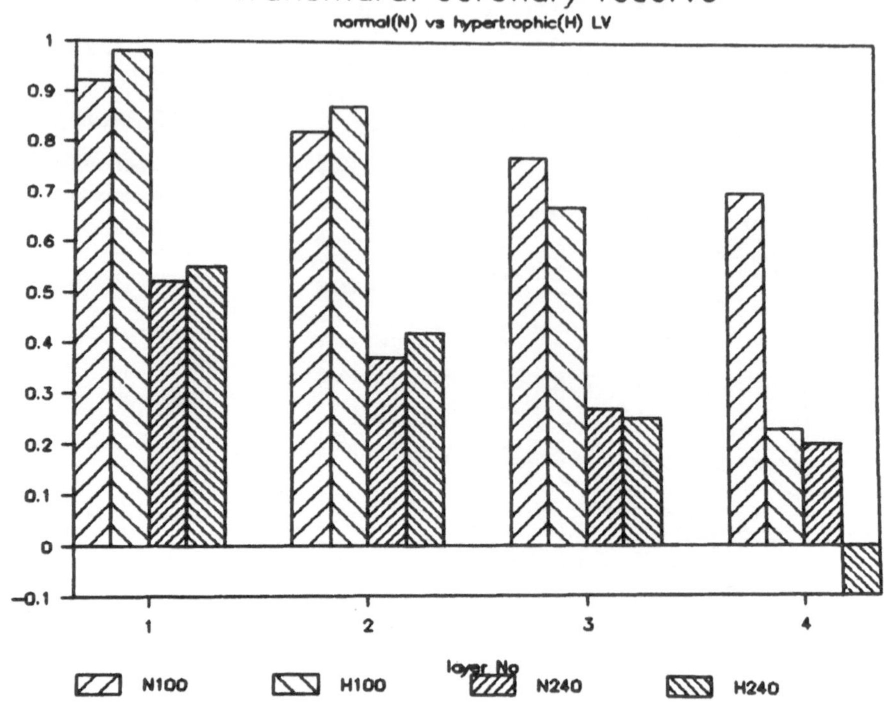

Figure 7. Comparison of the transmural (epicardium to endocardium) autoregulatory function which corresponds to the coronary reserve of normal and hypertrophic LV at two heart rates. N100: normal, HR = 100 bpm. H100: hypertrophy, HR = 100 bpm. N240: normal, HR = 240 bpm. H240: hypertrophy, HR = 240 bpm.

HR = 240 bpm. The negative endocardial value of Twf(y) shown in Fig. 7 for the hypertrophic case, at HR = 240 bpm, is only an illustrative aid to emphasize the fact that the autoregulatory capacity was exhausted at these conditions and that the subendocardial layers are hypoxic.

Discussion

A comprehensive model which combines transmural mechanics, perfusion and energetics was applied here to analyze and describe LVH due to pressure overload. Such a comprehensive model, which depends on a large number of parameters, requires that appropriate assumptions be made wherever knowledge is lacking. However, a continuous comparison between the calculated model results and experimental data is needed in order to verify the assumptions and elucidate various questions raised during the simulation process.

LVH was shown to be accompanied by many mechanical changes which help the heart to function and eject blood against a higher afterload. The few studies which examine the elastance during hypertrophy show an increased elastance and a leftward shift of the P-V relationship [6]. Such behavior may reflect either an increased fiber contractility, a decrease in the reference volume, or both. Although some data may suggest a decreased LV volume with compensated hypertrophy [14]. More experiments are needed to quantify this point.

An increase in LV source resistance is predicted by the model, based on data reporting a decrease in the unloaded shortening velocity of the fibers [1, 5], which evidently reflects a change in the myosin composition [23], at least in animals if not in humans [24]. May this change in resistance be used as a clinical parameter to evaluate myocardial function? More experiments are needed to answer this and other questions.

Inspection of the oxygen balance within the LV wall seems to indicate that hypertrophy tends to affect the endocardial flow more than the epicardial flow. This is evident only at high heart rates where the relative duration of the diastole is smaller. In addition to the increased compressive forces, the minimal coronary resistance is known to be higher in LVH [11, 12] and this fact may affect arterial changes related to hypertension. The oxygen demand distribution is opposite in direction to the coronary flow distribution. Higher rates of oxygen utilization is needed by the endocardial layer due to higher loads (and higher SLA's) of these layers. Thus, a chronic mismatch in oxygen demand and supply may lead to a chronic hypoxia and to the development of subendocardial fibrosis – a well known feature of long standing hypertension [31–33].

Conclusion

An analytic semiquantitative comprehensive approach was applied to a common disease of the LV. Mechanical energetical and perfusion aspects of the disease were simulated by utilizing a simulation model and the specific questions raised by the model were discussed. The model analysis may help in understanding the complex interaction within the cardiac system in health and disease and lead to better mathematical definition of the physiological laws which affect the cardiac system.

Acknowledgment

This study was supported by a grant from the Women's Division, MEP Group, American Technion Society, NY.

References

1. Burger SB, Strauer BE (1981): Left ventricular hypertrophy in chronic pressure load due to spontaneous essential hypertension, I. Left ventricular function, left ventricular geometry and wall stress, II. Contractility of the isolated left ventricular myocardium and left ventricular stiffness. In: Strauer BE (ed) The heart in hypertension. Springer, New York, p. 1352.
2. Devereaux RD, Reicheck N (1980): Left ventricular hypertrophy. Cardiovasc Rev Rep 1: 55–68.
3. Grossman W, Jones D, McLaurin LP (1975): Wall stress and patterns of hypertrophy in the human LV. J Clin Invest 56: 56–64.
4. Hess OM, Schneider J, Koch R, Bamer C, Grimon J, Krayenbuehl PH (1981): Diastolic function and myocardial structure in patients with myocardial hypertrophy. Circulation 63: 360–371.
5. Okada T, Okauyama H, Mashima H, Sato H, Kitamura K (1984): Left ventricular function and muscle mechanics in hypertrophied rabbit heart. Am J Physiol 247 (Heart Circ Physiol 16): H699–H706.
6. Nakamura T, Kimura T, Arai S, Motomiya M, Suzuki S (1984): Left ventricular function of concentric hypertrophied heart after chronic pressure overload as studied in the isolated canine heart preparation. Jpn J Physiol 34: 613–628.
7. Sasayama S, Ross J, Franklin D, Bloom CM, Bishop S, Dilley RB (1976): Adaptation of the left ventricle to chronic pressure overload. Circ Res 38: 172–178.
8. Harmell BB, Alpert NR (1977): The mechanical characteristics of hypertrophied rabbit cardiac muscle in the absence of congestive heart failure, The contractile and series elastic element. Circ Res 40: 20–25.
9. Marcus ML, Mueller TM, Gascho JA, Kerber RE (1979): Effects of cardiac hypertrophy secondary to hypertension on the coronary circulation. Am J Cardiol 44: 1023–1028.
10. Marcus ML, Koyanayi S, Harrison DG, Doty DB, Hiratza LF, Eastham CL (1983): Abnormalities in the coronary circulation that occur as a consequence of cardiac hypertrophy. Am J Med 75: 62–66.
11. O'Keefe DD, Hoffman JIE, Cheitlin R, O'Neill MJ, Allard JR, Shapkin E (1978): Coronary blood flow in experimental canine left ventricular hypertrophy. Circ Res 43: 43–51.
12. Bache RJ, Vrobel TR, Aretzen CE, Ring WS (1981): Effect of maximal coronary vasodilatation on transmural myocardial perfusion during tachycardia in dogs with left ventricular hypertrophy. Circ Res 49: 742–750.
13. Bache RJ, Vrobel TR, Ring WS, Emery RW, Anderson RW (1981): Regional myocardial blood flow during exercise in dogs with chronic left ventricular hypertrophy. Circ Res 48: 76–87.
14. Parrish DG, Ring WS, Bache RJ (1985): Myocardial perfusion in compensated and failing hypertrophied left ventricle. Am J Physiol 249 (Heart Circ Physiol): H534–H539.
15. Rembert JC, Kleinman LH, Fedor FM, Wechsler AS, Greenfield, JC (1978): Myocardial blood flow distribution in left ventricular hypertrophy. J Clin Inv 63: 379–386.
16. Mueller TM, Marcus ML, Kerber RE, Young TA, Barnes RW, Abboud FM (1978): Effect of renal hypertension and left ventricular hypertrophy on the coronary circulation in dogs. Circ Res 47: 543–549.
17. Beyar R, Sideman S (1984): Computer studies of left ventricular performance based on its fiber structure, sarcomere mechanics and transmural electrical activation propagation. Circ Res 55: 358–374.
18. Beyar R, Sideman S (1986): Left ventricular mechanics related to the local distribution of oxygen demand throughout the wall. Circ Res 58: 664–677.
19. Beyar R, Sideman S (1985): Effect of twisting motion on the nonuniformities of transmyocardial fiber mechanics and energy demand, A theoretical study. Special Issue on Modeling and Simulations, IEEE Trans. Biomed Eng, BME 32: 764–769.
20. Beyar R, Sideman S (1987): Time dependent coronary blood flow distribution in the left ventricular wall. Am J Physiol 252: (Heart Circ Physiol), H417–H433.

21. Beyar R, Sideman S (1985): A mathematical approach to interrelation between the coronary blood flow and the metabolic demands: In Sideman S, Beyar R (eds) Simulation and imaging of the cardiac system. Martinus Nijhoff Publ, Boston/Dordrecht, pp. 332–357.
22. Yoran C, Covell JW, Ross J Jr (1973): Structural basis for the ascending limb of left ventricular function. Circ Res 32: 293–303.
23. Hirtzel HO, Tuchschmid CR, Schnider J, Kraylnbuehl HP, Schaub MC (1985): A relationship between myosin isoenzyme composition, hemodynamics and myocardial structure in various forms of human cardiac hypertrophy. Circ Res 57: 729–740.
24. Holubarsch CH, Litten RZ, Mullieri LA, Alpert NR (1985): Energetic changes of myocardium as an adaptation to chronic hemodynamic overload and thyroid gland activity. Basic Res Cardiol 80: 582–593.
25. Nicolas A, Sciacca RR, Weis MB, Blood DK, Brennan DL, Canon PJ (1980): Effect of left ventricular hypertrophy on myocardial blood flow and ventricular performance in systemic hypotension. Circulation 62: 329–340.
26. Guazzi M, Giorentini C, Olivari MT, Polase A (1979): Cardiac load and function in hypertension, ultrasonic and hemodynamic study. Am J Cardiol 44: 1007–1021.
27. Suga H, Ryuichi H, Goto Y, Yamoda O, Igarashi Y (1983): Effect of positive isotropic agents on the relation between oxygen consumption and systolic pressure volume area in canine left ventricle. Circ Res 53: 306–318.
28. Burkhoff D, Yue D, Frantz M, Oikawa R, Schaefer J, Sagawa K (1985): Influence of contractile state on myocardial oxygen consumption. Circulation 72 (Suppl III) 298.
29. Beyar R, Sideman S (1986): The source parameters of the left ventricle related to the physiological characteristics of cardiac muscle. Biophys J 49: 1185–1194.
30. Shroff SG, Janicki JS, Weber KT (1983): Left ventricular systolic dynamics in terms of its chamber mechanical properties, Am J Physiol 245 (Heart Circ Physiol): H110–H124.
31. Lund DD, Twietmeyer TA, Schmid PG, Tomanek RJ (1979): Independent changes in cardiac muscle fibers and connective tissue in rats with spontaneous hypertension, aortic constriction, and hypoxia. Cardiovasc Res 13: 44–49.
32. Caspari PG, Necomb M, Gibbson K, Harris P (1977): Collagen content in the normal and hypertrophied human ventricle. Cardiovasc Res. 554–558.
33. Buccino RA, Harris E, Spann JR Jr, Sonnenblick EH (1969): Response of myocardial connective tissue to development of experimental hypertrophy. Am J Physiol 216: 425–428.

Discussion

Arts: Concerning the stress distribution in your model; you showed that at the start of the ejection phase there was a high stress in the subendocardial layers and a low stress in the subepicardial layers. In my study I do not see as large a difference as you have shown. I believe that this is due to the fact that the apex in your model is fixed and is not free to rotate, and thus you prevent torsion. The transmural distribution will then be different.
Beyar: We include torsion as an input parameter in the model and it greatly affects the transmural sarcomers length distribution as well as the stress distribution. In spite of this torsion, the endocardial sarcomere lengths at end-diastole are higher than the epicardial sarcomere lengths. Thus by local Starling law the endocardial layers will have a higher stress developed at the early stages of the cycle. Another factor contributing to the higher initial endocardial stress is the electrical activation velocity which starts at the endocardium and spreads to the epicardium. Thus, at the very beginning of the activation, the endocardial fibers are activated while the epicardial fibers are yet passive. Consequently, you have the 'endocardial kick' which then decreases due to the higher shortening of the endocardial layers throughout the ejection.
Sonnenblick: One of the most profound changes in hypertrophy is the prolongation of contraction and delayed relaxation that makes tremendous problems of early diastolic filling. Is your model going to deal with diastolic dysfunction? This is probably the primary limitation in many cases of cardiac disability.
Beyar: Very late relaxation can indeed impede the diastolic filling as well as the coronary circulation in hypertrophy more than in a normal heart, since you have less time left for both diastolic coronary flow and diastolic filling of the LV and more time for the systolic compression of the endocardial flow. We have started to model the effect of the rate of relaxation on the filling patterns in a normal heart. However, we have not as yet dealt with the problem of LV filling in hypertrophy.

36. Coronary reserves in myocardial hypertrophy

H.R. WEISS and G.J. GROVER

Abstract

The purpose of the present investigation was to determine the effects of thyroxine (T_4) induced myocardial hypertrophy on coronary flow reserve, O_2 extraction reserve and the reserve of unperfused capillaries. Studies were conducted in anesthetized open chest New Zealand white rabbits. One group had blood flow determined with radioactive microspheres and O_2 extraction determined microspectrophotometrically. Reserves were tested with hypoxia. In the other group, FITC-dextran was injected to label the perfused microvessels. An alkaline phosphatase stain was employed to locate the total microvascular bed. O_2 consumption increased 280% in the 16-day T_4 group and this was accompanied by significant increases in coronary flow and O_2 extraction. Blood flow further increased 101% for the hypoxic 16-day T_4 group. Venous O_2 saturation also decreased significantly in hypoxia. There were 2544 ± 210 capillaries/mm^2 and 5 ± 1 arterioles/mm^2 in control subendocardium. These decreased significantly to 1457 ± 65/mm^2 and 1 ± 1/mm^2 respectively after 16 days of T_4. In controls, 59 ± 2% of the capillaries and 56 ± 9% of the arterioles were perfused in the subendocardium. This increased significantly to 88 ± 3% and 79 ± 8% respectively by 16 days of T_4 treatment. Thus, the physiological response to the increased work and decreased capillary density is to increase the proportion of the capillary bed perfused to at least maintain physiological diffusion distances. The T_4 hypertrophied hearts were also able to increase their blood flow and decrease their venous O_2 saturation in response to further stress.

Introduction

Hyperthyroidism is associated with increases in heart work, heart rate, cardiac output, blood pressure and cardiac contractility [1, 2]. As we have previously shown this leads to an uniformly increased left ventricular O_2 consumption [3].

This increase in heart work can lead to cardiac hypertrophy [4–6]. Thyroxine (T_4) also leads to an increase in coronary blood flow [3, 6, 7]. Cardiac hypertrophy is often associated with a loss of flow reserves [8–10]. There can be decreased venous O_2 saturation and increased O_2 extraction [3]. This can cause a loss of O_2 extraction reserves [11]. One issue addressed in this report is the degree of flow and O_2 extraction reserves remaining in a T_4 hypertrophied heart. Hypertrophy also leads to a thickening of muscle fibers and cells although the number of microvessels providing O_2 to these fibers does not increase greatly [12–18]. This leads to a decrease in the number/mm^2 of capillaries in hypertrophy [12, 13, 15, 16, 18] compared to control [19, 20].

There is much evidence from both direct and indirect observations that a reserve of unperfused capillaries exists in the control state [21–25] although some contrary evidence exists [26, 27]. We have found that approximately half of the capillaries are perfused in control rabbit hearts [24]. This reserve can be utilized in various forms of O_2 supply stress [24, 28]. One purpose of this study was to determine whether a greater proportion of the capillaries were perfused under the stress induced by T_4 which leads to hypertrophy. In addition, we wished to determined the degree of loss of flow and O_2 extraction reserves during T_4 induced cardiac hypertrophy.

Methods

In this study New Zealand white rabbits (1–3 kg) were divided into three groups. One group served as control (saline control), one received 0.5 mg/kg l-thyroxine (T_4) subcutaneously daily for 3 days (3-day T_4 group), and another received this dose of T_4 daily for 16 days (16-day T_4 group).

The animals were anesthetized with 30 mg/kg of sodium pentobarbital via the circumflex ear vein. Polyethylene catheters were inserted into a femoral artery and vein. The venous catheter was employed in some animals for injection of 100 mg/kg of 150,000 MW dextran labeled with fluorescein isothiocyanate (FITC) and/or for supplemental anesthetic. The trachea was cannulated and artificial respiration was instituted using a Harvard respirator. A left thoracotomy was performed at the 5th intercostal space, and the pericardium was cut to expose the heart. In those animals in which blood flow was determined a catheter was placed in the left atrium.

In the animals in which blood flow was determined, a series of control measurements of hemodynamic and blood gas parameters was performed along with a coronary flow measurement using radioactive microspheres (7.5×10^5, $15 \pm 3\ \mu m$ in diameter). After these measurements, half of the hearts were rapidly removed by cutting the heart and dropping it into liquid N_2. The rest of the animals were subjected to 10–20 min of 8% O_2 in N_2. A second flow measurement was obtained and the hearts were then frozen.

To measure O_2 saturation in frozen arterial and venous blood vessels a three-wavelength microspectrophotometric method was used as described previously [29]. This technique involves the microspectrophotometric observation of blood in vessels ranging in size from 20 to 100 μm in diameter. Hearts were cut on a band saw at −20° C. Sections (20 μm) were cut on a rotary microtome at −20° C in a N_2 atmosphere. They were transferred to precooled glass slides and covered with degassed silicone oil and a coverglass. These slides were placed on a Zeiss microspectrophotometer fitted with a N_2-flushed cold stage to obtain readings of optical density at 560, 524, and 507 nm. The slit width was set at 5-nm band pass, and size of the measuring spot was 8 μm. Readings were obtained to determine O_2 saturation in five arteries and veins, 20–100 μm in diameter. Immediately adjacent areas were prepared for determination of blood flow. By use of the Fick principle, the paired product of O_2 extraction and blood flow was obtained to determine O_2 consumption on a regional basis within the heart.

FITC-dextran (Sigma, 150,000 m.W.) was injected into the venous catheter and flushed with 1 ml of saline in the rest of the experimental rabbits. After 14 sec, the hearts were removed and placed in liquid N_2.

The hearts were cut into wafers on a band saw at −20° C. The subepicardial and subendocardial regions of the left ventricular free wall were examined. Each frozen tissue sample was mounted on a microtome specimen holder and coated with embedding medium. 2 μm thick sections of tissue containing both regions were cut on a Slee automated microtome-cryostat set at −35° C. At least 100 μm of tissue were cut and discarded before preceding to the next tissue section.

Photographs were taken with a Zeiss fluorescent microscope equipped for automated photography. The slides were epi-illuminated with violet light by a 100 W halogen light source to excite the fluorescence of the FITC-dextran. A barrier filter was situated in the light path to allow only wavelengths greater than 495 nm to pass, thereby promoting optimal viewing of the fluorescence.

The slides were stained for alkaline phosphatase [24]. The region photographed previously was now relocated and photographed. This field had the total vessel endothelium stained while the fluorescent photograph exhibited only the perfused vasculature. Both negatives were matched and the alkaline phosphatase negative was marked to identify perfused and unperfused microvessels.

The marked alkaline phosphatase negative was projected onto a Weibel stereological device with appropriate counting grid for viewing and measurement. Fundamental principles of morphometry have been reviewed [30, 31]. These principles were applied to determine the capillary and arteriolar parameters of interest of the heart [12, 15, 24].

The volume fraction (Vv), in mm^3/mm^3, of capillaries and arterioles was calculated using a point counting technique and the following equation: $Vv = Pc/Pt$, where Pc and Pt are the number of test points within a profile of the vessel and the total number of test points in the grid, respectively. A probable error in Vv of less than ± 5% for capillaries and ± 7.5% for arterioles was accepted [31].

Table 1A. Hemodynamic and blood gas values in normoxia and hypoxia flow groups.

	Normoxia group			Hypoxia group					
	Saline control	3-day T_4	16-day T_4	Saline control		3-day T_4		16-day T_4	
				Before hypoxia	After hypoxia	Before hypoxia	After hypoxia	Before hypoxia	After hypoxia
N	7	7	7	8	8	8	8	8	8
Systolic BP (mm Hg)	85 ± 6	87 ± 8	107 ± 7[a]	78 ± 3	69 ± 2[b]	107 ± 6[a,b]	87 ± 6[a,b]	129 ± 8[a]	99 ± 5[a,b]
Diastolic BP (mm Hg)	65 ± 5	69 ± 7	88 ± 5[a]	64 ± 2	56 ± 3[b]	78 ± 6	62 ± 5[b]	97 ± 10[a]	66 ± 4[b]
Heart rate (beats/min)	222 ± 22	342 ± 27[a]	388 ± 25[a]	274 ± 20	256 ± 12	361 ± 8[a]	310 ± 8[a,b]	419 ± 19[a]	365 ± 19[a,b]
PaO_2 (Torr)	76 ± 4	68 ± 4	69 ± 2	72 ± 3	29 ± 1[b]	67 ± 2	27 ± 1[b]	65 ± 2	24 ± 1[a,b]
$PaCO_2$ (Torr)	38 ± 3	33 ± 3	32 ± 1	33 ± 1	31 ± 1	31 ± 1	30 ± 1	30 ± 1	30 ± 1
pH	7.41 ± 0.02	7.46 ± 0.02	7.43 ± 0.01	7.43 ± 0.01	7.39 ± 0.16	7.44 ± 0.05	7.39 ± 0.02	7.41 ± 0.01	7.37 ± 0.02

All values are means SE. N = 7. T_4, thyroxine; BP, blood pressure; PaO_2 and $PaCO_2$, arterial O_2 and CO_2 partial pressure, respectively.
[a] Significantly different from respective saline control.
[b] Significantly different from paired control (before vs. after).

The number of capillaries or arterioles per mm^2, Na, was calculated by the formula: Na = N/ area photographed, where N is the number of capillary or arteriolar profiles counted per grid.

Data was subjected to analysis of variance, both one-way and repeated measures to study differences between animals, groups and treatments with respect to hemodynamic parameters, blood gases, flow, O_2 consumption and morphometric parameters. Sources of differences were determined by Duncan's multiple range test. A value of $p<0.05$ was accepted as significant.

Results

The hemodynamic and blood gas values for the control, 3-day T_4 and 16-day T_4 groups are shown in Table 1A for the flow group and 1B for the FITC group. T_4 significantly increased heart rate and blood pressure when injected for 16 days and increased 3-day T_4 group heart rates when compared to controls. Blood gas and pH values did not differ significantly between the three nonhypoxic groups. In the animals made hypoxic, the low O_2 gas mixture caused a significant depression in blood pressure and heart rate. Arterial PO_2 was significantly lowered by PCO_2 and pH were unchanged.

Heart weights were 4.21 ± 0.29, 4.10 ± 0.17, and 5.23 ± 0.23 g for controls, 3-day, and 16-day T_4 animals, respectively. Only the 16 day-heart weight was significantly higher than control. Heart weight-to-body weight ratios were 2.59 ± 0.30, 3.69 ± 0.12, and 4.36 ± 0.10 g/kg for control, 3-day, and 16-day T_4 animals.

Myocardial blood flows are presented in Table 2. Before hypoxia, myocardial blood flow was higher in the 16-day T_4 group compared with the 3-day T_4 group, which was in turn greater than prehypoxic, saline controls. There were no differences noted between normoxic group animals and hypoxic group animals

Table 1B. Sytemic hemodynamic and blood gas parameters in control and thyroxine-treated FITC rabbits.

	Control	3-day T_4	16-day T_4
Systolic blood pressure, (mm Hg)	96 ± 17	98 ± 9	147 ± 30[a]
Diastolic blood pressure, (mm Hg)	72 ± 19	76 ± 8	100 ± 10[a]
Heart rate (beats/min)	260 ± 47	329 ± 40[a]	458 ± 63[b]
PaO_2 (mm Hg)	69 ± 9	70 ± 7	70 ± 7
$PaCO_2$ (mm Hg)	33 ± 4	35 ± 3	32 ± 3
pH	7.35 ± 0.05	7.32 ± 0.11	7.33 ± 0.04

Values are presented as mean ± S.D., N = 6.

[a] and [b] indicates, respectively, significantly different from control group and from both control group and 3-day T_4 group.

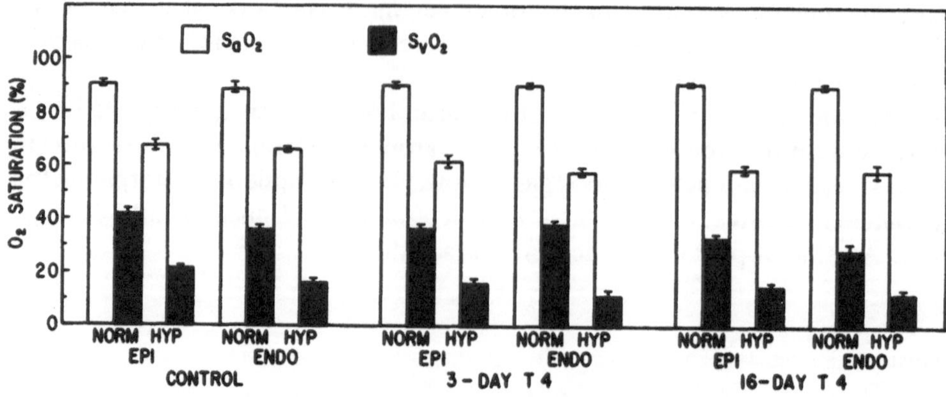

Figure 1. Arterial and venous O_2 saturation in the subepicardium (Epi) and subendocardium (Endo) of saline control and T_4-treated rabbits during normoxia and hypoxia. There was an Epi-Endo difference in venous O_2 saturation in saline controls during normoxia with Endo have a lower SvO_2. Endo SvO_2 was significantly lower than Epi for saline controls, 3-day T_4, and 16-day T_4 animals when subjected to hypoxia. Each value is mean ± SE (n = 7–8).

under normoxic conditions (before hypoxia). With hypoxia, the myocardial blood flow was higher in the 16-day T_4 group compared with the 3-day T_4 group, which was in turn greater than hypoxic saline controls. Hypoxia did not alter myocardial blood flow in saline controls when compared with their respective normoxia group. Hypoxia did result in a markedly increased flow in 3- and 16-day T_4 animals when compared with the 3- and 16-day T_4 normoxia groups, respectively.

In saline-treated normoxic control animals, the average left ventricular arterial O_2 saturation (SaO_2) was 89.0 ± 2.0%. Hypoxia significantly depressed SaO_2 in all three groups when compared with their respective normoxic group. No regional differences were observed in SaO_2 with hypoxia.

The average venous O_2 saturation (SvO_2) in the left myocardium of normoxic saline control animals was 38.7 ± 1.3%. The subendocardial region had a slightly but significantly lower SvO_2 than the subepicardium in the saline-treated normoxix controls (Fig. 1). Treatment with T_4 significantly decreased average SvO_2 only for the 16-day T_4 group. With hypoxia, SvO_2 was significantly lower for all treatments compared with their normoxic counterparts. With hypoxia, the 3- and 16-day T_4 animals had a significantly lower SvO_2 compared with hypoxic saline controls.

In both the normoxic and hypoxic groups, average myocardial O_2 consumption was significantly higher in the 16-day T_4 group compared with the 3-day T_4 group, which in turn was greater than saline controls (Table 2). Hypoxia did not alter myocardial O_2 consumption for any treatment compared with their respective normoxia group treatment. The only subepicardial-subendocardial difference

Table 2. Myocardial blood flows in saline control, 3-day T_4, and 16-day T_4 animals under normoxic and hypoxic conditions.

	Normoxia group			Hypoxia group					
	Saline control	3-day T_4	16-day T_4	Saline control		3-day T_4		16-day T_4	
				Before hypoxia	After hypoxia	Before hypoxia	After hypoxia	Before hypoxia	After hypoxia
Average, myocardial	166.8±15.5	332.1±27.2	465.9±30.93	180.9±10.5	198.5±8.3	299.2±15.2[a]	494.2±42.0[a,b]	561.4±28.8[a]	937.2±32.0[a,b]
Subepicardial	152.3±23.0	334.1±60.7	473.6±63.5	178.7±10.8	194.3±17.9	318.5±19.1[a]	509.2±92.6[a]	540.0±54.4	949.4±60.9[a]
Subendocardial	181.3±38.7	310.2±48.2	458.3±62.7	183.1±21.8	202.6±15.5	279.9±31.2	479.1±76.8[a]	581.8±61.2[a]	925.1±68.5[a]

All values are means SE.

[a] Significantly different from respective hypoxia group saline control.

[b] Significantly different from respective normoxia group treatment.

observed in O_2 consumption was in normoxic saline control animals with the subendocardium having a higher O_2 consumption.

The average values for the volume fraction (Vv) of the myocardium that contains capillaries or arterioles are presented in Table 3. The mean total capillary Vv averaged 0.196 mm^3/mm^3 for the control group and this was significantly greater than the value determined in the 16-day T_4 group. The value for the total arteriolar bed averaged 0.004 mm^3/mm^3 in controls which was significantly higher than both T_4 treated groups. Regional values are shown in Fig. 2. No significant subepicardial vs. subendocardial differences were found in either the arteriolar or capillary network in any group. All regional values for the 16-day T_4 group were lower than control.

Table 3. Average morphometric parameters of the total and perfused arteriolar and capillary network of control and thyroxine-treated FITC hearts.

	Vv (mm^3/mm^3)	Na(N/mm^2)
Arterioles		
Control		
Total	0.00429 ± 0.00236	4.1 ± 3.0
Perfused	0.00205 ± 0.00123	2.0 ± 1.1
(%)	51.71 ± 18.34	59 ± 21
3-day T_4		
Total	0.00159 ± 0.00114[a]	1.7 ± 1.09
Perfused	0.00126 ± 0.00070	1.6 ± 0.9
(%)	87.71 ± 16.11[a]	91 ± 139
16-day T_4		
Total	0.00104 ± 0.00074[a]	1.2 ± 0.79
Perfused	0.00093 ± 0.00066	1.0 ± 0.59
(%)	88.62 ± 17.93[a]	86 ± 189
Capillaries		
Control		
Total	0.1956 ± 0.0259	2369.37 ± 638.16
Perfused	0.1200 ± 0.0248	1438.58 ± 431.18
(%)	61.35 ± 8.76	60.41 ± 5.46
3-day T_4		
Total	0.1868 ± 0.0365	1844.91 ± 444.53
Perfused	0.1559 ± 0.339[a]	1540.52 ± 475.49
(%)	83.23 ± 4.89[a]	82.61 ± 6.02[a]
16-day T_4		
Total	0.1356 ± 0.0252[a]	1379.52 ± 198.66[a]
Perfused	0.1228 ± 0.0253	1239.71 ± 208.52
(%)	91.14 ± 4.92[b]	89.69 ± 5.45[b]

Values are presented as mean ± S.D., N = 6.

[a] and [b] indicate, respectively, significantly different from control group and from both control group and 3-day T_4 group.

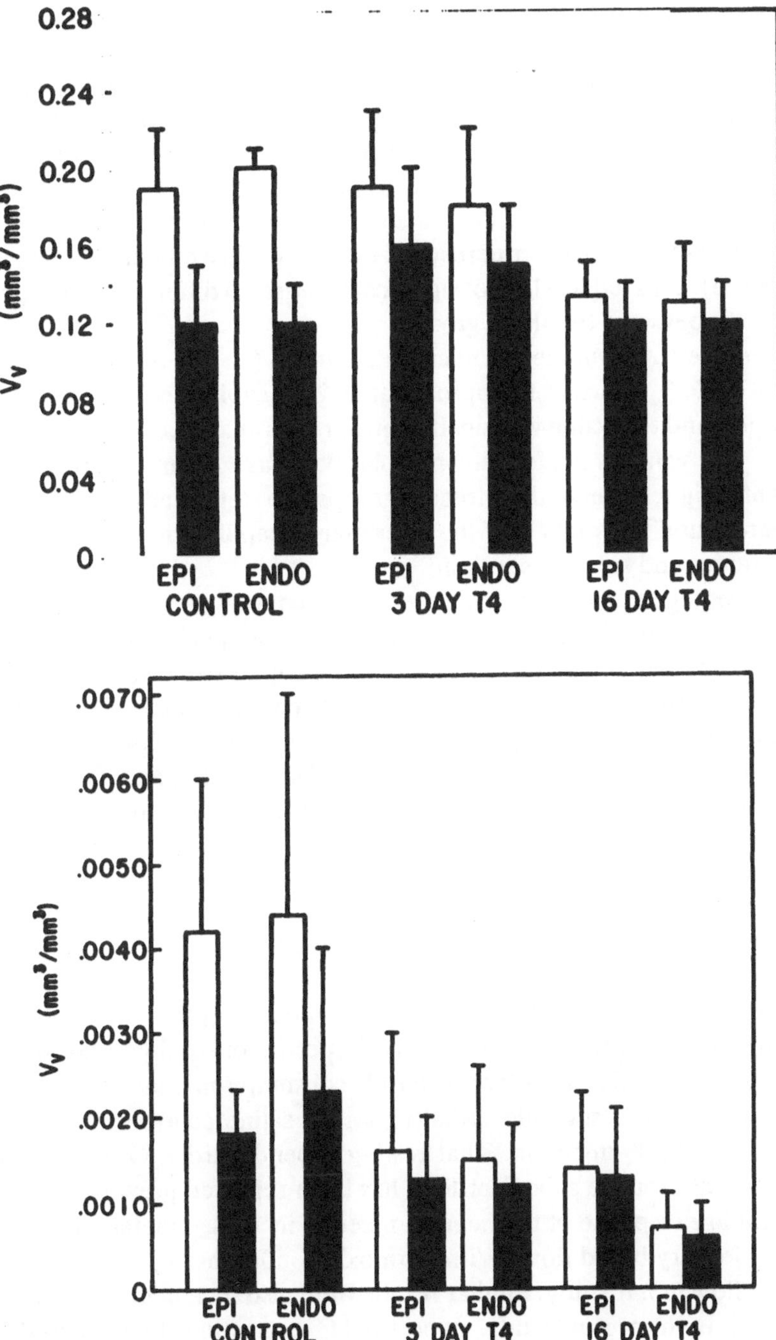

Figure 2. Subepicardial and subendocardial values of the capillary (Top) and arteriolar (Bottom) volume/mm³ for the total (light bars) and perfused (dark bars) portion of the microvasculature, Vv, for the control, 3-day T_4, and 16-day T_4 treated rabbits.

The percent perfused capillary Vv in controls was significantly lower than either group of T_4 treated animals (Fig. 3). The 3-day T_4 treated animals also had a lower percentage of their capillary beds perfused than the 16-day T_4 treated animals. These changes in the percentage of the total bed which were perfused prevented significant differences in the perfused Vv between the control and 16-day T_4 treated group, although 3-day T_4 perfused Vv was greater than control. Similar results were found for the percent of the arteriolar bed perfused in that the control group had a lower percent of the bed perfused than either T_4 treated group (Fig. 3). This led to a lack of significant statistical difference in the perfused Vv, Table 3, between the three groups.

The average total number of microvessels/mm^2 (Na) in the three groups are shown in Table 3. There were approximately 2369 capillaries/mm^2 in the control left ventricle and this value was significantly greater than that found in the 16-day T_4 group. The value of Na for the arteriolar bed was 4.1/mm^2 and this value was significantly higher than both T_4 treated groups. No statistically significant differences were found for total Na of the arteriolar or capillary network between the subepicardium and subendocardium.

The percentage of capillaries perfused in the control group (60%) was significantly less than either T_4 group. The 3-day T_4 percent perfused capillary Na was also less than that found in the 16-day T_4 group. There were no significant differences in the perfused capillary Na between the three groups. For the arteriolar bed, approximately 51% of the vessels were perfused in the control group, Table 3, and this was less than that found in the 3-day and 16-day T_4 group. The number of perfused arterioles was less in the control group than either T_4 treated series.

Discussion

T_4 injection markedly increased myocardial O_2 consumption. These results are similar to O_2 consumption increases seen in hyperthyroid or thyrotoxic subjects in other studies [2, 6, 7, 32]. Myocardial O_2 consumption was also found to be slightly higher in the subendocardial region in saline controls; this difference disappeared with T_4 injection. That resting subendocardial O_2 consumption is higher than that for the subepicardium has been reported previously [8, 29].

The primary response of the heart in meeting increased metabolic needs is to increase coronary blood flow. With normoxic conditions, T_4 increased myocardial blood flow in our study. Similar results were also seen in previous studies by others [6, 7]. In the present study, myocardial O_2 extraction also increased. This is similar to previous findings from this laboratory [3]. With cardiac hypertrophy induced by increased afterload, O_2 extraction is often increased, especially in the active developing stage of hypertrophy development [33].

Hypertrophy induced by other means also resulted in increases in myocardial

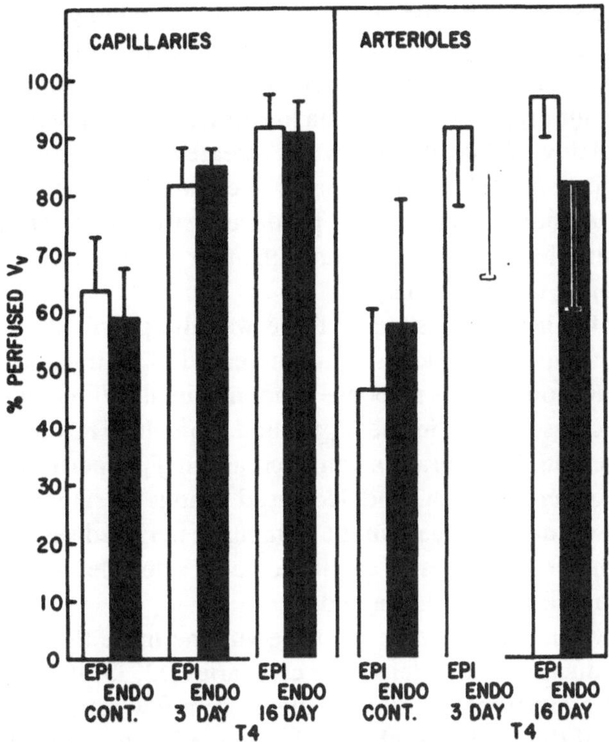

Figure 3. Subepicardial (light bars) and subendocardial (dark bars) values of the percentage of the capillary (left) and arteriolar (right) volume/mm³ perfused for the control, 3-day T_4, and 16-day T_4 treated rabbits.

blood flow acutely, although with time the flows return to control values as O_2 consumption returns to control values [9, 34].

Talafih et al. [3] showed that T_4-injected rabbits had a diminished coronary flow reserve. Reduced coronary reserves have also been noted in other types of cardiac hypertrophy [9, 10]. Reduced coronary reserves in T_4-induced hypertrophied hearts could diminish the ability of these hearts to handle an O_2 supply and/or demand stress imposed on them. This may be one mechanism for the increased incidence of cardiac failure or insufficiency observed in thyrotoxic subjects [1, 6]. We studied the effect of hypoxia on the ability of T_4-treated hearts to maintain an adequate O_2 supply/consumption balance.

To meet the O_2 supply deficit caused by hypoxia, coronary blood flow or more rarely O_2 extraction is increased [27, 34], despite decreases in blood pressure and heart rate. The stress of hypoxia if prolonged can lead to cardiac hypertrophy [35].

The increase in coronary blood flow with hypoxia in the T_4-treated animals occurred despite a marked reduction in vasodilator reserve found with these animals [3]. No subendocardial underperfusion was found with hypoxia in these animals. Vrobel et al. [36] found a normal distribution of perfusion in hypertrophied hearts but found subendocardial underperfusion with pacing at high heart rates. In our preparation, hypoxia lowers heart rate, potentially preserving subendocardial flow. While blood flow in T_4-treated animals is near the maximum found with adenosine [3], it still appears adequate to preserve myocardial O_2 consumption. Although hypoxia can produce a stress that can lead to cardiac hypertrophy, its effect appears less than with other stresses, e.g., exercise induces more hypertrophy than hypoxia [37].

In addition to the flow response, there was the possibility of increased O_2 extraction with hypoxia. T_4 leads to an increased O_2 extraction and decreased venous O_2 saturation but this response is not maximal. With hypoxia, venous O_2 saturations decreased even in the T_4 treated animals. Thus not only flow can increase but venous O_2 saturation can decrease in T_4 hypertrophic hearts. This could be due to increased flow and decreased venous O_2 saturations in the same number of vessels or an increase in the number of perfused vessels. The effect of T_4 on the number of perfused capillaries and arterioles was examined and alteration in capillary reserves studied.

Hypertrophy tends to increase myocyte volume more than vascular volume leading to a reduction in the density of capillaries [12, 13, 15–18]. This occurs in many types of hypertrophy, although there are a few reports of relatively full compensation of the microvasculature during cardiac hypertrophy [12]. Hyperthyroidism leads to an increase in myocardial blood flow and O_2 consumption [2, 3, 6, 32, 38]. Thyroxine also causes cardiac hypertrophy [3, 4, 5]. Hyperthyroidism should lead to a reduction in the number of myocardial capillaries/mm^2.

By 16 days of T_4 administration, we found a significant increase in minimal diffusion distances. This is consistent with reports of increased myocardial cell size with T_4 [4, 14]. With T_4 administration, O_2 extraction, consumption and flow in the heart were increased [3, 11]. There appears to be a smaller microvascular bed/mm^2 available to meet these increases.

Recently Chilian et al. [39] reported that administration of a lower dose of T_4 for three months led to a significant increase in the number of myocardial capillaries/mm^2 in the rat. This difference could be due to the dose of thyroxine or the species used. It is more likely, however, that the time of administration is critical. We looked during the early phase of hypertrophy (16 days) and they looked after 3 months. Thus, the early hypertrophic effects of T_4 may be like other forms of hypertrophy (lower capillary densities), while long-term thyroxine leads to angiogenesis.

There is much evidence for a reserve of unperfused capillaries in control hearts both from direct observation and indirect means [21–23, 25]. Recently, however, there have been some reports of a lack of capillary reserve in the rat heart [26, 27]. The question of whether a reserve of unperfused capillaries exists in T_4-hypertrophied hearts has not been addressed previously.

Under control conditions, studies have shown that approximately half of the capillaries are perfused at a given time [21–23, 25]. A similar reserve of unperfused arterioles has also been reported [24]. This reserve of unperfused vessels can be mobilized under conditions of O_2 supply stress [23, 24, 28]. In the present report, approximately 40–50% of capillaries and arterioles were unperfused in the control group.

After 3 days of T_4 administration, before significant hypertrophy, large increases in coronary blood flow and O_2 extraction have been reported [3]. From the present results, it appears that the number of perfused capillaries also increases by 3 days in compensation for the increased myocardial work. In addition to an increases in the absolute number of capillaries perfused at 3 days of T_4 administration, there was also an increase in the percentage of the total bed perfused. The number of perfused arterioles was not significantly different from control and the percentage of the total bed perfused increased.

With 16 days of T_4 administration, the reserve of unperfused arterioles and capillaries is significantly reduced. 80–90% of the microvessels were perfused in our 16-day T_4 group. In the 16-day T_4 group, with significant hypertrophy [3, 11], the reserve of unperfused microvessels is also reduced. Since the total microvascular bed per mm^3 is smaller, the number or volume of the perfused microvessels is similar to that found in control rabbit hearts. These changes were found in both the arteriolar and capillary beds.

In summary, after T_4 treatment we found great increase in coronary flow, O_2 extraction and O_2 consumption. There was, however, a flow reserve which could be mobilized by hypoxia. In addition, venous O_2 saturations could further decrease with hypoxia in an attempt to maintain O_2 consumption. 16 days of T_4 administration caused a significant reduction in the size/mm^3 of the microvascular bed. In partial compensation, there was a significant increase in the percentage of the arteriolar and capillary bed which was perfused. In the 3-day T_4 group, this led to an increase in the number of perfused microvessels. In the 16-day T_4 group, this led to a similar number of perfused microvessels as in the control group. Thus, there was an attempt to at least maintain physiological diffusion distances.

Acknowledgment

This study was supported by USPHS grant HL26919, Gary J. Grover was supported by an Individual National Research Service Award HL06803.

References

1. Graettinger JS, Muenster JJ, Selverstone LA, Campbell JA (1959): A correlation of clinical and hemodynamic studies in patients with hyperthyroidism with and without congestive heart failure. J Clin Invest 38: 1316–1327.

2. Skelton CL, Coleman H, Wildenthal K, Braunwald E (1970): Augmentation of myocardial oxygen consumption in hyperthyroid cats. Circ Res 27: 301–309.
3. Talafih K, Briden KL, Weiss HR (1983): Thyroxine-induced hypertrophy of the rabbit heart – effect on regional O_2 extraction, flow and O_2 consumption. Circ Res 52: 272–279.
4. Edgren J, von Knorring J, Lindy S, Torto H (1976): Heart volume and myocardial connective tissue during development and regression of thyroxine-induced cardiac hypertrophy in rats. Acta Physiol Scand 97: 514–518.
5. Gemmill CL (1956): Metabolic effects of thyroxine, 3,3′,5-triiodothyronine, 3,3′-diiodo-5-bromothyronine and 3,3′,5-diiodothyronine administered orally to rats. Am J Physiol 187: 323–327.
6. Piatnek-Leunissen K, Olson RE (1967): Cardiac failure in the dog as a consequence of exogenous hyperthyroidism. Circ Res 20: 242–252.
7. Leight L, DeFrazio V, Talmers FN, Hellems HK (1956): Coronary blood flow myocardial oxygen consumption, and myocardial metabolism in normal and hyperthryroid human subjects. Circulation 14: 90–99.
8. Holtz J, Grunewald A, Manz R, Restoroff WV, Bassenge E (1977): Intracapillary hemoglobin oxygen saturation of oxygen consumption in different layers of the left ventricular myocardium. Pflügers Archiv 370: 253–258.
9. Marcus ML, Mueller TM, Fascho JA, Kerber RE (1979): Effects of cardiac hypertrophy secondary to hypertension on the coronary circulation. Am J Cardiol 44: 1023–1038.
10. Wangler RD, Peters KG, Marcus ML, Tomenek RJ (1982): Effects of duration and severity of arterial hypertension and cardiac hypertrophy on coronary vasodilator reserve. Circ Res 51: 10–18.
11. Talafih K, Grover GJ, Weiss HR (1984): Effect of T_4-induced cardiac hypertrophy on O_2 supply-consumption balance during normoxia and hypoxia. Am J Physiol 246: H374–H379.
12. Anversa P, Olivetti G, Melissari M, Loud AV (1979): Morphometric study of myocardial hypertrophy induced by abdominal aortic stenosis. Lab Invest 40: 341–349.
13. Breisch EA, Bove AA, Phillips SJ (1980): Myocardial morphometrics in pressure overload left ventricular hypertrophy and regression. Cardiovasc Res 14: 161–168.
14. McCallister LP, Page E (1973): Effects of thyroxine on ultrastructure of rat myocardial cells. A stereological study. J Ultrastruc Res 42: 136–155.
15. Olivetti G, Anversa P, Loud AV (1980): Morphometric study of early postnatal development in the left and right ventricular myocardium of the rat. II. Tissue composition, capillary growth, and sarcoplasmic alterations. Circ Res 46: 503–512.
16. Rakusan K, Hrdina PW, Turek Z, Lakatta G, Spurgeon HA, Wolford GD (1984): Cell size and capillary supply of the hypertensive rat: quantitative study. Basic Res Cardiol 79: 389–395.
17. Tomanek RJ (1980): The relative distribution of coronary blood flow in rats with moderate and marked left ventricular hypertrophy. Can J Physiol Pharmacol 58: 830–835.
18. Tomanek RJ, Searls JC, Lachenbruch PA (1982): Quantitative changes in the capillary bed during developing, peak, and stabilized cardiac in the spontaneously hypertensive rat. Circ Res 51: 295–304.
19. Anversa P, Melissari M, Beghi C, Olivetti G (1984): Structural compensatory mechanisms in rat heart in early spontaneous hypertension. Am J Physiol 246: H739–H746.
20. Wright AJA, Hudlicka O (1981): Capillary growth and changes in heart performance induced by chronic bradycardial pacing in the rabbit. Circ Res 49: 469–478.
21. Crystal GJ, Downey HF, Bashour FA (1981): Small vessel and total coronary blood volume during intracoronary adenosine. Am J Physiol 241: H194–H201.
22. Duran WN, Marsicano TH, Anderson RW (1977): Capillary reserve in isometrically contracting dog heart. Am J Physiol 232: H276–H281.
23. Martini J, Honig CR (1969): Direct measurement of intercapillary distances in beating rat heart in situ under various conditions of O_2 supply. Microvasc Res 1: 244–256.

24. Weiss HR, Conway RS (1985): Morphometric study of the total and perfused arteriolar and capillary network of the rabbit left ventricle. Cardiovasc Res 19: 343–354.
25. Weiss HR, Winbury MM (1974): Nitroglycerin and chromonar on small vessel blood content of the ventricular walls. Am J Physiol 226: 838–843.
26. Steinhausen M, Tillmans H, Thederan H (1978): Microcirculation of the epimyocardial layer of the heart. I. A method for in vivo observation of the microcirculation of superficial ventricular myocardium of the heart and capillary flow pattern under normal and hypoxic conditions. Pflügers Archiv 378: 9–14.
27. Vetterlein F, Dal Ri H, Schmidt G (1982): Capillary density in rat myocardium during timed plasma staining. Am J Physiol 242: H133–H141.
28. Kleinert HD, Scales JL, Weiss HR (1980): Effect of carbon monoxide or low oxygen gas mixture inhalation on regional oxygenation, blood flow, and small vessel blood content of the rabbit heart. Pflügers Archiv 383: 105–111.
29. Weiss HR, Sinha AK (1978): Regional oxygen saturation in small arteries and veins in the canine myocardium. Circ Res 42: 119–126.
30. Underwood EE (1970): Quantitative stereology. Addison-Wesley Publishing Co, Reading.
31. Weibel ER (1979): Stereological methods, vol. 1, Practical methods for biological morphometry. Academic Press, London.
32. Gunning JF, Harrsion CE, Coelman HN (1974): Myocardial contractility and energetics following treatment with d-thyroxine. Am J Physiol 226: 1166–1171.
33. Malik AB, Abe T, O'Kane HO, Geha AS (1973): Cardiac function, coronary flow, and oxygen consumption in stable left ventricular hypertrophy. Am J Physiol 225: 186–191.
34. White FC, Badke FR, Covell JW, LeWinter M, Bloor CM (1979): Regional myocardial blood flow in volume overload hypertrophy. J Mol Cell Cardiol 11 (Suppl 1): 66.
35. Powers ER, Powell WJ (1973): Effect of arterial hypoxia on myocardial oxygen consumption. Circ Res 33: 749–756.
36. Vrobel TR, Ring WS, Anderson RW, Emery RW, Bache RJ (1980): Effect of heart rate on myocardial blood flow in dogs with left ventricular hypertrophy. Am J Physiol 239: H621–H627.
37. Guski H, Meerson FZ, Wassilew G (1981): Comparative study of ultrastructure and function of the rat heart hypertrophied by exercise or hypoxia. Exp Pathol 201: 108–126.
38. Goldman S, Olajos M, Friedman H, Roeske WR, Morkin E (1982): Left ventricular performance in conscious thyrotoxic calves. Am J Physiol 282: H113–H121.
39. Chilian WM, Wangler RD, Peters KG, Tomanek RJ, Marcus ML (1985): Thyroxine-induced left ventricular hypertrophy in the rat: Anatomical and physiological evidence for angiogenesis. Circ Res 57: 591–598.

Discussion

Spaan: Are there functional capillaries that are considered non-perfused? You count capillaries but maybe other capillaries would have shown up if you would have counted at different times at different places.

Weiss: Yes, we think that the functional capillaries are sometimes perfused and sometimes not, and that this state changes rapidly. This is sometimes called 'twinkling'; a rapid opening and closing of the microvessels. It was shown that, in dog, the cycle time for temporal heterogeneity is about 45 seconds in the heart. What we are showing is essentially a moment in time. We are looking at spatial heterogeneity. Obviously, if we waited an additional 10 seconds, injected our dye and then killed the animal, we would see different microvessels filled. But in examination of hundreds of capillaries we always see about 50–60 percent of them filled. We get a steady state between 8–15 seconds. At 30 seconds we observe about 80–90% filled and at 45 seconds almost all are filled. We believe the cycle time in rabbits is more rapid than in dogs.

Van der Vusse: In one of your slides there was no difference in oxygen consumption between the endocardial and epicardial layers in the normal heart.

Weiss: In a normal rabbit heart, there is a significant O_2 consumption difference between subepicardium and subendocardium. That difference disappears when the hearts become hyperthyroid and cardiac hypertrophy occurs. Rabbits in ischemia do not tend to show the same kind of subepicardial vs. subendocardial differences that dogs show. The wall is thinner and there seems to be less problems. At rest, though, the oxygen consumption difference is identical for rabbits and dogs: about 20% higher in the subendocardial layers.

Basic phenomena in transport and metabolism

37. Making mathematical descriptions of metabolic reaction networks manageable

B. PALSSON

Abstract

The dynamics of complex systems can be effectively analyzed by judicious use of intrinsic time constants. Order of magnitude estimation based on time constants has been used successfully by engineers to examine behavior of complicated processes and the main goal of this paper is to introduce this approach for the analysis of complex metabolic systems.

Time constants for the common rate processes are introduced and the use of their relative magnitude to simplify several simple but important physiological transport problems is illustrated. Time constants and dynamic modes of motion are then rigorously defined within the context of well established linear algebra. Extension of the order of magnitude estimation is then introduced into the systemic frame work. The main goals of the analysis are:

1. to provide improved understanding of biochemical dynamics and their physiological significance and
2. to yield reduced dynamic models that are physiologically realistic but tractable for practical use. Applications to important physiological systems are discussed.

Introduction

The basic biochemistry that underlies the living process is now well documented as evidenced by the biochemical reaction pathway maps that are commonly found on laboratory walls. The major metabolic pathways are well characterized in terms of stoichiometry and biochemical kinetics. One of the challenges that faces metabolic research today is to develop the capability to deal with these complex reaction networks as integrated systems. An enzyme by itself is 'just' a catalyst and the living process is only observed when all the enzymes are put together: the living process is a holistic one.

There are several important difficulties associated with the study of large and organizationally complex systems:

conceptualization: the human mind can only keep track of a few variables simultaneously and understanding the complex patterns of interaction in large metabolic networks is difficult. Several basic physiological and teleological questions also arise. Is there a physiological structure intrinsic to metabolic dynamics? Large dynamic systems have the tendency to become unstable, how do metabolic networks overcome this difficulty? etc.;
simplification: what factors are important to describe a given metabolic process? What degree of complexity is needed?, what enzymes are crucial?, how do the metabolite concentrations move?, etc. This issues can be successfully addressed using temporal decomposition;
parameters: there are two key issues associated with the parameters involved. First the large number of them that appear and the difficultes associated with estimating them. Secondly how are the overall dynamics affected by parameter variations (e.g. arising from genetic defects);
computations: keeping track of a large number of dynamically interconnected variables is numerically difficult. This difficulty has, however, essentially vanished with the rapid advances in computer technology;

In this article we shall address the first two issues: how does one conceptualize metabolic dynamics and once that is accomplished how can the complex dynamic descriptions be reduced into manageable but physiologically realistic models. Partial answers are obtained via simple straight forward linear analysis accompanied with judicious examination of the dynamic structure. We begin by presenting the thinking that goes into order of magnitude analysis: an approach that engineers have used successfully to deal with complicated systems.

Approaching simplified dynamic descriptions

Time constants: key to the understanding of rate processes

It is normally desirable to begin dynamic analysis by examining the orders if magnitude of key rate processes and estimate their effects on the system under consideration. Order of magnitude estimation leads to identification of problems requiring detailed analysis and elimination of processes of little consequence, gaining improved insight into system characteristics and the important factors that contribute the most to the solution Furthermore classification of many systems and problems fall naturally within order of magnitude framework. The hierarchical character of biological systems lends itself naturally to such schemes. Hierarchy is found in: time, space and physiological function. Here we are particularly interested in temporal decomposition.

Time constants: definitions

A time constant is a measure of the time it takes to observe significant changes in a given process. More specific definitions are to be described.

Linear systems
The definition of a time constant is perhaps most rigorous and well understood for linear systems. Lets consider a simple first order system (higher order systems are discussed below):

$$\frac{dx}{dt} = -ax, \ x = x_0 \text{ at } t = 0, \Rightarrow x(t) = x_0 \exp(-at). \tag{1}$$

The response shown in Figure 1 is characterized by the constant a. Equation 1 can be written as

$$x(t)/x_0 = \exp(-t/\tau), \text{ where } \tau = 1/a. \tag{2}$$

The quantity τ is the time constant for the system. When time, $t = \tau$, has lapsed then about 63% of the motion has relaxed. For times greater than about 3 to 4 times τ essentially full relaxation has occurred.

Half-lives
A common measure of process duration is the half-live, referring to how long it takes a process, i.e. isotope decay, enzyme inactivation, to reach its half point of completion. For first order linear systems the half life is given by

$$t_{1/2} = \ln(2)\tau. \tag{3}$$

Note that the closely related doubling time is a frequent measure of microbial growth and the generation time used in cell kinetics.

More general definition [1]
One way of characterizing the time scale of a process is to use the time it takes for relaxation from one extreme value to the other assuming that the process is proceeding at its maximum rate, see Figure 2. This definition gives

$$t_{char} = \frac{|f_{max} - f_{min}|}{|df/dt|_{max}}. \tag{4}$$

Note that this definition is consistent with linear systems for first order processes.

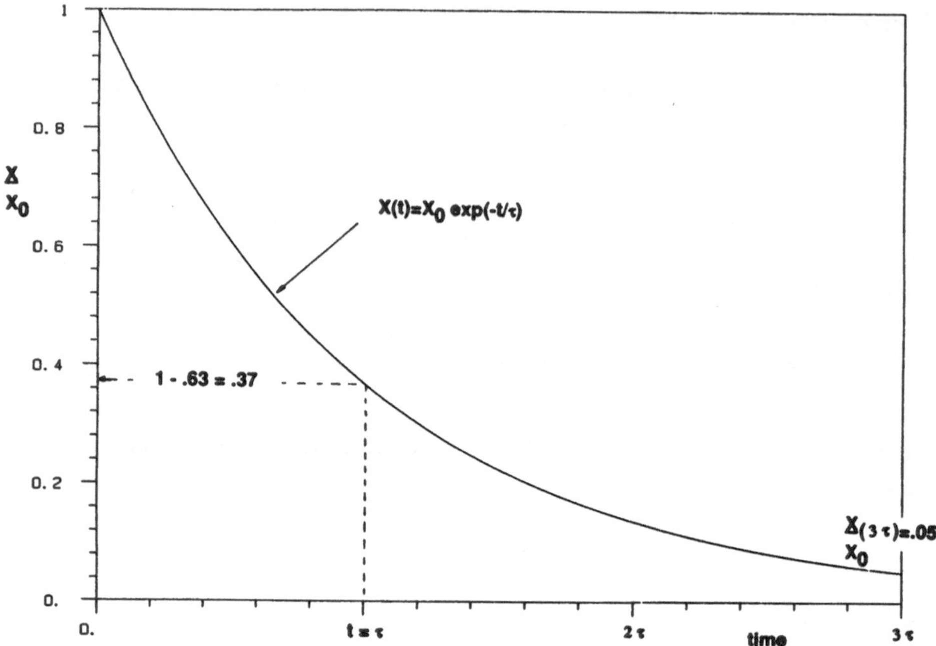

Figure 1. An exponential decay.

Characteristic time constants for the rate processes

We will now discuss the time constants that characterize biologically important rate processes. Five key time constants are shown in Table 1.

Convection

Convection refers to the motion of bulk fluid. The commonly used measure of fluid transit time is the average residence time defined as the ratio between system volume, V, and the volumetric flowrate, Q, as

$$t_{conv} = V/Q. \tag{5}$$

This is the time it takes to turnover volume V at a volumetric flowrate Q. For systems of constant cross sectional area, A, as for a flow down a tube, it is often useful to use

$$t_{conv} = V/Q = AL/Av_m = L/v_m \tag{6}$$

as the characteristic time for fluid transit.

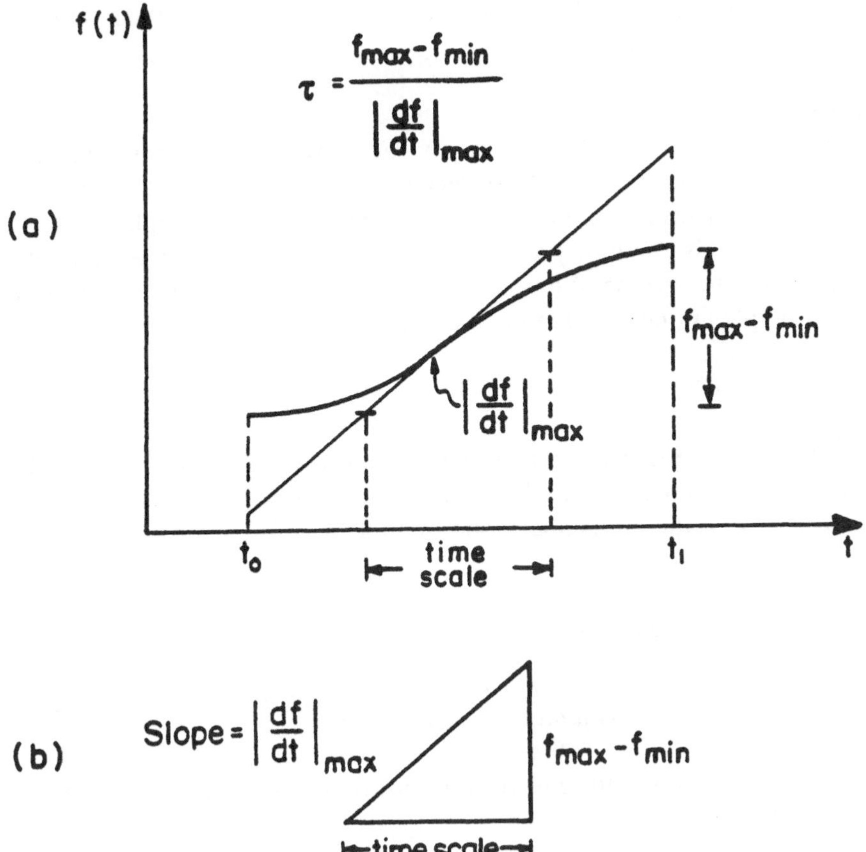

Figure 2. Definition of time scale. (a) The ingredients needed to define the time scale. (b) The time-scale triangle (from Segel [1].

Perfusion

The perfusion time constant, t_{per} is closely related to the convectional time constant. The perfusional time is the characteristic time for saturation of a tissues with a given solute via perfusion with solute containing blood under flow-limited conditions. For a homogeneous tissue of volume V_T perfused by blood flowing at rate Q_B through a single artery the perfusion time constant is given by:

$$t_{per} = KV_T/Q_B, \tag{7}$$

where K is the partition coefficient defined by

$$K = \frac{\text{equilibrium tissue concentration}}{\text{concentration is afferent blood}}. \tag{8}$$

This time constant is readily justified by analyzing simplified limits of the Krogh tissue cylinder model [2].

Diffusion
Einstein developed in 1910 [3] a theory for Brownian motion which can used directly to describe diffusion. Diffusion is basically a random motion of molecules analogous to Brownian motion of macroscopic particles in simple systems. The net effect of this random process is motion of solute from regions of high concentration to regions of low solute concentrations. It may be shown on the basis of simple arguments that the diffusional response time is on the order of

$$t_{diff} = L^2/D, \tag{9}$$

where L is the distance between the two least favorable points in the system and D is the diffusion coefficient. Analysis of several specific cases [5] shows that t_{diff} is a good estimate of the diffusional response time.

Reaction
The characteristic time constant for reaction is taken as the turnover rate

$$t_{rxn} = \frac{\text{average concentration}}{\text{average volumetric reaction rate}} = C/R. \tag{10}$$

This is the time it takes to remove concentration C at the reaction rate R.

Growth
The time constants of growth are biological time constants that unlike diffusion, convection and reaction, cannot be predicted by simple analysis of an idealized

Table 1. Some important biological time constants.

Process	Time constant	
Bulk fluid motion (convection)	$t_{res} = V/Q$	
	$= L/v_m$	(for constant area)
Perfusion	$t_{per} = KV_T/Q_B$	
Molecular motion (diffusion)	$t_{diff} = L^2/D$	
Reaction	$t_{rxn} = C/R$	
	$= 1/k$	(first order reaction)
Growth	$t_{growth} = \ln(2)/k$	(doubling time)
Observation	t_{obs}	(time span of observation)

Symbols used: Q: Volumetric flowrate, V: volume, L: length, v_m: average velocity, K: partition coefficient, D: the diffusion coefficient, C: concentration, R: volumetric reaction rate, k: first order rate constant.

physical situation. On the contrary the growth time depends, in part, on the rates of mass transport and reaction. Growth times range from 20 min doubling time for rapidly growing bacteria, to 24 hours for mammalian cells to doubling times of 20–30 years for mammals.

Observation
This is the time span over which we intend to analyze and observe the system. The basis of the analysis is in fact to a significant extent formed by this time scale. We need first and foremost to consider system transients that overlap with the time span of observation; we only concern ourselves with those processes that change significantly over the time span of observation, Figure 3.

Comparing two rate processes

In this subsection we illustrate how the relative order of magnitude of the time constants can be used to identify dominant effects and how to eliminate less important processes. Several of the examples found in this subsection originate from [2].

Model topology
Before we discuss specific physical examples we make the following observation on system structure. For two processes in series, Figure 4, we readily see that the slower of the two will dominate the overall behavior and the faster process will become unimportant. Contrary for two process occurring in parallel the faster process dominates the overall behavior and the slower process becomes unimportant.

Mechanism of mixing-pharmacokinetic modeling [2]
It is very often assumed that diffusional transport within a organ is so effective that blood leaving the organ is in equilibrium with the entire tissue mass. Careful analysis, however, suggests such rapid internal dispersion to be unlikely, and yet the assumption of rapid equilibration has been quite successful in many applications.

This apparent paradox, much discussed in the physiological literature, can be explained on the basis of simple order-of-magnitude arguments. If, as is frequently observed, characteristic organ response times, t_{organ}, are short compared to those describing changes in average composition over the whole body, t_{body}, departures of organ concentrations from the assumed equilibrium will be small, whatever the internal transport kinetics.

Order of magnitude analysis. Consider the response of the simple system of Figure 5 to a time varying input concentration of tracer from the standpoint of

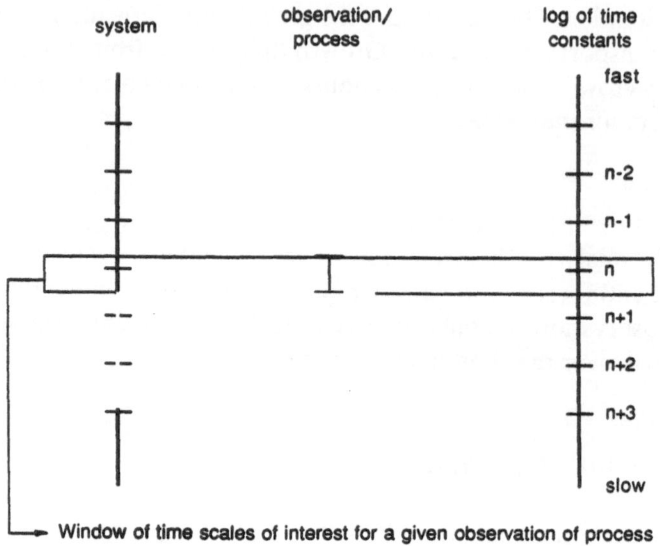

Figure 3. Schematic illustration of overlapping systems and observation/process time scales.

a) Processes in series

Process 1 τ_1 → Process 2 τ_2

if τ_1 is much larger than τ_2 then the second process is fast and will not influence the overall dynamics significantly.

b) Process in parallel

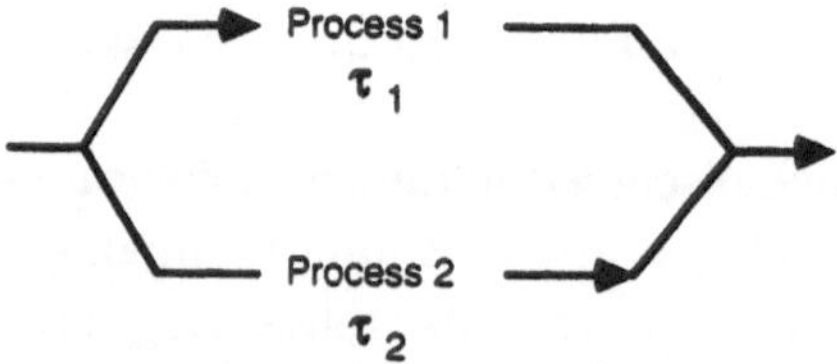

If τ_1 is much larger than τ_2 then process 1 is unimportant with respect to overall dynamics since all the 'flow' will be through process 2

Figure 4. Model topology and dominant time scales.

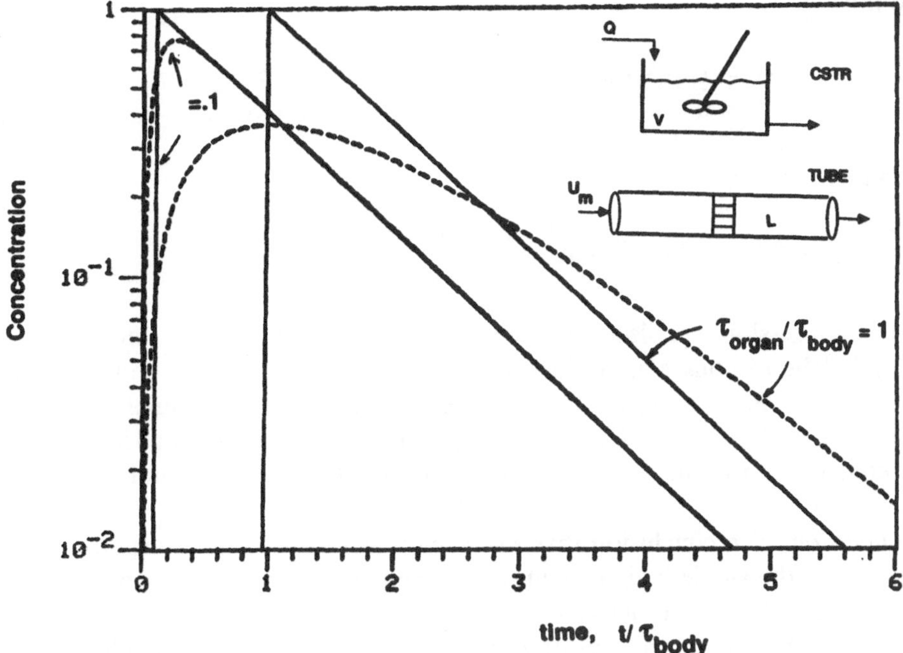

Figure 5. Effect of input time constants on responses for perfect mixing (---) and plug flow (—), modified from [4].

system time constants. Shown in the figure is a closed system of volume V through which an incompressible fluid is flowing at constant volumetric rate Q. Solute is entering at a concentration falling off exponentially with time with a time constant of t_{body}. Once in the system mean solute residence time t_{organ} is V/Q. Hence we expect the dimensionless ratio:

$$a = \frac{t_{organ}}{t_{body}} \tag{11}$$

to be the key parameter in determining the overall dynamic response.

Formal treatment. We wish to determine how much we can learn about this system without specific knowledge of the solute residence time distribution, and we therefore consider two limiting cases of the internal mixing process:

no mixing (plug flow): solute leaves the organ at a time t_{organ} after entry;

complete and instantaneous mixing (the CSTR assumption): the probability of a solute molecule leaving at a time t after it enters is $\exp(-t/t_{organ})$.

We choose to express the response as the differences between outlet and inlet concentrations, and can be shown that these are:

no mixing:

$$c_o - c_i = \exp(-t/t_{body})(\exp(t_{organ}/t_{body}) - 1) \text{ for } t>t_{organ},$$
$$= 0 \qquad \text{for } t<t_{organ}; \qquad (12)$$

complete mixing:

$$c_o - c_i = \exp(-t/t_{body})(\frac{1-\exp(t/t_{body} - t/t_{organ})}{1-t_{organ}/t_{body}} - 1). \qquad (13)$$

These expressions are plotted in Figure 5 (from [4]) for $t_{organ} = t_{body}$ and for $t_{organ} = t_{body}/10$. The responses are quite different for t_{organ} equal to t_{body}, and this is not unexpected since the types of behavior modelled are very dissimilar. However, for t_{organ} equal to one-tenth of t_{body} the differences become very small indeed after a relatively short time: the longer time constant dominates system behavior.

Conclusion. The conclusion that we reach is that if the organ response is fast relative to the whole body response then the mechanism of mixing in the organ has a negligeble effect on overall system behavior.

This is a very important result from a practical standpoint and tends to justify the rather casual approach engineers frequently take to modeling complex systems. The assumption of perfect mixing within organs is often used to model drug distributions in the body (pharmacokinetics). Body organs do not really act like perfect mixers, but their response times tend to be short relative to the time scales of drug absorption or elution. The assumption of perfect mixing is quite convenient computationally.

Convection and diffusion in parallel: the axial Peclet number [2]
'We next consider the superposition of diffusion and flow in the simple one-dimensional system of Figure 6. Situations of this general type occur in membrane transport, boundary-layer transport at high net mass transfer rates and in a variety ducts. We wish to determine the relative importance of diffusional transport and convection, and when if ever we can ignore one of the two.

Order of magnitude analysis. We begin by noting that the time required to transport solute down the duct with diffusion is:

$$t_{diff} = L^2/D, \qquad (14)$$

and, similarly, the time for convective removal is

$$t_{conv} = L/v_m. \qquad (15)$$

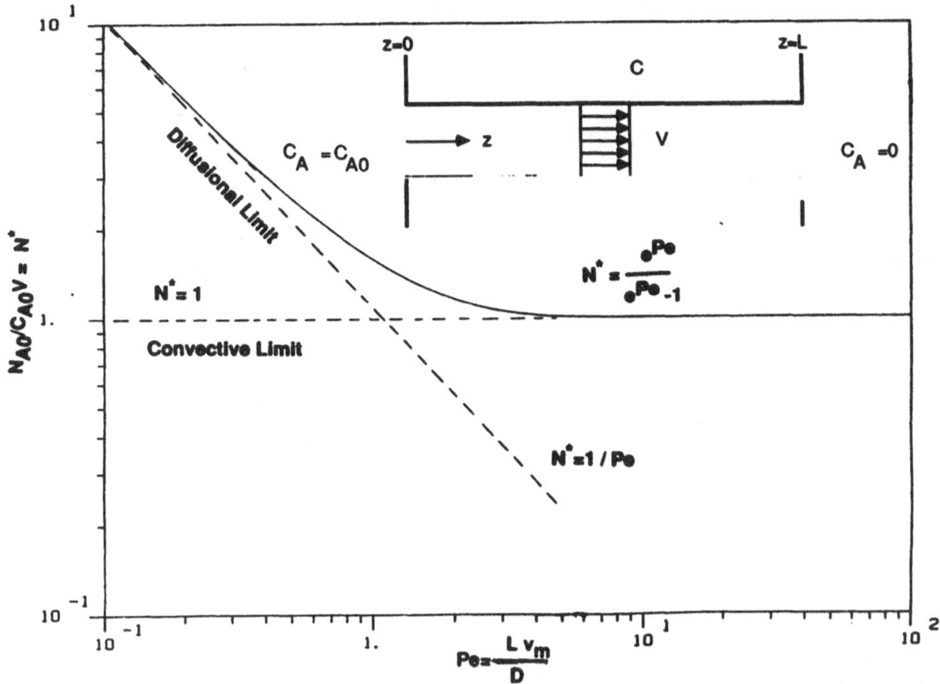

Figure 6. Convection and diffusion taking place in parallel down a duct.

The processes do occur in parallel so the faster of the two will dominate overall behavior. We expect the two transport mechanisms to be of comparable importance when these two times are equal, or when the ratio

$$\frac{t_{diff}}{t_{conv}} = \frac{L^2/D}{L/v_m} = \frac{Lv_m}{D} = \text{Pe (the axial Peclet number)} \tag{16}$$

is near unity. Furthermore we would expect this ratio, known as the Peclet number to be a measure of the relative importance of diffusion and convection. Both these expectations are readily verified.

Formal treatment. The equation of continuity for component A in our system is:

$$v_m \frac{dC_A}{dz} = D\frac{d^2C_A}{dz^2}, \tag{17}$$

which can be integrated twice to give

$$C^* = \frac{C_A}{C_{Ao}} = \frac{\exp(Pe) - \exp(Pe\xi)}{1 - \exp(Pe)}, \tag{18}$$

where ξ is the dimensionless axial coordinate z/L. The flux through the duct is given by

$$N^* = \frac{N_A}{C_A v_m} = \frac{\exp(Pe)}{\exp(Pe) - 1}. \tag{19}$$

This result is graphed in Figure 6.

Conclusion. It may be seen that solute fluxes approach the limits

$$N_A = C_{Ao} v_m \quad t_{conv} \ll t_{diff} \text{ (convection dominated)}, \tag{20}$$

and

$$N_A = C_{Ao} D/L \quad t_{diff} \ll t_{conv} \text{ (diffusion dominated)} \tag{21}$$

for low and high Pe, respectively. Only for the (approximate) range of

$$1/3 < Pe < 3 \tag{22}$$

is the full solution necessary. In other words if there is about threefold difference between the time constants then the slower process is unimportant (recall that for first order systems 95% relaxation has occurred when three time constants have lapsed). As a rule of thumb three to five fold differences in the time constants are sufficient to justify elimination of a process as a first approximation.

Reaction and diffusion in series: the Thiele modulus [2, 6]
We now turn our attention to reactions taking place within a phase with at least one reactant diffusing in from the phase boundary. The general problem is to determine the effect of diffusion on reaction rates and we are primarily concerned here with determining the range of conditions for which diffusional resistance can be effectively ignored. This is a very difficult problem to solve properly and has occupied a large number of outstanding researchers for many years [7]. We will look at the simple case of a first order reaction taking place in a spherical particle. The results obtained are relatively independent of geometry and reaction order.

Order of magnitude analysis. As before the diffusional response time is:

$$t_{diff} = R^2/D, \tag{23}$$

where R is the radius of the sphere. The reaction response time is:

$$t_{rxn} = C_A/R_A = C_A/kC_A = 1/k, \tag{24}$$

where k is the first order reaction rate constant. The magnitude of diffusional resistance is normally gauged in terms of the effectiveness factor η which is defined as:

$$\eta = \frac{\text{overall reaction rate with diffusion}}{\text{overall reaction rate without diffusion}}. \tag{25}$$

Following our previous discussion we expect diffusion and reaction to be of comparable importance when the two time constants are approximately equal and that effectiveness factors under these circumstances should not be far below unity. Furthermore we might expect effectiveness factors to depend primarily upon the ratio of these time constants:

$$\eta = \text{fn}(\varphi), \tag{26}$$

where φ is defined as

$$\varphi = \frac{t_{diff}}{t_{rxn}} = \frac{R^2 k}{D}. \tag{27}$$

Formal treatment. The reaction diffusion characteristics of the sphere are described by:

$$\frac{D}{r^2}\frac{d}{dr}\left(r^2\frac{dC_A}{dr}\right) = kC_A. \tag{28}$$

This equation can be solved with the boundary conditions that the surface concentration is C_{Ao} and that the profile is symmetric around the center to give

$$\frac{C_A}{C_{Ao}} = \frac{\sinh\sqrt{\varphi}\,\xi}{\xi\sinh\sqrt{\varphi}}, \tag{29}$$

where $\xi = r/R$ and the effectiveness factor is given by:

$$\eta = \frac{3}{\varphi}\left(\sqrt{\varphi}\coth(\sqrt{\varphi}) - 1\right). \tag{30}$$

This curve is shown in Figure 7.

Conclusion. When the Thiele modulus exceeds unity the reaction rate begins to be limited by diffusion. The overall rate is reaction controlled if the Thiele modulus is less than unity.

The expectations from the order of magnitude analysis borne out to a remarkable degree and are found in general to be relatively independent of particle shape and the details of the chemical kinetics. In a provocative article Weisz [6]

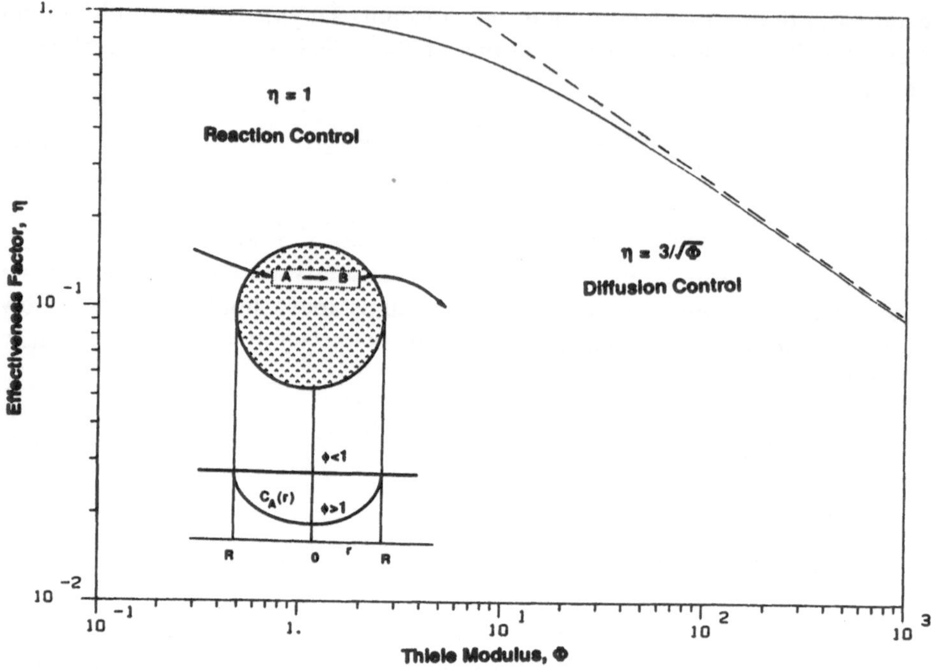

Figure 7. Reaction and diffusion in a spherical pellet.

suggests, and supports by a number of examples, that biological systems behave through evolutionary design at the edge of diffusional limitations.

Axial convection vs. radial diffusion: the Graetz problem [2]

We consider here laminar steady flow of a fluid through a hollow cylinder of circular cross-section as shown in Figure 8. We wish to estimate how long this cylinder must be to remove a solute uniform distributed in the feed stream if solute concentration can be maintained at zero on the tube wall by some unspecified process. To do this we must estimate the relative importance of solute diffusion to the tube wall and flow, or convection, in the axial direction.

Order of magnitude analysis. The radial diffusion time is given by

$$t_{diff} = R^2/D. \tag{31}$$

The average the time available for diffusion from any fluid element to the wall is the mean hold-up time

$$t_{conv} = L/v_m, \tag{32}$$

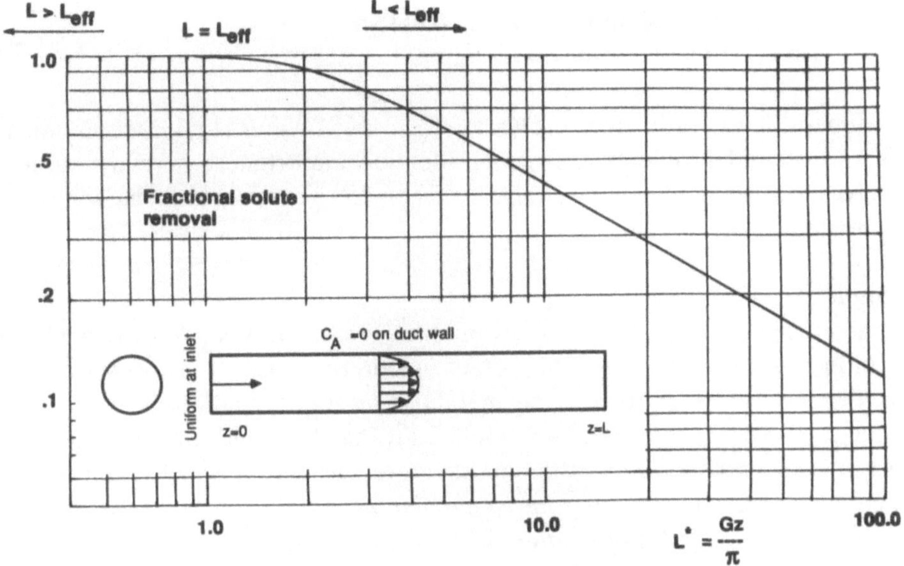

Figure 8. The Graetz problem.

where L is tube length and v_m is flow mean velocity. Then to a first approximation the required length L_{eff} can be estimated by setting these two response times equal to each other:

$$t_{diff} = t_{conv} \Rightarrow L_{eff} = v_m R^2/D; \tag{33}$$

in which case a molecule can on the average diffuse from the center to the wall during an average transit time. Furthermore, we would expect fractional solute removal to be a function primarily of the dimensionless length

$$L^* = \frac{L_{eff}}{L} = \frac{v_m R^2}{LD} = \frac{t_{diff,\ radial}}{t_{conv,\ axial}}. \tag{34}$$

Formal treatment. Solving the Graetz problem

$$v_z(r)\frac{\partial C_A}{\partial z} = \frac{D}{r}\frac{\partial}{\partial r}\left(r\frac{\partial C_A}{\partial r}\right) \tag{35}$$

with the appropriate boundary conditions, is not easy and we only show results from exact calculations, Figure 8. The order of magnitude estimate is consistent with the detailed results.

Conclusion. The conclusion that we reach is that L_{eff} is a good measure of the effectiveness of solute removal:

$$L<L_{eff} \text{ incomplete removal of solute,} \quad L>L_{eff} \text{ effective removal of solute.} \tag{36}$$

The dimensionless ratio $tR^2v_m/LD(=t_{diff}/t_{conv})$ is known as the Graetz number. This and related problems are of considerable importance, here we content ourselves with using the above analysis to characterize transport behavior of the mammalian blood circulation.

Example
Characterizing the transport behavior of blood vessels. It is generally recognized that blood vessels perform two important functions: transport of solute over the large distances between the actively metabolizing zones of adjacent organs, and exchange of mass by diffusion between the flowing blood and surrounding tissue mass. It is also recognized that the exchange vessels are the small vessels which are generally referred to as the *micro-circulation.*

Using the above order of magnitude results one can argue that the exchange vessels must indeed be those of the micro-circulation, and that their mass-transfer behavior is markedly different from that of the large vessels. To do this, we use as a measure the ability of solute in the flowing blood to diffuse to the vessel wall by assessing the relative time spans of axial convection and radial diffusion. The results are shown in Table 2.

Table 2. Mass transport effectiveness of blood vessels. First data set is for a 13-kg dog [8] and the second is for a canine [9].

Vessel	R (cm)	L (cm)	v_m (cm/sec)	Gz
Aorta	0.5	40	50	31250
Large arteries	0.15	20	13.4	30195
Main arterial branches	0.05	10	8	200
Terminal arteries	0.03	1.0	6	540
Arterioles	0.001	0.2	0.32	0.16
Capillaries	0.0004	0.1	0.07	0.0112
Venules	0.0015	0.2	0.07	0.0788
Terminal veins	0.075	1.0	1.3	731
Main venous branches	0.12	10	1.48	213
Large veins	0.3	20	3.6	1620
Venae cavae	0.625	40	33.4	32617
Aorta	0.75	5	20	225000
Large arteries	0.25	12	10	5200
Arterioles	0.0025	0.15	0.5	2.0
Capillaries	0.0003	0.06	0.1	0.015
Venules	0.002	0.15	0.35	1.0
Venae cavae	0.5	30	25	20800

It is immediately clear the three classes of vessels stand out from all the rest: the arteries, capillaries and venules, which are the smallest three classes of blood vessels. These vessels, especially the capillaries, exhibit transit times that are many times longer than needed to transport solute to their walls and thereby provide effective diffusional contact between blood and tissue. These have historically been called collectively the micro-circulation, and Table 2 gives a quantitative functional significance to this term. None of the larger vessels is within a factor of one hundred of this required length.

Research

There is an interesting postface to this discussion for the active researcher. There exists a pronounced time scale hierarchy in research work. The most important time scales are:

1. idea generation – minutes-hours,
2. simple analysis – hours-days,
3. numerical computation – days-months,
4. experimental work – months-years.

One of the goals of this chapter is to try to help researchers to gain as much progress on the second and third time scale so that minimal time is wasted on the long time scale of laborious and expensive experimental work.

Dimensional analysis – scaling

The simplification procedure can be broken down into three basic steps [10]:

1. somehow identify a 'small' term,
2. delete the small term from the equations and obtain a simplified solution, and
3. check the simplified solution for consistency.

The first step is the most difficult one since it relies on physical insight which may, in part, be obtained by examination of the time constants as discussed above. To facilitate this process it is customary to put the equations into a dimensionless form. The parameters in the equations appear in minimum number of dimensionless propery ratios. The same dimensionless groups appear regardless of how the equations are made dimensionless, and the number of dimensionless groups is given by the well known Buckingham Pi theorem. The dimensionless groups can in fact be interpreted as ratios of the time constants discussed above, see Table 3.

The process by which the equations are made non-dimensionless is nonunique. The 'correct' way of putting the equations into a dimensionless where judgements of relative orders of magnitude can be made is called *scaling*. More formally the process of scaling is defined by Lin and Segel [10] as:

> in the process of scaling one attempts to select intrinsic reference quantities so that each term in the dimensional equations transforms into a product of a constant dimensional factor which closely estimates the term's order of magnitude and a dimensionless factor of unit order of magnitude.

In other words if one has an equation which is a sum of terms,

$$T_1 + T_2 + \ldots = 0, \tag{37}$$

one tries to scale the variables involved so that they are of unit order of magnitude t_i, and the multiplier π_i will indicate the order of magnitude of the product, i.e. write the above equation as

$$\pi_1 t_1 + \pi_2 t_2 + \ldots = 0. \tag{38}$$

The difficult part of the procedure is to identify good reference scales for the variables. The time constant discussion above aids in obtaining the required physical insight so that this selection can be properly done.

Table 3. Important dimensionless numbers.

Fluid dynamics		
the Reynolds number	Re =	$\dfrac{\text{time of momentum diffusion } (l^2/v)}{\text{characteristic time for convection } (l/v_m)}$
Heat transfer		
the Prandtl number	Pr =	$\dfrac{\text{time for thermal diffusion } (l_2/\alpha)}{\text{time for momentum diffusion } (l^2/v)}$
the Peclet number	Pe =	$\dfrac{\text{time of heat transport by conduction } l^2/\alpha)}{\text{time of heat transport by convection } (l/v_m)}$
the Nusselt number	Nu =	$\dfrac{\text{thermal diffusion response time } (l^2/\alpha)}{\text{heat transfer response time } (l\varrho C_p/h)}$
Mass transfer		
the Schmidt number	Sc =	$\dfrac{\text{time for mass diffusion } (l^2/D)}{\text{time for momentum diffusion } (l^2/v)}$
the Peclet number	Pe =	$\dfrac{\text{time of mass transport by diffusion } (l^2/D)}{\text{time of mass transport by convection } (l/v_m)}$
the Graetz number	Gz =	$\dfrac{\text{characteristic radial diffusional response time } (R^2/D)}{\text{mean transit time for the fluid } (L/v_m)}$
the Sherwood number	Sh =	$\dfrac{\text{diffusional response time } (l^2/D)}{\text{mass transfer response time } (l/k_c)}$
Reaction		
the Thiele modulus	φ =	$\dfrac{\text{time constant for diffusion } (l^2/D)}{\text{time constant for reaction } (C/R_A)}$
the Damkohler number	Da =	$\dfrac{\text{time of fluid flow } (V/Q)}{\text{time of reaction } (C/R_A)}$

Example

Equation 17 in dimensionless form is

$$\text{Pe}\,\frac{dC^*}{d\xi} = \frac{d^2C^*}{d\xi^2}, \tag{39}$$

where the Peclet number is a direct measure of the relative importance of the two terms (i.e. if Pe is small then ignore convection).

Time constants in higher order systems

We now turn our attention to systems which have more than one state variable [11–14]. The main difficulty in extending the order of magnitude estimation procedure to systems with more than one variable is to assess the dynamic interaction between the variables.

Linear analysis

One can by simple linear analysis obtain good qualitative/quantitative information about the dynamics of a system described by a large number of equations. If the describing equations are linear then linear analysis is exact and quantitative information can be extracted. Otherwise one has to linearize the set of equations around a reference point as:

$$\frac{dx}{dt} = f(x) = f(x_o) + J(x - x_o) + \ldots, \tag{40}$$

where x is a vector of concentrations, f(x) is a n-dimensional non-linear function describing the rate processes, J is the Jacobian matrix (df_i/dx_j) and the subscript o denotes the reference conditions. The Jacobian matrix is then diagonalized $J = M^{-1}\Lambda M$ where the matrix Λ has the eigenvalues of J on the diagonal, and M^{-1} and M are matrices comprised of the eigenrows and the eigenvectors respectively. The linearized system is then transformed into a set of dynamically independent variables as

$$\frac{dm}{dt} = \Lambda m,\ m = M^{-1}x',\ x' = x - x_o. \tag{41}$$

Here x' is a vector of deviation variables from steady state x_o. The new variables, m, are called the *modes* and they move independently of each other on time scales defined by the corresponding eigenvalue. The negative reciprocal of the eigenvalues are the time constants. This procedure therefore transforms a large system of interacting variables into a set of decoupled variables where each motion can be considered independently of the rest of the system.

The information obtained through linear analysis is:

a. the time constants which give the distribution of time scales inherent in the system. Knowing the distribution of time constants one can systematically eliminate transients that are faster and slower than the time scale of interest: i.e. the process time scales;
b. the dynamically independent modes. The modal matrix, M^{-1} maps the systems variables onto the time scales and therefore gives valuable information about the motion of the various components.

Furthermore one can assess the influence of the reaction rates on the modes as follows

$$\frac{dx}{dt} = Sv \Rightarrow \frac{dm}{dt} = M^{-1}Sv = Wv, \tag{42}$$

where S is the stoichiometric matrix, v is a vector of reaction rates and W is a matrix of weights that indicates the enzymes that move any given mode.

Although the modes are abstract mathematical quantities, they lead to elegant physical interpretations when linear analysis is applied to chemical kinetics [11, 12]. The use and meaning of the modes is illustrated by a simple and readily understandable example.

Example
Let us consider the simple reaction scheme

$$A \underset{k_{-1}}{\overset{k_1}{\rightleftharpoons}} B \overset{k_2}{\rightarrow} C. \tag{43}$$

The mass action kinetic model for this reaction mechanism is:

$$\frac{dC_A}{dt} = -k_1C_A + k_{-1}C_B, \tag{44}$$

$$\frac{dC_B}{dt} = k_1C_A - (k_{-1} + k_2)C_B. \tag{45}$$

This is a linear model with a Jacobian matrix

$$(J = \begin{pmatrix} -k_1 & k_{-1} \\ k_1 & -(k_{-1} + k_2) \end{pmatrix}). \tag{46}$$

The dynamic characteristics of the Jacobian are given in terms of:
The eigenvalues: the eigenvalues of the Jacobian matrix (46) are the roots of the

characteristic equation:

$$\lambda^2 - \text{tr}(J)\lambda + \det(J) = 0, \tag{47}$$

which are

$$\lambda_1, \lambda_2 = \frac{\text{tr}(J)}{2} \pm \sqrt{\frac{\text{tr}(J)^2}{4} - \det(J)}, \tag{48}$$

and the time constants are

$$\tau_1 = -1/\lambda_1 \quad \tau_2 = -1/\lambda_2. \tag{49}$$

The modes: the dynamically independent modes are

$$m_1 = C_A + c_1 C_B, \; m_2 = c_2 C_A + C_B, \tag{50}$$

where the interaction coefficients, c_1 and c_2, are [11, 12]

$$c_1 = \frac{\lambda_1 - j_{11}}{j_{21}}, \tag{51}$$

$$c_2 = \frac{j_{21}}{\lambda_2 - j_{11}}. \tag{52}$$

Order of magnitude analysis: time scale separation occurs when [11, 12]

$$\det(J) \ll \text{tr}(J)^2. \tag{53}$$

The ratio between the determinant and trace squared for the above reaction mechanism is

$$\frac{\det(J)}{\text{tr}(J)^2} = \frac{a}{(1 + K + a)^2}, \tag{54}$$

where

$$a = k_2/k_1, \; K = k_{-1}/k_1, \tag{55}$$

and the eigenvalues take the asymptotic values

$$\lambda_1 \to \det(J)/\text{tr}(J), \; \lambda_2 \to \text{tr}(J) \tag{56}$$

when condition (53) is met.

If the time span of observation is longer than the faster time constant we would like to eliminate these rapid transients and simplify the dynamic description. Two limiting parameter values are of interest:

a. The binding step faster than product release, $a \to 0$, while K is a constant. The limiting values of the eigenvalues and the interaction coefficients are

$$\begin{aligned} &\tau_1 \to (1+K)/k_2 \;\; c_1 \to 1, \\ &\tau_2 \to 1/(k_1 + k_{-1}) \;\; c_2 \to -1/K, \end{aligned} \tag{57}$$

and hence the dynamically independent modes are

$$\begin{aligned} &m_1 = C_A + C_B, \text{ slow mode}, \\ &m_2 = -C_A/K + C_B \text{ fast mode}. \end{aligned} \tag{58}$$

Relaxing the fast dynamics leads to the quasi-equilibrium assumption since

$$\frac{dm_2}{dt} = 0, \; \Rightarrow \frac{C_A}{C_B} = K \tag{59}$$

or equilibrium for the binding step of the reaction. On the slower time scale C_A and C_B are dynamically equivalent and move as an aggregate pool as $C_A + C_B$. Relaxing the fast transients leads to a single differential equation describing the reaction dynamics as

$$\frac{dC_A}{dt} = \frac{-k_2 C_A}{1+K} = -k_{app} C_A. \tag{60}$$

This prediction is ascertained via full numerical integration, Figure 9. Note that from the simplified model one can only determine k_{app} but not both k_2 and K.

b. Intermediate breaks down much more rapidly than it is formed. $K \to$ large while. $K/a = k_2/k_{-1}$ is finite. Under this limiting condition we can obtain the dynamically independent modes, through an analogous process as the one illustrated above, as

$$\begin{aligned} &m_1 = C_A + \frac{K}{K+a} C_B, \text{ slow mode}, \\ &m_2 = C_B, \text{ fast mode}. \end{aligned} \tag{61}$$

Relaxing the fast dynamics in this limit correspond to the quasi-steady state assumption since

$$\frac{dm_2}{dt} = \frac{dC_B}{dt} = 0, \; \frac{C_B}{C_A} = \frac{k_1}{k_{-1} + k_2}, \tag{62}$$

and

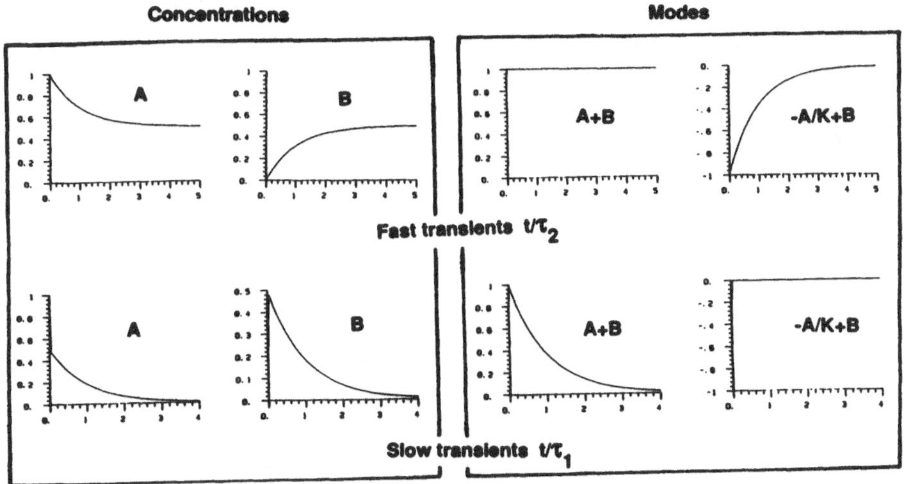

Figure 9. Dynamic response of $A \rightleftarrows B \rightarrow C$ for $K = 1$, $a = 1$ and $A_0 = 1$.

$$\frac{dC_A}{dt} = \frac{-k_1 k_2}{k_{-1} + k_2} C_A = -k_{app} C_A. \tag{63}$$

This prediction is confirmed by numerical integration.

This simple example shows how the use of modal analysis yields insight into reaction dynamics and furthermore leads to simplification of the dynamic description. The simplification in the limits discussed above is identical to commonly used kinetic assumptions: the quasi-equilibrium and quasi-steady state assumptions.

Red cell metabolism

A comprehensive kinetic model of glycolysis and the associated adenosine phosphate reactions in mammalian red blood cells has been developed [15]. The model consists of 17 differential equations which are simply dynamic mass balances on the 17 metabolites considered, Table 4. The equations are not repeated here but are found in the original reference. We will now examine the dynamic character of this model using the linear analysis described above.

Glycolysis

The time constants and the modal matrix for red cell glycolysis show that the three slowest modes move on the order of minutes. The other modes are fast and lead

Table 4. In vivo kinetic model of red cell metabolism (Schauer, Heinrich and Rapoport [15]).

Glycolysis

$$\frac{dG6P}{dt} = V_{HK} - V_{PGI} \qquad \frac{d3PG}{dt} = V_{PGK} + V_{DPGase} - V_{PGM}$$

$$\frac{dF6P}{dt} = V_{PGI} - V_{PFK} \qquad \frac{d2PG}{dt} = V_{PGM} - V_{EN}$$

$$\frac{dFDP}{dt} = V_{PFK} - V_{ALD} \qquad \frac{dPEP}{dt} = V_{EN} - V_{PK}$$

$$\frac{dDHAP}{dt} = V_{ALD} - V_{TPI} \qquad \frac{dPYR}{dt} = V_{PK} - V_{PYR} - V_{LDH}$$

$$\frac{dGAP}{dt} = V_{ALD} + V_{TPI} - V_{GAPDH} \qquad \frac{dLAC}{dt} V_{LDH} - V_{LAC}$$

$$\frac{d1,3DPG}{dt} = V_{GAPDH} - V_{PGK} - V_{DPGM} \qquad \frac{d2,3DPG}{dt} = V_{DPGM} - V_{DPGase}$$

Adeninenucleotides

$$\frac{dA}{dt} = V_{AMPase} + V_{A} - V_{ADA} - V_{AK}$$

$$\frac{dAMP}{dt} = V_{AK} + V_{ApK} - V_{AMPDA} - V_{AMPase}$$

$$\frac{dADP}{dt} = V_{HK} + V_{PFK} + V_{AK} + V_{ATPase} - V_{PGK} - V_{PK} - 2V_{ApK}$$

$$\frac{dATP}{dt} = V_{PGK} + V_{PK} + V_{ApK} - V_{HK} - V_{PFK} - V_{AK} - V_{ATPase}$$

NADH

$$\frac{dNADH}{dt} = V_{GAPDH} - V_{LDH}$$

Abbreviations – Enzymes

HK	Hexokinase
PGI	Phosphoglucoisomerase
PFK	Phosphofructokinase
ALD	Aldolase
TPI	Triosephosphateisomerase
GAPDH	Glyceraldehydephosphate dehydrogenase
PGK	Phosphoglyceratekinase
PGM	Phosphoglyceromutase
EN	Enolase
PK	Pyruvatekinase
LDH	Lactatedehydrogenase
DPGM	Diphosphoglyceratemutase
DPGase	Diphosphoglyceratephosphatase

Table 4. (Continued).

ATPase	Adenosinetriphosphate phosphohydrolase
AMPase	Adenosinemonophosphate phosphohydrolase
ADA	Adenosinedeaminase
AMPDA	AMPdeaminase
AK	Adenosinekinase
ApK	Adenylatekinase
Abbreviations – Intermediates	
G6P	Glucose6-phosphate
F6P	Fructose6-phosphate
FDP	Fructose1,6-diphosphate
DHAP	Dihydroxyacetonephosphate
GAP	Glyceraldehyde3-phosphate
3PG	3-phosphoglycerate
2PG	2-phosphoglycerate
PEP	Phosphoenolpyruvate
PYR	Pyruvate
LAC	Lactate
1,3DPG	1,3-Diphosphoglycerate
2,3DPG	2,3-Diphosphoglycerate
ATP	Adenosinetri-phosphate
ADP	Adenosinedi-phosphate
AMP	Adenosinemono-phosphate
A	Adenosine

to the formation of the following metabolic pools:
the hexose monophosphate pool: HP = G6P + F6P,
the triose phosphate pool: TP = 2FDP + DHAP + GAP + 1,3DPG,
the phospoglycerate pool: PG = 3PG + 2PG + PEP,
the end product pool: EN = PYR + LAC.
These three modes are primarily moved by three enzymes, HK, PFK and PK; these enzymes are generally considered to be the 'irreversible' steps in glycolysis.

After applying the series of kinetic assumptions predicted by the modal matrix one gets the following model:

$$\xrightarrow{\text{HK}} \text{HP} \xrightarrow{\text{PFK}} \text{TG} + \text{PG} \xrightarrow{\text{PK}} \text{EN} \xrightarrow{\text{exit}} . \qquad (64)$$

Rapoport-Luebering shunt

Glycolysis in red cells has a unique side branch:

$$\begin{array}{ccccc} & \text{DPGM} & & \text{DPGase} & \\ \text{1,3-DPG} & \rightarrow & \text{2,3-DPG} & \rightarrow & \text{3PG} \end{array}, \tag{65}$$

which is not found in other cells. 2,3-DPG is used to regulate the binding of oxygen to Hemoglobin.

The time constant that we calculate for this loop by itself is about half a day which is well in agreement with experimental observations. Note that this side loop has much slower transients than glycolysis.

Adenosine phosphate metabolism

The time constants and the modal matrix of the adenosine metabolism reveal that there is a slowly moving pool ATP + ADP + AMP + A that governs the behavior of this sytem on the slowest time scale that is on the order of days. This pool is moved the two deaminases and the exchange rate of AMP.

Overall metabolism

Coupling together all the three parts discussed above one finds, Table 5, a modal structure that has three slow time scales, .64, 11, and 61 hours. The metabolites aggregate into the following pools:
$P_1 = 2{,}3DPG$;
$P_2 = 3HP + 2TG + PG$;
$P_3 = 3ATP + 2ADP + AMP$;
$P_4 = AMP + ADP + ATP + A$.
The composition of the three slow modes in terms of these pools is:

$$m_{15} = P_2 + P_3 - 2.5P_4, \tag{66}$$

$$m_{16} = 3P_1 + P_2 + P_3 + 13P_4, \tag{67}$$

$$m_{17} = P_4. \tag{68}$$

The following interpretation follows:
a. *pools:*
P_1: is only the physiologically important compound 2,3-DPG;
P_2: summation of all high energy bonds in glycolysis;
P_3: summation of the high energy bonds on adenosine;
P_4: summation of all the adenosines present;
b. *modes:*
mode 15 represents the energy content of the cell and changes in the energy

Table 5. A modal matrix of the red blood cell.

τ	G6P	F6P	FDP	DHAH	GAP	1,3DPG	3PG	2PG	PEP	PYR	LAC	2,3DPG	NADH	A	AMP	ADP	ATP
msec to sec						1.0											
							−0.1	1.0	−0.4								
					−0.1	−0.5				0.3			1.0				
	−0.4	1.0															
					0.1	−0.1	−0.3	0.5	1.0								
			−0.1		1.0	0.4		−0.1	−0.1	0.1				−0.1			
														1.0			
	−0.1	−0.1	1.0		−0.2	−0.1	−0.1	−0.1	−0.1	0.1			−0.1	−0.2	−0.2	0.1	
mins	0.2	0.2	−0.1	0.1	−0.3		−0.4	−0.4	−0.4	0.3			−0.3	0.4	0.8	−0.4	
	−0.2	−0.2	1.0	−0.4	1.0	0.6	0.2	0.2	0.2	−0.4			0.4	−0.1	0.2	−0.4	0.1
	−0.3	−0.3	−0.4	−0.2	−0.1	−0.1	−0.2	−0.2	−0.2					−0.7	−0.6	−0.1	0.1
	0.7	0.7			−0.2	−0.4	−0.3	−0.3	−0.3	−0.2			0.2	0.7	0.8		−0.1
	0.6	0.6	−0.3	−0.2		0.6	1.0	1.0	1.0	0.7	0.1		−0.6	0.7	0.4	0.2	−0.1
	0.8	0.7	0.1	0.1		−1.0	−0.6	−0.6	−0.6	−0.1	1.0		1.0	1.0	0.6	0.2	−0.2
40 min	1.5	1.5	2.0	1.0	1.0	1.0	0.5	0.5	0.5					−1.1	−0.7	−0.2	0.3
12 hr	1.5	1.5	2.0	1.0	1.0	1.0	0.5	0.5	0.5			1.5		6.0	7.0	7.5	8.0
2.5 d														1.0	1.0	1.0	1.0

metabolism are expected to happen on this time scale; on the order of 40 min;
mode 16 represents the motion of 2,3-DPG and its interactions with the energy metabolism; recall that formation of 2,3-DPG bypasses and ATP producing step. The motion of the concentration of 2,3-DPG is known to move on a time scale with a time constant of approximately 12 hrs;
mode 17 represents the decay of the total adenosines in the cell. This decay has been postulated as an important contributing factor in the decay of red cells under storage conditions. Here the loss of adenosines falls out as a natural slow motion in the cell occurring with a time scale of about 2.5 days;

Only a few reaction rates are required to describe the motion of the four pools [16].

These results illustrate how the overall dynamic structure of a 'complete' metabolic network differs from its components. Note here that physiologically meaningful pools form that move on different time scales. Although not detailed here the predictions made by linear analysis are found to be accurate and are ascertained via full numerical integration.

In vitro model of red cells

A kinetic model of red cell metabolism under in vitro conditions has been formulated [17]. The additional factors included are important inorganic ions, osmotic pressure and pH. Analogous treatment as above indicates that the important motion over the time scales of blood storage have to do with changes in the transmembrane potential and in the relative amounts of sodium and potassium in the cell. These transients are also on the order of days.

Growth of bacterial populations

Oversimplified descriptions, like the simple Monod growth model that describe the state of the organism with a single variable, have been extensively used. The increasing focus of currently developing biotechnology on intracellular events signifies an impetus for developing physiologically rational growth models that account for the underlying well documented biochemistry. Pioneering steps in this direction have been taken [18–20] and an exponential growth single cell model (SCM) for E. coli has been formulated, Figure 10. The model consists of detailed description of about 18 key metabolites and it contains about 88 kinetic parameters. This complexity makes it difficult to assess the role of the basic biochemistry in the overall growth process and furthermore this degree of complexity is likely to hamper the practical utility of this model. A balance between physiological reality and simplicity is needed to develop tractable models of practical utility.

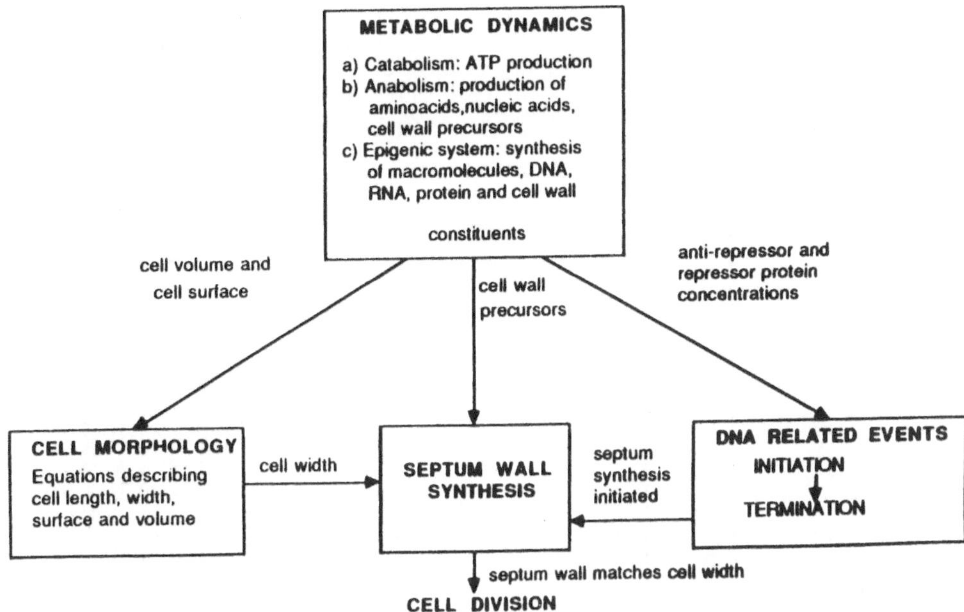

Figure 10. Topological structure of *Escherichia coli* growth model.

The SCM can serve as a starting point for the development of a simplified but physiologically rational E. coli growth model and we will now extract the dynamic essentials from the complex model that are necessary to describe the growth process itself. Judicious interpretation leads to a simple three pool growth model that basically describes the main classes of macromolecules in the cell. The material in this section is taken form [21].

Time scale hierarchy and modal structure

A representative modal matrix and time constants for a newly born E. coli cell with a doubling time of 45 minutes is shown in Table 6. The information displayed in this table immediately gives important information about the dynamic characteristics of this model.

The first column in Table 6 shows the inherent time constants in the system and inspection of those reveals that the metabolic transients can be divided into three time regimes:

Transients in the order of tens of minutes to an hour. These transients comprise the set of modes which characterize the dynamics over the growth time scale and are of key importance here.

The first mode in the Table 2 has a positive eigenvalue resulting in an exponential growth pattern. The relationship between the linearized growth time constant

Table 6. Modal matrix of a 45 minute cell of *Escherichia coli.*

Mode no.	Time constant	A1	A2	P1	P2	P3	P4	M1	M4	M5	E3	RNA1	RNA2	RNA3
1	−0.95 hr	0.5		0.1	−0.1	−0.1	0.9	0.1	1.0		0.6	−0.1	−0.1	−0.1
2	<min	0.5	1.0				0.2							
3		0.3		−0.2			1.0							
4		1.0		−0.1										
5		1.0												
6		1.0		0.1	−0.2	0.5								0.1
7		−0.2			0.1	1.0								−0.1
8		0.8		0.1	0.1	0.2	−0.1		−0.1					1.0
9		1.0		0.2	0.4	0.6	−0.2		−0.2			−0.4	0.1	1.0
10	hr	0.2		0.1	0.4	0.4	−0.8	0.1	−0.9	−0.1		0.5	0.5	0.4
11		0.2		0.1	−0.2	−0.2	0.4	0.2	0.5		0.9	−0.2	−0.2	−0.2
12	>10 hrs					−0.1		−0.1	−0.3	1.0	0.1			
13							−0.1		−0.1	−0.3	1.0	0.1		

A1 = ammonium ions, A2 = glucose, P1 = amino acids, P2 = ribonucleotides, P3 = deoxy ribonucleotides, P4 = cell envelope precursors, M1 = proteins, M4 = cell envelope constituents, E3 = septation enzyme, RNA1; RNA2; RNA3 = different forms of RNA. This modal matrix is calculated for a freshly born cell with a cycle time of 45 minutes.

and the doubling time of the cell is given by the relation:

$$t_{double} = -\ln(2)t_{growth}, \tag{69}$$

where t_{growth} is the time constant of the unstable growth mode. This time constant gives an excellent prediction of the cycle time of the cell. Figure 11 shows that the predicted doubling time and the doubling time obtained through simulation of the full model are in good agreement.

Furthermore, careful inspection of modes 1, 10 and 11 which describe the motion of the order of hour shows that these modes are comprised of physiologically significant pools:
$pool_1$ = ribonucleotides + deoxy ribonucleotides + RNA,
$pool_2$ = amino acid + protein,
$pool_3$ = cell envelope precursors + cell envelope constituents.
Fast transients (order of seconds to minutes). The modal matrix tells us that the fast transients can be associated with reactions that equilibrate rapidly resulting in the formation of steady state pools. These pools represent low molecular weight metabolism [21].
Slow transients (in the order of days). The slowest dynamics in this model represent a slowly changing mass balance on septation enzyme on the order of 15 to 35 hours. This time span is longer than the time scale of interest here.

Dynamics of the growth process

The events happening on the time scales of about an hour are essentially those associated with the motion of macromolecules. The interactions between the lower molecular weight precursors and the macromolecules lead to the formation of elegant pools that are comprised of macromolecules and their precursors, e.g., proteins and amino acids.

Table 2 shows that the proteins and amino acids move in a fixed ratio on these times and are dynamically equivalent. similar observations are made for the pools of cell envelope and its constituents and Ribonucleotides, Deoxy-Ribonucleotides and RNA. This implies that on the order of tens of minutes to hours, these three key metabolite pools represent the essential behavior of E. coli metabolism during growth. Consequently, the whole system can be reduced to describe the movement of key concentration variables during the exponential growth phase of the cell. From these results one can construct a simple 3 pool model as shown below.

These pools are known to form the growth determining factors [22]. Similar observations are made when the modal matrices for the E. coli cells with other doubling times.

Since the dynamics of cell morphology and certain decision making events are

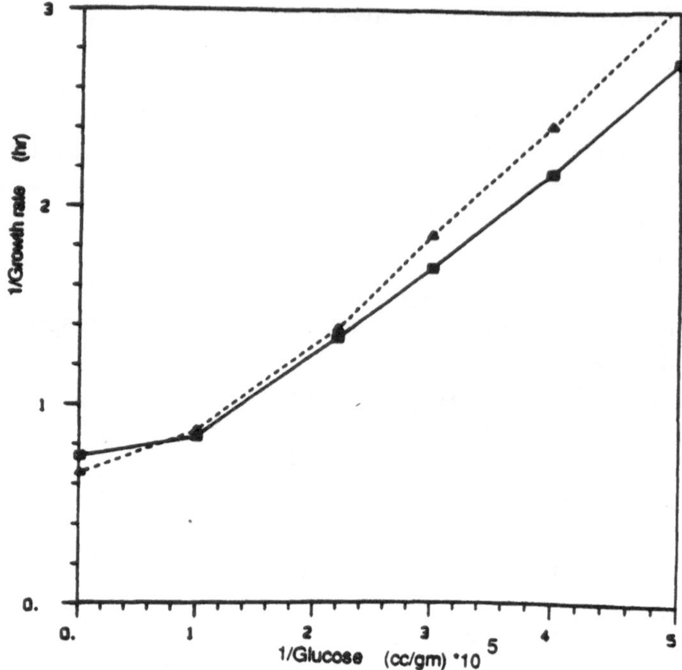

Figure 11. Calculated doubling time as a function of external glucose concentration (△ = predicted, □ = simulated).

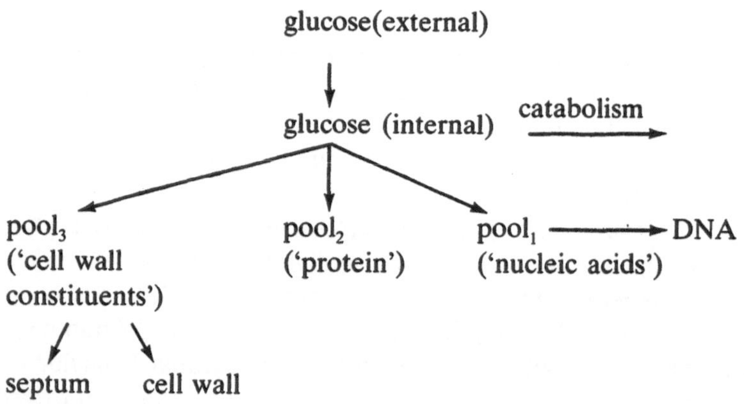

functions of the amount of macromolecules present, i.e., the significant pools, this reduced model would have the ability of simultaneously predicting the cell morphology and cellular composition. Hence the number of parameters is reduced to a significant few and that simplifies making a priori predictions of transient behavior of cell growth.

Recapitulation

Systemic approach to large metabolic reaction networks is becoming increasingly important. Better integrated view of the physiological role metabolic dynamics is needed. Reduction in model complexity is essential to make metabolic models attractive for practical use.

The results in this chapter indicate that all these issues can be addressed within the framework of straight forward application of order of magnitude estimation and judicious use of linear analysis. We see that the dynamic order reduces naturally and logically within the framework of linear analysis to give an insight into the physiological function of key concentration variables. Further applications of traditional engineering systems science to complex biological systems should prove fruitful.

Acknowledgment

Numerous discussions with Professor E.N. Lightfoot influenced this paper, in particular the section on *Approaching simplified dynamic descriptions*, significantly. Sadettin Ozturk helped to prepare the figures and text. Financial support, in part, was provided by the Whitaker Foundation.

References

1. Segel LA (1984): Modeling dynamic phonemena in molecular and cellular biology. Cambridge University Press, Cambridge.
2. Lightfoot EN (1980): Mass transport and reaction in living systems. Class Notes, University of Wisconsin.
3. Einstein A (1910): Investigations on the theory of Brownian motion, Methuen, London Engl. Trans by Cowper.
4. Lenhoff AM (1984): Convective dispersion and interphase mass transfer, Ph.D. thesis. University of Wisconsin, Madison.
5. Carslaw HS, Jaeger JC (1959): Conduction of heat in solids, 2nd edition. Oxford University Press, Oxford.
6. Weisz PB (1973): Diffusion and chemical transformation. Science 179: 433–440.
7. Aris R (1975): The mathematical theory of diffusion and reaction in permeable catalysts, Vol I., Clarendon Press, Oxford.
8. Lightfoot EN (1974): Transport phenomena and living systems. John Wiley and Sons, New York.
9. Caro CG, Pedley TJ, Seed WA (1974): Mechanics of the circulation. In: Guyton AC (ed) Cardiovascular physiology, ch. 1. Medical and Technical Publishers, London.
10. Lin CC, Segel LA (1974): Mathematics applied to deterministic problems in the natural sciences. Macmillan Publishing Co., Inc, New York.
11. Palsson BO (1984): Mathematical modeling of dynamics and control in metabolic networks, Ph.D. thesis. University of Wisconsin, Madison.
12. Palsson BO, Lightfoot EN (1984): Mathematical modeling of dynamics and control in metabolic networks. I. On Michaelis – Menten Kinetics. J Theor Biol 111: 273–302.

13. Palsson BO, Jamier R, Lightfoot EN (1984): Mathematical modelling of dynamics and control IN metabolic networks: Part II Dimeric Enzymes. J Theor Biol 111: 303.
14. Palsson BO, Palsson H, Lightfoot EN (1985): Mathematical modelling of dynamics and control in metabolic networks: Part III Linear Reaction Sequences. J Theor Biol 113: 231.
15. Schauer M, Heinrich R, Rapoport SM (1981): Mathematische Modellierung der Glykolyse und des Adeninnukleotidstoffwechsels menschlicher Erythrozyten. Acta Biol Med Germ 40: 1659.
16. Palsson BO, Joshi A, Ozturk SS (1987): Reducing complexity in metabolic networks: making metabolic meshes manageable. Fed Proc 46.
17. Werner A, Heinrich R (1985): A kinetic model for the interaction of energy metabolism and osmotic states of human erythrocytes. Biomed Biochim Acta 44: 185–212.
18. Shuler ML, Leung S, Dick CC (1979): A mathematical model for the growth of a single bacterial cell. Ann NY Acad Sci 326: 35–55.
19. Domach MM, Leung SK, Cahn RE, Cocks GG, Shuler MM (1984): Computer model for glucose - limited growth of a single cell of Escherichia coli B/r-A. Biotech Bioeng 26: 203–216.
20. Domach MM (1983): Refinement and use of a structured model of a single cell of Escherichia coli for the description of Ammonia – limited growth and asynchronous population dynamics, Ph.D thesis. cornell University, Ithaca, New York.
21. Palsson BO, Joshi A (1987): On the Dynamic order of Escherichia coli structured growth models/ Biotech & Bioeng 29.
22. Ingraham JL, Maaloe O, Neidhart FC (1983): Growth of the bacterial cell. Sinauer Associates, Inc. Sunderland, MA.

Discussion

Sideman: You have showed a number of time constants. What is the criterion used to determine the time constants?

Palsson: Everything we did is according to a standard procedure. We wrote the dynamic equations and then solved for the steady state by using a Newton routine, and got the eigenvalues and eigenvectors from a program called 'Eispack'. Computationally, this is not too difficult. The difficulty comes in the interpretation of the results. The modes are mathematically abstract quantities, but when applied to metabolic networks they obtain some physiological meaning which makes them interesting. The question is why do all the high energy phosphate bonds in glycolysis group together on the slower time scales. The answer lies in the stoichiometric structure of the system plus the activity of the different enzymes. The study represents the fundamental aspect of studying metabolic dynamics. We try to see if there is a physiological meaningful dynamic structure here. The practical use of this analysis is that it gives a way to extract the essential kinetic information for metabolic networks.

Bassingthwaighte: In a large set of enzymatically coupled reactions, you have the slow ones which are the controlling ones. You presented a mechanism for linearizing a sequence of reactions into one linear differential operator which describes the transfer function between control points. This is the basis for linearizing the whole system. Then, presumably, one can modulate the transfer functions between these control points or shift between them if necessary.

Palsson: Slow is a relative term. For instance, changes in the red cells energy metabolism during circulation is relatively slow, while changes in the adenosine pool during blood storage may not be relatively slow, although the absolute time scales for the two cases indicate otherwise. What intrigues me in particular is that we can now identify the enzymes that act on these different time scales and are therefore responsible for controlling the different aspects of the dynamics of the system. Also, the linear analysis is only a prediction, an approximation, of the dynamic behavior of the non-linear model. We do not use the linear equation to simulate the full transients.

Now we return to the point which Dr Bassingthwaighte made. If you are looking at, say, glycolosis in the myocytes, under anoxia, the glycolytic rate will be very different than when you have the TCA cycle active, and maybe the model of structure will change in two different physiological states. The control may then shift from one enzyme to another, and in that case you would have to look at the two steady states separately.

Hoffman: One of the real advantages of the analysis would be in the area of structured identifiability. Once one can look at the time constants, one can choose the order of the system and decrease the complexity, reduce the order of the system and decide the set of equations you are going to solve.

Palsson: Yes. That is one of the major goals of this analysis. And as a result of my analysis, it is perhaps better to look at the pools of metabolities rather than at the individual concentrations as the dynamic variables in a reduced model. These pools may be dynamically coupled. Furthermore, you can identify the enzymes that are responsible for the slow motion, or the motion over the time scales of interest, and those are the ones for which you will have to know the kinetic characteristics very well. The other enzymes may be much less important and approximate knowledge is enough.

38. Integrated phenomenology of transport, permeation, and metabolic reactions in the heart

J.B. BASSINGTHWAIGHTE, L. NOODLEMAN, R.T. EAKIN
and R.B. KING

Abstract

The delivery of substrate to the cells of an organ by flow, membrane permeation and diffusion may be independent of or coupled to the intracellular metabolic reactions. Modern imaging techniques permit quantitative detection of the time course of tracers within individual small regions of an organ which can be interpreted in terms of the transport and reaction phenomena. The use of models for the interpretation puts explicit demands upon the investigators to provide sufficient data so that parameters can be realistically constrained by the evidence. Integrative models which give realistic descriptions are the vehicles for providing these constraints and for evaluating the state of the cellular events. Most important, the models are predictive,thereby aiding in the design of subsequent studies.

Introduction

Substrate transport and intracellular reaction sequences need to be considered together in the context of the governance of the intracellular milieu. The capacities of cellular systems are designed with multiple orders of redundancy in both structure and function. These 'redundancies' provide flexibility, control, and resiliency in the face of stress. From the point of view of the control system theorist, there are few or no set points for intracellular regulation, but rather the internal milieu is controlled via a highly complex system of transport and reaction phenomena which tend to balance each other to provide relatively tight control over the critically important constituents. Such 'balance point' control systems exhibit deviations in concentrations that are less than proportional to the imposed loads on the system. The absence of set points is understandable since inbuilt reference standards are not a normal feature of biological systems, but nevertheless such systems are susceptible to analysis using standard engineering analysis and control system theory.

While this philosophical viewpoint can be illustrated via studies at the molecular level or the whole body level, we will concentrate on applying it to studies of substrate and ion transport and regulation at the level of the cells and tissues of the myocardium. The specific kinds of relationships that one might examine are those between rates of transport and rates of metabolism, or between rates of reactions at different points along a sequence of reactions. Some, but not all, reactions must be regulated. For the sake of parsimony in equipping the cell, the capacity for specialized transporter mechanisms should be roughly matched to the capacity for intracellular enzymatically facilitated reactions. Since both may be regarded as resistances to a flux, there is little point in one being radically different from the other under the conditions in which the cell is operating. This is a pretty loose definition however, because the cell must normally be able to handle a wide range of situations, e.g. the cardiac myocyte must function over a wide range of heart rates, cardiac work levels, and do so in spite of variability in the amounts and even the types of substrates delivered.

It is the purpose of this review therefore to illustrate some of these issues in the course of describing current activity in the field of transport and exchange in the myocardium, and in attempting to suggest some research needs for the future.

Background

The modern developments in the regulation of myocardial substrate utilization are built by combining knowledge gained in at least four fields. These four are loosely termed

1. circulatory mass transport and flow regulation,
2. tracer kinetics and pharmacokinetics,
3. biochemistry of intermediary metabolism, and
4. membrane transport.

In combining these one needs to include the basic aspects of cell biology, bioenergetics, membrane phenomena, diffusional processes, circulatory physiology, and endocrine regulation. An overview relating these to positron emission tomography covers the convective and transport processes [1].

In all of these fields the use of tracer methodology has been a key tool. Studies with single tracers have been used for estimating the rates of formation of intermediates in reaction sequences, for observing the rates of trans-membrane transport, for measuring the exchange between blood and the tissues of an organ, and for determining whole body pharmacokinetics. In some cases it has been critical to assure that the tracer remained on the original substrate molecule, but in others it has been equally important to follow the tracer label through a set of reactions in which it was transferred from one molecule to another. The distinction between branches in biochemical pathways has in some cases relied on the use of dual tracer labeling, two labels on different parts of a molecule.

A particularly powerful tool for assessing blood tissue exchange processes has been the multiple indicator dilution technique. In this technique several tracers are introduced simultaneously into the blood entering an organ, and their separation in passing through the organ provides a means for estimating rates of barrier penetration and intracellular reaction. An overall description of the technique has been provided by Bassingthwaighte and Goresky [2]. This technique was introduced by Chinard and co-workers [3] and extended by Goresky [4]. These early applications of the multiple indicator dilution technique made use of 'flow-limited' tracers, which by definition are tracers which traverse barriers and diffuse into tissue so rapidly that the flow limits the exchange. The studies were designed to measure the volumes of distribution and the transit times of the several tracers through an organ. In particular, the technique was applied to measuring lung water [3, 5], originally with tritiated water, later with other solutes such as iodoantipyrine that distributed within the water space, and more recently with thermal indicator [6]. The measurement of lung water was useful in the assessment of the state of the organ, providing an on-the-spot measure of the degree of pulmonary edema.

The use of the multiple indicator dilution technique for measuring barrier permeability was initiated by Crone [7]. He made pulse injections into the inflow to the brain, making observations of the outflow concentration time curves for albumin and glucose, and calculated the permeability-surface area for glucose across the blood brain barrier. The experiments were conceptually akin to those of Renkin [8] in which a steady tracer infusion of potassium, which was taken up by the cells of the skeletal muscle, resulted in the continuous arteriovenous difference and allowed an estimate of the composite barrier permeability between the blood and the cells. The difference was that the Crone technique, by virtue of using an intravascular reference substance simultaneously with the substrate, provided during each second a measure of the flux from blood into tissue over the first several seconds; the steady state infusion used by Renkin however could only provide a measure of net extraction influenced by permeation of the capillary and the sarcolemmal barriers in series. (Neither technique accounted for reduction in apparent extraction by backflux from the tissue into the outflowing blood, but the rapid sampling technique of Crone legitimized the assumption that for the first seconds the backflux was small.) Crone's refinement therefore set the stage for later investigators to use more fully developed models for the interpretation of outflow dilution curves (see Figure 1). A partial accounting for back diffusion was provided by Martin and Yudilevich [9] and Johnson and Wilson [10], considering the extravascular region as a lumped mixing pool.

Sangren and Sheppard [11] defined a capillary tissue model consisting of a central cylindrical capillary surrounded by a cylindrical extravascular region (Figure 1, middle). By neglecting axial diffusion and assuming radial diffusion to be instantaneous they obtained an analytical solution for the impulse response of this system. This model was used by Goresky et al. [13] for the analysis of dilution

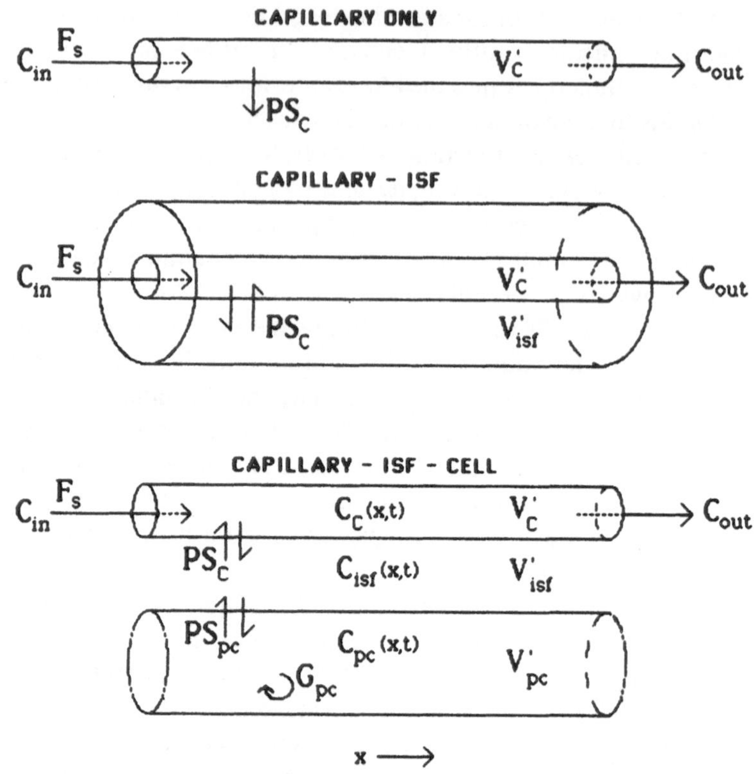

Figure 1. Capillary-tissue exchange models with infinitely radial diffusion and zero axial diffusion. Upper panel: The Crone-Renkin model for tracer escape from the capillary with no 'back-diffusion', reflux from tissue to blood. Middle panel: The 2-region, mass-conservative model of Sangren and Sheppard [11], allowing reflux. Lower panel: The 3-region capillary-interstitial fluid-cell model of Rose et al. [12], which is also mass-conservative when the consumption, G_{pc}, is zero. Terms are: F_s, flow $ml\,g^{-1}min^{-1}$; C, concentration, molar; V′, volume of distribution, ml/g; PS, permeability-surface area product, $ml\,g^{-1}min^{-1}$; G, consumption, $ml\,g^{-1}min^{-1}$. Subscripts are: C for capillary, isf for interstitial fluid, pc for parenchymal cell. (Reprinted with permission of Academic Press, New York.)

curves in the myocardium. A conceptually similar model was developed by Bassingthwaighte [14], adding axial diffusion terms and incorporating the blood tissue exchange model into a whole organ model. The use of these models which provided a complete accounting for all of the tracer which entered the organ not only allowed the calculation of volumes of distribution in the tissue, as Chinard et al. [3] had pioneered, but also allowed for bi-directional flux of tracer across the membranes, i.e., accounted for 'back diffusion', or reflux from tissue to blood. In actuality, the numbers obtained for barrier permeability-surface area products were not very different from those obtained by Martin and Yudilevich [9] and by Alvarez and Yudilevich [15] but were somewhat higher and more theoretically satisfying. The improved accuracy of estimation of the barrier permeability for a variety of solutes also provided new insight, namely evidence from the tracer kinetics that there was indeed some steric hindrance to molecular passage across the capillary wall. The degree of hindrance provided an estimate of the average dimension of the channels between endothelial cells. Assuming these to be uniform, which appears to be the case by electron microscopy, the effective width of an approximating slit between adjacent endothelial cells appears to be 100 to 110 Å [16, 17].

These approaches have provided measures of the capillary permeability and, with extensions of the modeling to a two-barrier system, to sarcolemmal permeability-surface area products for substrates of interest (Figure 1, lower panel). Rose and Goresky [18] obtained estimates of palmitate extraction by the myocardium and interpreted these in terms of the permeability-surface area product for the capillary, for the sarcolemma, and for intracellular consumption. While the distinction between sarcolemmal permeation and intracellular consumption was perhaps not clear, this was the first study on the rates of fatty acid uptake by myocardium that attempted to distinguish between transport and reaction. The work did not provide insight into the mechanisms of transport, nor distinguish carrier-mediated from other transport, but nevertheless did provide estimates of rates of permeation and uptake that were compatible with the observable arteriovenous differences across the heart. It is important to be able to compare estimates of transport rates by two totally different techniques, one using tracers for providing intimate details, and the other a chemical technique for measuring overall myocardial consumption. However, because the experiments were done in intact, closed chest animals with rapid recirculation, the tails of the indicator dilution curves were obscured, which marred the estimation of transport rates and of volumes of distribution. Accounting for recirculation is not an insurmountable problem, but requires continuous measurement of the inflow dilution curve as well as the outflow dilution curve, and the use of models constructed with differential operators. Solutions to model equations in the form of the unit impulse response are less useful because they have to be convoluted with the input function in order to derive an output function to be fitted to the data.

Some of these difficulties were resolved by the development of the same type of concentric cylinder modeling of blood tissue exchange units but expressed in terms of differential operators. The earliest version of Bassingthwaighte et al. [19] included both axial and radial diffusion, but the latter was omitted in the faster algorithms of Bassingthwaighte [14] and extended by Bassingthwaighte et al. [20]. The use of the differential operator provided two benefits. One was an immense reduction in computation time, which for a three region model amounted to about a one million times faster computation compared to the analytic solution of Rose et al. [12] which was used by Rose and Goresky [18] for palmitate extraction studies. Kuikka et al. [21] applied a multicapillary version of a three-region, two barrier model to the assessment of glucose transport in the myocardium. They used three glucoses, D-, L-, and 2-deoxy-D-glucose, using albumin as the intravascular reference tracer. The L-glucose served as an extracellular reference tracer, allowing relatively precise measurement of the sarcolemmal permeation rate. Flow heterogeneity was accounted for in the modeling by the use of multiple blood tissue units in which the flow was determined from the regional flows in the myocardium, as measured by microsphere depositions. The use of the actually measured flow distributions to analyze the data avoided the systematic errors that accompany usage of a single capillary model. Bassingthwaighte and Winkler [22], and Bassingthwaighte and Goresky [2] showed that the use of the single capillary model instead of the more appropriate multicapillary model results in systematic errors in the estimate of capillary permeability, underestimating it by a minimum of 25% and usually more. This is the kind of error anticipated by Zierler [23] and is simply a consequence of the idea of using linear averages to approximate non-linear situations.

The flow heterogeneity was accounted for by Kuikka et al. [21] and by Bassingthwaighte et al. [24] by considering the organ to be composed of a set of capillary tissue units in parallel with the flow through each of these sets determined from the flow distributions through the organ (Figure 2). The input function for all of the capillary tissue units was assumed to be the same, namely a dispersed function that arrived at the entrances to the capillary tissue units after traversing the arterial inflow; it was assumed likewise that the venous outflow pathways all resulted in the same degree of dispersion from each of the capillary tissue units. Although good fits to the data of the model solutions were obtained, this does not prove the accuracy of this particular heterogeneity model. An alternative model was proposed by Rose and Goresky [25] and has been utilized in their subsequent publications. Transport by flow was assumed to be non-dispersive in large vessels and through capillary tissue units. (It is this lack of dispersiveness in any vessels that makes us reluctant to accept this model.) This model also fits dilution curves well over the first 15 to 20 seconds, although the test is limited by the fact that Goresky and colleagues acquire their data in closed chest animals for only 20 to 30 seconds, principally because of the early recirculation. An evaluation of the relative accuracy of the two models versus each other, or versus an intermediate formulation, has not yet been accomplished. The question of how to formulate a correct heterogeneity model in the myocardium is therefore still open.

Current generation modeling

Models are merely working hypotheses, doomed to transient service. Problems with past models become evident when high resolution data are obtained in situations which stretch the models beyond their limits. For example, when transport rates are not very high, as for glucose where the capillary permeability-surface area product and the sarcolemmal PS are both low, then the 3-region 2-barrier multiple capillary versions of the organ suffice. So far as one can tell, they provide excellent estimates of the capillary PS, moderately accurate esti-

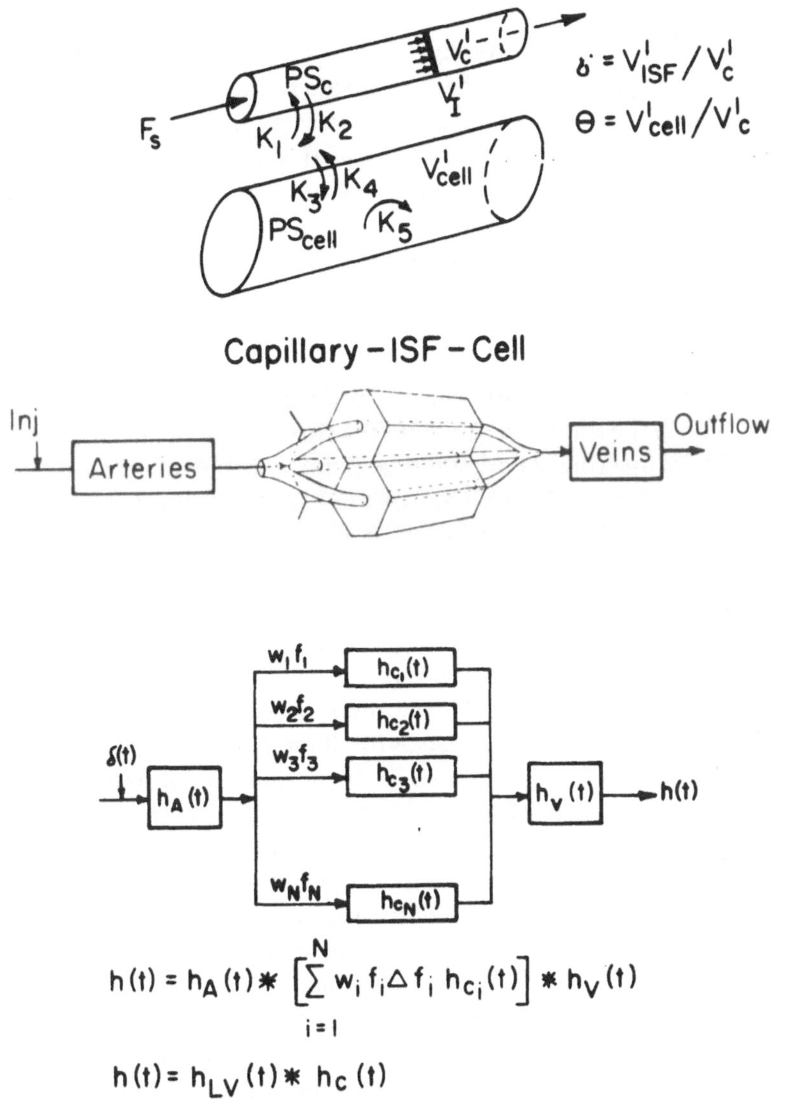

Figure 2. Model configuration to account for heterogeneity of regional flows and transit times. (Reprinted from Mathematical Computer Simulation 24: 502, 1982.)

mates of the sarcolemmal PS, but not very good estimates of the intracellular reaction rates. That is easily understood when one appreciates that in order for estimates of intracellular reaction to be ascertained from the outflow dilution curves for untransformed tracer-labeled substrate there must be reflux of unmetabolized tracer from the organ. Therefore, estimates of intracellular transformation rate may be improved by making measurements of the rate of appearance of tracer in a metabolite. For glucose the prominent metabolites available in the outflow would be carbon dioxide and water, the same metabolites which would appear for fatty acids, but via totally different pathways. In special cases only a single metabolite appears, and when it appears rapidly in the outflow, then the rate of transformation can be accurately measured. Such is the case for the conversion of angiotensin-I to angiotensin-II during transcapillary passage through the lung; there is no pulmonary retention of either. In this instance the conversion is so rapid that there is no delay at all between the substrate (angiotensin-I) and the product (angiotensin-II); the sum of the two forms in the outflow are superimposable on the reference albumin outflow dilution curve, indicating complete recovery for the tracer labeled hormone in one form or the other [26]. This, however, is an exceptional case.

The situations which have proven more difficult to analyze in the myocardium are those in which the transport rates into the tissue are high, and for which there is also substantial metabolism or retention in the tissue. Two particular examples that are quite revealing of the situation are those for fatty acids and for adenosine. The studies of these substrates require extensions from the current state of the art.

The analysis of fatty acid dilution curves requires extension of the modeling in two directions, and simultaneously requires substantial refinement of the standard experiments. These demands occur not only because of the nature of the substrate itself and its handling by the myocardium, but also because of the extraordinarily high binding of fatty acids by albumin in the blood; approximately 99.94% of fatty acid is albumin bound under normal circumstances. In spite of this high binding, 40 to 70% of the total fatty acid may be extracted during single transcapillary passage, meaning that removal of fatty acid from its binding site on the albumin must be occurring very rapidly. Further complicating the modeling is the observation that fatty acid extraction is much higher for its molecular weight than can be accounted for by permeation through the clefts between endothelial cells. Figure 3 diagrams the possibilities. In other words, there must be transport through the endothelial cells themselves, and because of the tight binding to albumin, there is every reason for believing that almost all of the transport is through endothelial cells and little or none through the clefts, simply because the albumin-bound fatty acid cannot traverse the clefts.

The first extension of the modeling, which has already been accomplished [24, 1] is to account for the greater detail in the capillary barrier itself. Instead of using a simple passive membrane treated as a linear conductance represented by the permeability-surface area product, PS_c, the capillary barrier is treated more realistically as a composite barrier as in Figure 4 [27]. The passive leak conductance is indicated in the diagram by PS_g, which represents the permeation through the interendothelial cellular gaps or clefts together with any passive symmetrical conductance across the plasmalemma of the endothelial cells between the lumen of the capillary and the interstitial fluid region. (For hydrophilic solutes the latter is negligible so that PS_g represents the clefts only. For highly

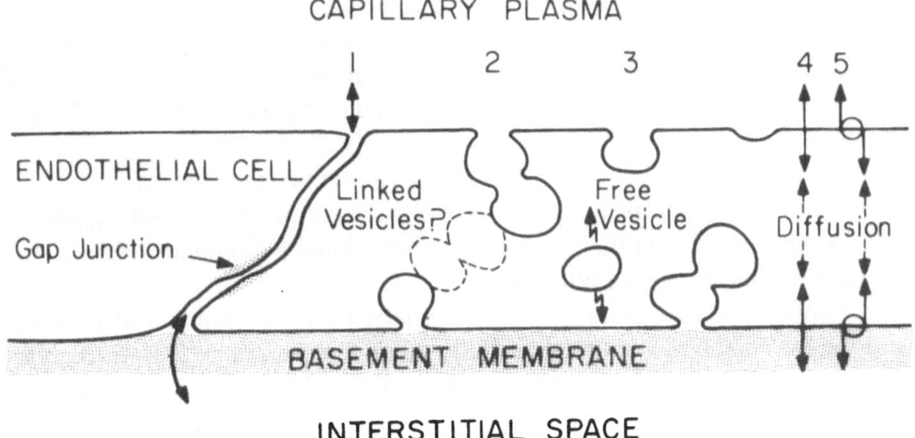

Figure 3. Routes of transendothelial transport. (Reprinted from Bassingthwaighte and Goresky [8] with permission from the American Physiological Society.)

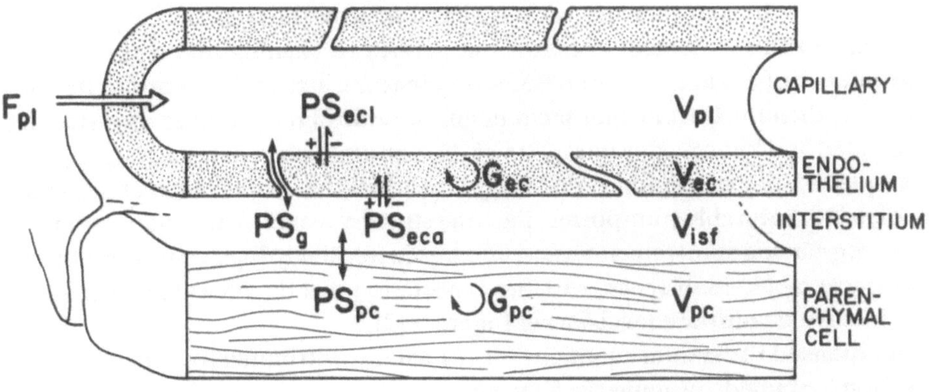

Figure 4. Capillary-tissue transendothelial transport. (Reprinted from Gorman et al. [27] with permission of the Am Physiol Soc)

penetrating solutes such as ethanol or highly lipid solute substances that do not bind within the endothelial cells, PS_g might be governed mainly by transendothelial diffusion.) The conductances across the two sides of the endothelial cell are diagrammed as possibly asymmetric. There is no a priori reason for thinking of PS_{ecl} as being equal to that on the abluminal surface, PS_{eca}. For the purposes of analyzing data, the investigator must make a choice. The possibilities go beyond passive symmetrical conductances. Carrier-mediated conductances may be inherently symmetrical or equilibrative. The fluxes will ordinarily be influenced by the actual chemical concentrations on both sides of the membrane, and are therefore asymmetric even when equilibrative whenever the steady state is not an equilibrium state. A third possibility is energetically coupled transport, which is ordinarily asymmetrical, and can lead to accumulation or depletion within the cell. The same possibilities exist for the sarcolemmal permeability-surface area product PS_{pc}.

Consumption within the cells is diagrammed and represents the first intracellular reaction with a clearance constant G_{cc} for the endothelial cell and G_{pc} for the parenchymal cell. The model has the equations given by Bassingthwaighte et al. [28] and Bassingthwaighte [29].

The application of this model to the analysis of adenosine transport was described by Bassingthwaighte et al. [28] and by Gorman et al. [27] through the myocardium, where linear coefficients were used for both the conductances and the consumption terms, G_{cc} and G_{pc}. This was considered appropriate for the situation because tracer adenosine transport in the presence of constant concentrations of native substrates was what was being examined by the experimental technique. The principle involved is that the tracer concentrations are many orders of magnitude lower than the chemical concentrations, so that the rate constants are determined by the non-tracer chemical concentrations and are uninfluenced by the passage of a tracer transient through the system. The corollary to this statement is that if one wishes to examine the concentration dependence of a transport or consumption mechanism, to demonstrate its non-linearity, then the tracer experiment might be done in the presence of varied but controlled and known concentrations of the non-tracer labeled substrate [2]. For example, if the expectation is that PS_{ccl} represents the conductance of a carrier-mediated or saturable transporter, then the strategy would be to obtain estimates of tracer-labeled substrate at a succession of increasingly high concentrations of non-tracer labeled substance, with the expectation that the PS would decrease as one increased substrate levels, as in Figure 5 [2].

Solutions to the system equations for the axially distributed four region model are best obtained by numerical techniques. An analytical solution has been developed by C.Y. Wang [28], but solving numerically for impulse responses of two minutes duration is approximately 10^8 times faster than calculating the analytic solution. The reason for this remarkable gain in efficiency is that the numerical solutions can be set up to account for the radial exchange during the initial conditions so that during each time step only multiplication is used, whereas the analytical solutions require the use of three single convolution integrations over Bessel functions, and one double convolution integration, all of which are most time consuming.

A typical solution is shown in Figure 6 for the case in which a brief pulse injection was made at the input to the capillary tissue region. The response a short time later when the pulse had traversed about two thirds of the way through the capillary is shown in the left panel. The leading pulse has been slightly spread by axial diffusion and material has entered all of the extravascular regions, but is

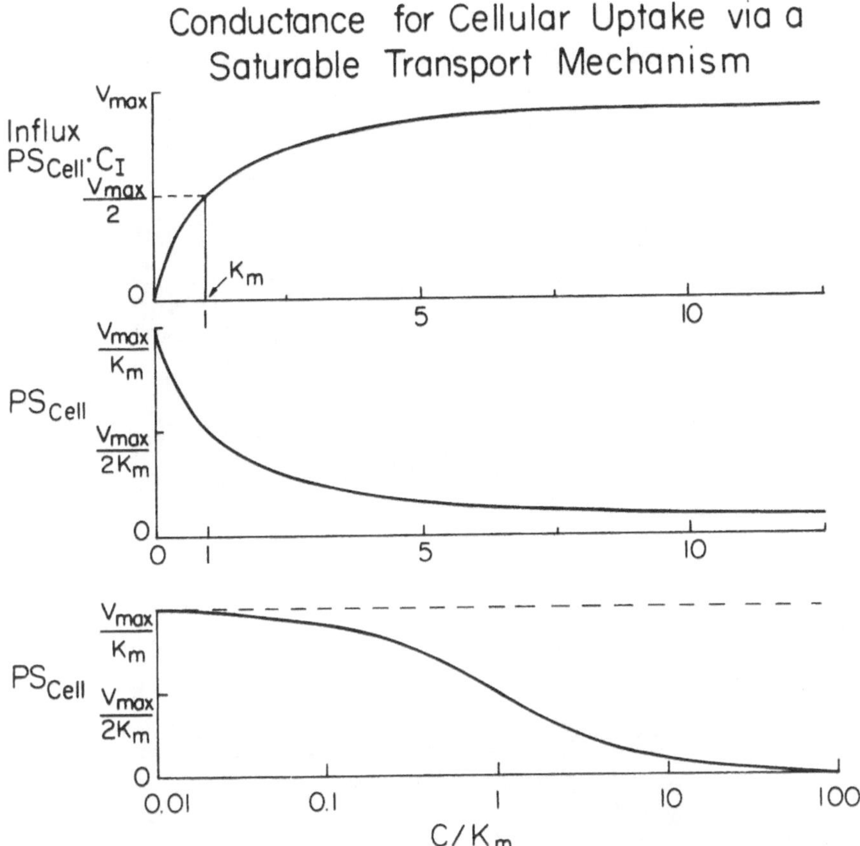

Figure 5. Concentration-dependent PS products for carrier-mediated transport. Cellular influx and PS_{Cell} versus concentration. PS_{Cell} diminishes as a function of concentration if the transport mechanism is saturable. The mechanism here is analogous to a first-order Michaelis-Menten reaction for enzyme kinetics. More complex reactions would be expected to give curves of different form. C_I, interstitial concentration; V_{max}, maximum transport rate; K_m, concentration at which transport rate is half maximal. S_{Cell} is not affected by changes in concentration and in the heart is ~2,000 cm^2/g. (Reprinted from Bassingthwaighte and Goresky [2] with permission from the American Physiological Society.)

seen to be most concentrated at the upstream end of the capillary. The profile within the capillary shows the slightly dispersed leading spike of non-extracted material, maximal at two thirds of the capillary length. It is followed by a secondary and much broader peak of concentrations in the capillary with a maximum at about one third of the distance along. The spike and trailing wave are characteristic of these solutions for medium to high ratios of PS/F. If the PS is very high the leading spike of unextracted tracer vanishes quickly via loss into the surrounding tissue. In this particular solution the spike actually vanishes before the end of the capillary is reached. The trailing wave is due to reflux from the tissue back into the blood with medium to high permeabilities. The probability of

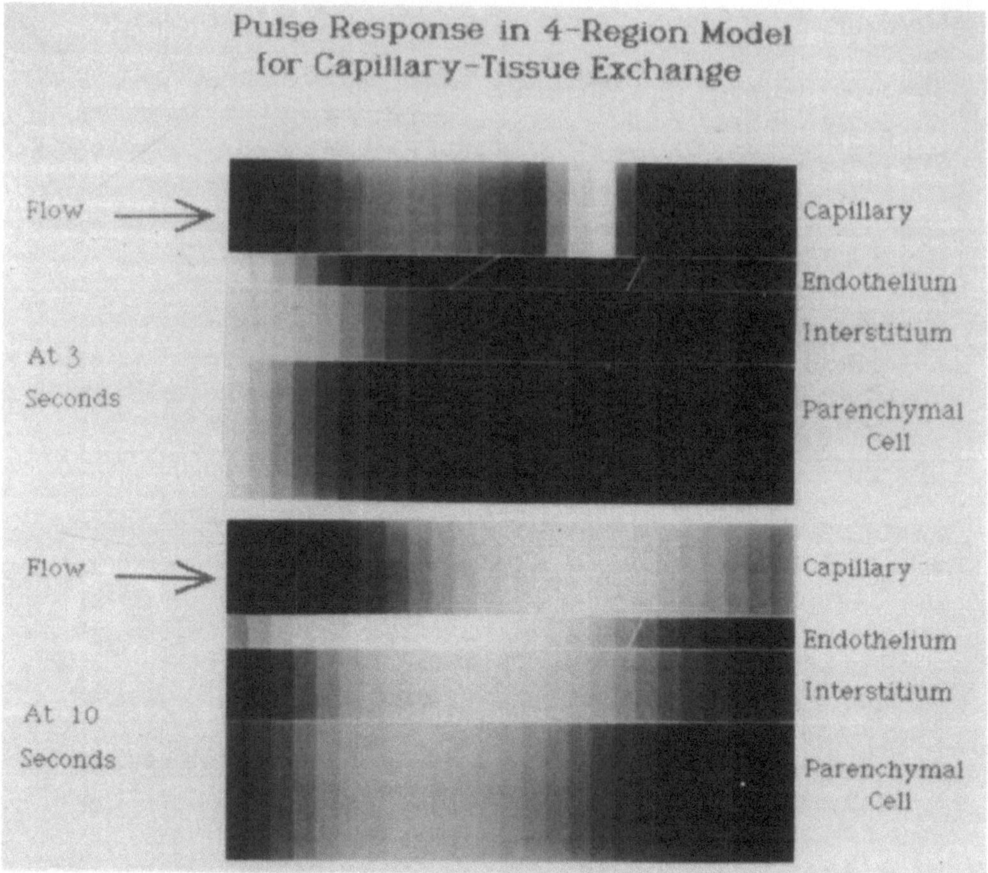

Figure 6. Display of a solution to a 4-region capillary-tissue exchange model, using a Lagrangian-based numerical solution. Upper panel: Concentration profiles at 3 seconds after introduction of a brief pulse injection into the inflow. Lower panel: At 10 seconds. Parameters are: $F_s = 0.6$ ml g^{-1}min^{-1}; the volumes, ml g^{-1}min^{-1}, were $V_c = 0.04$; $V_{ec} = 0.01$; $V_{isf} = 0.15$; $V_{pc} = 0.1$. The PS products, ml g^{-1}min^{-1}, were $PS_g = 3.0$; $PS_{ecl} = 0$; $PS_{eca} = 0.3$; $PS_{pc} = 3.0$. The consumption terms, G, were zero.

re-escape from blood into tissue is high and so this wave represents delivery of material from the upstream end of the tissue into the more downstream elements of the tissue, and does not go straight into the outflow. When the permeabilities are low then the spike persists until it reaches the outflow and the tail is relatively small, and instead of being a wave as in this figure, is of more or less an exponential form, the concentrations just following the spike in the outflow being the highest and diminishing thereafter.

In the lower panel is shown the progression of the same solution as in the left panel but at 7 seconds later. By this time there has been very little loss of tracer from the system, but the material is moving as spreading waves trailing behind the broadly spread concentration profile in the capillary. In this solution the value for PS_g is high and for PS_{ecl} is 0, so that entry into the endothelial cell is gained from the abluminal surface with conductance PS_{eca}. Thus the concentration peaks in the endothelial cell and the parenchymal cell lag behind that in the ISF. The parenchymal must always lag behind that in the ISF since it cannot have direct contact with the capillary blood, but if the permeability surface area product for the luminal surface of the endothelial cell is high then the endothelial cell might actually precede the interstitial profile. Because there are two separate pathways from capillary to ISF, the endothelial cell may be either trailing or leading compared to the ISF. In no case can the extravascular concentrations lead compare to the capillary concentrations when the flow in the neighboring capillaries is concurrent. This appears to be a reasonable descriptor for hydrophilic solutes, for it is never observed that a hydrophilic solute which can escape into the interstitial fluid or the cells reaches the outflow before a vascular indicator such as albumin or erythrocytes. This conclusion contradicts the model formulation of Johnson and Wilson [10] in which they consider the extravascular region to be an instantaneous mixing pool.

The present status is that these models, with up to four radial regions, have been incorporated into multicapillary models designed to represent an intact organ. The mathematical formulation is given in Figure 2 from Levin et al. [30], the configuration indicating that the individual capillary tissue units are considered to be independent of each other (no exchange across the interface between neighbors), and that the input to all of them is the same, dispersed, as it were, by a single supplying artery. It is this configuration that should be improved in subsequent versions. A more general one is given in Figure 7, in which there is a set of several large vessels, each one having a different flow or transit time. Each is connected to one or more capillary tissue units, the apportionment of the flow from each large vessel to each unit being assigned either arbitrarily or from data such as the distribution of flows or the observed outflow dilution curves. The constraining expressions provide assurance of mass balance in the system. The difficulty in applying this formulation is in assigning the distributions of the large vessel flow amongst the capillaries; the flow distributions, observed with microspheres [31] or with a molecular marker, IDMI [32] must match the products $w_i f_i$ for the capillary tissue units, but do not specify the large vessel distributions since these flow markers are deposited almost completely in capillaries.

Next developments

The simple descriptors defined above work well for most tracer experiments, because linear descriptions are adequate, certainly for steady states. For application to the analysis of 3-dimensional images, further simplifications are an aid to practical use in estimating regional flows and metabolic rates [33]. These may

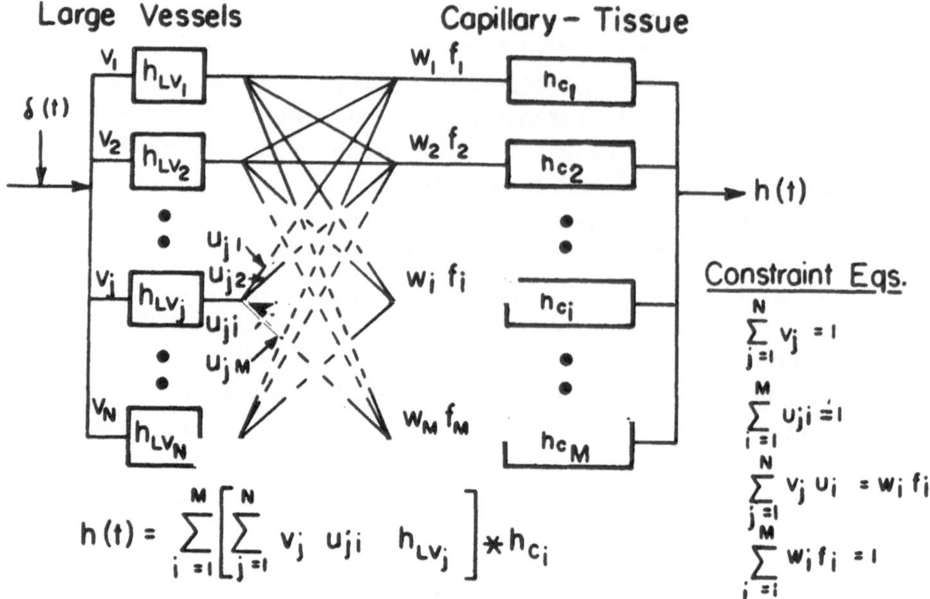

Figure 7. Capillary-tissue transport model with variable degree of association between transport functions of large vessels and capillaries. The large-vessel transit times, with fractions of flow v_j through the N independent pathways, may be non-dispersive [i.e., $h_{LVj}(t) = \delta(t - \tau_{LV_j})$] or dispersive. Flow from the jth large-vessel pathway is distributed among M capillary tissue units, the distribution being defined by the u_{ji} to the ith of the M capillary-tissue units. The distribution functions, the u_{ji}'s may differ from each other in the most general case. (Reprinted from Bassingthwaighte and Goresky [2] with permission from the American Physiological Society.)

be algebraic approximations, table look-up operations, or the uses of similarity and interpolation. A particular desire is to avoid time-consuming integrations whenever possible, something which is partially accomplished by using differential operators instead of convolutions, as discussed earlier.

To obtain a more realistic description, the complexity must be increased to incorporate new features. The fundamental problem is the lack of data. How to handle heterogeneity of parameters other than flow, for example, in PS or in volumes of distribution, is not clear. While these are recognized experimentally, for permeability by Rous et al. [34] and for vascular and interstitial volumes by Gonzalez et al. [35], the problem in using even good estimates of the distributions of values of these features is that it is not known how or whether there is an association (or dissociation) within regions between these and the known local flows. More data are required in a variety of situations before useful attempts can be made in incorporating multifactorial heterogeneity into the modeling.

Features that can be handled reasonably by taking advantage of the power of the modern computing technology are the following:

1. sequences of metabolic products, some of which remain intracellular and

others of which escape into the interstitium and effluent plasma;
2. axial and radial diffusion effects;
3. non-linear binding to surfaces or to mobile or immobile molecules;
4. non-linear facilitated transport and countertransport.

Sequences of metabolites require the development of multispecies models each of which has a minimal complexity similar to that of Figure 4. For adenosine, the immediate metabolites that can be identified in the outflow dilution samples are inosine, hypoxanthine, and uric acid, the products of degradation. Highly polar compounds, such as ATP, into which most of the tracer adenosine is incorporated, do not penetrate the cell membrane very rapidly and for short term studies can be modeled as if remaining in the cells. The corollary to this analytical undertaking is that the experimental data must be acquired; for adenosine tracer injections, the outflow samples must be analyzed for the concentration of the tracer-labeled metabolites in each of a sequence of outflow samples. A set of data acquired by Gorman et al. [27] are shown in Figure 8; a similar set of model outflow dilution curves from the multispecies modeling is shown in Figure 9. Solutions of the form shown in Figure 9 can only be obtained by incorporating endothelial cells into the model, and even then only by allowing the transformations to occur in the endothelial cells. Similar rates of transformation within myocytes cannot produce inosine and hypoxanthine curves with the peaks almost synchronous with that of adenosine and with such a brief time course. The modeling thereby provided the first evidence on these points, and predicted the observations of Nees et al. [36] that 90% or more of the retained tracer found by autoradiography in the heart is in the endothelial cells.

Axial and radial diffusion are generally avoided in such modeling because for well-perfused organs two approximations are reasonably accurate:
1. radial concentration gradients are dissipated very rapidly compared to capillary transit times and can therefore be neglected under most circumstances, and
2. axial diffusivity within the tissue is too slow to have a significant effect on the exchange process.

For the heart and liver, there is little question about radial diffusivity being fast, as estimated from the diffusion coefficients of Safford et al. [37, 38], and the intercapillary distances of Bassingthwaighte et al. [39], but there is some evidence that the outflow dilution curves are mildly influenced by axial diffusion, perhaps as much in the capillary lumen as in the tissue. Both were incorporated in an early model for blood tissue exchange, as shown in Figure 10, but this is impractical for analyzing dilution curves because the computation times are exceedingly long and the effects small.

Non-linear binding, to surfaces or to soluble macromolecules within the tissue, can be accounted for by using concentration-dependent volumes of distribution when the equilibration between the solute and the binding sites is in more or less continuous equilibrium. The effective volume of distribution, V'_d is the sum of

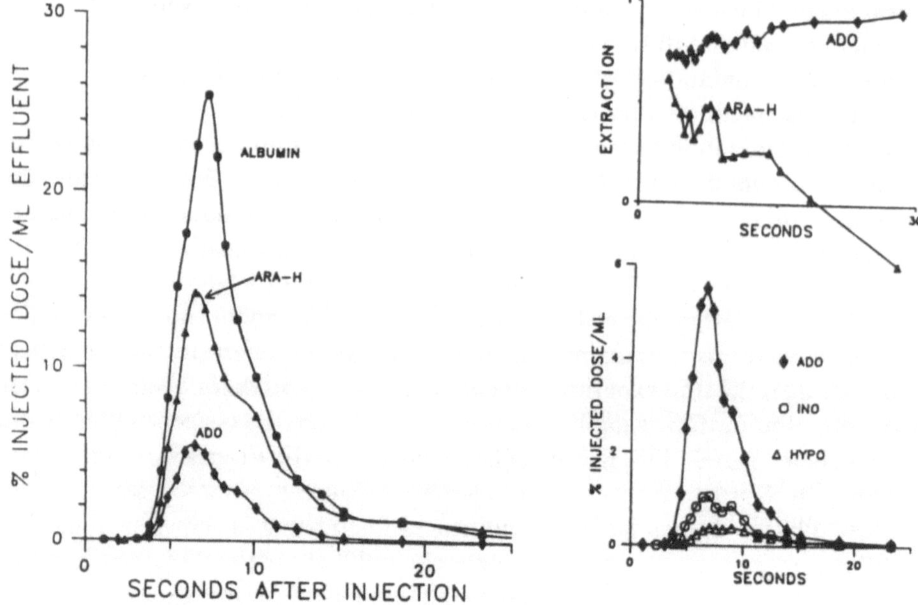

Figure 8. Appearance of adenosine (Ado), arabino furanosyl hypoxanthine (AraH), and albumin in venous effluent following multiple-tracer injection. Note relatively low concentration of Ado in venous effluent when compared with AraH. This leads to high extraction for Ado relative to AraH shown in upper right graph. Also note that extraction of Ado is steady, whereas extraction of AraH falls off due to back diffusion of this extracellular tracer from interstitial space. Lower right panel shows expanded view of Ado, inosine (ino), and hypoxanthine (hypo) curves. (Reprinted from Gorman et al. [27] with permission of the Am Physiol Soc.)

the volume of distribution for an equivalent unbound solute, V_d, plus a concentration-dependent term for the bound solute. When the binding is first order, at equilibrium the expression is:

$$V_d' = V_d \left[1 + \frac{B_T}{(K_b + C_{solute})}\right],$$

where K_b is the binding constant, molar, and B_T is the molar concentration of the binding site [37]. When the non-tracer concentrations are in steady state, the value for V'_d can be calculated during the initial conditions, but when they are changing, then these calculations must be made for each time step as the solution progresses, a costly calculation when many regions are involved.

Nonlinear or saturable transporters provide mechanisms for allowing hydrophilic molecules to move across lipid bilayers. Because the number of transporter molecules on a membrane is limited, and the conformational change required for translocation takes finite time, there is a maximal capacity for solute flux. The usual transporter carries solute in both directions; commonly the rate of con-

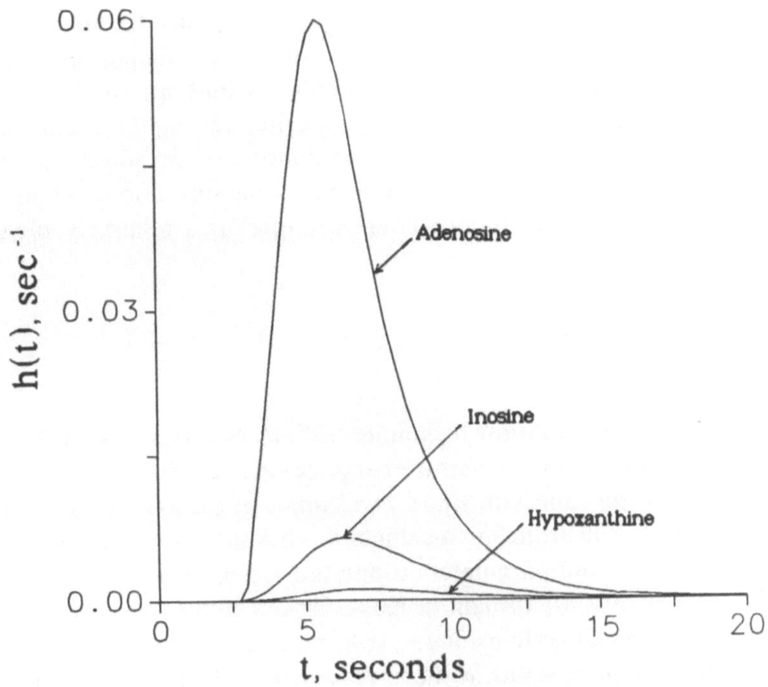

Figure 9. Multispecies model solutions for tracer adenosine, inosine, and hypoxanthine following adenosine entry into the inflow. The metabolites inosine and hypoxanthine come entirely from the endothelial cell. Metabolites released from myocytes have a delayed, more dispersed washout curve even if the capillary barrier is considered to be an inert passive one. (Reprinted from Bassingthwaighte et al., in Yudilevich DL, Mann GE (eds) Carrier-mediated transport of solutes from blood to tissue; Longman, London, 1985, pp. 191–203.)

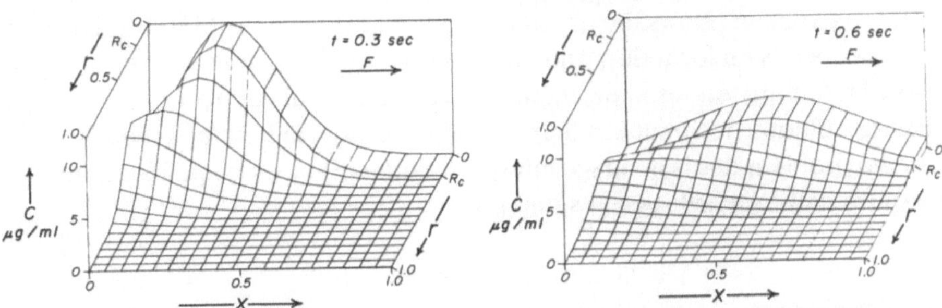

Figure 10. Concentration profiles in capillary and tissue when exchange is diffusion limited. Parameters for the solution were $rc = 4\,\mu$, $R = 20\,\mu$, $L = 100\,\mu$, $F = 3$ ml/g/min, $D_{Tx} = D_{Tr} = 2 \times 10^{-7}$ cm²/sec, $dp = 1 \times 10^{-6}$ cm²/sec, $P = 1000 \times 10^{-5}$ cm²/sec. The xr plane is labeled 1.0, 1.0 at $x = L$, $r = R$. 'Snapshots' of the concentration matrix at 0.3 sec (left panel) and 0.6 sec (right panel) after introduction of a 0.01 sec pulse injection at the input show that resistance to passage through the capillary wall at this high P is negligible but that the low tissue diffusion coefficient results in a 'trailing wave' of concentration in the tissue. (Reprinted from Bassingthwaighte et al. [19] with permission from the Benzon Foundation.)

formational change allowing the translocation is faster when a solute molecule is complexed with the transporter than when it is free. This combination of features has the corollary that countertransport should be facilitating, which is to say, the presence of transportable solute on the opposite side of the membrane will accelerate the transport of tracer. This possibility sets the stage for designing experiments that can characterize the transporter via flux studies while limiting the substrate, inhibitor, or agonist concentrations to a relatively physiologic range.

Conclusions

The multiple indicator dilution technique utilizes Nature's design for a rapid reaction apparatus by using the perfused organ as the vehicle for rapid passage of the substrate past the cells with short dwell times in the system. The exposure time of cells to the substrates or reactants is what occurs in nature and so the measurements made and parameters estimated are relevant to the physiologic state. Such statements are difficult to make for cell culture systems or perfused columns, since artificial systems have yet to be designed to provide packing as dense and void volumes so low as those provided by the natural organ.

A problem with using the natural organ is that several cell types are present. The separation of their influences must be accomplished by analysis of the kinetics of exchange and reaction. When two cell types have similar geometric positions and kinetic behavior they can only be lumped together in the analysis. In such cases their individual kinetics must be elucidated with other tools, such as sequential sample autoradiography, which has the spatial resolution to make distinction between neighboring cells.

Imaging of metabolic events by positron emission tomography depends on kinetic analysis but allows the use of only one tracer at a time [33]. Minimization of error depends on local flow and metabolism remaining constant throughout a series of tracer injections a few minutes apart. This is in contrast to the multiple indicator dilution technique where tracers are injected simultaneously. How serious a problem this is in image interpretation must be evaluated for individual substrates and for each special situation.

Acknowledgment

The authors greatly appreciate the expertise of M. McKay in the preparation of the manuscript and of B. van Steenwyk and R. Clay in the preparation of Figure 6.

References

1. Bassingthwaighte JB (1985): Overview of the processes of delivery: flow, transmembrane transport, reaction and retention. In: McMillin-Wood JB, Bassingthwaighte JB (eds) Cardiovascular metabolic imaging: physiological and biochemical dynamics in vivo. Circulation 72: IV39–IV46.
2. Bassingthwaighte JB, Goresky CA (1984): Modeling in the analysis of solute and water exchange in the microvasculature. In: Renkin EM, Michel CC (eds) Handbook of physiology, Sect. 2 The cardiovascular system, Vol IV, The microcirculation, Ch. 13 American Physiological Society, Bethesda, MD pp. 549–626.
3. Chinard FP, Vosburgh GJ, Enns T (1955): Transcapillary exchange of water and of other substances in certain organs of the dog. Am J Physiol 183: 221–234.
4. Goresky CA (1963): A linear method for determining liver sinusoidal and extravascular volumes. Am J Physiol 204: 626–640.
5. Goresky CA, Cronin RFP, Wangel BE (1969): Indicator dilution measurements of extravascular water in the lungs. J Clin Invest 48: 487–501.
6. Gray BA, Beckett RC, Allison RC, McCaffree DR, Smith RM, Sivak ED, Carlile PV Jr (1984): Effect of edema and hemodynamic changes on extravascular thermal volume of the lung. J Appl Physiol 56: 878–890.
7. Crone C (1963): The permeability of capillaries in various organs as determined by the use of the 'indicator diffusion' method. Acta Physiol Scand 58: 292–305.
8. Renkin EM (1959): Transport of potassium-42 from blood to tissue in isolated mammalian skeletal muscles. Am J Physiol 197: 1205–1210.
9. Martin P, Yudilevich DL (1964): A theory for the quantification of transcapillary exchange by tracer-dilution curves. Am J Physiol 207: 162–168.
10. Johnson JA, Wilson TA (1966): A model for capillary exchange. Am J Physiol 210: 1299–1303.
11. Sangren WC, Sheppard CW (1953): A mathematical derivation of the exchange of a labeled substance between a liquid flowing in a vessel and an external compartment. Bull Math Biophys 15: 387–394.
12. Rose CP, Goresky CA, Bach GG (1977): The capillary and sarcolemmal barriers in the heart: An exploration of labeled water permeability. Circ Res 41: 515–533.
13. Goresky CA, Ziegler WH, Bach GG (1970): Capillary exchange modeling: Barrier-limited and flow-limited distribution. Circ Res 27: 739–764.
14. Bassingthwaighte JB (1974): A concurrent flow model for extraction during transcapillary passage. Circ Res 35: 483–503.
15. Alvarez OA, Yudilevich DL (1969): Heart capillary permeability to lipid-insoluble molecules. J Physiol 202: 45–58.
16. Grabowski EF, Bassingthwaighte JB (1976): Capillary transport and exchange: An osmotic weight transient model for estimation of capillary transport parameters in myocardium. In: Grayson J, Zingg W (eds) Microcirculation Vol. 2 (Proc First World Cong. for the Microcirculation). Plenum Publ Corp, New York pp. 29–50.
17. Yipintsoi T, Tancredi RG, Eakin RT, Bassingthwaighte JB (1986): Permeation of myocardial capillary membranes shows restricted diffusion to hydrophilic solutes. (unpublished data)
18. Rose CP, Goresky CA (1977): Constraints on the uptake of labeled palmitate by the heart: The barriers at the capillary and sarcolemmal surfaces and the control of intracellular sequestration. Circ Res 41: 534–545.
19. Bassingthwaighte JB, Knopp TJ, Hazelrig JB (1970): A concurrent flow model for capillary-tissue exchanges. In: Crone C, Lassen NA (eds) Capillary permeability (Alfred Benzon Symp II). Munksgaard, Copenhagen pp. 60–80.
20. Bassingthwaighte JB, Lenhoff AM, Stephenson JL (1984): A sliding-element algorithm for rapid solution of spatially distributed convection-permeation models. Biophys J 45: 175a (Abstract).
21. Kuikka J, Levin M, Bassingthwaighte JB (1986): Multiple tracer dilution estimates of D-, and

2-deoxy-D-glucose uptake by the heart. Am J Physiol 250: H29–H42.

22. Bassingthwaighte JB, Winkler B (1982): Kinetics of blood to cell uptake of radiotracers. In: Columbetti LG (ed) Biological transport of radiotracers. CRC Press, pp. 97–146.
23. Zierler KL (1961): Theory of the use of arteriovenous concentration differences for measuring metabolism in steady and non-steady states. J Clin Invest 40: 2111–2125.
24. Bassingthwaighte JB, Kuikka JT, Chan IS, Arts T, Reneman RS (1985): A comparison of ascorbate and glucose transport in the heart. Am J Physiol 249: H141–H149.
25. Rose CP, Goresky CA (1976): Vasomotor control of capillary transit time heterogeneity in the canine coronary circulation. Circ Res 39: 541–554.
26. Ryan JW (1983): Assay of peptidase and protease enzymes in vivo. Biochem Pharmacol 32: 2127–2137.
27. Gorman MW, Bassingthwaighte JB, Olsson RA, Sparks HV Jr (1986): Endothelial cell uptake of adenosine in canine skeletal muscle. Am J Physiol 250: H482–H489.
28. Bassingthwaighte JB, Chaloupka M, Wang CY (1983): Transport by endothelial cells in vivo: Model analysis from indicator dilution after single transcapillary passage. Fed Proc 42: 580 (Abstract).
29. Bassingthwaighte JB (1985): Constraints in the interpretation of dynamic images of metabolic events. In: Sideman S, Beyar R (eds) Simulation and imaging of the cardiac system. Martinus Nijhoff, Dordrecht pp. 378–390.
30. Levin M, Kuikka J, Bassingthwaighte JB (1980): Sensitivity analysis in optimization of time-distributed parameters for a coronary circulation model. Med Prog Technol 7: 119–124.
31. King RB, Bassingthwaighte JB, Hales JRS, Rowell LB (1985): Stability of heterogeneity of myocardial blood flow in normal awake baboons. Circ Res 57: 285–295.
32. Little SE, Link JM, Krohn KA, Bassingthwaighte JB (1986): Myocardial extraction and retention of 2-iododesmethylimipramine: a novel flow marker. Am J Physiol 250: H1060–H1070.
33. McMillin-Wood JB, Bassingthwaighte JB (eds) (1985): Cardiovascular metabolic imaging: physiological and biochemical dynamics in vivo. Circulation 72: IV1–IV171.
34. Rous P, Gilding HP, Smith F (1930): The gradient of vascular permeability. J Exp Med 51: 807–830.
35. Gonzalez F, Harris C, Bassingthwaighte JB (1980): Volumes of distribution of intact rabbit hearts. Physiologist 23: 78 (Abstract).
36. Nees S, Herzog V, Bock M, Gerlach E (1984): Vasoactive adenosine (AR) perfused through isolated hearts is selectively trapped within the coronary endothelium (CE). Fed Proc 43: 900 (Abstract).
37. Safford RE, Bassingthwaighte JB (1977): Calcium diffusion in transient and steady states in muscle. Biophys J 20: 113–136.
38. Safford RE, Bassingthwaighte EA, Bassingthwaighte JB (1978): Diffusion of water in cat ventricular myocardium. J Gen Physiol 72: 513–538.
39. Bassingthwaighte JB, Yipintsoi T, Harvey RB (1974): Microvasculature of the dog left ventricular myocardium. Microvasc Res 7: 229–249.

Discussion

Clark: You pointed out some of the model parameter values that were used, and how they were obtained. Did you use an automatic parameter estimation scheme to obtain the remainder of the model parameters that were not directly specified? Secondly, in the reactor problem, what was the form of the system describing equation; was it a parabolic partial differential equation in r, z and time?
Bassingthwaighte: We have used automated parameter adjustment routines. The strategy is, first, to reduce the degrees of freedom as much as possible by obtaining several different types of data simultaneously (mean flow, distributions of flows, outflow responses for 3 or more tracer-labelled solutes). Secondly, we use a highly efficient optimizer based on sensitivity functions. This also helps in the experimental design by aiding the investigator in choosing appropriate input forms and data sampling protocols. The equations were parabolic partial differential equations, but normally account for only the axial position and time. Although we have obtained solutions accounting for radial diffusion (Bassingthwaighte, Knopp, et al., 1970), the radial distances in well-perfused organs are small enough so that gradients are negligible.
Beyar: In extreme situations of the system, like in very fast heart rates or high metabolic rates, or maybe in some diseases like hypertrophy when the intercapillary distance is increased, can the diffusion processes be limiting in terms of transferring metabolites to the cells, and maybe limit the rate of metabolism that can be achieved?
Bassingthwaighte: Such a limitation does not appear to be very likely for fatty acids and glucose, whose rates of transport across membranes appear adequate, but could be borderline with very large cells and high metabolic demand. A more likely limiting factor is oxygen delivery, because high consumption in the periphery of a cell may reduce delivery to the cell's central regions.
Spaan: Capillary lengths and flow through a capillary network are quite heterogeneous, so there may be shunting of molecules from one capillary through the tissue to another one. Shunting is more likely to occur for molecules that are not metabolized or bound. How would that affect your computations?
Bassingthwaighte: Our standard blood-tissue exchange models do not account for shunting of metabolized solutes. However, we have developed a crude model for diffusional arteriovenous shunting (Bassingthwaighte JB, Yipintsoi T, Knopp TJ, Microvasc Res 28: 233–253, 1984). It shows qualitatively appropriate behavior, but more development is needed.
Spaan: Peter Wieringa did some modelling on oxygen transfer. His work shows that, because of shunting, there is much less heterogeneity for oxygen than you would expect if shunting was absent.
Bassingthwaighte: I do not presently visualize how arteriovenous shunting can reduce heterogeneity in local oxygen tension. Capillary-to-capillary diffusion could assist, very locally, in this regard, but it would appear from the photographs

of NADH fluorescence by C.H. Barlow and B. Chance of ischemic areas in perfused rat hearts (Science 193, 909–910, 1976) that the heterogeneity is at a macroscopic level, namely at microvascular unit sizes approaching 1 mm^3, which means about 3000 capillaries per unit.

39. Transport between myocardial capillaries and cardiac lymphatics

U. DINNAR

Abstract

The significance of coronary venous pressure on coronary perfusion was clearly demonstrated in an earlier analysis [1] which showed that capillary flow is strongly affected by increased levels of both arterial and venous pressures generated by the contracting heart during systole. Another result of that analysis was the importance of cardiac lymphatics. Although it has a very low flow rate, which is a small fraction of the coronary perfusion, cardiac lymphatics may influence the delicate balance of metabolic demands, regional levels of blood flow, oxygen extraction and transvascular and lymphatic flows.

The present study extends the mathematical consideration to include variations in lymphatic resistance to flow, and its effect on coronary perfusion and transcapillary exchange. The model also predicts variations in enzyme concentration in the blood serum, interstitial space and the cardial lymph system, which are caused by pathophysiological conditions in the heart.

Introduction

Despite the extensive study of the heart, there is very little knowledge on the exact contribution of cardiac lymphatics to overall physiological behavior of the heart [1]. In fact, all the analytical descriptions of cardiac mechanics and coronary perfusion ignore cardiac lymphatics. Studies of the lymphatics of the heart were mainly aimed at its anatomical structures and the differences in the concentration of various substances between coronary blood serum and lymph. The reason for this negligence is probably the difficulties involved in the study and the lack of knowledge on all contributing parameters. Those who measured the influence of various pathophysiological conditions on cardiac lymph flow used different measuring techniques and different set-ups, hence reaching, in some instances, different and conflicting results. For example, Szabo [2] and Drinker [3] reported decreased lymphatic flow following acute myocardial ischemia, while Patek [4], Bradham [5] and Cellis [6] reported increased lymph flow.

It is generally accepted that there is a fall in the lymph pH 2 hours after myocardial ischemia [7–9], associated with an increase in lactate concentration. In addition, other substances show a very definite change in concentration between coronary blood serum and lymphatic fluid. Also, there is an increase in WBC and RBC count in cardiac lymph shortly after ischemia. It is known that ischemic events will alter cellular membrane integrity, leading to a higher permeability and an increased quantity of larger macromolecule and enzyme which pass into the lymphatic drainage system and back to the systemic circulation. In case of lymphatic obstruction it is expected that those macro-molecules will remain in the interstitial space leading to higher concentration in the myocardium, which will not be detected by regular measurements of blood constituents. It is also expected that a detailed study of the time course of various concentration will be valuable in the determination of inter-relationships and the definitions of pathophysiological conditions in the etiology of myocardial dysfunction.

There is a strong relation between coronary perfusion and cardiac lymph formation. It is well documented that coronary artery ligation will promote lymphatic concentration of creatine phosphokinase, dehydrogenase, glumatic-oxalocetic transaminase, lyosenzymes, lipid, protein and others [10–12]. This is highly significant in the overall performance and prognosis of the damaged heart. As reported by Szlavy et al. [13], the 'cardiac lymph collected 2–4 hours after coronary artery occlusion and subsequently injected into the coronary vessels of control dogs, caused ventricular fibrillation in 3 out of 5 animals within 90 minutes'. This clearly demonstrates the significance of the cardiac lymphatic system, especially the relation between cardiac lymphatic and other myocardial parameters such as intra-myocardial pressure which generates lymphatic ligation during systole and may be helpful in generating lymphatic pump effects during diastole. The relations between transcapillary exchange and the retaining of enzymes and other substances released during myocardial ischemia, and of course the relationship between cardiac lymph flow and coronary perfusion are discussed here. A short summary of the formation and flow of cardiac lymphatics is given in Table 1.

Mathematical model of coronary perfusion

The model used here for the coronary perfusion is essentially the same model described earlier [1], except for an additional parameter of lymphatic resistance to flow. It is known that the flow generation in the lymphatic system is not the same as in the other blood vessels due to the existence of the lymphatic pump and the lymphatic valves. However, the rate of lymphatic flow is less than 1% of the incoming coronary perfusion and the results obtained by a numerical simulation scheme are very similar to the results obtained in the previous paper by a closed form expressions. The model assumes that a single capillary embedded in the myocardium is exposed to four different pressures:

1. the coronary arterial pressure,
2. the coronary venous pressure,
3. the transmural hydrostatic pressure difference, and
4. the transmural colloiosmotic pressure, as determined by the concentration of the various substances and the oxygen tension.

The values of the pressures, shown at the top of Fig. 1, are based on the measurements of many investigators published in the literature. The exact values of the myocardial venous pressure are based on the published data of Armour and co-workers [21–24].

The coronary arterial and venous pressures, shown in Fig. 1, already reflect the effect of the intramyocardial systolic pressure. The capillaries were taken as rigid tubes with a very small diameter that does not change under the influence of the transmural pressure. The flow across the wall is determined by the well known Starling hypothesis.

$$V = k\ (P - P_t - \pi_1 + \pi_2), \tag{1}$$

where V is the velocity across the wall, k is the filtration coefficient, P is the intraluminal blood pressure, P_t is the intramyocardial tissue pressure, π_1, and π_2 are the effective osmotic pressures, inside and outside the capillary, respectively, and assuming the blood is an homogenous incompressible Newtonian fluid flowing in a laminar and axisymmetric flow with no body forces and with negligible inertia, the governing equations, in cylindrical coordinates, are given by *continuity,*

$$\frac{1}{r}\frac{\partial}{\partial r}(rv_j) + \frac{\partial u_j}{\partial z} = 0, \tag{2}$$

Table 1. Cardiac lymphatics: formation and flow.

Increases with	Decreases with
Catecholamines and cardiac and sympathetic nerve stimulation [3]	Ischemia, less than 20 minutes, with increase after reperfusion [14]
Left ventricular pressure [16]	
Ischemia, more than 1 hour [19] (effect of collateral flow?)	
Coronary sinus ligation [20]	
Hypoxia [15, 18]	
Hypertonic mannitol or saline infusion [17]	
Isoproterenol, verapamil (in conscious dogs) [14]	

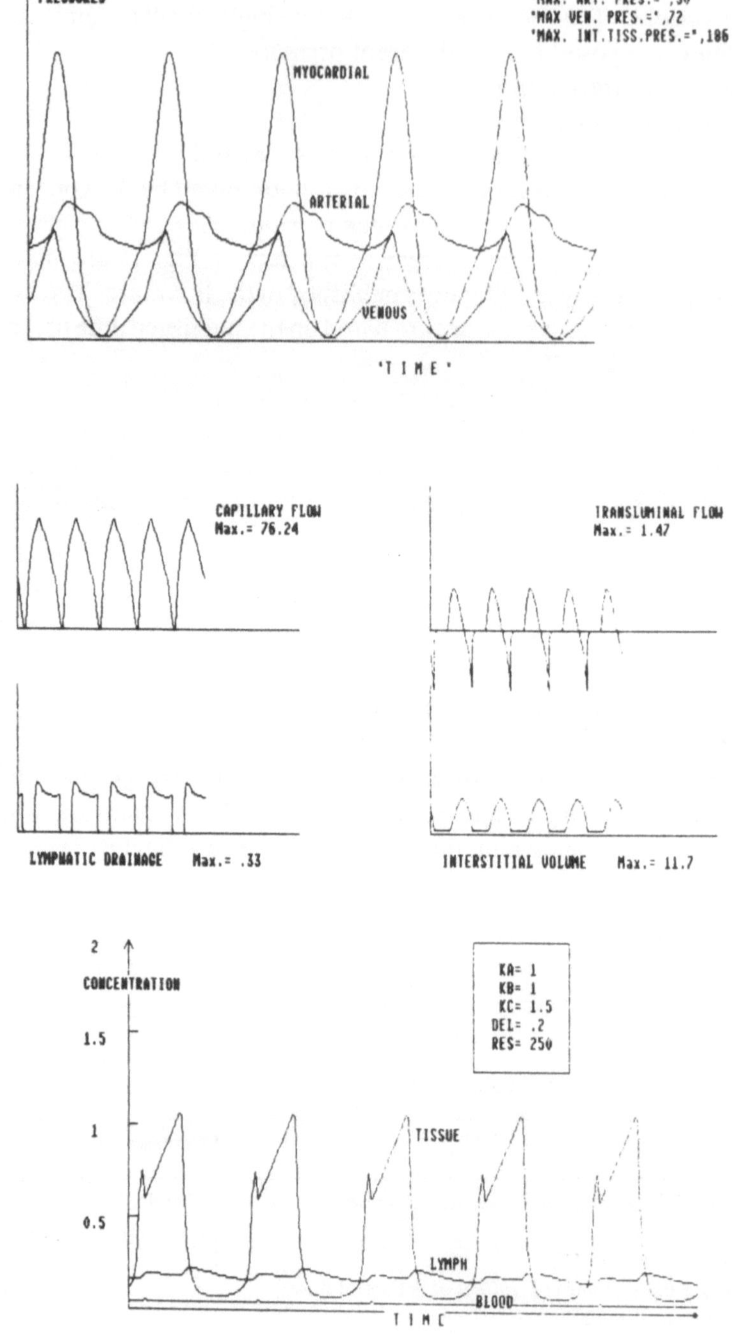

Figure 1. Pressures (upper portion), flows and intramyocardial fluid volumes (middle portion) and enzyme concentration (lower portion) in the myocardium in 'normal' physiology.

and *momentum*,

$$\frac{\partial P_j}{\partial r} = \eta\left(\frac{\partial^2 v_j}{\partial r^2} + \frac{1}{r}\frac{\partial v_j}{\partial r} - \frac{v_j}{r} + \frac{\partial^2 v_j}{\partial z^2}\right),$$

$$\frac{\partial P_j}{\partial z} = \eta\left(\frac{\partial^2 u_j}{\partial r^2} + \frac{1}{r}\frac{\partial u_j}{\partial r} + \frac{\partial^2 u_j}{\partial z^2}\right), \qquad (3)$$

subjected to the following boundary conditions:

$$\frac{\partial u_1}{\partial r} = 0 \text{ and } v_1 = 0 \text{ at } r = 0,$$

$$u_1 = 0 \text{ and } u_2 = 0 \text{ at } r = R,$$

$$v_1 = v_2 = k(P_1 - P_2 - \alpha) \text{ at } r = R,$$

$$P_1 = P_a \text{ and } u_2 = 0 \text{ at } z = 0,$$

$$P_1 = P_v \text{ and } u_2 = 0 \text{ at } z = L, \qquad (4)$$

where u is the longitudinal velocity, v is the radial velocity, α is the transmural colloid osmotic pressure difference, P_a is the incoming arterial pressure and P_v the venous pressure, and η is the viscosity. j = 2 denotes the intramyocardial external domain and j = 1 the intravascular domain. The pressures at z = 0 and z = L are averaged over the cross-section.

The flow can be solved using the assumptions of homogeneous incompressible Newtonian fluid, a laminar and axisymmetric flow with no body forces, and a negligible inertia. The flow equations (1–4) are solved simultaneously with the equations for the transcapillary exchange of fluid and for the lymphatic drainage. These parameters will determine the rate of change of interstitial fluid within the myocardium.

The solution yields the following expressions for the inlet and outlet flow rates from a single capillary, (q_{in}) and (q_{out}), respectively:

$$q_{in} = \frac{\pi R^4}{8\eta L}\,\frac{\delta}{\sinh\delta}\left(1 - \frac{\delta^2\varepsilon^2}{6}\right)[P_a \cosh\delta - P_v - P_t(\cosh\delta - 1)],$$

$$q_{out} = \frac{\pi R^4}{8\eta}\,\frac{\delta}{\sinh\delta}\left(1 - \frac{\delta^2\varepsilon^2}{6}\right)[P_a - P_v \cosh\delta + P_t(\cosh\delta - 1)]. \qquad (5)$$

The difference between the two flows gives the transmural flow rates:

$$q_{tm} = q_{in} - q_{out} = \frac{\pi R^4}{8\eta L}\,\frac{\delta}{\sinh\delta}\left(1 - \frac{\delta^2\varepsilon^2}{6}\right)(\cosh\delta - 1)\;(P_a + P_v - 2P_t). \qquad (6)$$

During systole, at certain instances, the driving intramyocardial pressure may generate sufficient forces to nearly dry the myocardium of interstitial fluid. It is assumed that a minimal value of the interstitial volume of fluid exists. Upon reaching this value the transluminal flow into the capillaries is stopped. Results of the numerical calculation for the 'normal' case are presented at the center of Figure 1, showing the changes with time of capillary and transluminal flows, the lymphatic drainage and the changes of the interstitial fluid volume.

The 'normal' conditions were determined by equating the values of peak flows and pressures to those published in the literature, with the lymphatic drainage taken as 0.5% of the incoming coronary flow. Integrations of the flow gives, for the normal case, that 1.12% of the incoming flow is passed through the capillary walls and into the interstitial space, while only 0.62% is returned through the wall. The rest must return to the circulatory system via the lymphatic system.

The model can now be used to study transcapillary exchange of various substances. From the previous results it is clear that under conditions of unequal permeabilities of substances across the capillary wall, into and out of the interstitial volume, the lymphatic system will have the responsibility of carrying excessive amount of the substances, in order to maintain steady state. Indeed, measurements reported in the literature demonstrate different values for substance concentration between blood serum and lymphatic fluid. Cardiac lymphatic concentrations of various substances, and the changes associated with pathophysiological conditions, are given in Tables 2 and 3. Table 4 summarizes the differences in enzyme concentration between blood serum and lymph. The changes of these values due to changes in cardiac capillaries permeability, lymph resistance to flow and other parameters may thus be highly significant in the diagnosis of myocardial ischemia, when based on enzyme evaluation. This point is incorporated into the model, and presented below.

Analysis of enzyme concentration

Myocardial infarction is considered as the result of insufficiant coronary perfusion and subsequent defficiency of oxygen. Hence, it is coupled with accumula-

Table 2. Sodium, potassium and chloride concentrations in cardiac lymphatics.

Sodium	142–162 meq/l	Decreases after more than one hour of ischemia Increases in congestive heart failure
Potassium	2.8–4.9 meq/l	Increases with: more than 1 hour of ischemia, coronary sinus ligation
Chloride	113–129 meq/l	Decreases with: congestive heart failure, coronary sinus ligation Increases with more than 1 hour of ischemia

tion of products of anaerobic metabolism. In addition to problems related to coronary blood flow one must consider the changes in interstitial composition of these products and especially those which play a larger role in pathophysiology. These changes result not only from anaerobic metabolism and myocardial cell injury, but from changes of the capillary permeability as well. Hence, it is of utmost importance to study the nature of transcapillary exchange on one hand (input into the interstitial subsystem) and the lymphatic drainage (its output) on the other. For example, interstitial edema tends to aggravate ischemia, by mechanically affecting the capillary flow, while a decrease in interstitial fluid PH tends to increase intercapillary sludging and thrombosis. In addition, the buildup of potassium ions and lysosomal enzymes tend to enhance the vulenerability of ischemic nyocardium to fibrilation and tissue destruction.

Measurements of blood enzymes concentration do not yield immediate infor-

Table 3. Protein, wbc and rbc in the cardiac lymph

PROTEIN:	[g/100 ml]	normal	3.6–4.9
		albumin	2.2
		globulin	1.6
		long term ischemia	slight increase
		congestive heart failure	slight decrease
WBC*	[1/mm³]	normal	800–5400
		1 hour ischemia	elevated
		CHF	decreased
RBC	[1/mm³]	normal	16000–205000
		2 hour ischemia	elevated
		CHF	elevated
PLATELETS	[1/mm³]	normal	10000–20000

* about 80% are lymphocytes

Table 4. Various enzyme concentrations.

	Normal heart serum	Normal heart lymph
GOT	7.2	31.0
GPT	6.9	5.3
LDH	42	130
MDH	80	180
ICDH	6.9	3.8

GOT = aspartate aminotransferase (glutamic oxalacetic transaminase); GPT = alanine aminotransferase (glutamic pyruvic transaminase); LDH = lactate dehydrogenase; GLDH = glutamic dehydrogenase; MDH = malate dehydrogenase; ICDH = isocitrate dehydrogenase; CPK = creatine phosphokinase.

mation. Szabo et al. (2) showed that induction of experimental myocardial infarction resulted in elevation of enzyme concentration (LDH, MDH, GOT and CPK) in the cardiac lymph during the first hour after ligation of the coronary branch, while the corresponding rise in serum activity occured only 2 to 6 hours later.

To study the pattern of various enzyme concentration the compartamental system shown in Fig. 2 was used. Figure 3 describes the parameters as related to the various compartments described in Fig. 2. The coronary arterial flow Q(t) is reaching the capillary bed with the same enzyme concentration as that of the systemic blood pool $C_B(t)$. Because of the transluminal pressure drive and the capillary wall permeability, 'DEL', fluid will flow either into or out of the interstitial space. Enzyme permeability is assume to have different values for flow in these different directions; d_1 denotes wall permeability from the capillary bed into the interstitial space, and d_2 represents the reversed direction. The larger quantity of the incoming flow is passed via the coronary venous system, S(t), with a concentration of $C_t(t)$, into the systemic blood pool. The amount of transcapillary flow, together with the lymphatic flow, L(t), will change the volume of the interstitial fluid $V_L(t)$ and the concentrations of the various substances. In addition there is a uniform production, 'PR', of enzyme in the interstitial volume. The assumption of uniform production can be changed by any other assumption, but is preferred here due to lack of knowledge on rates of enzyme release. The lymphatic volume V_l is taken as constant, thus resulting in time dependent enzyme concentration $C_L(t)$. The amount of lymphatic drain into the systemic blood pool, is determined by the lymph resistance to flow 'RES'. Process of enzyme reabsorption, denoted by 'RE', assumed proportional to the compartment volume, is assumed in all the compartments.

Applying the law of conservation to the different compartments gives the following results:
Lymphatics:

$$d(V_L C_L)/dt = V_L C_t - V_L C_L - RE(1). \tag{7}$$

Interstitial space:

$$d(V_t C_t)/dt = d_1 V_c - d_2 V_c - V_L C_l - RE(tissue) + PR, \tag{8}$$

where $d_2 = O$ for $V_c > O$, and $d_1 = O$ for $V_c < O$.

Capillary:

$$V_a C_B + d_2 V_c - d_1 V_c = V_u C_u. \tag{9}$$

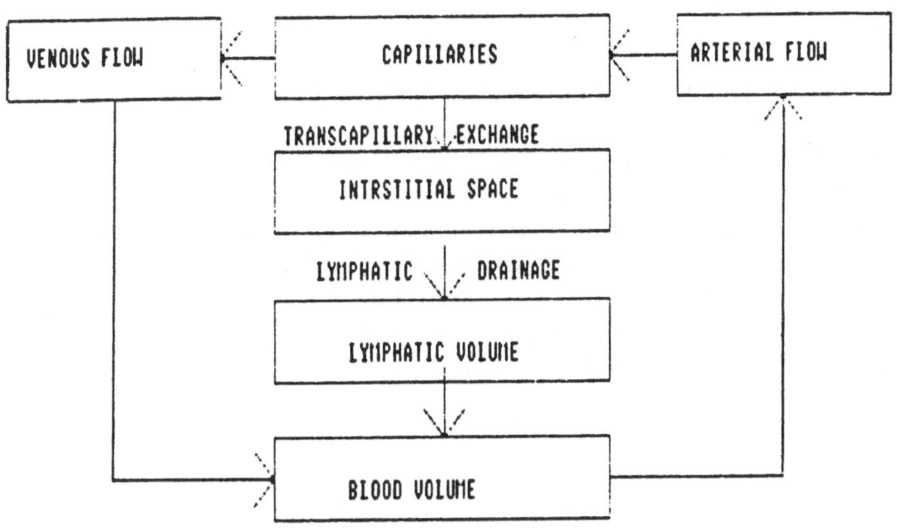

Figure 2. Compartmental model of the myocardial circulation.

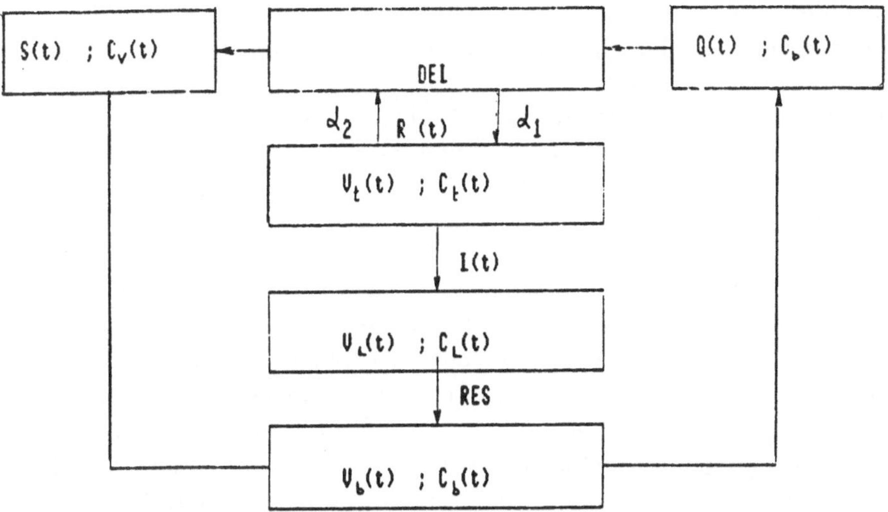

Figure 3. Defenitions of compartmental parameters.

Blood:

$$d(V_B C_B)/dt = V_L\ C_L + V_u\ C_u - V_a\ C_B - RE(B), \tag{10}$$

where $V_C = R(t)$; $V_a = Q(t)$;. $V_u = S(t)$; $V_t = Vol(t)$ and $V_L = L\ (t)$.

Mathematical simulation using this set of equations, up to a steady state, gives the pattern of change in enzyme concentration in the various compartments as a function of time. The results for the 'normal' case with a specific values of PR and RE, are described in the next section. The values of PR and RE were determined from the conditions of a steady-state value for the normal ratio of concentration between blood serum and cardiac lymphatics.

Results

Coronary arterial perfusion pressure

Figure 4 describes the pressures, flows and enzyme concentration for a 50% increase in coronary arterial perfusion pressure. Figure 5 shows the same descriptions for a 50% decrease in arterial pressure. In both cases the other pressures remain the same.

The results show that an increased coronary perfusion increases capillary flow significantly with a continuous flow throughout the cardiac cycle. However, the larger quantities of capillary flow would not be handled by the lymphatic drainage system and a steady state solution required a 25% decrease in capillary permeability, which caused a decrease in the transluminal fluid exchange and in the maximal interstitial fluid volume. The increased lymphatic drain caused a significant decrease in tissue concentration of enzyme. (However, in reality, there is no anaerobic activity under this conditions.) Decreased coronary perfusion pressure, on the other hand, caused a significant decrease in transcapillary and lymphatic flow, and a much smaller value of maximal interstitial volume of fluid. This will lead to insufficient supply of oxygen and myocardial ischemia. Under this conditions the values of enzyme concentration, in both lymph and intramyocardial tissue, reach almost twice their normal level. The values taken for this demonstration may be extreme, but it is used to stress the interrelation between the various parameters. The results of continuous changes in coronary perfusion pressure are described in Figure 6. The discontinuities in the line are due to a need to change the value of the capillary permeability to maintain steady state. The results show a very sharp increase in enzyme concentration, both in the lymphatic system and the intramyocardial tissue. However, these changes will not be significant when measured in the systemic blood.

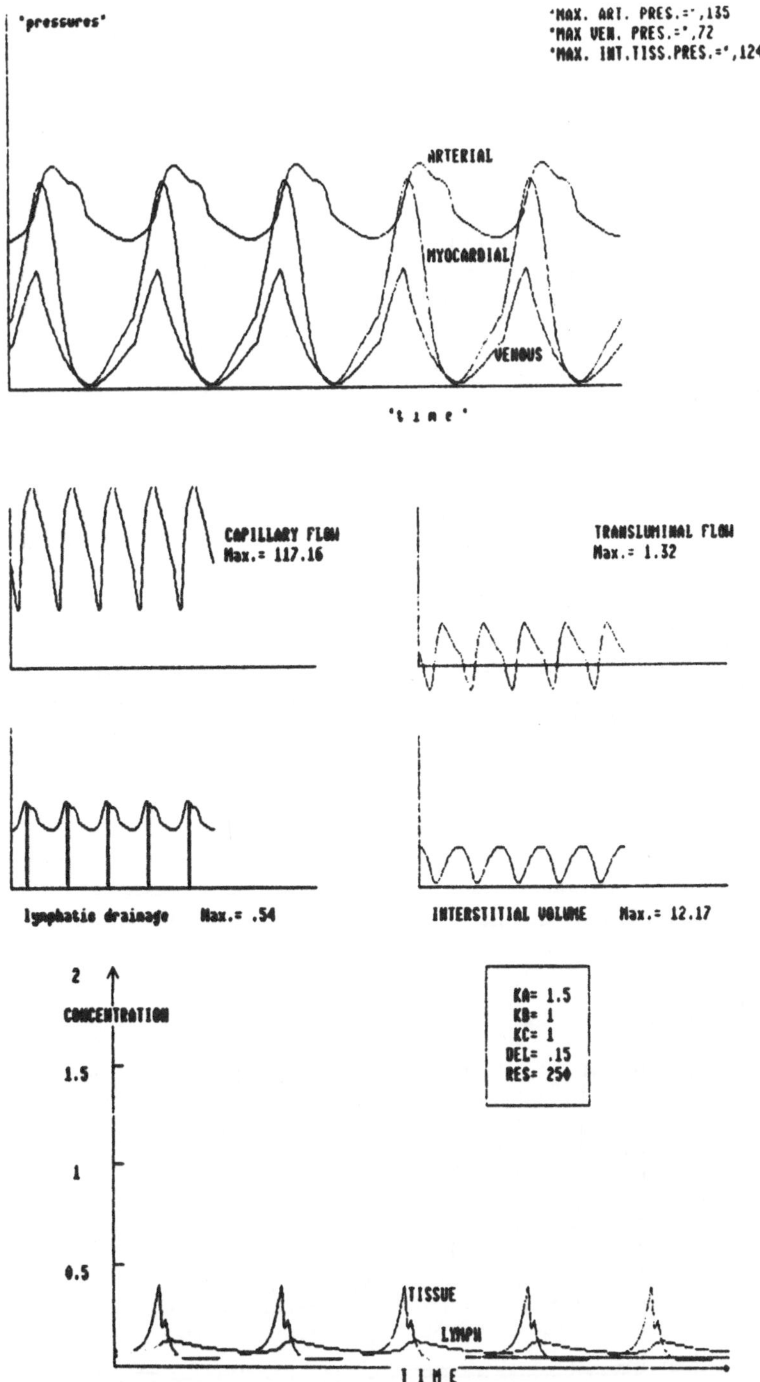

Figure 4. Pressures (upper portion), flows and intramyocardial fluid volumes (middle portion) and enzyme concentration (lower portion) in the myocardium for 50% increase in arterial coronary perfusion pressure.

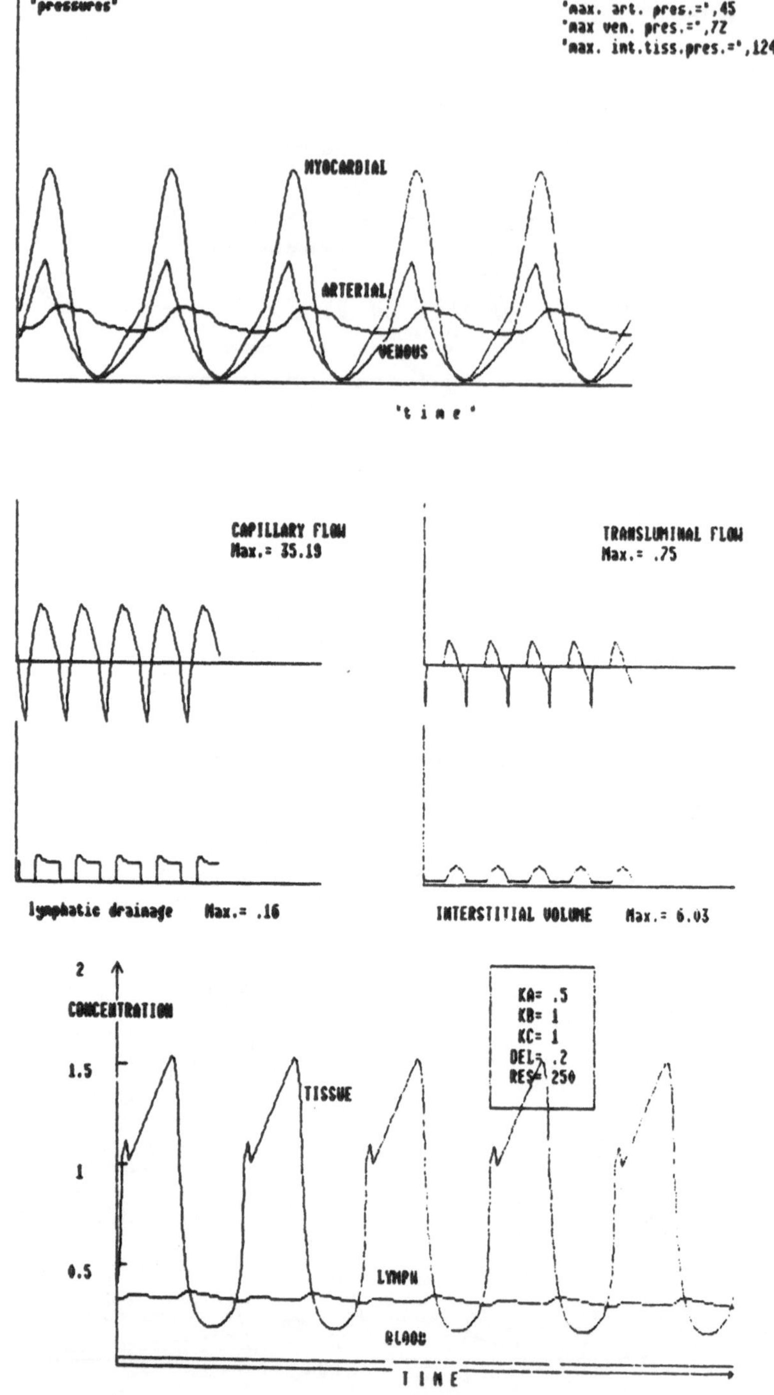

Figure 5. Pressures (upper portion), flows and intramyocardial fluid volumes (middle portion) and enzyme concentration (lower portion) in the myocardium for 50% decrease in arterial coronary perfusion pressure.

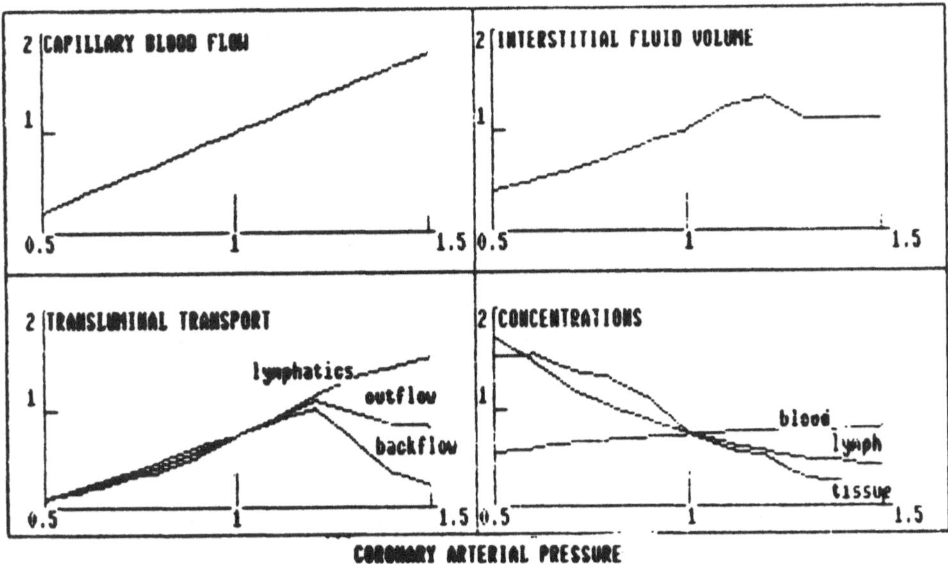

Figure 6. Variations of myocardial parameters as a function of arterial coronary perfusion pressure.

Intramyocardial pressure peak

Similar patterns are obtained for a change in intramyocardial pressure peak, shown in Figures 7 and 8. It is obvious from the results that the system can stand with very small changes any increase in intramyocardial pressure which will result from stronger contractions of the myocardium. However, any weakening of myocardial contractions which leads to smaller values of intramyocardial pressures will change significantly the values of transluminal exchange of fluid and the volume of interstitial fluid in the myocardium. This reduction in the amount of fluid transfered through the capillary wall may alter the metabolic energy supply to the myocardial tissues, which may lead to a further decrease in the strength of contraction and intramyocardial pressure. As can be seen from Figure 9, a decrease of 25% in intramyocardial pressure leads to a 50% reduction in transcapillary flow and consequentially to 67% reduction in interstitial fluid volume. The reason for this drastic change is the need to change capillary permeability. Again the changes in enzyme concentration will not be detected if measured in the lymphatic drainage vessels of the heart. These results point to the important role of the contracting myocardium in the control of transcapillary exchange.

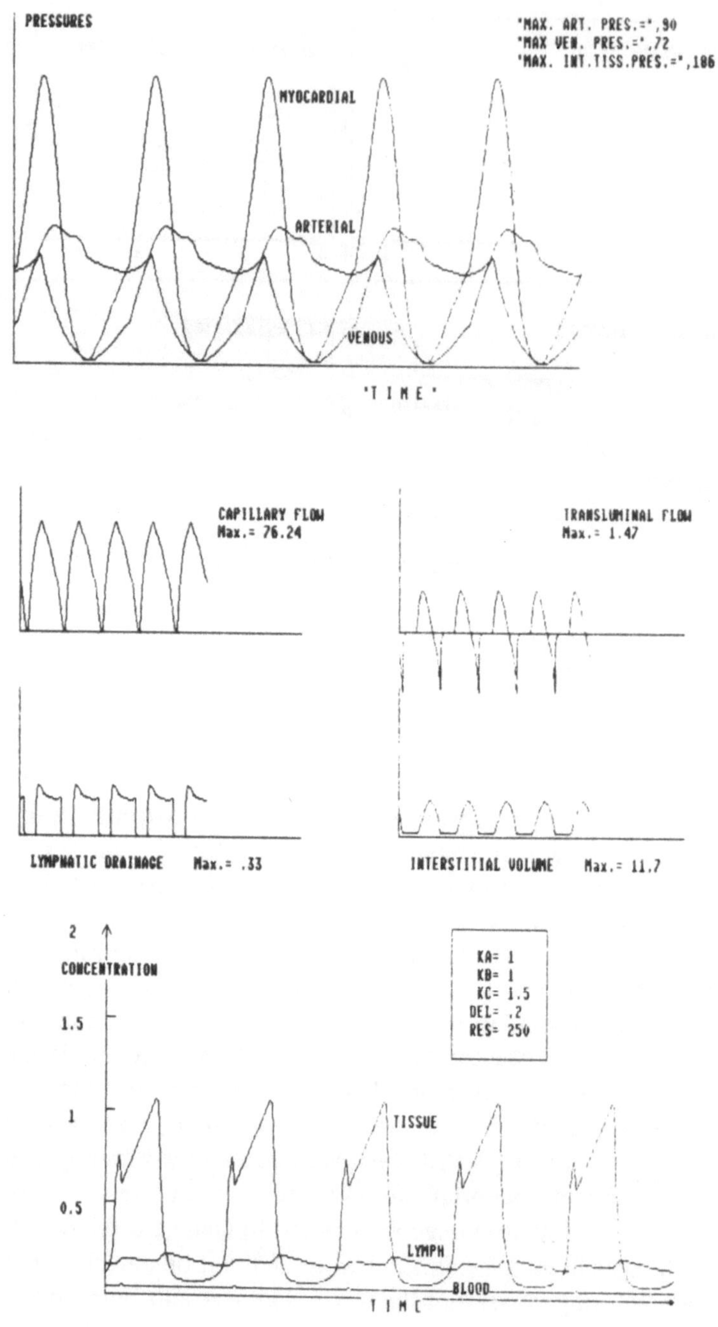

Figure 7. Pressures (upper portion), flows and intramyocardial fluid volumes (middle portion) and enzyme concentration (lower portion) in the myocardium for 50% increase in the intramyocardial pressure.

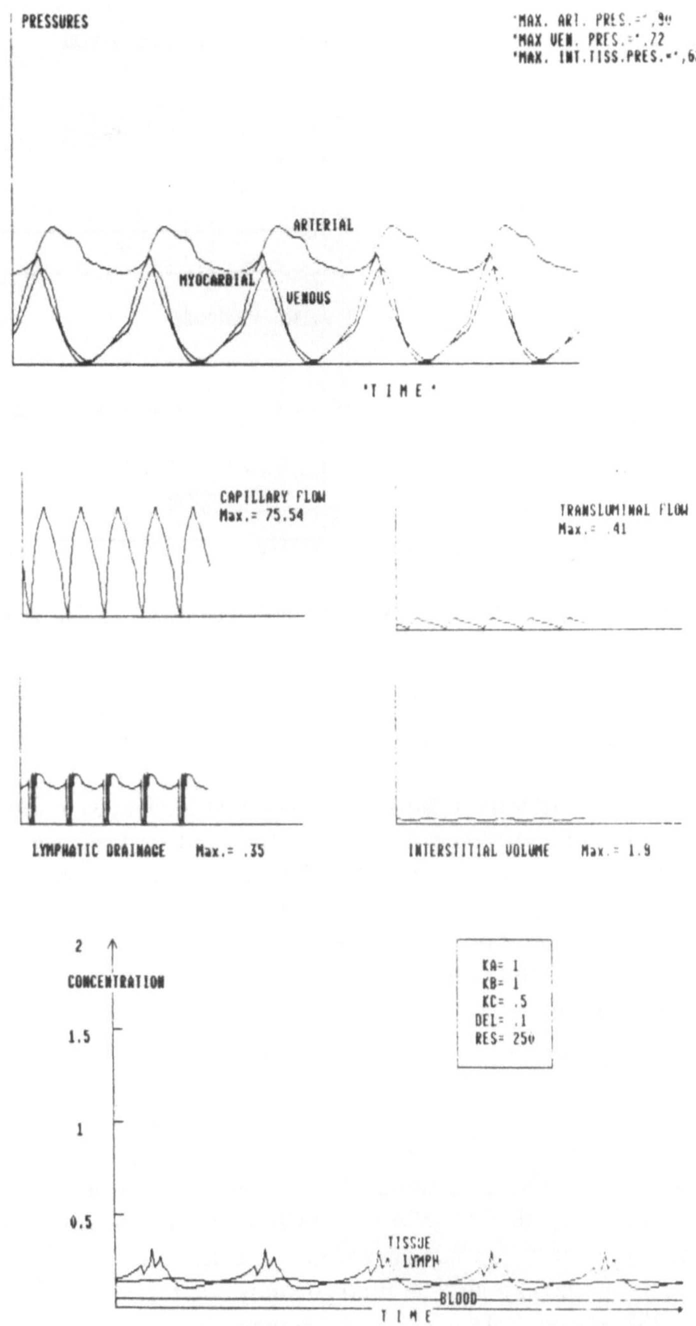

Figure 8. Pressures (upper portion), flows and intramyocardial fluid volumes (middle portion) and enzyme concentration (lower portion) in the myocardium for 50% decrease in intramyocardial pressure.

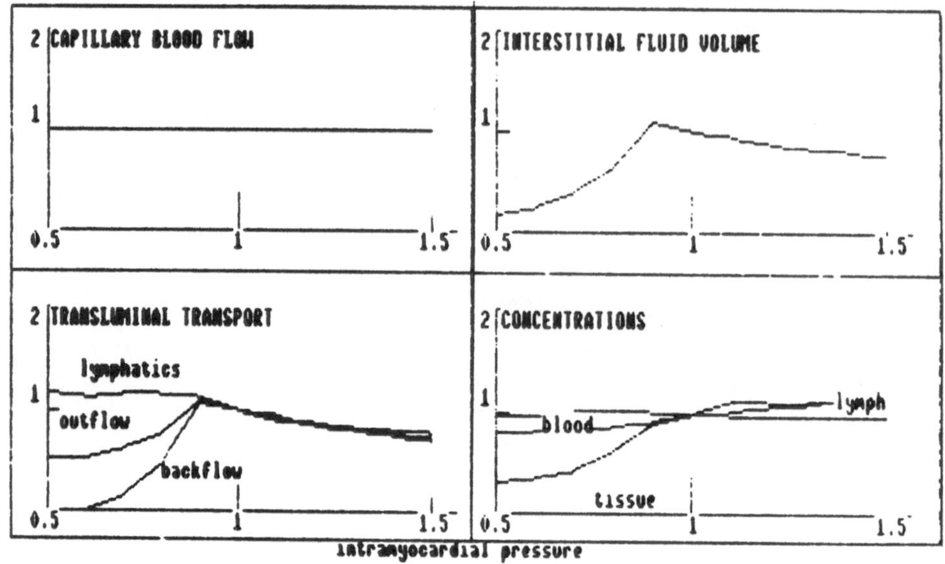

Figure 9. Variations of myocardial parameters as a function of intramyocardial pressure.

Additional changes

Figures 10 and 11 describe the changes associated with changes in the lymphatic resistance to flow and with the permeability of the capillary wall. Again, as in the previous case, these changes will not affect the coronary perfusion but will significantly alter the transluminal exchange values and the value of interstitial fluid volume. It is important to note that the model predicts that changes in transcapillary permeability will be visible in measurements of systemic blood enzyme concentrations.

Discussion

The model described here is capable of predicting the overall behavior of the coronary perfusion and the intramyocardial variables, such as volume of interstitial fluid, lymphatic and transcapillary flows, and the concentration of various substances. The model can also be used to study the transfer of various blood substances to the myocardial tissue and, from there, into the lymphatic system. It should be noted that there is a lack of knowledge on the physiological range of these values and, more important, on the range of variation of these parameters under normal and pathophysiological conditions. Yet, the model shed light on the relationship between change in one of the parameters and all the others. A study

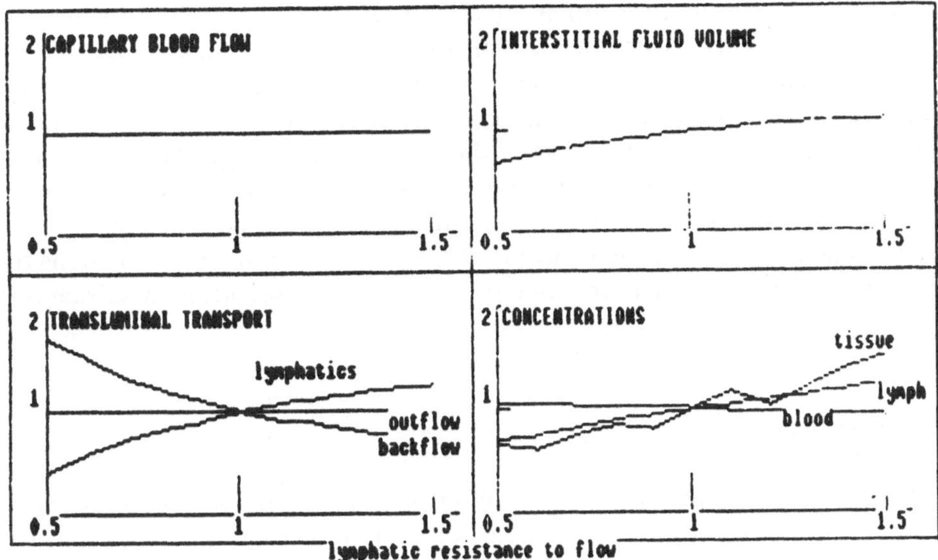

Figure 10. Variations of myocardial parameters as a function of lymphatic resistance to flow.

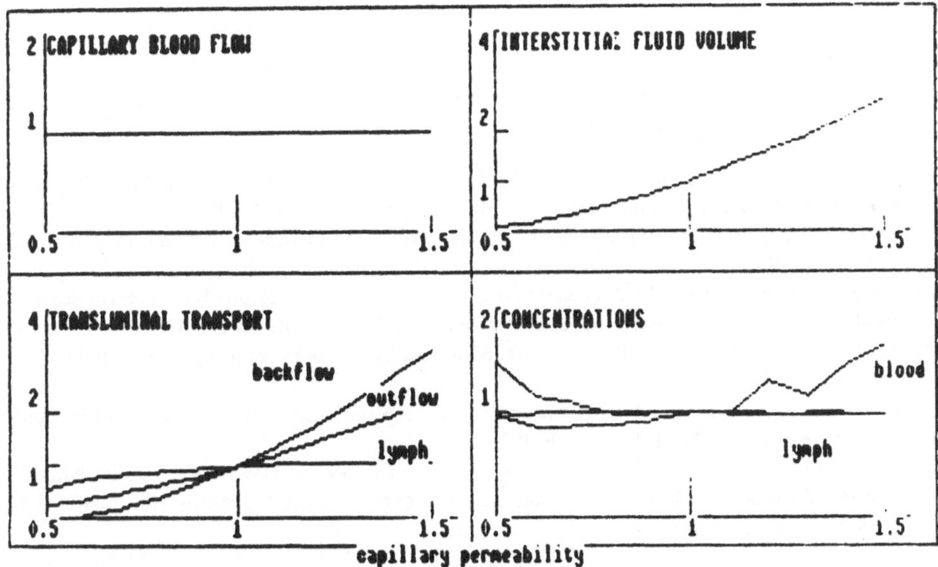

Figure 11. Variations of myocardial parameters as a function of capillary permeability.

currently under way at the Julius Silver Institute at the Technion is aimed at measuring the range of these parameters for a detailed evaluation of the model.

Another important feature of the model is in the study of physiological and mechanical variations between the subendocardial and subepicardial layers, where the intramyocardial pressure is different and the anatomical picture, like capillary count and consequently the interstitial volume surrounding each capillary, are different. It also shows the importance of studying the lymphatic system to the understanding of the behavior of the heart and a better evaluations of clinical parameters which are determined by the measurements of substances present in the blood.

Acknowledgment

The author thanks the support of the Women's Division of the American Technion Society (MEP) to the heart research center at Technion.

References

1. Dinnar U (1987): Interaction between intramyocardial pressure and transcapillary exchange – a possible control of coronary circulation. In: Sideman S, Beyar R (eds). CRC Press.
2. Szabo G, Magyar Z, Reffy A (1974): Lymphatic transport of enzymes after experimental myocardial infarction. Lymphography 7: 37–44.
3. Drinker CK, Warren MF, Maurer FW, et al (1940): The flow pressure and composition of cardiac lymph. Am J Physiol 130: 43–45.
4. Patek PR (1939): The morphology of the lymphatics of the mammalian heart. Am J Anatomy 64: 203–249.
5. Bradham PR, Parker EF, Barrington BA (1970): The cardiac lymphatics. Ann Surg 171: 899–902.
6. Cellis A, Cicero R, Del Castilo H (1969): Cardiac lymphography in human subjects. Acta Radiol Diag 8: 177–182.
7. Uhley HN, Leeds SE, Elevitch FR (1976): Canine cardiac lymph potassium, pH and flow after experimental myocardial infarction. Proc Soc Exp Biol Med 151: 146–148.
8. Feola M, Glick G (1975): Cardiac lymph flow impairment and myocardial ischemia in dogs. Am J Physiol 229: 44–48.
9. Araki H, Takenaka F (1975): An increase in cathepsin D activity in cardiac lymph and pericardial fluid induced by experimental myocardial ischemia in the dog. Life Sci 17: 613.
10. Feola M, Lefer AM (1977): Alterations in cardiac lymph dynamics in acute myocardial ischemia. J Surg Res 23: 299–305.
11. Garlick DG, Rankin EM (1970): Transport of large molecules from plasmas to interstitial fluids and lymph in Dogs. Am J Physiol 219: 1595–1605.
12. Osbakken MD, Kopiwoda SY, Swan A, Castronovo EP, Strauss HW (1982): Cardiac lymphoscintigraphy following closed chestcatheter injection of radiolabelled colloid into the myocardium of dogs: Concise communication. J Nuclear Med 23: 883–889.
13. Szlavy L, Adams DF, Hollenberg NK, Abrams HL (1980): Cardiac lymph and lymphatics in normal and infarcted myocardium. Am Heart J 100: 323–331.
14. Michael L, Lewis R, Brandon T, Entman M (1979): Cardiac lymph flow in conscious dogs. Am J Physiol 327: H311–H317.

15. Miller AJ, Ellis E, Katz L (1964): Cardiac lymph flow rates and composition in dogs. Am J Physiol 206: 63–66.
16. Taira A, Matsuyama M, Morishita Y, Terashi I, Kawashima Y, Maruko M, Arikawa K, Murata K, Akita H (1976): Cardiac lymph and contractility of the heart. Jpn Circ J 40: 665–670.
17. Dobbs W (1974): The flow of lymph to the cardiac node following saline infusion in the dog. Microvasc Res 8: 14–19.
18. Maurer FW (1940): The effects of decreased blood oxygen and increased blood carbon dioxide on the flow and composition of cervical and cardiac lymph. Am J Physiol 131: 331–348.
19. Ali M, Ellis A, Glick G (1977): Effects of methylprednisolone on cardiac lymph in acute myocardial ischemia in dogs. Am J Physiol 232: H602–H607.
20. Leeds SE, Uhley HN, Sampson JJ, et al (1970): The cardiac lymphatics after ligation of the coronary sinus. Proc Soc Exp Biol Med 135: 59–62.
21. Armour J, Klassen G (1981): Epicardial coronary venous pressure. Can J Physiol Pharmacol 59: 1250–1259.
22. Klassen G, Armour J (1982): Epicardial coronary venous pressure: autonomic responses. Can J Physiol Pharmacol 60: 696–707.
23. Klassen G, Armour J (1983): Canine coronary venous pressure response to positive inotropism and vasodilation. Can J Physiol Pharmacol 61: 213–221.
24. Armour J, Klassen G (1984): Pressure and flow in epicardial venus of the dog heart: responses to positive inotropism. Can J Physiol Pharmacol 62: 38–48.

Discussion

Hoffman: Although the interstitial lymphatic flow is very small, I agree with you that the heart tolerates increases in the interstitial fluid very badly and that a very small increase in the total percentage of water has a marked effect on flow in the heart. So I think it really has an importance quite beyond its magnitude.
Dinnar: Maybe I ought to point out that results of Sabo et al. show the significance of the high concentration of lymphatic substances. They took lymphatic fluid and injected it back into the coronary circulation of dogs. In four out of five dogs injected with the lymphatic fluid they caused ventricular fibrillations within a few minutes. Thus, lymphatic fluid is very important, especially in cases where we have pathophysiological problems such as an obstruction of the lymphatic system. In some cases where surgeons do not pay any attention to the lymphatic fluid, and let the lymphatic system drain into the chest, the result can be very traumatic.
Beyar: One point which is difficult to understand is the high venous pressures of 70–80 mm Hg in your model based on Armour and Klassen (Can. J. Physiol. Pharmacol. 59: 1250–1259, 1981) reported venous pressures. If you assume such pressures to exist at the venous side of the microcirculation, it follows that there is a very high pressure gradient between the veins and the coronary sinus. Where does such a pressure gradient occur and by what mechanism?
Dinnar: I assume here that during the peak of the intramyocardial pressure, the effect of this pressure in the coronary arterial pressure must definitely be imposed on the venous side. The extent, whether it is 50, 70 or 80 mm Hg, is only an hypothesis. We do not have exact data because measurements are very scarce. Logically, it must be a high value because it is vulnerable to the increased intramyocardial pressure, and we know that the myocardial pressure is very high.
Hoffman: The pressures that Klassen and his group have recorded in the veins are real. For a long time many of us thought that they were artifacts, but they are not. But their interpretation is different. Basically, what you are seeing is an impulse response. You are getting a huge amount of blood suddenly pushed out of the myocardium in systole and you are getting a change from kinetic to potential energy which then builds up in the veins, which are not built to take this huge flow without a rise in pressure. That does not mean what the pressure is in the myocardium, and there is, in fact, a substantial gradient between the venous pressures in the small veins and the coronary sinus. That probably is exactly the same effect. I think you have to interpret it very carefully. The pressure is real but the interpretation is different.
Spaan: It is important that you consider the mass transfer over the capillary and include the lymphatics. It is an important step. I would like to come back to the venous pressure measurement. As a standard procedure in our experiments we measure the pressure in an epicardial vein, not in a coronary sinus, but in a small vein. What we see is that the pressures in that vein are steady, at around 2, 3, or

4 mm Hg. As soon as you have a little occlusion of venous flow, then you are going to see those large amplitudes. And with complete sinus occlusions you can indeed have those high pressures build up. But in normal situations and at low venous pressures you do not see them. It is just a ripple in the pressure.
Dinnar: There is question about the exact value, its relation to intramyocardial pressure and the variations between subepicardial and epicardial vessels. I agree that the values in the epicardial vessels are much smaller than the values I used here for subendocardial layers. But if you can make the appropriate measurement, you may be able to detect backward flow which is squeezed into the capillary, or squeezed from the capillary back into the interstitial space. We still do not have the way to measure it.

40. Disturbances in myocardial lipid homeostasis during ischemia and reperfusion

G.J. VAN DER VUSSE, F.W. PRINZEN and R.S. RENEMAN

Abstract

Fatty acids are essential for myocardial functioning. They play a pivotal role as oxidizable substrates for cellular energy production. In addition, maintenance of the integrity of membrane phosphoglycerides, consisting in part of polyunsaturated fatty acids, is crucial for adequate cellular performance. Evidence is accumulating that the normal level of nonesterified fatty acids (NEFA) in normoxic cardiac tissue is extremely low, i.e. in the order of 20–50 nmol · g^{-1} wet weight. During ischemia, lasting for longer than 10 minutes, NEFA accumulated in the flow-deprived tissue. Accumulation was most outspoken in the subendocardial layers, if residual flow was below 0.3 ml · min^{-1} · g^{-1} wet weight and ATP levels dropped below 5–7 μmol · g^{-1} dry weight. Arachidonic acid showed the highest relative increase. A concomitant increase of lysophosphoglycerides has been measured. Arachidonic acid and lysophosphoglyceride levels decreased during the first 5 minutes of reperfusion following 60 minutes of ischemia, and tended to increase thereafter. The present findings clearly indicate that fatty acid homeostasis in myocardial tissue is disturbed during ischemia and reperfusion. Possible mechanisms underlying these derangements are discussed.

Introduction

As in most other organs, fatty acid homeostasis in the heart is a complex system, characterized by a variety of fatty acid pools, lipid-converting enzymes and transport routes for fatty acids and their derivatives. In general, free fatty acids or nonesterified fatty acids (NEFA) are delivered to the heart cells complexed with albumin in the blood. Through not completely elucidated mechanisms, NEFA are transported across the luminal and abluminal membranes of the endothelial cells via the interstitial space, across the sarcolemma into the sarcoplasma of the heart musle cells. The majority of the NEFA molecules will be oxidized in the mitochondria to deliver energy for electro-mechanical activity. Part of the NEFA will be incorporated into esterified fatty acid pools such as triacylglycerol, phosphoglycerides and cholesteryl esters.

Under flow restricted conditions resulting in oxygen deprivation of myocardial cells, fatty acid homeostasis will be disturbed [1, 2, 3]. Lack of oxygen will reduce or abolish mitochondrial β-oxidation. In turn, accumulation of fatty acid derivatives such as acylCoA and acylcarnitine will occur [1]. In addition, impaired turnover of phosphoglycerides will be most likely the cause of the well-established accumulation of arachidonic and other polyunsaturated fatty acids in ischemic myocardial tissue [2, 3].

In contrast to glucose metabolism in the heart, reports on modeling of cardiac fatty acid metabolism are scarce. This is probably due to the complexity of the metabolic patterns of fatty acid homeostasis. Conflicting results on, for instance, the content and turnover of the various fatty acid pools under normoxic and ischemic circumstances have to be considered as well [4, 5].

In the present study we have investigated the content of the various lipid pools in normoxic cardiac tissue and their relative fatty acid composition. Knowledge about the exact content of lipids in the heart is required for a proper understanding of *in vitro* findings indicating regulatory and even deleterious effects of lipids on myocardial functioning [5].

In addition, the time course of changes in the NEFA content in ischemic and reperfused myocardial tissue has been investigated. Special attention was paid to a possible relationship between the extent of underperfusion and the reduction of tissue ATP levels on the one hand, and myocardial NEFA content, with special reference to arachidonic acid, on the other. Since changes in tissue phosphoglyceride content can be expected when arachidonic acid accumulates, the effect of ischemia and reperfusion on the most relevant myocardial phosphoglyceride moieties has been investigated as well.

Methods and procedures

The experiments were performed on open-chest mongrel dogs, premedicated intramuscularly with 10 mg fluanisone and 200 μg fentanylcitrate per kg body weight. Anesthesia was induced intravenously with sodium pentobarbital (10 mg/kg body weight) and, after endotracheal intubation, was maintained with nitrous oxide in oxygen (60/40, vol/vol) in combination with a continuous infusion of sodium pentobarbital (2 mg/kg per hr). The lungs of the animals were artificially ventilated with a positive pressure respirator (Pulmonat). Body temperature was kept constant at 37.5° C. After incision of the chest, the pericardium was opened over the anterolateral aspect of the heart. In the dogs submitted to ischemia alone (without reperfusion of the affected area) regional myocardial ischemia was induced by stenosis of the left anterior interventricular coronary artery using an inflatable silastic cuff. The mean coronary artery pressure distal to the stenosis was about 3.0 kPa and was kept constant with an autoregulating feedback system [2]. In the dogs submitted to ischemia followed by reperfusion, the left anterior interventricular coronary artery was completely occluded with the use of a small titanium clamp for 60 min. Reperfusion of the affected area was allowed for another 60 min by removing the clamp. A subgroup of 10 dogs served as controls. Flow in their coronary arteries remained unimpeded throughout the experimental period.

Insertion of catheters for hemodynamic measurements and for collection of blood have been described in detail before [2]. Regional myocardial blood flow was measured with radioactively labeled microspheres [2, 6]. Transmural biopsies for lipid analysis, and for determination of ATP, were taken from the ischemic and normoxic area at time intervals indicated in the Results section below. The experiment was terminated after taking the biopsies at given time intervals after induction of ischemia. Blood was collected from the femoral artery and the local cardiac vein, draining the area perfused by the left anterior interventricular coronary artery, to measure AV differences of arachidonic acid and lysophosphoglycerides during the pre-ischemic, ischemic and reperfusion phase.

Tissue ATP was measured in freeze-dried tissue specimen with a fluorometric method as previously described [7]. Extraction and determination of myocardial lipids have been described in detail before [2, 8]. Routinely, after storage of the biopsies at −80° C, aliquots of deeply frozen tissue (150–300 mg) were pulverized in an aluminum mortar with a stainless steel pestle, previously cooled in liquid nitrogen. The tissue powder was transferred to test tubes cooled with liquid nitrogen. The test tubes were placed at −21° C and the tissue powder was wetted with 2 ml of methanol at −21° C. The content of the test tubes was allowed to warm to room temperature and was subsequently weighed. Chloroform was added until a mixture of chloroform and methanol of 2 : 1 (vol/vol) was obtained. The anti-oxidant butylated hydroxytoluene (0.01%) was present in the methanol and chloroform. Subsequently, a mixture of heptadecanoic acid, cholesteryl heptadecanoate, and triheptadecanoine was added to the extraction mixture to correct for losses during the assay procedure. NEFA, triacylglycerol, cholesteryl esters, and total phospholipids were isolated from the extracts by thin-layer chromatography using TLC plates coated with Silica gel F254 (Merck, FRG). The plates were predeveloped with chloroform: methanol: H_2O: acetic acid (10 : 10 : 1 : 1 vol/vol) until the liquid front had reached a level 1 cm above the site of application of the lipid spots. Hexane:diethyl ether:acetic acid (24 : 5 : 0.3 vol/vol) was used as devoloping solvent. The lipid spots were made visible with Rhodamine G, scraped from the plate and transferred into test tubes, containing 0.5 ml BF_3-methanol solution (7% BF_3). The fatty acid moieties of the various lipid classes were methylated at 20° C for 15 minutes (NEFA), at 100° C for 30 minutes (triacylglycerol), and at 100° C for 45 minutes (cholesteryl esters and phospholipids). The methyl esters were extracted from the methylating mixture with pentane. After evaporation of the pentane, under a stream of N_2 at 37° C, the methyl esters originating from NEFA, triacylglycerol, and phospholipids were dissolved in trimethyl pentane, containing appropriate amounts of methyl pentadecanoate as an internal standard. The methyl esters of the cholesteryl esters were rechromatographed on silica gel plates to remove the anti-oxidant butylated hydroxytoluene. In case the phosphoglyceride subgroups were measured, the original chloroform/methanol tissue and blood extracts were chromatographed with the use of a silica gel column [8]. The neutral lipid containing fraction was subsequently separated into NEFA, triacylglycerol and cholesteryl ester fractions using the TLC system described above. The phosphoglyceride containing fraction was chromatographed applying a two-dimensional TLC technique [8]. Further details of the quantitative estimation of phosphoglyceride subgroups in cardiac tissue have been published before [8].

Results

The values of the content of NEFA, triacylglycerol, cholesteryl esters and total phosphoglycerides in normoxic dog myocardium are summarized in Table 1. No significant differences in the content of these lipids could be detected between subepicardial, mesocardial and subendocardial layers, with the exception of triacylglycerol (data not shown). The content of the latter lipid group was about 2 times higher in the subepicardial layer than in the more inner layer of the left ventricle. Since, in most animals, fat could be observed macroscopically in the

Table 1. Lipid content and relative fatty acid composition of normoxic dog myocardium. The values measured in the meso layer of the free wall of the left ventricle are shown (mean ± SD, n = 6–10) and expressed as nmoles fatty acid equivalents g^{-1} wet weight.

Lipid group	NEFA	Triacyl-glycerol	Cholesteryl esters	Phospho-glycerides
Amount (nmol/g wet weight)	28 ± 14	5,530 ± 4,384	203 ± 175	43,068 ± 2,048
Relative fatty acid composition (%)[a]				
14:0	0.4	2.2	1.0	0.5
16:0	29.8	21.5	9.8	8.6
16:1	10.6	5.0	3.4	1.6
18:0	28.2	9.6	3.2	16.4
18:1	14.2	41.2	21.2	18.0
18:2	8.8	16.6	41.3	25.2
20:4	5.0	0.7	14.4	28.3

[a] The various fatty acids are indicated by their chemical notation.

vicinity of the superficial epicardial coronary arteries, it is likely that the gradient of triacylglycerol is caused by fat cells at the epicardium and does not necessarily reflect differences in the content of esterified fatty acids in the myocytes of the various layers. The amount of non esterified fatty acids (NEFA) in heart muscle represents only about 0.06% of the total amount of fatty acids present in heart tissue. The majority of fatty acids is incorporated into phosphoglycerides (88.2%). Palmitic acid (C 16 : 0) and stearic acid (C 18 : 0) are the main constituents of NEFA. Oleic acid (C 18 : 1) accounts for about 41% of all fatty acids incorporated in triacylglycerol. Linoleic acid (C 18 : 2) and arachidonic acid (C 20 : 4) are the main constituents of fatty acid in the total phosphoglyceride pool. The data presented in Table 2 show that phosphatidylcholine (PC) and phosphatidylethanolamine (PE) are the main phosphoglycerides moieties in this lipid group. Lysophosphoglycerides such as lysophosphatidylcholine (LPC) and lysophosphatidylethanolamine (LPE) were present in very small amounts, representing 0.5 and 0.4% of the total amount of phosphoglyceride molecules, respectively.

After 2 hours of ischemia induced by narrowing of the left anterior interventricular coronary artery total NEFA content was significantly increased in subendocardial and mesocardial layers of the affected area (Fig. 1). The increased tissue content of the individual NEFA in the subendocardial layer is depicted in Figure 2. The longer chain, unsaturated fatty acids, such as linoleic acid (by about 600%) and arachidonic acid (by about 1000%), showed the highest relative increase. The relationship between residual blood flow and the extent of accumulation of NEFA has been delineated in more detail in Figure 3. This graph clearly indicates that NEFA accumulates in cardiac tissue underperfused for 2 hours if residual flow in that area is reduced to less than 40% of that in the normoxic areas of the heart. The accumulation of NEFA has been found to be a relatively slow process. No significant increase of total NEFA in the subendocardial layers at 10 min after the onset of ischemia could be detected. Fifty minutes later the accumulation of NEFA in these ischemic layers was significant, e.g. $168\,nmol \cdot g^{-1}$ in comparison with $25\,nmol \cdot g^{-1}$ wet weight in the non-ischemic areas. The data in Table 3 show the time course of the accumulation of arachidonic acid (C 20 : 4) in the ischemic subendocardial layer in more detail. A time delay of at least 10 min following the start of ischemia is clearly present.

A possible relationship between the decrease in tissue ATP levels and accumulation of arachidonic acid has been explored in two ways. First, the content of arachidonic acid in the subepicardial, mesocardial and subendocardial layers, rendered ischemic for 120 min, has been compared with the ATP content measured in the same layer in the vicinity of the lipid sample (Figure 4). This figure indicates that arachidonic acid readily accumulates when the tissue ATP level drops below 5–7 $\mu mol \cdot g^{-1}$ dry weight. In Table 3 the time course of the decrease in tissue ATP in the ischemic subendocardial layers is shown. Comparison with the pattern of arachidonic acid accumulation observed in the same layer indicates

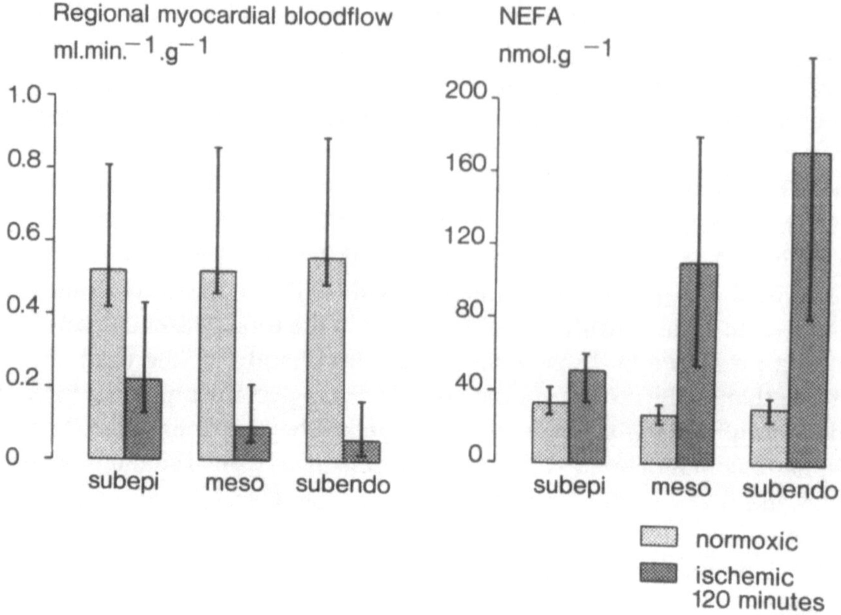

Figure 1. Regional myocardial blood flow and NEFA content in subepi, meso-, and subendocardial layers of normoxic and ischemic regions of dog left ventricular myocardium. Values shown in this figure are median values and 95% confidence limits of 16 biopsies from the area perfused by the partially occluded left interventricular coronary artery (ischemic region, dark bars) and of 16 biopsies from the area perfused by the left circumflex coronary artery (normoxic region, light bars) obtained in eight dog hearts. * Significantly different from the values in the corresponding layers of the normoxic area of the heart ($P<0.05$). (Reprinted with permission from the American Heart Association from [2].)

that the decrease of ATP precedes the rise of arachidonic acid. Ischemia of a duration of 120 min had no significant effect on the tissue triacylglycerol, cholesteryl ester and total phosphoglyceride content of the ischemic area.

The effect of reperfusion of previously ischemic heart tissue on tissue levels of arachidonic acid and (lyso)phosphoglycerides has been investigated in a subgroup of 15 dogs. In these open-chested, anesthetized animals, the left anterior interventricular coronary artery was completely occluded for 60 min. After removal of the clamp reperfusion of the affected area was allowed for another 60 min.

Total NEFA was significantly increased in the subendocardial layers at the end of the ischemic period and following reperfusion (Table 4). It should be noted that the lipid content shown in this table has been expressed as nmoles of fatty acid equivalents per gram of dry weight of tissue instead of wet weight as in the previous tables and figures. The reason to do so was the observation that the percentage wet weight of ischemic and, in particular, reperfused myocardial tissue, increased significantly. Expressing the tissue content of lipids on the basis

Table 2. Content and relative fatty acid composition of various phosphoglyceride subgroups such as phosphatidylcholine (PC), lysophosphatidylcholine (LPC), phosphatidylethanolamine (PE), lysophosphatidylethanolamine (LPE), phosphatidylinositol (PI), phosphatidylserine (PS) and cardiolipin (DPG) in normoxic dog myocardium.

The total amount (nmol of fatty acid equivalents g^{-1} wet weight) and percentage fatty acid composition (%) are presented. The various fatty acids are indicated by their chemical notation. DMA refers to the dimethyl acetal form of the corresponding fatty aldehyde. Mean values and S.E.M. are shown (n = 7).

Fatty acid	Lipid subgroups						
	PC	LPC	PE	LPE	PI	PS	DPG
Total amount	19,212 ± 992	112 ± 20	13,986 ± 771	85 ± 14	2,243 ± 102	1,218 ± 67	6,212 ± 281
Relative composition (%)							
14:0	–	2.2 ± 1.3	–	4.6 ± 1.3	–	–	0.5 ± 0.1
14:0 DMA	1.9 ± 0.6	n.m.	–	n.m.	n.m.	n.m.	n.m.
16:0	14.2 ± 0.7	21.1 ± 2.4	2.2 ± 0.2	5.4 ± 2.4	1.7 ± 0.2	1.2 ± 0.1	1.4 ± 0.3
16:0 DMA	20.8 ± 0.9	n.m.	6.9 ± 0.9	n.m.	n.m.	n.m.	n.m.
16:1	0.5 ± 0.1	1.1 ± 0.6	0.2 ± 0.1	–	0.2 ± 0.1	0.2 ± 0.1	1.3 ± 0.1
18:0	6.8 ± 0.4	32.4 ± 3.3	24.4 ± 0.7	37.4 ± 2.1	50.6 ± 0.4	48.3 ± 0.3	1.4 ± 0.2
18:0 DMA	1.5 ± 0.2	n.m.	6.4 ± 0.4	n.m.	n.m.	n.m.	n.m.
18:1	23.7 ± 0.6	11.0 ± 1.4	5.5 ± 0.4	11.9 ± 1.9	3.7 ± 0.2	10.2 ± 0.4	5.3 ± 0.3
18:1 DMA	2.6 ± 0.2	n.m.	4.4 ± 0.4	n.m.	n.m.	n.m.	n.m.
18:2	13.6 ± 0.8	20.4 ± 5.3	5.6 ± 0.3	22.0 ± 1.9	13.3 ± 0.8	14.6 ± 1.0	87.6 ± 0.9
18:3	0.3 ± 0.1	–	0.1 ± 0.1	–	–	–	0.7 ± 0.2
20:0	–	5.4 ± 1.1	–	–	0.2 ± 0.1	0.4 ± 0.1	–
20:4	14.0 ± 1.1	4.8 ± 1.7	42.1 ± 1.4	16.5 ± 1.5	29.8 ± 0.9	22.0 ± 1.0	0.1 ± 0.1
22:4	0.2 ± 0.1	–	0.5 ± 0.1	–	0.3 ± 0.1	1.7 ± 0.3	–
22:6	0.2 ± 0.1	–	0.7 ± 0.1	–	–	–	–

n.m. = not measured; – = not detectable.

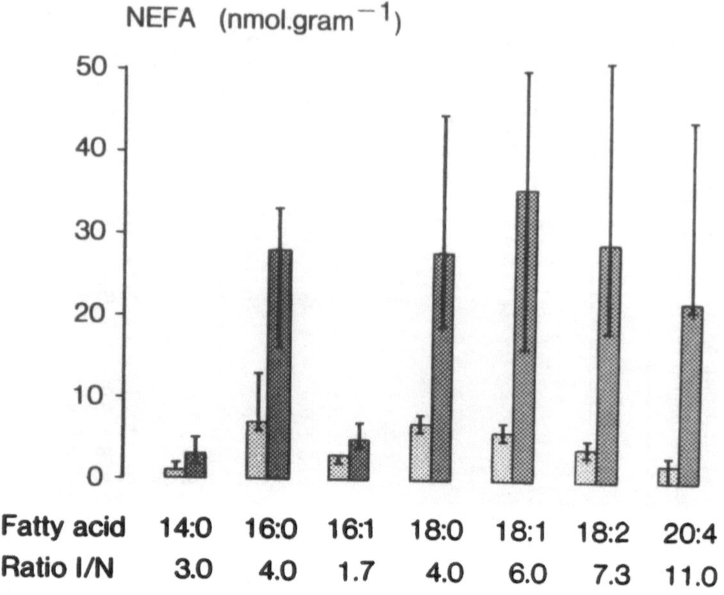

Figure 2. Content of individual NEFA in the subendocardial layer of the normoxic and ischemic area of dog left ventricular myocardium. Median values and 95% confidence limits of 16 biopsies from the subendocardial layer of the normoxic region (light bars) and the ischemic region (dark bars) in eight dog hearts are shown. Biopsies were taken after 120 minutes of ischemia. Data are expressed as individual fatty acid per gram of net tissue. 14 : 0 refers to myristic acid, 16 : 0 to palmitic acid, 16 : 1 to linoleic acid, 18 : 0 to stearic acid, 18 : 1 to oleic acid, 18 : 2 to linoleic acid, and 20 : 4 to arachidonic acid. * Significantly different from the values in the corresponding layer in the normoxic region of the left ventricle at $P<0.05$. (Reprinted with permission from the American Heart Association from [2].)

of wet weight might therefore mask small changes in tissue content of the material under investigation. Upon reperfusion total NEFA remained elevated with a tendency to increase further at 60 min after restoration of flow.

Arachidonic acid levels increased significantly during ischemia, but decreased

Table 3. Time course of the changes of subendocardial ATP and arachidonic acid contents during ischemia. Median values and 95% confidence limits are given.

Substance	Control	Ischemia (min)		
		10	60	120
ATP	17	13[a]	6[a]	5[a]
(μmol · g^{-1} wet weight)	12–19	10–15	4–12	3–13
Arachidonic acid	2	2	8.5[a]	16[a]
(nmol · g^{-1} wet weight)	0–3	1.5–3	4–12	8–40

[a] Indicates significantly different from control values by paired analysis (n = 5–30).

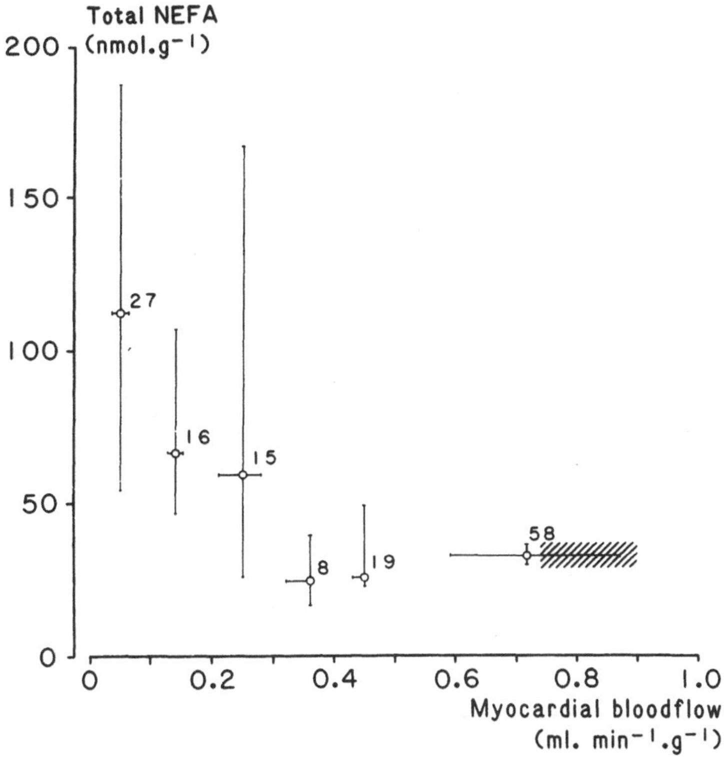

Figure 3. Relationship between content of nonesterified fatty acid (NEFA) and myocardial blood flow in samples from ischemic and nonischemic myocardium 120 min after onset of stenosis of the left anterior interventricular coronary artery. Myocardial blood flow was determined in tissue directly surrounding the site where biopsies for determination of NEFA content were taken. Values were obtained in tissue specimens from all 3 myocardial layers. Data were grouped according to myocardial blood flow and divided into cohorts of 0.1 ml · min^{-1} · g^{-1}. Median values and 95% confidence limits of each cohort are presented. Figures near the median values refer to number of observations. Dashed area represents the 95% confidence limits of data of all samples from non-ischemic areas. (Reprinted with permission from the American Physiological Society from [6].)

during the initial reperfusion phase. Fifty-five minutes thereafter the measured values were found to be increased again. LPC levels were significantly increased at 60 min of ischemia. During the initial reperfusion period the content of this lysophosphoglyceride returned to normoxic values. However, the content started to increase again after prolonged reperfusion. No significant changes in the tissue level of LPE could be detected during ischemia and reperfusion.

Analysis of arterial and local cardiac venous blood (from the area perfused by the left anterior interventricular coronary artery) collected during normoxia, ischemia and reperfusion revealed that no significant uptake or release of arachidonic acid and LPE occurred throughout the experimental period. With respect to LPC, a small but significant release could be measured during the pre-ischemic

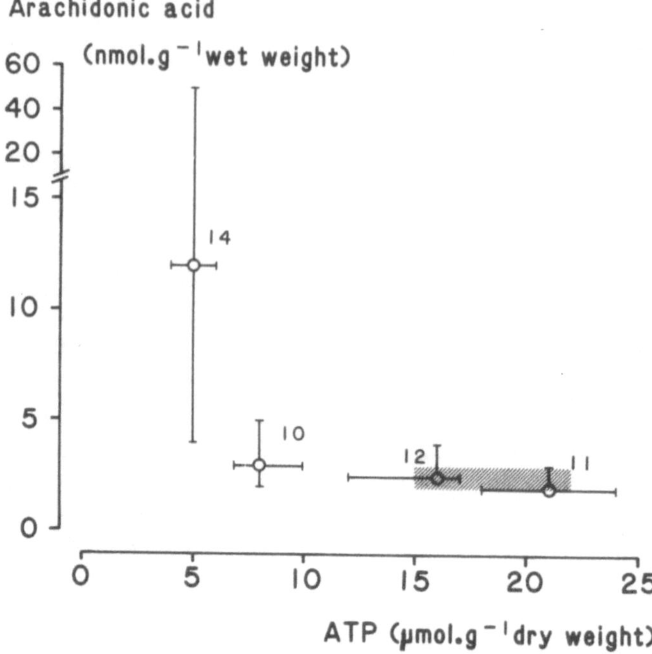

Figure 4. Relationship between the contents of arachidonic acid and ATP in samples taken from ischemic and non-ischemic subepicardial, mesocardial and subendocardial layer 120 minues after onset of stenosis of the left anterior interventricular coronary artery. ATP content was determined in tissue specimen taken in the vicinity of the biopsies for fatty acid determination. The data were grouped according to ATP content and divided into cohorts with ATP values ranging from 4–6, 7–10, 11–17 and 18–25 μmol · g^{-1} dry weight. Median values and 95% confidence limits of each cohort are presented. The figures near the median values refer to the number of observations. The dashed area represents the 95% confidence limits of the data of all samples from the non-ischemic area.

Table 4. Content of nonesterified fatty acids (NEFA), arachidonic acid (AA), lysophosphatidylcholine (LPC) and lysophosphatidylethanolamine (LPE) in normoxic, ischemic and reperfused subendocardial tissue. Mean values and standard deviations are given. Values are expressed as nmoles fatty acid equivalents g^{-1} of dry weight of tissue.

Time	Normoxic value (n = 15)	60 min of ischemia (n = 6)	5 min of reperfusion (n = 4)	60 min of reperfusion (n = 5)
Lipid group				
NEFA	175 ± 30	608 ± 102[a]	615 ± 354[a]	1400 ± 1152[a]
AA	8 ± 2	96 ± 33[a]	43 ± 40[a]	154 ± 126[a]
LPC	395 ± 150	608 ± 218[a]	372 ± 105	543 ± 229[a]
LPE	519 ± 412	548 ± 276	390 ± 198	765 ± 371

[a] Significantly different from corresponding normoxic values ($P \leq 0.05$).

period. However, after the onset of ischemia and reperfusion no significant difference between arterial and local venous concentrations could be observed (data not shown).

Discussion

Content of lipids in normoxic myocardial tissue

The content of NEFA in normoxic myocardial tissue has been a subject of continuous debate [5]. Although the values published range from 25 to at least 22,000 nmols per gram of wet weight of tissue, results of recent carefully conducted studies are in favor with the notion that the level of nonesterified fatty acids in myocardial tissue is extremely low [2, 5]. On the basis of the present investigation we can conclude that less than 0.1% of all fatty acid in the heart is present in the nonesterified form. After correction for NEFA present in blood and interstitial fluid, a concentration of about 10 nmoles NEFA/ml sarcoplasmic fluid has been calculated as a reasonable value for heart cells.

High levels of NEFA, as measured in normal heart tissue, are most likely caused by technical imperfections during the assay procedure [5]. Storage of tissue specimens at temperatures above −80° C, incorrect extraction procedures, and assay techniques with low specificity for NEFA will readily increase the values of NEFA measured. In addition to technical considerations, a variety of findings have indicated that low NEFA levels have to be expected in normoxic heart tissue with respect to normal function. Rose and co-workers [9] estimated on basis of their multiple indicator dilution experiments an intracellular NEFA concentration in the order of 20 nmol/gram intracellular fluid. *In vitro* studies with isolated enzymes [5] and mitochondrial fractions [10] have indicated that NEFA concentrations above 100 nmol/ml are detrimental to an appropriate function of cellular intermediate metabolism. Groot and colleagues [1] have reported that the K_m of the fatty acid activating enzyme system (fatty acylCoA synthetase) is in the order of 8 μM. Since fatty acids are avidly oxidized by heart cells under aerobic conditions and the V_{max} of the enzyme system is substantially higher than the flux of fatty acids through the oxidative pathway [2, 12], a low intracellular level of NEFA is compatible with the measured K_m of fatty acylCoA synthetase as mentioned above.

In contrast with NEFA, less information is available about the physiological content of lysophosphoglycerides in cardiac tissue. Table 5 shows that, for instance, the content of lysophosphatidylcholine varies from 25 to about 1200 nmol $\cdot$ g^{-1} wet weight of tissue in the various studies reported in the literature. A similar range was found for lysophosphatidylethanolamine. Shaikh and Downar [13] have shown that inappropriate extraction procedures will readily result in artificially elevated lysophosphoglyceride levels in cardiac tissue specimens. In addition, the presence of a variety of lysophosphoglyceride converting enzymes in the myocytes [16, 17] makes high concentrations of these phosphoglyceride species in normoxic tissue less likely.

It has been well established that maintenance of the integrity of membrane phosphoglycerides is a prerequisite for adequate cellular functioning [18]. Enzymatic degradation of phosphoglycerides by phospholipase A_2, present in myocardial structures, will primarily result in the formation of nonesterified fatty acids and lysophosphoglycerides. Since the majority of the fatty acids incorporated on the A_2 (β) position of phosphoglycerides are polyunsaturated long chain fatty acids, accumulation of arachidonic and linoleic acid can be anticipated. Whether substantial amounts of lysophosphoglycerides accumulate in the cardiac cell is still a matter of debate [3, 13–15] since the presence of, for instance, lysophospholipase will promote degradation lysophosphoglycerides into nonesterified fatty acids (mainly saturated and mono-unsaturated fatty acids) and glycerol 3-phosphatides.

Evidence is accumulating that irreversible myocardial cell damage due to ischemic insult is associated with loss of integrity of cellular membranes [19, 20]. The accumulation of polyunsaturated NEFA such as arachidonic and linoleic acid in ischemic myocardial tissue (Figure 2) is in favor of the idea that myocardial phosphoglyceride homeostasis is disturbed during oxygen deprivation [2, 3, 6, 14, 21]. Canine subendocardial layers are very sensitive to ischemic insults, most likely due to a relatively more severe reduction of flow in these layers as compared to the middle and subepicardial ones. In this respect, the observation that NEFA accumulation is more pronounced in subendocardial than subepicardial layers (Figure 1) is in accordance with a functional relationship between ischemic damage and NEFA accumulation. Prinzen et al. [6] and Chien et al. [3]

Table 5. The content of lysophosphoglycerides in normoxic cardiac tissue.

Lysophosphoglyceride	Content ($nmol \cdot g^{-1}$ wet weight)	Species	References
Lysophosphatidylcholine	1400	rabbit	Sobel et al. 1978 [14]
	40	pig	Shaikh and Downar, 1981 [13]
	414[a]	cat	Corr et al., 1982 [15]
	25[b]	dog	Chien et al., 1984 [13]
	112	dog	Roemen and Van der Vusse, 1985 [8]
Lysophosphatidylethanolamine	1200	rabbit	Sobel et al., 1978 [14]
	60	pig	Shaikh and Downar, 1981 [13]
	315[a]	cat	Corr et al., 1982 [15]
	85	dog	Roemen and Van der Vusse, 1985 [8]

[a] With the assumption that 1 gram of tissue contains 150 mg protein.
[b] With the assumption that 1 gram of tissue contains 2 mg DNA.

have reported that the time course of NEFA accumulation resembles the time course of the onset of irreversible loss of cell function in ischemic myocardial tissue as reported by Jennings et al. [19]. Both groups of investigators have shown that accumulation of NEFA is a relatively slow starting process (Table 3). Despite a very rapid cessation of fiber shortening in the subendocardial layers (within seconds) as well as a rapid decrease of creatine phosphate and pH (within 2 minutes) and a fast increase of inorganic phosphate and lactate in myocardial tissue [22], all indicating a severe disturbance in mechanical and biochemical function of the affected cells, accumulation of NEFA in the myocardium was not measurable during the first 10 to 20 minutes of the ischemic insult [3, 6]. Thereafter accumulation of these fatty acids gradually occurred. Since the first signs of irreversible damage to myocardial cells has been reported to take place between 30 and 60 minutes [19] after the onset of ischemia the similarity of both time courses is quite suggestive.

From the experimental work of Jennings and colleagues [19], the notion emerges that loss of function of ischemic myocytes is strongly related to the decrease in cellular ATP level. They have shown that changes in ultrastructure and membrane function occurred when myocardial ATP content was below $5\,\mu mol \cdot g^{-1}$ dry weight. This value corresponds to about 25% of the normoxic level of ATP. We found (Table 3 and Figure 4) that ATP reduction preceded NEFA accumulation and that arachidonic acid significantly accumulated when ATP levels were below $5\text{–}7\,\mu mol \cdot g^{-1}$ dry weight of ischemic tissue, a value in good agreement with the above mentioned observations of Jennings et al. [19]. In addition, recently Chien et al. [23] and Gunn et al. [24] have shown that when ATP levels in myocytes are reduced by other than ischemic means (in their experiments by reducing metabolic activity with specific inhibitors), arachidonic acid will be specifically released from phosphoglycerides when the ATP level will drop below 25% of its original value. Although these findings might suggest a causal relationship between a fall in tissue ATP levels and degradation of membrane phosphoglycerides, at this moment no definite mechanism can be proposed to explain this relationship in full detail. The depletion of ATP will hamper the formation of arachidonyl CoA, an intermediate required for the incorporation of arachidonic acid into phosphoglycerides. In addition, the accumulation of AMP (due to impaired ATP regeneration under ischemic circumstances) will also block the enzymatic process involved in the formation of arachidonyl CoA. Enhanced degradation of phosphoglycerides has to be considered as well. In this case, a direct relationship between ATP depletion and arachidonic acid release is less evident, since myocardial phospholipases are ATP independent enzymes. The activity of the last mentioned enzymes may be enhanced in ischemic tissue by increased intracellular Ca^{2+} levels due to impaired ATP dependent Ca^{2+} pump activity or by better contact between the phosphoglyceride substrates and the enzyme proteins due to morphological changes in the affected cells.

Accumulation of long chain non esterified fatty acids in ischemic myocardial tissue can be detrimental by itself. Beside the vulnerability of various cytoplasmic and mitochondrial enzyme systems to increased NEFA concentrations (for recent survey see [5]), intercalation of NEFA into cellular lipid bilayers can occur resulting in marked effects on membrane Ca^{2+} ATPase and permeability [25]. Increased eicosanoid synthesis from arachidonic acid can be expected as well, possibly giving rise to the formation of substances, with either protective or deleterious effects on the ischemic myocardial structures [26].

The acceptance that the increase of tissue arachidonic acid levels is a sensitive marker of enhanced phosphoglyceride degradation raises the question whether other degradation products accumulate as well. After the publication of Sobel and co-workers [14], reporting a substantial increase of lysophosphoglycerides in ischemic rabbit myocardial tissue, a variety of investigators have studied this phenomenon with contrasting results. Shaikh and Downar [13] have reported a quantitatively very small, but significant increase in porcine hearts. Chien et al. [3] failed to observe any change in lysophosphatidylcholine content in ischemic dog hearts. Corr and coworkers [15] reported a significant increase in both lysophosphatidylcholine and lysophosphatidylethanolamine in feline hearts made ischemic for 10 minutes. Recently, we found a significant increase in lysophosphatidylcholine in dog hearts oxygen deprived for 60 minutes (Table 4). Chien et al. [3] have explained the lack of stoichiometric relationship between arachidonic acid and lysophospholipaside accumulation by subsequent action of lysophospholipases, present in myocardial tissue [16, 17]. The concomitant increase of saturated long-chain fatty acid favors this idea, although release of these fatty acids from other endogenous sources such as triacylglycerol cannot be excluded [27].

From the data presented in Table 4, we can calculate that during 60 minutes of ischemia the increase of total NEFA amounted to 433 nmol $\cdot$ g^{-1} dry weight in the subendocardial layer. The sum of LPC and LPE increased with 242 nmol $\cdot$ g^{-1} dry weight during the same period of time. If we assume that both NEFA and lysophosphoglycerides are degradation products of phosphoglycerides and no further conversion of NEFA has taken place, the present findings indicate that less than half of the lysophosphoglycerides generated in ischemic myocardial tissue will be degraded by virtue of lysophospholipase activity.

It should be noted that the increase of both NEFA and lysophosphoglycerides is small in comparison with the total amount of phosphoglycerides in heart tissue. An increase of about 400 nmoles lysopohosphoglycerides or NEFA per g dry weight of tissue corresponds with degradation of about 0.37% of all phospholipid molecules present per hour. Although this amount represents only a small fraction of the total content of phosphoglycerides in myocardial tissue, this change might have a great qualitative impact on the function of the tissue affected.

Reperfusion of ischemic tissue is a prerequisite to save the tissue from a certain death. However, reperfusion in itself might be deleterious to the previously ischemic area when no special precautions are taken [28]. Although reperfusion-induced damage is still a matter of debate, aggravation of disturbed lipid homeostasis has been proposed as a possible mechanism. On the one hand, restoration of flow to the ischemic area causes the washaway of NEFA and lysophosphoglycerides leading to the loss of these important substances which will prevent adequate resynthesis of the degraded phosphoglyceride molecules. On the other hand, reperfusion will promote the supply of ions such as Ca^{2+} to the previously ischemic cells which has been shown to result in increased Ca^{2+} levels inside the cell [29]. As a consequence, phospholipase A_2 might be activated and phosphoglyceride degradation will continue or will even be enhanced. On the basis of the present results no definite conclusion can, however, be made. Although total NEFA content remained unchanged during the first 5 minutes of reperfusion, the levels of arachidonic acid decreased to 45% of the ischemic value. Since analysis of local venous blood did not show a change of the arachidonic acid concentration as compared with control or ischemic blood [Van der Vusse et al., unpublished observations], release of this fatty acid from the reperfused tissue is less likely. Although significant production and release of 6-keto $F_{1\alpha}$ during the initial reperfusion has been found [Engels and Van der Vusse, unpublished observations], the amount produced accounted for maximally 5% of the arachidonic acid accumulated. On the basis of these findings resynthesis of phosphoglycerides during the initial period of reperfusion has to be considered. The simultaneous decrease of lysophosphoglycerides is in favor of this idea, since we were unable to measure a significant increase of the concentration of lysophosphoglycerides in venous blood, draining the reperfused area of the heart [Van der Vusse et al., unpublished observations]. Since the decrease of tissue contents of arachidonic acid and lysophosphoglycerides were found to be transient, enhanced hydrolysis of phosphoglycerides probably occurred during prolonged reperfusion. The mechanism of the late-onset phosphoglyceride degradation remains to be elucidated.

References

1. Liedtke AJ (1981): Alternations of carbohydrate and lipid metabolism in the acutely ischemic heart. Prog Cardiovasc Dis 23: 321–336.
2. Van der Vusse GJ, Roemen THM, Prinzen FW, Coumans WA, Reneman RS (1982): Uptake and tissue content of fatty acids in dog myocardium under normoxic and ischemic conditions. Circ Res 50: 538–546.
3. Chien KR, Han A, Sen A, Buja LM, Willerson JT (1984): Accumulation of unesterified arachidonic acid in ischemic canine myocardium. Circ Res 54: 313–322.
4. Van der Vusse GJ, Reneman RS (1983): Glycogen and lipids (endogenous substrates) In: Drake-Holland AJ, Noble MIM (eds) Cardiac metabolism. J. Wiley & Sons, Chicester, U.K., pp. 215–237.
5. Van der Vusse GJ, Reneman RS (1984): The myocardial non-esterified fatty acid controversy. J Cell Mol Cardiol 16: 677–682.

6. Prinzen FW, Van der Vusse GJ, Arts T, Roemen THM, Coumans WA, Reneman RS (1984): Accumulation of nonesterified fatty acids in ischemic canine myocardium. Am J Physiol 247: H264–H272.
7. Van der Vusse GJ, Coumans WA, Van der Veen E, Drake AJ, Flameng W, Suy R (1984): ATP, creatine phosphate and glycogen content in human myocardial biopsies: markers for the efficacy of cardioprotection during aorto-coronary bypass surgery. Vasc Surg 18: 127–134.
8. Roemen THM, Van der Vusse GJ (1985): Application of silicagel column chromatography in the assessment of non-esterified fatty acids and phosphoglycerides in myocardial tissue. J Chromatography 344: 304–308.
9. Rose CP, Goresky CA (1977): Constraints on the uptake of labelled palmitate by the heart. The barriers at the capillary and sarcolemmal surfaces and the control of intracellular sequestration. Circ Res 41: 534–545.
10. Piper HM, Sezer O, Schwartz P, Huetter JF, Spieckermann PG (1983): Fatty acid-membrane interactions in isolated cardiac mitochondria and erythrocytes. Biochim Biophys Acta 732: 193–203.
11. Groot PHE, Scholte HR, Huelsmann WC (1976): Fatty acid activation: specificity, localization and function. Adv Lipid Res 14: 75–126.
12. Aas M (1971): Organ and subcellular distribution of fatty acid activating enzymes in the rat. Biochim Biophys Acta 231: 32–47.
13. Shaikh NA, Downar E (1981): Time course of changes in porcine myocardial phospholipid levels during ischemia. Circ Res 49: 316–325.
14. Sobel BE, Corr PB, Robinson AK, Goldstein RA, Witkowski FX, Klein MS (1978): Accumulation of lysophosphoglycerides with arrhythmogenic properties in ischemic myocardium. J Clin Invest 62: 546–553.
15. Corr PB, Snyder DW, Lee BI, Gross RW, Keim CR, Sobel BE (1982): Pathophysiological concentrations of lysophosphatides and the slow response. Am J Physiol 243: H182–H195.
16. Gross RW, Sobel BE (1982): Lysophosphatidylcholine metabolism in the rabbit heart. J Biol Chem 257: 6702–6708.
17. Nalbone G, Hostetler KY (1985): Subcellular localization of the phospholipases A of rat heart: evidence for a cytosolic phospholipase A_1. J Lipid Res 26:104–114.
18. Van den Bosch H (1974): Phosphoglyceride metabolism. Ann Rev Biochem 43: 243–277.
19. Jennings RB, Hawkins JE, Lowe JE, Hill ML, Klotman S, Reimer KA (1978): Relation between high energy phosphate and lethal injury in myocardial ischemia in the dog. Am Pathol 92: 187–215.
20. Willerson JT, Seales F, Mukherjee A, Platt MR, Templeton GH, Fink GC, Buja LM (1977): Abnormal myocardial fluid retention as an early manifestation of ischemic injury. Am J Pathol 87: 159–188.
21. Weglicki WB, Owens K, Urschel CW, Serur JR, Sonnenblick EH (1973): Hydrolysis of myocardial lipids during acidosis and ischemia. Recent Adv Stud Cardiac Struct Metabol 3: 781–793.
22. Prinzen FW, Arts T, Van der Vusse GJ, Coumans WA, Reneman RS (1986): Gradients in fiber shortening and metabolism across ischemic left ventricular wall. Am J Physiol 250: H255–H264.
23. Chien KR, Sen A, Reynolds R, Chang A, Kim C, Gunn MD, Buja LM, Willerson JT (1985): Release of arachidonate from membrane phospholipids in cultured neonatal rat myocardial cells during adenosine triphosphate depletion. J Clin Invest 755: 1770–1780.
24. Gunn MD, Sen A, Chang A, Willerson JT, Buja LM, Chien KR (1985): Mechanisms of accumulation of arachidonic acid in cultured myocardial cells during ATP depletion. Am J Physiol 249: H1188–H1194.
25. Katz AM, Messineo FC (1981): Lipid-membrane interactions and the pathogenesis of ischemic damage in the myocardium. Circ Res 48: 1–17.
26. Berger HJ, Zaret BL, Speroff L, Cohen ES, Wolfson S (1976): Regional cardiac prostaglandin release during myocardial ischemia in anesthetized dogs. Circ Res 38: 566–571.

27. Bilheimer D, Buja LM, Parkey RW, Bonte FJ, Willerson JT (1978): Fatty acid accumulation and abnormal lipid deposition in peripheral border zones of experimental myocardial infarcts. J Nucl Med 19: 276–283.
28. Van der Vusse GJ, Reneman RS (1985): Pharmacological intervention in acute myocardial ischemia and reperfusion. Trends Pharmacol Sci 6: 76–79.
29. Ferrari R, Di Lisa F, Raddino R, Bigoli C, Curello S, Ceconi C, Albertini A, Visioli O (1984): Factors influencing the metabolic and functional alterations induced by ischemia and reperfusion. In: Ferrari R, Katz AM, Shug A, Visioli O (eds) Myocardial ischemia and lipid metabolism. Plenum Press, NY, pp. 135–157.

Discussion

Sideman: If you were to define the limiting metabolic reaction in the heart, so that you could model the metabolism of the heart, what would be the limiting component you would choose?
Van der Vusse: With respect to lipid metabolism, no unambiguous answer to that question can be given at present. Lipid metabolism is not only governed by the activities of enzymes involved in metabolic pathways but also by transport of fatty acids and their derivatives across membrane barriers. In addition, the regulatory role of Z-protein has to be considered as well.
Downey: A comment concerning the relationship between residual blood flow and infarction. In our dog model of 48 hours of coronary occlusion, we find that the transition between living and dead tissue occurs at a blood flow of about 0.4 ml/min/gm. Tissue with more flow survives while that with less dies.
Van der Vusse: I like to admit that the agreement between your findings and ours (i.e. accumulation of NEFA in ischemic areas with a residual blook flow lower than 0.4 ml/min g) is remarkable. We have also noticed that NEFA accumulates in the affected area when ATP levels drop below 5–7 μmol/g dry weight. It is noteworthy that Jennings and co-workers (Am J Pathol 92: 187–215, 1978) have reported that myocardial cell function is greatly impaired when ATP levels are reduced to 6 μmol/g dry weight and lower due to ischemia. On the basis of these parallels we may conclude that accumulation of NEFA in general and arachidonic acid in particular is involved in the process of ischemic myocardial injury.

41. Heat transfer and temperature profiles during ischemia and infarction in the left ventricular wall

E. BARTA, S. SIDEMAN, H. ADACHI and R. BEYAR

Abstract

A theoretical analysis and an experimental procedure for determining the temperature fields in the left ventricular (LV) wall are presented. The bio-heat equation which accounts for heat conduction, convection and heat production in the LV wall is formulated and solved to yield the transmural as well as the epicardial temperature distributions at a variety of operating conditions.

A typical hyperbolic temperature distribution across the myocardium, with a maximum near the midwall, is predicted for the normal heart. The temperature profiles in an ischemic or infarcted zone deviate from the normal behavior, displaying a gradual decrease in the midwall temperatures and a tendency for a monotonous endocardial to epicardial temperature decrease in the transmural necrotic region. The calculated epicardial circumferential temperature distribution map of an acute infarcted LV is in agreement with the experimental epicardial temperatures measured by using a thermal imaging technique. The data show a typical decrease in temperature in the infarcted zone with a relatively narrow (approx. 1 cm) border zone between the infarct and the normal tissue. The model may thus be used as a tool to evaluate the static and dynamic features of the myocardial flow distribution in normal and pathological situations.

Introduction

The problem of the heat transfer in the LV wall is interesting from the theoretical, experimental and clinical points of view. However, only limited experimental data exist regarding the temperature distribution within an infarcted segment of the LV wall [1]. Extending an earlier theoretical analysis of the healthy heart [2], the problem of the irregular heart has recently been presented [3], demonstrating that the temperature distribution of the LV wall is a function of the local heat production, the local energy metabolism, the heat convected by blood perfusion and the heat conducted through the muscle tissue.

Recent developments in imaging systems for measurements of the temperature distribution at the epicardium in open chest preparations suggest the clinical application of thermocardiography as a tool for assessing the performance of the injured myocardium during ischemia and perfusion. Extending previous studies wherein the bio-heat equation is solved for a symmetric 'normal' LV [2] and infarcted asymmetric LV [3], we now formulate and solve the asymmetric heat transfer problem associated with an infarcted or ischemic segment of the LV, relating particularly to the epicardial temperature maps which can be obtained experimentally.

As reviewed by Bowman [4], the solution of the bio-heat equation in various tissues has long been used as a tool to evaluate tissue perfusion. However, with few exceptions, lumped rather than distributed local values were considered. The purpose of this work is to evolve the solution of the problem of heat transfer in an infarcted myocardium based on the distributed parameters of transmural flow and oxygen consumption and to compare it to experimental measurements (in dogs) of epicardial temperatures before, during and after acute coronary occlusion. If successful, this procedure may be reversed so as to evaluate the regional perfusion by non-invasive measurements of the epicardial temperature field during open heart surgery so as to determine the instantaneous local perfusion throughout, and following, a by-pass operation.

The mathematical formulation

The bio-heat equation which accounts for the conduction, convection by blood perfusion and heat production due to metabolic activity is applied here to the equatorial cross-section of a thick-walled spheroid (Fig. 1). Assuming a constant and uniform thermal diffusivity constant $\alpha = k/\varrho c$ where k is the thermal conductivity constant, ϱ the density of the tissue, and c its heat capacity constant, the general form of the bio-heat equation is given by:

$$\frac{1}{\alpha}\frac{\partial u}{\partial t} = \frac{\partial^2 u}{\partial r^2} + \frac{1}{r}\frac{\partial u}{\partial r} + \frac{1}{r^2}\frac{\partial^2 u}{\partial \varphi^2} + C_1(r,\varphi,t)u + C_2(r,\varphi,t) \tag{1}$$

for

$$R_1 \leq r \leq R_2, \quad 0 \leq \varphi < 2\pi, \quad 0 \leq t < \tau,$$

where u is the difference between the instantaneous local temperature of the tissue, T, and T_b, the blood temperature; R_1, R_2 are the radii of the endocardial and epicardial layers, respectively; φ is the circumferential angle and τ is the time duration of one heart beat cycle

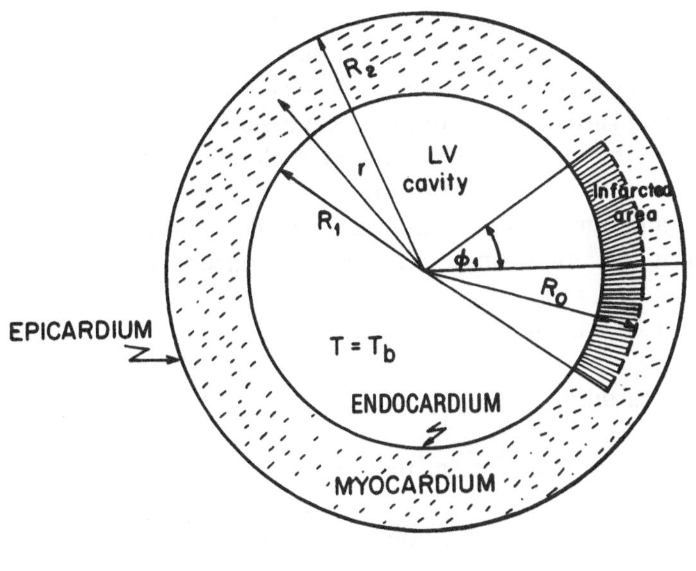

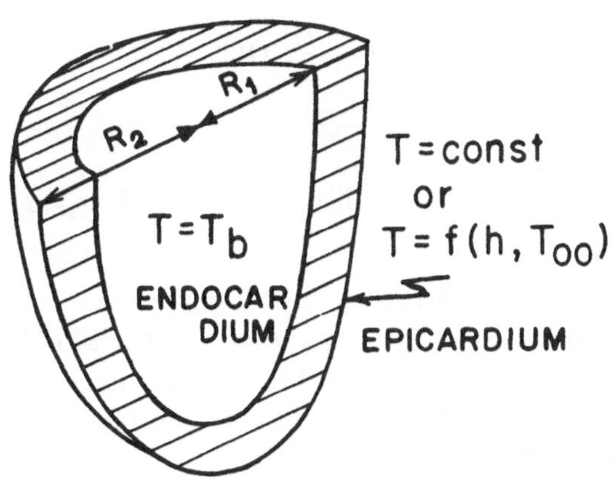

Figure 1. Spheroidal presentation of the LV.

$$C_1(r,\varphi,t) = \frac{m(r,t) \cdot \varrho \cdot \varrho_b \cdot c_b}{k} \cdot k_1(r,\varphi), \tag{2}$$

$$C_2(r,\varphi,t) = \frac{q_m(r,t)}{k} k_2(r,\varphi). \tag{3}$$

The subscript b denotes the blood; m(r,t) is the instantaneous local perfusion rate per unit mass of muscle, $q_m(r,t)$ is the metabolic heat production rate, evaluated by utilizing Beyar and Sideman's analysis of cardiac mechanics [5], myocardial perfusion [6] and energetics [7, 8]. As described earlier [2, 3] $q_m(r,t)$ is cycle-time averaged here and, assuming that 75% of the calculated local oxygen consumption $MVO_2(r)$ is converted to heat, $\bar{q}_m(r) = 14.75\,\varrho\, MVO_2(r)$ [J/g tissue · sec]. $k_1(r,\varphi)$ and $k_2(r,\varphi)$ are weight factors that may assume any value between zero and one and denote the local inactivity of the muscle due to flow or oxygen insufficiency, respectively, in cases of infarction and ischemia.

The initial and boundary conditions are given as follows:

a. A periodicity equation, since each beat is assumed to be identical:

$$u(r,\varphi,0) = u(r,\varphi,\tau);\ R_1 \leq r \leq R_2,\ 0 \leq \varphi < 2\pi. \tag{4}$$

b. At the endocardium:

$$u(R_1,\varphi,t) = 0;\ 0 \leq \varphi < 2\pi,\ 0 \leq t < \tau, \tag{5}$$

i.e., the temperature of the endocardial layer equals the temperature of the blood in the LV cavity.

c. At the epicardium the temperature may be given either by:

$$u(R_2,\varphi,t) = u_A;\ \varphi_0 \leq \varphi \leq \varphi_1,\ 0 \leq t < \tau \tag{6}$$

or by

$$-k\frac{\partial u}{\partial r}(R_2,\varphi,t) = h[u(R_2,\varphi,t) - u_\infty];\ \varphi_1 \leq \varphi < \varphi_2,\ 0 \leq t < \tau, \tag{7}$$

where h is the free convection heat transfer constant; u_∞ is the difference between the surrounding (room)temperature and the blood temperature; φ_0, φ_1, φ_2 (all between 0 and 2π) are defined for the specific case under consideration.

Equation (6) represents an external constant temperature, as may be the case at the septum (which is in contact with the blood that fills the RV cavity) or at the free wall of the LV in an intact, closed, thorax. Equation (7) describes an open chest case where the heart is in contact with air and the epicardial temperature is set according to free convection heat transfer.

Finally, the continuity condition for the circumferential direction is given in accordance with the specific problem under consideration.

Symmetrical cases

If a circumferential symmetry for the healthy LV is assumed, the φ-dependence is eliminated. Solutions of (1)–(7) are obtained by using central differences for the spatial derivatives and a forward difference for the time derivative. As described earlier [2], the numerical network is defined so as to fit the blood flow and oxygen consumption network given by the solutions of Beyar and Sideman [5, 6, 8].

As determined for the normal healthy heart [2], the time dependence of the local temperature is very weak and a time averaged equation may be formulated by integrating (1) over the whole cycle without introducing a significant error, yielding

$$0 = \frac{\partial^2 \bar{u}}{\partial t^2} + A(r)\frac{\partial \bar{u}}{\partial r} + C_1(r)\bar{u} + C_2(r), \tag{8}$$

where $\bar{u}$ is the local temperature averaged over one cycle (which is solved by the shooting method) and

$$A(r) = \frac{1}{\tau}\int_0^{\tau} \frac{1}{r(t)}\, dt, \tag{9}$$

$$C_1(r) = \frac{1}{\tau}\int_0^{\tau} C_1(r,\ t)dt. \tag{10}$$

Asymmetrical cases

The occurrence of a regional pathology negates the assumed symmetry of the LV muscle since the gradient of the temperature now has a circumferential as well as a radial component. Another situation of asymmetry is defined by accounting for the inhomogeneous boundary conditions when studying the effect of the RV on the LV myocardial temperature. Equations (6) and (7) apply then at the different regions of the epicardium.

The time averaged equation for the asymmetric LV is given by:

$$0 = \frac{\partial^2 \bar{u}}{\partial r^2} + A(r)\frac{\partial \bar{u}}{\partial r} + B(r)\frac{\partial^2 \bar{u}}{\partial \varphi^2} + C_1(r,\varphi)\bar{u} + C_2(r,\varphi), \tag{11}$$

where

$$B(r) = \frac{1}{\tau}\int_0^{\tau} \frac{1}{r^2(t)}\, dt. \tag{12}$$

Central differences are used for computation of all the derivatives and (11) turns out to be block tridiagonal system equations (or a block tridiagonal plus two terms that result from the circumferential periodicity conditions). A detailed description of the mathematical solution are given elsewhere [3]. Briefly, the general scheme of the solution procedure is as follows:

a. The system of equations is written in a block form.

b. The special structure of the matrix is utilized to get a fast (and elegant) LU decomposition.
c. The resolved two triangular linear systems are then solved.

The physiological constants

The physical constants used in this study are summarized in Table 1. The relevant hemodynamic parameters of the normal heart function under restig conditions are summarized in Table 2 for man and dog.

Experiments

Materials and equipment

Healthy normal dogs were used to study intact open chest by thermocardiography. Heart exposure was gained by left thoractomy under general anesthesia. The dogs were intubated and ventilated. The proximal left anterior descending (LAD) coronary artery was ocluded by an atraumatic vascular clip for 90 minutes, followed by 210 minutes of reperfusion. Regional subendocardial and subepicardial blood flows were determined by using radioactive microspheres. Heart rate was maintained at 120 bpm.

Real-time infrared imaging was used (Probeye Series 400 Thermal Video Systems with a 6-element indium antimonide detector) to map the epicardial and surface temperature differences with a thermal resolution of 0.1 °C. A Hughes Thermal Video System was used. The camera head was 60 to 70 cm from the heart. A high speed rotating mirror within the camera head scanned the heart. Temperature was detected by using indium antimonide. The temperature signal was sent from the camera to an image processor, where the infrared image was created and updated 20 times per second. The signals could also be recorded on discs or video tapes.

After 5 minutes of LAD occlusion, the myocardial surface temperature in the

Table 1. Contants used in the model [9].

Parameter	Value
k	$0.0058\ W\ cm^{-1}\ °C^{-1}$
ϱ_b	$1.02\ g\ cm^{-3}$
ϱ	$1.07\ g\ cm^{-3}$
c_b	$3.725\ J\ g^{-1}\ °C^{-1}$
c	$3.725\ J\ g^{-1}\ °C^{-1}$

affected region decreases rapidly, with color changing from red to orange to green. Typically, the change from a normal area to the center of an hypotermic area is 37.0–34.2 = 2.8 °C. Immediately after reperfusion the blood flow can be followed by the real time images with colors going from green to orange to red.

Four measurements of flow and temperature distribution were taken during the experiment:

a. Control measurements of the healthy myocardial surface.
b. After 90 minutes occlusion of the LAD.
c. After 2 minutes of reflow with release of the occlusion.
d. 210 minutes after reopening of the artery and reperfusion.

Calculation procedure

To simplify the analysis of the data from the different dogs, we assumed that the dogs were of an average size; that the oxygen consumption at each point was proportional to the blood perfusion value there, normalized with respect to the normal values of oxygen consumption given by Beyar and Sideman [8]. The difference between the right ventricle and the LV blood temperatures was taken as 0.3 °C [10]. The LV blood temperature and the free convection heat transfer coefficient were determined by the requirement that the model calculated average of the epicardial temperatures along the circumference will equal the experimental results for the control preocclusion state.

These assumptions give the values of the coefficients A(r), B(r), $C_1(r, \varphi)$, $C_2(r,\varphi)$ in the bio-heat equation (11). The numerical net is changed so that points fit the measured data points. The solution is found by using (5) and (7) and the continuity condition at the circumferential direction as boundary conditions. Notice that small spatial changes in the blood perfusion causes m(r,t) and $q_m(r,t)$

Table 2. Hemodynamic parameters at rest for human and dog data [2, 5, 6, 8].

Parameter	Human HR			Dog HR
	60	90	120	90
Initial short semiaxis (cm)	2.3	2.3	2.3	1.91
Initial (end diastolic) volume (ml)	101.9	101.9	101.9	52.0
End systolic volume (ml)	33.7	28.0	24.0	21.0
Stroke volume (ml)	68	74	78	31
Cardiac output (ml min^{-1})	4096	6654	9349	2844
Ejection fraction (%)	67	72	76	60
Arterial pressure (mm Hg)	131/85	128/85	129/85	126/85
Average oxygen consumption (ml s^{-1} g^{-1})	0.0013	0.0019	0.0026	0.0017
Average coronary perfusion (ml s^{-1} g^{-1})	0.011	0.013	0.018	0.011

to be φ-dependent. This dictates that two blocks be added to the compact tri-diagonal block form of the system of equations. The mathematical procedure is the same as described above.

Results

Temperature distribution in the healthy heart

A symmetric approximation

The temperature distribution within a healthy LV wall, which is assumed to be a symmetrical body, is characterized by the following features [2]:

a. The endocardial temperature is usually higher than the epicardial temperature.
b. The temperature attains its maximum value near the midwall (Fig. 2).
c. The local temperature is practically constant over one cardiac cycle, showing changes with time that are usually smaller than 0.005 °C. The transmural changes with location are more than a hundred times greater.

The agreement with reported experimental data [1, 11–13] is rather satisfactory.

An asymmetrical – healthy heart

Accounting for the effect of the temperature in the right ventricle (RV) on the LV wall leads, by definition, to an asymmetrical problem. This situation is formulated by introducing different epicardial circumferential temperature domains, (6) and (7), i.e., the boundary conditions posed on the external surface are inhomogeneous, with the septal temperature taken as the temperature of the RV blood and a free convection heat transfer coefficient controls the remaining free wall. The detailed configuration and the detailed mathematical analysis is given elsewhere [3].

Similar to the case of a transmural infarct (see below), it is seen in Fig. 3 that the effect of the septal boundary conditions on the LV transmural free wall temperature is restricted to a very narrow border zone. Clearly, solving for the temperature profile in a segment of the LV by utilizing the symmetrical assumption, while neglecting the effect of adjacent segments subjected to different conditions, is justified.

Temperature distribution in a diseased heart

Transmural infarction

As seen in Fig. 4, the temperature profile in the center of an infarcted area is a monotonically decreasing, almost linear, curve between the relatively high endocardial temperature and the lower epicardial temperature.

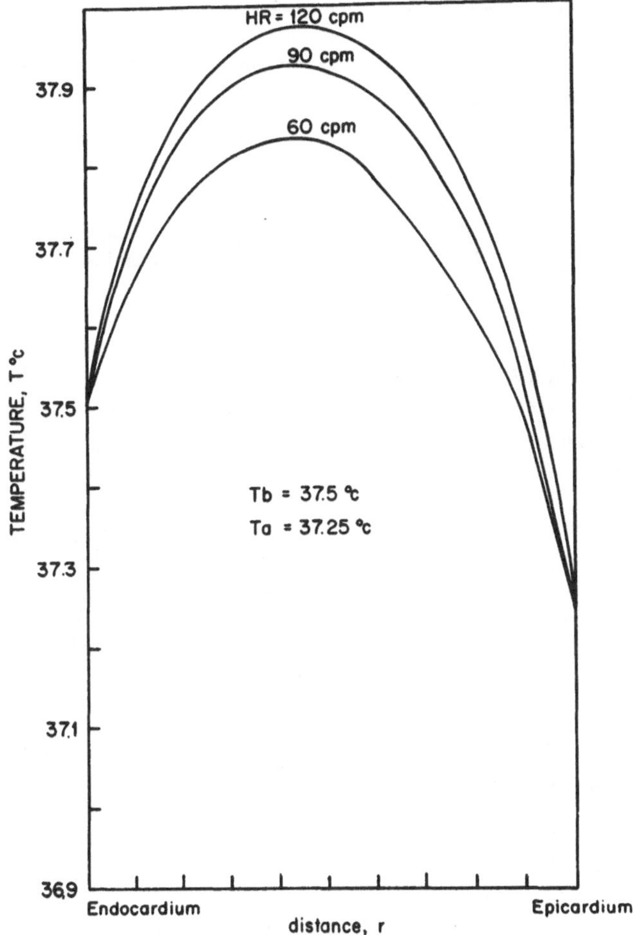

Figure 2. Myocardial temperature distribution for several values of heart rates, HR. A healthy, close chest, case with $T_b = 37.5\,°C$.

Although an infarct has a very pronounced effect on the transmural temperature distribution, the boundary between the normal and the infarcted tissue is confined to a relatively narrow zone. This is demonstrated in Fig. 4 where the epicardial temperature curves for $\varphi = 3\pi/20$ and $\varphi = 4\pi/20$, which represent two adjacent points 2.5 cm apart on the epicardial layer, differ by 2.75 °C.

Subendocardial infarction

As shown in Fig. 5, the transmural temperature distribution through a subendocardial infarction of up to 50% of the wall thickness is not markedly different from that for the normal tissue. Thus, as long as the subepicardial layers maintain

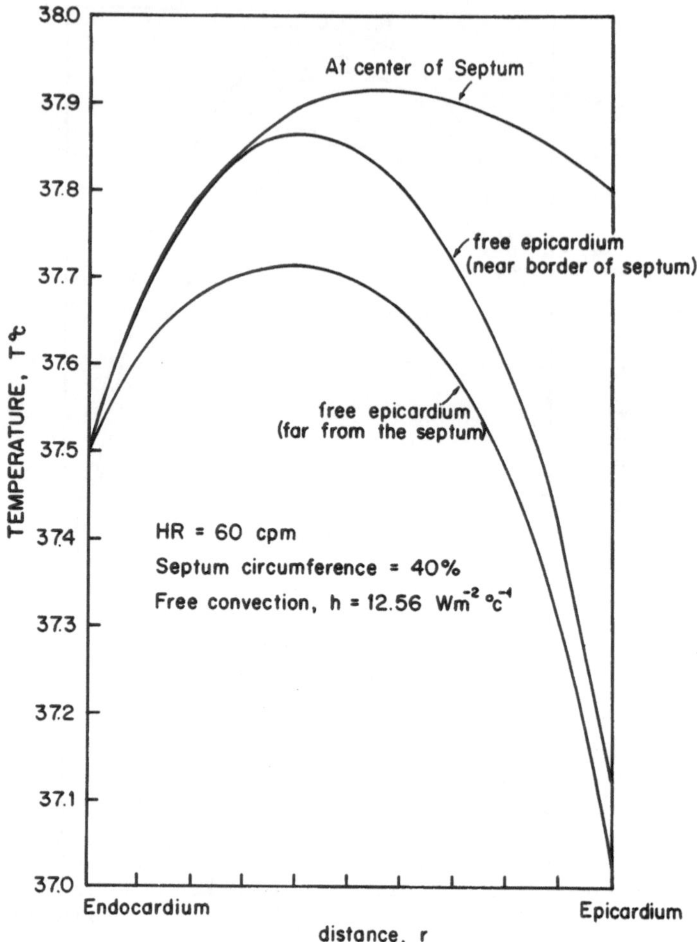

Figure 3. Effect of transmural infarct on the temperature distribution at various circumferential cross-sections.

their function (and flow), the subendocardial ischemia seem to have a negligible effect on the epicardial temperature. This rather surprising result is easily explained by the relative importance of the heat conduction mechanism as compared to the heat removed by convection in the healthy muscle tissue as well as in the infarcted one.

Figure 6 represents the dependence of the temperature on the severity of the transmural ischemia and the associated reduction in perfusion and metabolic heat production. Clearly, a relatively mild ischemia associated with a small reduction in regional oxygen consumption has only a minor effect on the temperature at the epicardium at this region.

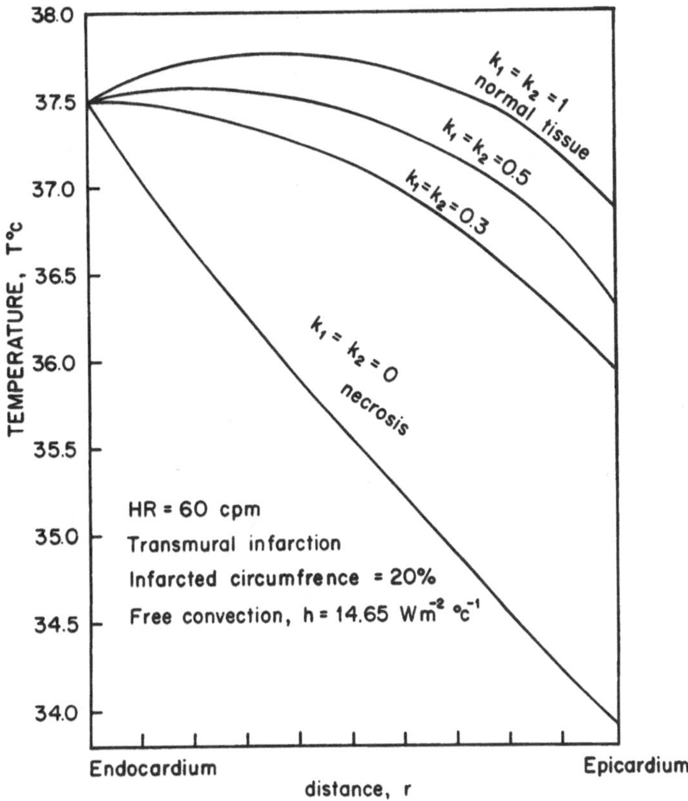

Figure 4. Effect of the depth of the infarcted region on the myocardial temperature distribution.

Discussion

Sensitivity to various parameters

The effect of various parameters on the temperature distribution in the LV myocardium are summarized below:

a. The heart rate strongly affects the temperature distribution within the healthy LV wall (Fig. 2), with higher transmural temperatures at the higher heart rates. As expected, the temperature distribution in the infarcted region does not depend on the heart rate since both the heat production and blood perfusion at the infarcted zone are close to zero and the effect of the adjacent tissues on the infarcted zone is minor.

b. The LV cavity blood temperature, T_b, has almost no effect on the reduced myocardial temperature since changing the blood temperature by ΔT leads to the same change in the muscle temperature.

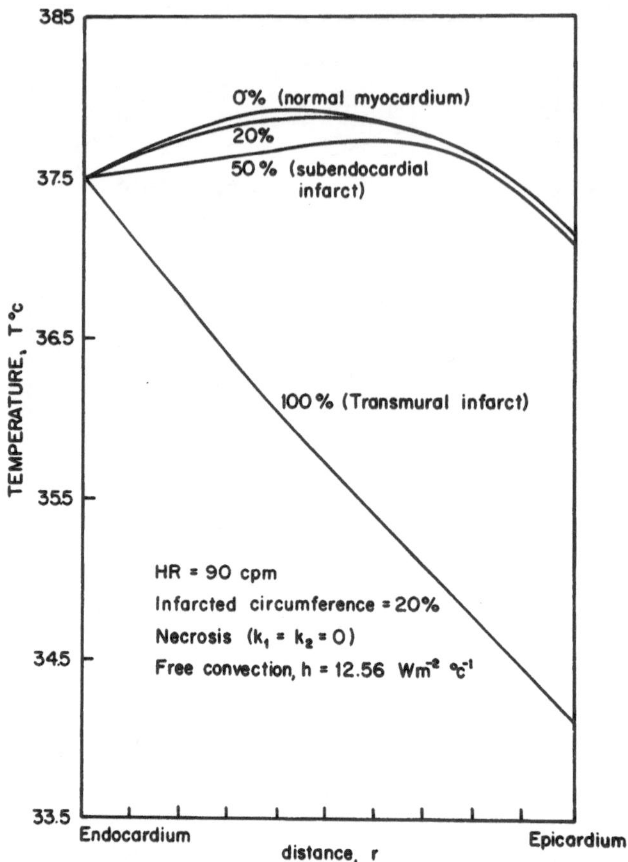

Figure 5. Temperature distribution as a function of the physiological performance of the infarcted area.

c. The RV blood temperature has but little effect on the temperature profile in the free LV wall region, because the RV effects are limited only to the septum.
d. The air temperature u_∞ in the free convection open chest case affects the epicardial temperature in an almost linear manner; a change of 1 °C in u_∞ changes the epicardial temperature by about 0.1 °C.
e. The free convection coefficient, h, affects the epicardial temperature in an almost linear manner. Increasing h by 4.2 W/m^2 °C affects a decrease of 0.1 °C in the epicardial temperature.
f. The severity of the ischemia leading to decreased heart production, as manifested by manipulating the values of k_1 and k_2 in (2) and (3), has a strong effect on the local temperature distribution. However, the effect of the injured region on adjacent regions is minor. Similarly, a subendocardial infarct or ischemia has a minor effect on the epicardial temperature provided that the blood flow in the epicardial muscle, and its function, remain unchanged.

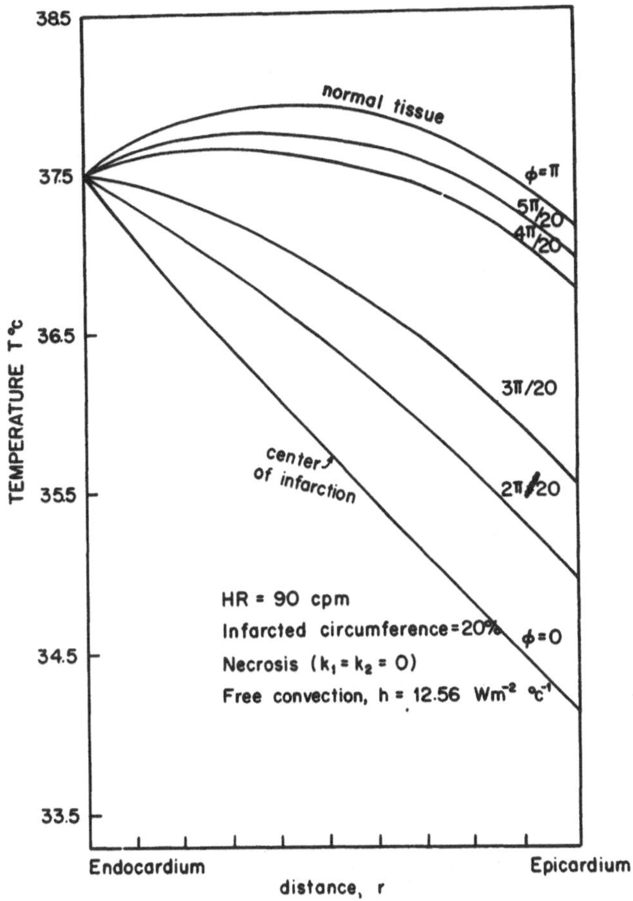

Figure 6. Temperature distribution in the septum and the free LV wall.

Comparisons with experimental results

The temperature distributions for the healthy 'symmetric' heart are consistent with experimental results of ten Velden et al. [9, 10] and Elzinga et al. [1] and are given in detail elsewhere [2]. The data of the LV temperature distribution in an infarcted region are incomplete [1] and thus a direct comparison of our model results is yet impossible. However, the measurement of the epicardial temperatures before, during and post-infarction by the thermal imaging technique described here makes it possible to relate the model predictions to experimental results. A circumferential temperature distribution was combined with circumferential flow distribution, as measured by radioactive microspheres.

The net of measurement points used in this experiment necessitates to define a new numerical net and spoils the compact block tri-diagonal structure of the

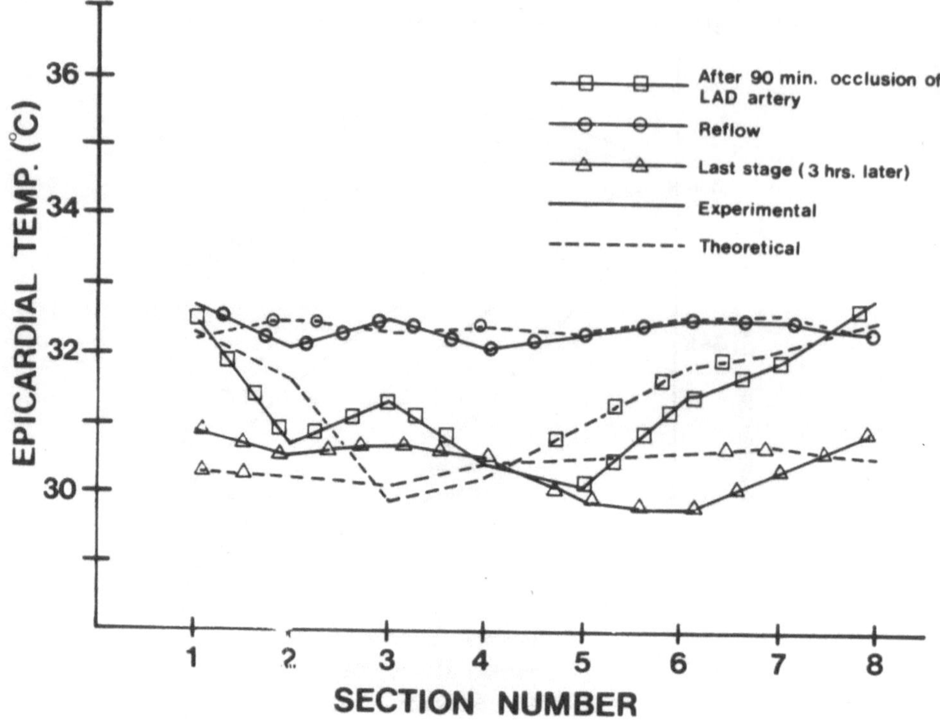

Figure 7. Comparison of theoretical and experimental epicardial temperatures for three different dogs.

system of equations. Here, two blocks are added in both corners of the matrix to the former three diagonals and a new LU factorization algorithm is formulated especially for this structure of the matrix.

The results of the comparison with different canine hearts are shown in Fig. 7, with a fairly good agreement between the model calculations and the measurements.

Conclusions

a. The temperature distribution within the healthy LV wall is characterized by a maximum in the midwall region.
b. The temperature in the infarcted necrotic wall shows a monotonic temperature decrease from the endocardial to the epicardial surfaces.
c. The temperature distribution in an ischemic tissue has an intermediate pattern between healthy and infarcted tissues.
d. The temperature distribution within the wall and at the epicardium is highly dependent on the surrounding conditions like the room temperature and free

heat convection constant, the heart rate, the blood perfusion rate and the metabolic rate.
e. The effect of infarcted tissue on the temperature distribution, although very pronounced locally, do not extend its effect to normal tissues thus demonstrating a narrow border zone and justifying the application of symmetrical models to calculate the temperature distribution in the LV.

Acknowledgment

This study was supported by a grant from Mr. Y. Schneider, Las Vegas, Nevada, USA, and sponsored by the MEP Group, Women's Division, American Technion Society, USA.

References

1. Elzinga G, Ten Velden GHM, Westerhof N (1983): Temperature distribution and transport of heat in the canine myocardium in heart perfusion. In: Dintenfaas DGJ, Seaman GVF (eds) Energetics and ischemia. NATO ASI Series No. 1 62. Plenum Publ Corp, NY, pp. 577–593.
2. Barta E, Beyar R, Sideman S (1985): Temperature distribution within the left ventricular wall of the heart. Int J Heat Mass Transfer 28: 663–673.
3. Barta E, Sideman S, Beyar R (1986): Spatial and temporal temperature distribution in the healthy and locally diseased wall of the heart. Int J Heat Mass Transfer Warren Rohsenow Festschrift 29: 1253–1261.
4. Bowman HF (1985): Estimation of tissue blood flow in heat transfer. In: Shitzer A, Medicine and biology. Eberhart RC (eds) Plenum Press, NY, pp. 193–230.
5. Beyar R, Sideman S (1984): A computer study of the left ventricular performance based on fiber structure, sarcomere dynamics and transmural electrical propagation velocity. Circ Res 55: 358–374.
6. Beyar R, Sideman S (1987): Time dependent coronary blood flow distribution in the left ventricular wall. Am J Physiol Heart 252: H417–H433.
7. Beyar R, Sideman S (1986): Spatial energy balance within a structural model of the left ventricle. Annals Biomed Eng 14: 467–487.
8. Beyar R, Sideman S (1986): Left ventricular mechanics related to the local distribution of oxygen demand throughout the wall. Circ Res 58: 664–677.
9. Hernandez EJ, Hoffman JK, Fabian M, Siegeel JH, Eberhart RC (1979): Thermal quantification of regional myocardial perfusion and heat generation. Am J Physiol 236: 345–355.
10. Neill WA, Krasnow N, Levine HJ, Gorli R (1963): Myocardial anaerobic metabolism in intact dogs. Am J Physiol 204: 427–432.
11. Ten Velden GHM, Elzinga G, Westerhof N (1982): Left ventricular energetics: heat loss and temperature distribution of canine myocardium. Circ Res 50: 63–73.
12. Ten Velden GHM, Westerhof N, Elzinga G (1984): Heat transport in the canine left ventricular wall. Am J Physiol 247 (Heart Circ Physiol 16): H295–302.
13. Westerhof N, Duijst P, Elzinga G, Ten Velden GHM (1987): Relation between transmural temperature, metabolism and coronary blood flow in the canine left ventricle. In: Sideman S, Beyar R (eds) simulation and control of the cardiac system. CRC Press, NY, in press.

Discussion

Clark: Vascularization of the ventricular wall is very seldom uniform and homogeneous. For example, in a relative sense the subendocardial layer of the wall is often generously vascularized compared with the mid and outer layers of the wall. The temperature distribution within the wall will undoubtedly be affected by the vascular distribution pattern. Given such a nonuniform distribution, could this point be easily accounted for in your model?
Barta: We can indeed account for this point, but we did not do it for lack of data to compare to. Other possible changes concern the non-symmetric geometry. It can be done and will be done when more data become available.

Clinical implications

42. Long-term assessment and management of chronic cardiac failure

E.H. SONNENBLICK and T.H. LEJEMTEL

Abstract

In the long-term management of chronic heart failure, the aim is to reduce morbidity and thus, improve quality of life on one hand, while not increasing mortality on the other. Unfortunately, these two end points are not closely related and, indeed, may even be dissociated. Morbidity, while initially caused by limited pump function, depends ultimately on intactness of the peripheral circulation and specific organ function [1]. Pump performance can be altered by either systolic or diastolic dysfunction, or both. Systolic dysfunction can be characterized by a lowered ejection fraction, but this does not correlate with morbidity as characterized by a decrease in exercise duration. Diastolic dysfunction may be characterized by inordinately elevated filling pressures which may result from a thickened left ventricular wall, and/or inordinately delayed ventricular relaxation which interferes with left ventricular filling. Indeed, all of these abnormalities may be combined in these circumstances, while systolic function may be well preserved. Obviously, management is different when systolic function is abnormal than when diastolic function alone is impaired. Mortality provides a very discrete end point and is best predicted by both the reduced level of ventricular performance (ejection-fraction) and the degree of exercise impairment (VO_2-Max).

The initial aims of therapy are to increase cardiac output while lowering ventricular filling pressure acutely. This is generally not associated with an enhancement of maximum exercise performance. Moreover, the acute improvement in pump function does not predict the extent of improvement in exercise performance observed during chronic therapy. Once acute improvement in left ventricular performance has been obtained with either unloading agents, for example, angiotensin converting enzyme inhibitors, or inotropic agents, such as, phosphodiesterase inhibitors, it generally fails to translate immediately into an increase in exercise performance which appears to be limited by inability of the peripheral muscular vasculature to dilate adequately in response to exercise [2, 3]. However, over a period of time that is measured in weeks, with the persistence of hemodynamic improvement, there is a readjustment of the peripheral circulation to allow an improvement in peripheral skeletal muscle blood flow during exercise, and this improvement in skeletal muscle blood flow is the predication upon which improved exercise performance occurs [4]. As a matter of fact, on a chronic basis, improvement in peripheral blood flow and exercise performance may take place *independent* of alterations in left ventricular performance as characterized by the ejection fraction [5].

Accordingly, in the assessment of long term management, one uses indices of exercise performance to judge an improvement in quality of life and this tends to occur in response to either vasodilators or inotropic agents. However, this improvement in exercise performance which also correlates reasonably well with an improved quality of life does not require an improvement in ejection fraction, and indeed, the ejection fraction may stay the same or fall, while improvement in exercise performance is sustained. In contrast, long-term survival appears to correlate with the ejection fraction, independently of what happens to quality of life. Thus, there is a great discrepancy in the long term outcome of therapy, in that quality of life may be enhanced by an improvement in the peripheral circulation while duration of life remains limited by the persistence of the primary cardiac damage and a persistently lowered ejection fraction [6].

The long term aims of therapy may well be different, depending on the stage of the disease. With mild cardiac dysfunction and reasonably intact myocardium, the long term aim should be preservation of myocardial tissue since this may significantly impact on patient survival. Once substantial myocardial destruction has already occurred with tissue loss, fibrosis, and severe reactive hypertrophy, therapy is essentially palliative, and combinations of vasodilators, and when needed, inotropic agents, offers one approach to the optimal improvement of quality of life. Current data would not support the view that very substantial improvement in prolonging life can be obtained. However, such palliative cardiac therapy may stabilize a rapidly deteriorating process and therefore, reduce mortality for a limited period of time.

At earlier stages and with milder disease, vasodilators may be of help by producing a sustained reduction in cardiac size and central congestion, which may positively effect the progression of the disease. On the other hand, protection of the myocardial tissue with calcium channel antagonists and/or β-blocking agents may potentially produce greater therapeutic benefits than that of vasodilators. This remains to be evaluated.

References

1. Mancini DM, LeJemtel TH, Factor S, Sonnenblick EH (1986): Central and peripheral components of cardiac failure. Am J Med 80 (Suppl 2B): 2–13.
2. Kugler J, Maskin C, Frishman WH, Sonnenblick EH, LeJemtel TH (1982): Regional and systemic metabolic effects of angiotensin-converting enzyme inhibition during exercise in patients with severe heart failure. Circulation 66: 1256–1261.
3. LeJemtel TH, Maskin CS, Mancini D, Sinoway L, Feld H, Chadwick B (1985): Systemic and regional hemodynamic effects of captopril and milrinone administered alone and concomitantly in patients with heart failure. Circulation 72: 364–369.
4. Mancini D, Davis L, Wexler JP, Chadwick B, LeJemtel TH (1984): Long-term therapy with captopril improves maximal oxygen uptake by increasing skeletal muscle blood flow in patients with heart failure. Circulation 70 (4): 11–1983.
5. Maskin CS, Forman R, Klein NA, Sonnenblick EH, LeJemtel TH (1982): Long-term amrinone therapy in patients with severe heart failure. Am J Med 72: 113–118.
6. LeJemtel TH, Sonnenblick EH (1984): Should the failing heart be stimulated? New Engl J Med 310: 1384–1385.

Discussion

Palsson: You were talking about reduced cardiac output, but you did not see any reduction in the oxygen uptake . . . I wonder if the oxygen transport characteristic of the red cell may be adapting to the diseased state. Namely, do you have evidence for a shift in the hemoglobin binding curve?
Sonnenblick: The maximum oxygen uptake is substantially limited in heart failure relative to the normal individual. Whether there is a shift in the Hg dissociation curve is not clear, an increase in oxygen extraction does occur.
Palsson: The red cells may have the ability to adapt by changing the concentration of 2,3-DPG and producing a right shift in the oxygen curve.
Sonnenblick: It may contribute but it will not give you that much more oxygen.
Weiss: I would like to ask about the α-receptor blocking experiments. Have you ever tried local α-blockades, on the assumption that perhaps the general blockades would be so severe that there was no possibility for cardiac output buildup?
Sonnenblick: Local blockade was the approach used by Dr T. LeJemtel.
Baan: Maybe I misunderstood but in your studies you saw quite an increase in cardiac output. Where does it go if it does not go to the muscles?
Sonnenblick: In our opinion, there is no acute improvement in maximal exercise performance with any medication but some increase in sub-maximal performance may occur. With dobutamine, some increase in flow goes to the skin and the gut. With captopril, the increase in flow goes to the kidney. Improvement in the muscle blood flow does occur acutely with phosphodiesterase inhibitors such as milruione, and modest improvement in exercise tolerance can be seen early.
Spaan: How much does the improvement of the muscular peripheral circulation improve the performance of the heart? Is it a drawback to the improvement of the heart by exercise?
Sonnenblick: It is not necessarily a drawback, but there is an elemant of disappointment which reflects ventricular performance. The ejection fraction correlates very well with the long-term survival. Unfortunately, in severe, late failure we fail to see an improvement in the ejection fraction, despite improvement in exercise performance. Thus symptoms are ameliorated while the basic function of the heart, namely the ejection fraction is not improving but may even be getting worse.
Lab: If you were able to halt or reverse the functional deterioration of the heart, then presumably, chronically, the whole system will reverse itself. In other words the patient will get better.
Sonnenblick: That would theoretically be true but unfortunately most of the forms of heart failure are not highly reversible. In a sense a massive myocardial infarction creates a work overload associated with a reactive hypertrophy of the remaining normal muscle. Were the reactive hypertrophy controlled and volume remodelling of the wall prevented, progression might be altered.
Kostis: The problem starts with the heart. If you take care of the heart, would the periphery adapt itself?

Sonnenblick: I believe that you can manipulate and improve the periphery without much effect on the heart. Improvement in symptoms is predicated largely not by an alteration of what the heart does, but by enhanced muscle flow delivery (i.e., recapacity to dialate the periphery). Thus symptomatic improvement is independent of any improvement of the cardiac function, although the cardiac output remains a limiting factor. What leads to that initial abnormality? This tremendous discrepancy in terms of exercise performance is still in the limitation of peripheral blood flow. The cause of the normal extent of peripheral dilatation and sustained arteriolar vascular resistance in heart failure remains unclear. The increased sodium content in the peripheral vascular bed may lead to the swelling of the endothelial cells, associated with a decrease in capacity to dialate. The mechanism does not appear to be neurogenic.

Lab: Is there a case for natural hormone here?

Sonnenblick: A role for ANF has not been established.

Gallagher: What happens to peripheral vascular control if you put 'a new engine' in?

Sonnenblick: Improvement in exercise still requires time and the adaptation requires weeks to occur. It is an interesting question that deserves further study.

43. Acute and chronic cardiac failure: the oxygen transport system gone awry

K.T. WEBER and J.S. JANICKI

Abstract

The cardiopulmonary unit is the body's oxygen transport system which links the metabolizing tissues to the atmosphere and its supply of oxygen. As an obligate aerobic organism, man is critically dependent on this metabolic unit to sustain oxidative metabolism and life itself.

Cardiac disease which may lead to an acute and/or chronic failure of the heart to supply the tissues with oxygen at a rate which is commensurate with their aerobic requirements, disrupts the functional integrity of the cardiopulmonary unit. In understanding the concepts of oxygen transport one has a means to better understand the evaluation and management of the patient with cardiac failure, as well as to characterize the pathophysiologic behavior of the oxygen transport system that has gone awry.

Introduction

Oxidative metabolism is the principal source of energy for the body to maintain its various biologic functions. The human body therefore is an obligate aerobic organism. As a result, its metabolizing cells must not only be linked to the atmosphere and its source of oxygen, but oxygen must be delivered to the cells at a rate which is commensurate with their aerobic requirements. The heart, lungs and circulation, together with hemoglobin, function as the body's oxygen transport system. This Symposium has focused principally on the heart and its electrical and mechanical characteristics. Specific disorders in cardiac rhythm and myocardial perfusion have been considered in the context that they disrupt the orderly process of muscle contraction. From a broader clinical perspective, diseases of the heart interfere with the integrity and functional integration of the heart and lungs which form the cardiopulmonary unit, responsible for subserving the body's requirements for oxygen. In health as well as in disease it is the cardiopulmonary unit that will guarantee that the body's obligatory dependence on oxidative metabolism is satisfied. Whenever the heart falters and does not sustain oxygen delivery, it has failed its purpose. Acute and chronic cardiac failure represent circumstances where the oxygen transport system has gone awry. The purpose of this report will be to consider each of these broad clinical entities and how their accompanying pathophysiologic features compromise the inter-relationship and the interdependence that exists between the cardiopulmonary unit and the metabolizing tissues. We begin by first examining man's oxygen requirements.

Mammalian oxygen requirements and oxygen transport

The methods for obtaining oxygen were altered as animal life evolved from an aquatic to a terrestrial existence [1]. Oxygen could no longer be obtained from water; instead, it had to be derived from the atmosphere. The pattern of respiration also had to be altered. At the same time, the overall need for oxygen was increased as land-living animals became warm blooded. The mobility of land-living mammals depended on their ability to perform muscular work and the energy required to do so was derived from oxidative sources. An oxygen transport system evolved to meet these enhanced oxygen requirements; a system which could both provide oxygen at a rate commensurate with the aerobic requirements of the tissues and which could do so on a moment to moment basis. The cardiopulmonary unit serves this purpose.

The oxygen requirements of mammals are considerable and mandate that not only is their cardiac output and minute ventilation much larger than those of fish [1], but that their tissues' need for oxygen controls the performance of the heart and the lungs. The precise nature of the control logic for the oxygen transport system remains to be elucidated, but input signals appear to arise from a variety of sources, including skeletal muscle, the sympathetic nervous system, and the cardiovascular, respiratory and central nervous systems.

Table 1 depicts the oxygen requirements for the body's various organs as well as the oxygen they extract and the proportion of the cardiac output they receive in sustaining their oxidative metabolism [2]. Overall, the body receives more oxygen each minute than its organs' require. Moreover, blood flow distribution bears little relationship to the oxygen requirements of these organs. The kidneys exemplify this dicotomy in that the portion of the cardiac output they receive, and thereby the oxygen delivered, is not proportional to their oxygen uptake. The function of the kidneys in maintaining the osmotic pressure of the extracellular space supercedes its need for oxygen. A high glomerular filtration rate has a greater priority than the oxygen utilized by the kidney and thus renal blood flow represents 20% of systemic blood flow.

At rest, the human body consumes approximately 3.5 ml/min/kg of oxygen.

This level of oxygen uptake ($\dot{V}O_2$), which for an averaged sized individual equals 250 ml/min, requires that the lungs bring 8 to 10 l/min of fresh air into the lungs each minute and that the heart circulates 4 to 6 l/min of blood through the lungs and to the tissues each minute. From the arterial blood the tissues extract a portion of the oxygen they receive (see Table 1). The oxygen delivered to the tissues each minute can be calculated from the product of the cardiac output and the arterial oxygen content, where oxygen content is equal to the concentration of hemoglobin, its percent saturation and the oxygen combining capacity of the blood [2]. For a cardiac output of 5 l/min and an average arterial oxygen content of 19 ml/dl (i.e., 14 g hemoglobin/dl × 0.96 × 1.34 ml/g), the tissues receive 950 ml of oxygen each minute. Thus, oxygen delivery is normally four times greater than the prevailing oxygen requirements and as a result overall tissue oxygen extraction need only be 25% (Table 1).

With muscular work cardiac output and minute ventilation each rise in proportion to the prevailing $\dot{V}O_2$. Ventilation can normally increase 8 to 10 fold above its resting level to preserve oxyhemoglobin saturation and arterial oxygen content even in the face of heavy muscular work. Hence, ventilation normally poses no limitation to performing aerobic work. In untrained individuals cardiac output increases but 4 to 5 fold above its resting level and therefore it is the limit of the heart's ability to raise oxygen delivery that determines the body's aerobic capacity.

In physiologic terms, heart failure may be defined as that circumstance in which the heart is unable to provide the metabolizing tissues with oxygen at a rate which is in keeping with their aerobic requirements [3]. *Cardiac* failure refers to disorders of the myocardium that account for this defect in pump function while

Table 1. Oxygen utilization, transport, and extraction in normal human subjects at rest.

	Blood flow		Arterio-venous O_2 difference (ml/dl)	O_2 extraction[a] (%)	O_2 uptake		
	(l/min)	(% total)			(ml/min)	(ml/min/ 100 g)	(% total)
Viscera	1.40	24	4.1	21	58	2.3	25
Skeletal muscle	1.20	21	8.0	41	70	0.2	30
Kidneys	1.10	19	1.3	7	16	5.3	7
Brain	0.75	13	6.3	31	46	3.1	20
Skin	0.50	8	1.0	5	5	0.2	2
Other organs	0.60	10	3.0	15	12	-	5
Heart	0.25	3	11.4	59	27	9.0	11
Overall	5.80	-	4.0	25	234	3.5	-

[a] Using assumed arterial O_2 content of 19.4 vols % and body surface area of 1.75 m^2 (taken from [2] with permission).

circulatory failure relates to disorders extrinsic to the myocardium which compromise resting and exercise cardiac output. Acute cardiac failure is present when there is an abrupt reduction in oxygen delivery (e.g., acute myocardial infarction). In chronic cardiac failure, the severity of the impairment in oxygen delivery relative to prevailing oxygen requirements will determine the severity of failure. With a severe reduction in cardiac output, the body's $\dot{V}O_2$ at rest may not be satisified. Less severe expressions of disease require the physiologic stress of exercise and the increased $\dot{V}O_2$ attendant with muscular work to elicit this defect in oxygen delivery. Hence, chronic cardiac failure may be characterized as mild, moderate or severe depending on the level of muscular work which is required to elicit this defect in oxygen supply and demand. The clinical syndrome of congestive heart failure need not be present even though the patient has chronic cardiac failure [4]. Congestive heart failure represents a constellation of signs and symptoms that arise from hypoperfused tissues and congested organs and which is mediated by salt avid kidneys, expanded intravascular and extravascular volumes, and by the activation of the neurohumoral system (e.g., the adrenergic and renin-angiotensin systems).

Acute cardiac failure

Acute cardiac failure is most commonly seen following an acute myocardial infarction, with an exacerbation of chronic cardiac failure, or following open heart surgery. The one characteristic that is common to each state is the reduction in systemic blood flow. As cardiac output falls, metabolizing tissues extract greater quantities of oxygen to sustain oxygen availability. One can simultaneously estimate the severity of failure, the reduction in cardiac output, and the elevation in oxygen extraction by monitoring the oxygen saturation of the mixed venous blood found in the pulmonary artery [3]. Because the amount of hemoglobin in venous and arterial blood is the same, the amount of oxygen leaving the capillaries is represented by the oxygen saturation of venous blood. In operating on the steep portion of the oxyhemoglobin dissociation curve, the oxygen saturation of mixed venous blood is a sensitive indicator of oxygen availability in patients with acute heart failure. Hence, oxygen saturation in the pulmonary artery can be used to estimate systemic blood flow and systemic oxygen extraction. Figure 1 depicts the relationship between cardiac output and mixed venous oxygen saturation. It can be seen that as cardiac index falls, so does oxygen saturation indicating the greater extraction of oxygen which has occurred within the tissues. Figure 2 depicts the relationship between systemic arteriovenous oxygen difference and mixed venous oxygen saturation.

The ability of the tissues to extract more oxygen in the face of declining oxygen delivery serves as the cell's reserve in oxygen availability. Anaerobic sources of energy are not utilized until systemic oxygen extraction approaches 60% or more.

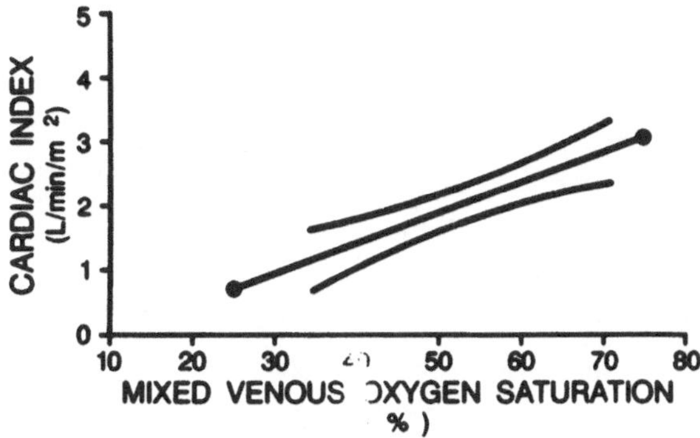

Figure 1. The relationship between cardiac index and mixed venous oxygen saturation in the pulmonary artery. Reproduced from [3] with permission.

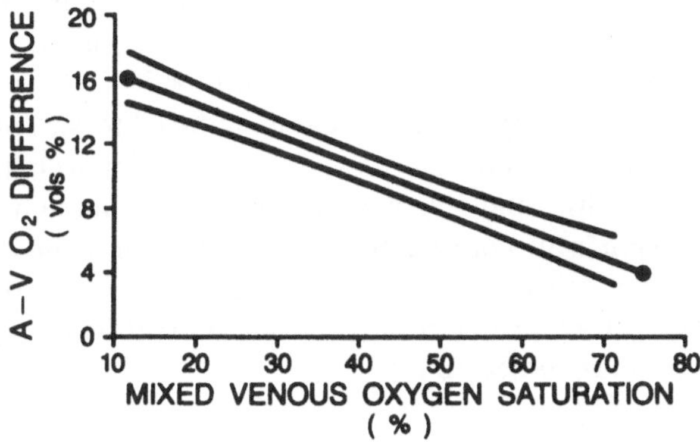

Figure 2. The relationship between systemic arteriovenous (A–V) oxygen difference and mixed venous oxygen saturation. Reproduced from [3] with permission.

Thus, oxidative metabolism is sustained until the cardiac output has fallen rather markedly. Lactate production, heralding the onset of anaerobiosis occurs when the mixed venous oxygen saturation is <40% corresponding to systemic blood flow of approximately <1.5 l/min/m^2 or less.

Other hemodynamic features of acute cardiac failure include an elevated left ventricular filling pressure, generally >15 mm Hg, an elevated systemic vascular resistance of >1600 dynes · sec · cm^{-5}, and a mean arterial pressure of 70–80 mm Hg. Right atrial pressure may or may not be elevated above normal (>5 mm Hg) depending on the state of the right heart, intravascular volume, and pulmonary vascular resistance.

The treatment of acute cardiac failure focuses on raising cardiac output and thereby oxygen delivery [3]. A reasonable therapeutic target for most patients is to raise cardiac index to 2 l/min/m^2 or more. For an averaged sized individual this

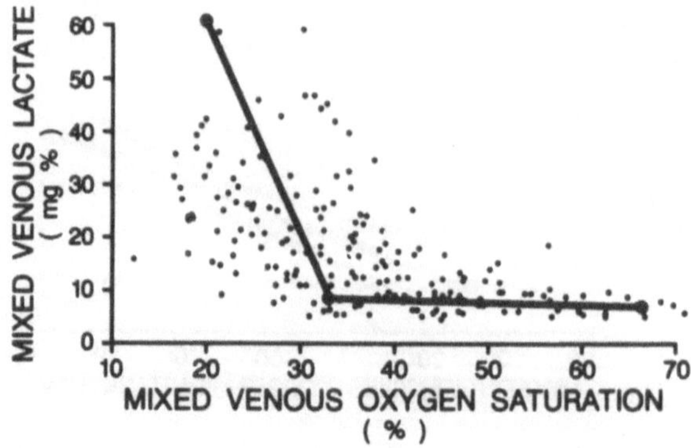

Figure 3. The relationship between lactate concentration of mixed venous blood and its oxygen saturation. Reproduced from [3] with permission.

amounts to a systemic blood flow of 3.5 l/min and an oxygen delivery of 500 ml/min or more. Under these conditions mixed venous oxygen saturation will rise to >50% and systemic oxygen extraction will fall to <50%. Left ventricular and thereby pulmonary venous pressure should be reduced to <20 mm Hg to alleviate pulmonary congestion and any oxygen transfer abnormality that may be attendant with interstitial and alveolar edema. In a certain number of patients, systemic hypotension is also present to further confound tissue oxygen delivery. Under these circumstances, pharmacologic agents which promote arteriolar vasoconstriction, restore mean arterial pressure, and preserve oxygen delivery to the heart and brain are indicated [3].

Chronic cardiac failure

In chronic cardiac failure, cardiac output is also reduced oftentimes to levels seen with acute heart failure. The chronic hypoperfusion state, however, is accompanied by enhanced tissue oxygen extraction and compensatory responses within the peripheral circulation, neurohumoral system, and intravascular space which permit the patient to adjust to the low flow state. Because of these compensatory responses from compartments outside the heart, parameters of cardiac performance such as the cardiac output, left ventricular filling pressure, ejection fraction or heart size, may not be distinguishable between patients at rest having severe versus milder expressions of cardiac failure [4]. In order to bring out differences in cardiac performance and to estimate the severity of chronic cardiac failure we utilize incremental muscular work to progressively raise O_2 requirements and which provides a physiologic stress. We specifically determine the impairment in aerobic capacity, measured from the noninvasive monitoring of breath-by-breath respiratory gas exchange, as an index of cardiocirculatory reserve [4]. The

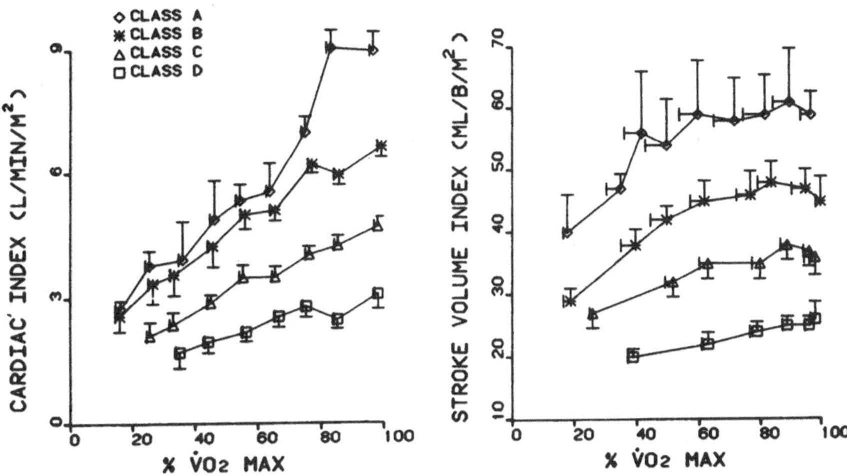

Figure 4. The cardiac index and stroke volume index response to incremental treadmill exercise is shown for each functional class with chronic cardiac failure and as a function of normalized aerobic capacity (% $\dot{V}O_2$ max). Reproduced from [4] with permission.

maximal oxygen uptake, or plateau in $\dot{V}O_2$ seen during incremental treadmill exercise ($\dot{V}O_2$ max), is used to grade the severity of chronic cardiac failure as follows [2, 4]: little or no failure is present when $\dot{V}O_2$ max is >20 ml/min/kg, which we term class A; mild to moderate failure is present when $\dot{V}O_2$ max falls between 16 and 20 ml/min/kg (class B); moderate to severe failure exists if the $\dot{V}O_2$ max is 10 to 16 ml/min/kg (class C); and severe failure is represented by a $\dot{V}O_2$ max of <10 ml/min/kg (class D). The maximum exercise cardiac index and stroke volume index which are seen in these different classes are shown in Figure 4. Maximum cardiac index averages >8, 6–8, 4–6 and <4 l/min/m² for class A, B, C and D patients, respectively. Thus, the noninvasive determination of $\dot{V}O_2$ max also predicts the cardiac reserve. It should be apparent that the stroke volume response to exercise is lost in class D patients; they have no pumping reserve.

Studies of systemic oxygen extraction performed in our laboratory during incremental treadmill exercise do not indicate that there is an abnormality in the ability of the tissues, specifically muscle, to extract oxygen. Systemic oxygen extraction rises to values in excess of 70%. Figure 5 depicts the response in mixed venous oxygen saturation and systemic oxygen extraction to graded treadmill exercise in classes A to D.

Anaerobiosis with lactate production occurs during exercise at different levels of muscular work for each exercise class based on their impairment in oxygen delivery. Figure 6 indicates that mixed venous lactate concentration exceeds 12 mg% (2 SD above the normal resting value for this laboratory) when $\dot{V}O_2$ is <8, 8–11, 11–14 and >14 ml/min/kg in class D, C, B, and A patients, respectively. The appearance of lactate production can be detected noninvasively from the

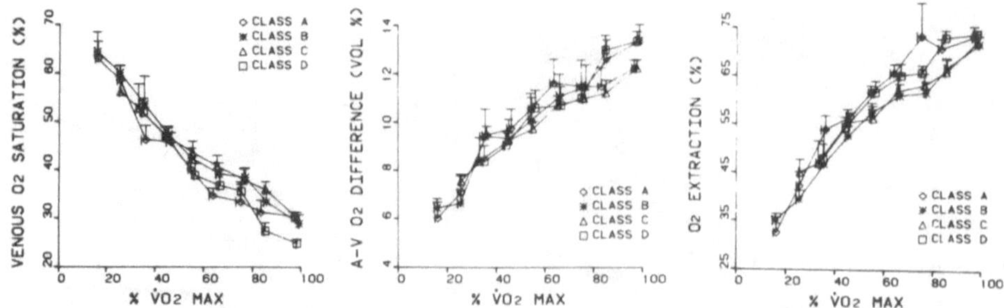

Figure 5. The response in mixed venous oxygen saturation, systemic arteriovenous (A-V) oxygen difference, and in systemic oxygen extraction (i.e., the ratio of AV oxygen difference to arterial oxygen content) to incremental treadmill exercise for the four exercise classes. The percent of maximal oxygen uptake (% $\dot{V}O_2$ max) which each level of work represents is indicated. Reproduced from [4] with permission.

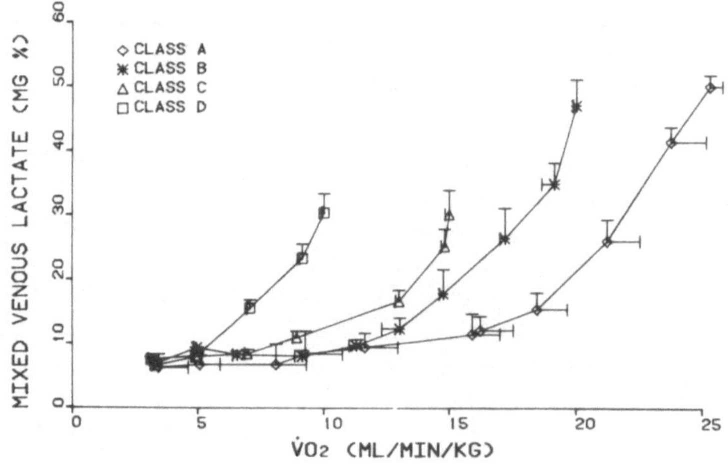

Figure 6. The response in mixed venous lactate concentration to incremental treadmill exercise and oxygen uptake ($\dot{V}O_2$) is shown for each functional class. Lactate production is present when lactate concentration exceeds 12 mg%. Reproduced from [4] with permission.

response in respiratory gas exchange as previously reported [2, 4]. Thus, as is the case for acute heart failure, concepts of oxygen transport are applicable to a better understanding of chronic cardiac failure which arise as a result of ischemic or myopathic heart disease.

The treatment of chronic cardiac failure is focused on improving the systolic performance of the failing heart, particularly during physical activity. In particular, a sensible target is to raise resting cardiac index by 30% to 35%. In addition, however, and quite distinct from the bedridden, hospitalized patient with acute cardiac failure, the central issue for the ambulatory patient with chronic cardiac

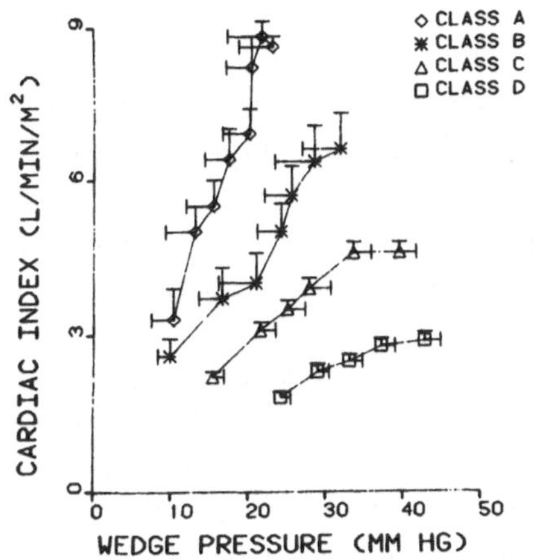

Figure 7. The relationship between cardiac index and left ventricular filling, or wedge, pressure to incremental treadmill exercise is shown for each functional class. Reproduced from [4] with permission.

failure is focused on where the enhanced systemic blood flow should be directed. The answer of course is to the metabolizing tissues in accordance with their aerobic requirements. To divert blood flow and oxygen to less metabolically active tissues is wasteful and counterproductive. Chronic elevations in left ventricular filling pressure to >20 mm Hg are present at rest and particularly during physical activity (see Figure 7). Nevertheless, these patients do not experience arterial oxygen desaturation with exercise [5]. Treatment should be focused on reducing the resting filling pressure by 30% or more and attenuating the rise in filling pressure during exercise.

References

1. Harris P (1983): Evolution of the cardiac patient. Cardiovasc Res 17: 315–319.
2. Weber KT, Janicki JS (eds) (1986): Cardiopulmonary exercise testing: physiologic principles and clinical applications. WB Saunders, Philadelphia.
3. Weber KT, Janicki JS, Maskin CS (1985): Pathophysiology of cardiac failure. Am J Cardiol 56: 3B–7B.
4. Weber KT, Janicki JS (1985): Cardiopulmonary exercise testing for evaluation of chronic cardiac failure. Am J Cardiol 55: 22A–31A.
5. Rubin SA, Brown HV, Swan HJC (1982): Arterial oxygenation and arterial oxygen transport in chronic myocardial failure at rest, during exercise and after hydralazine treatment. Circulation 66: 143–148.

Discussion

Sonnenblick: You subtly equate cardiac index to contractility but ejection fraction is more adequate to describe contractility, and cardiac index is not equal to ejection fraction.
Weber: I have not equated contractility with the cardiac index; I would even question whether the ejection fraction is an index of contractility in view of its dependence on loading.
Sonnenblick: We as well as others have shown that ejection fraction does not correlate at all with exercise performance. A major limitation to exercise in heart failure is an inability to supply oxygen to the exercising muscles. In the process of severe peripheral vascular desease the inability to exercise is due to malfunction of the arteries which deliver oxygen to the exercising muscles and not to a fixed increase in cardiac output.
Weber: Blood and O_2 will not get to the given organ, such as the working limb, because of various causes of circulatory failure (hypervolemia, anemia, mitral or aortic valve stenosis) or because of myocardial failure. I have focused only on cardiac or myocardial failure and the impairment in oxygen delivery. Several studies have shown that even when cardiac output is raised pharmacologically, there may be a redistribution of blood flow and therefore no change in O_2 delivery to the limb. On the other hand, certain drugs have been shown to acutely raise oxygen delivery to the working limb and to lower its rate of lactate production. In a study conducted in your laboratory by Siskind, it was shown that it was possible to delay the onset of lactate production when the cardiac output was raised with a drug that was a bipyridine derivative. We have also shown this to be true for this inotropic agent. There is a delicate balance between the heart's performance and the periphery, and this varies from patient to patient. Nevertheless, cardiac output is the major determinant of O_2 delivery. In the case of the peripheral circulation, we may also have contrasting or counter opposing effects during exercise. On the one hand, for example, we have a distended left atrium which leads to the release of atrial natriuretic factor which leads to vasodilatation of the renal circulation. On the other hand, and at the same time, we release norepinephrine into the circulation during exercise and this will promote renal vasoconstriction. These are contrasting effects and we do not know which is activated more than the other. We need more studies to address this issue. It is my view that while regional differences in blood flow and O_2 extraction occur to limit the aerobic capacity of the limb, cardiac output is the major factor responsible for this impairment.
Spaan: If you have pulmonary problems, will your analysis work?
Weber: This is beyond the intended scope of this presentation. However, we can summarize it briefly here. A patient with lung disease utilizes the majority of their ventilatory reserve with exercise. If you determine the maximum voluntary ventilation, you have some idea of this reserve. How much of this reserve do you

use in exercise? If you are normal or if you have heart failure, you use less than 50%. If you have primary ventilatory impariment, you use more than 50% of this reserve. Another point: you develop arterial oxygen desaturation more frequently in ventilatory disease, but not in heart failure. Next, your ability to reach the anaerobic threshold and a plateau in maximum oxygen uptake is generally prohibited in the ventilatory group, but not the cardiac patient. With these three criteria you can separate the ventilatory from the circulatory cases of dyspnea.

Beyar: If you have a cathetar in the coronary sinus measuring PO_2 and lactate production, you can evaluate the differential effect of the periphery and the heart.

Weber: We always wanted to place a catheter in the coronary sinus and exercise our patients to assess the heart's metabolic reserve, but the sinus catheter is a little stiff and may perforate the coronary sinus. So we have looked at using other forms of stress in a supine patient, at rest. Certainly, the metabolic reserve of these hearts, what we called 'the aerobic limit' of these hearts, may in fact be a major issue which leads to the inappropriate cardiac output response. Moreover, Dr Janicki has shown that the right atrium and the wedge pressure track one another in class D patients which suggests that the pericardium may also contribute to the abnormal exercise in stroke volume. Why does the ejection fraction (EF) not relate to aerobic capacity? I cannot say. We have also reported on this disparity. Perhaps it is related to the fact that we cannot predict who is going to develop a segmental wall motion abnormality or mitral regurgitation during exercise. Such an event can lead to a disparity between EF and maximum $\dot{V}O_2$ uptake.

LeJemtel: You are saying that the cardiac efficiency is the limitation but it is not. If you implant a new heart, it would take the patient two months to regain a $\dot{V}O_2$ above 25 ml/kg · min.

Weber: The cardiac output response to exercise is a major problem. You will agree that the problem starts with the heart. Congestive heart failure is a symdrome or constellation of signs and symptoms that arise from hypoperfused tissues and congested organs. The periphery, the kidney, and the lungs all participate in producing congestive heart failure. We can transplant the pump but it will take a certain time to change the periphery, the renal circulation, the neurohumoral system, etc. All are important. In addition and with the transplant, we have a dennervated heart, I am just trying to emphasize the important factor which relates to the inability of the heart to raise the cardiac output adequately with exercise. I do not see an essential disagreement.

Kostis: The disagreement is on how many variables come into play. Why the same LV disfunction does not always cause the same decrease in cardiac output and why the same decrease in cardiac output does not cause the same decrease in renal or muscle flow.

Sonnenblick: The transmission between the engine (heart) and the wheels (circulation) is complex and this is what becomes disordered.

Weber: But what will happen under exercise?

General discussion

44. Interactions: mechanics, metabolism and perfusion

MODERATOR: H. WEISS

Weiss: I would like to comment about mechanics, oxygen consumption and cardiac metabolism during infarction or ischemia. It's clear that the myocardial response to a reduction in blood flow is a loss of mechanical function and a decrease in oxygen consumption. I have studied this problem for many years, as have many other people. It is clear that during coronary artery blockage there is a large rapid drop in oxygen consumption and many changes within the cell such as loss of high energy phosphates. Because the matabolic rate drops to 20% of the control, the mechanical function also stops. Dr Gallagher and Dr Li have shown the loss of mechanical function within the area of ischemia and pointed out again the very sharp mechanical disfunction which seems to be coupled with very sharp differences in metabolism. One of the aspects of this is in alterations of lipid metabolism and mechanical properties. It would be very useful to couple those. We have been measuring oxygen consumption in the ischemic zone for many years and it would be interesting to see what happens to myocardial efficienty. Maybe not in the center, but in less ischemic tissue there are probably going to be large changes in the mechanical efficiency or in oxygen cost of doing work. This has not been extensively studied. Finally there have been several studies, of Perl and others, trying to model the mechanical aspects of ischemia. These can, if they pose experimental questions, be extremely useful for the experimentalists. It is my hope that this interaction of metabolic rate, local metabolic factors within the heart, the mechanical events, efficiency and modeling will eventually lead to some synthesis which gives a better understanding of what is occurring within the ischemic zone.

Klocke: In relation to perfusion, two points may be worthy of continued discussion. The first concerns our understanding of autoregulation. A number of laboratories have now demonstrated that autoregulation can be modulated importantly by factors not previously considered in detail. We used to say that when flow was reduced below resting levels by coronary arterial constriction, the flow reduction began only after the distal bed was maximally vasodilated. It is now clear this is not always true. Dr Weiss and others have elegantly demonstrated that metabolic influences are not always overriding in autoregulation. I would identify factors modulating (or potentially modulating) autoregulation as an area needing further attention.

My second point concerns chronic rather than acute responses to interventions which can limit flow. Chronic models of some of the pathophysiologic states that we are studying, e.g., coronary stenosis, need to be developed. I have an open mind as to the possibility that adaptations of the sort that Dr Sonnenblick suggested earlier in the peripheral circulation may occur in the heart as well.

Gallagher: In line with what Dr Klocke has just mentioned, I suggest that another area that has not received sufficient investigation is control of blood flow to the right ventricle. The issue was raised briefly during Dr Hoffman's presentation on how coronary blood flow on the right side of the heart is controlled but as far as I can tell there really is not any resolution to the question. There are a few reports suggesting that autoregulation, as seen on the left side of the heart, does not occur in the right ventricle, and that the response of the right ventricular vasculature to different pharmacologic agents and possibly nerve simulation is also different. This is a potentially wide open area for investigation.

Sideman: The interactions between the right and left sides should definitely be related. I am sure that much work is being done, and we have heard more than one related presentation here. Dr Barta's presentation was briefly concerned with the effect of the right ventricular temperature on the left ventricular muscle. These interactions are definitely to be tackled in force and, hopefully, we will do it in the future.

Spaan: I would like to make a comment on coronary perfusion. It is clear that if you determine the time constant from the venous side of the circulation you find it to be larger than if you determine the time constant from the arterial side. This means that if one tries to estimate, from experiments, the myocardial compliance from the arterial side one finds it one order of magnitude lower than if you do it from the venous side. It seems that there is a discrepancy that has to be understood one way or the other. Some work on that has to be done in the coming years.

Beyar: I would like to come back again to hypertrophy and the subendocardial layers under conditions of hypoxia. We would like to know what is the relationship between the stress developed within a certain layer in the LV wall, the oxygen demand and the possible diminished supply. What are the mechanical parameters which govern the development of cardiac fiber force under limited oxygen supply? There is probably a very complex relationship. Is the tension that each fiber develops during ischemia proportional to its local flow, consistant with experiments that show a linear relationship between the flow and the tension which develops in the muscles? Or is it a much more complex relationship which relates to other numerous metabolic factors?

45. Relating models to experiments

MODERATOR: S. SIDEMAN

Sideman: It is important to emphasize that modeling and simulation are not, and should never be, the ultimate goal of our efforts. In its best expression, a simulation model should reflect clinical and other basic physiological data and, by the power of logic, mathematics and computers, allow us to gain insight into the multivariable, multi-parameter, complex system under study. 'Modeling' is a normal thought-process in which we use some facts and a few assumption to evaluate a certain phenomenon and predict some characteristic trends of the system. Since the physiological data which serve to validate our models are independent of our stipulations, we face the danger of believing and validating our assumptions by relying on the sometimes fortunate agreement between facts and model predictions. It is obviously adviceable to follow Albert Einstein's statement that the best model has the least number of assumptions and the most experimental confirmations. As we can only approach this ideal, one has to view the 'confirmed' concepts and assumptions, based on 'general agreement with data', with the proper measure of respect and suspicion.

Perfection notwithstanding, the sheer act of constructing a model propagates new concepts which, when proven true, elucidate and highlight part of the complex physiological system. Not least important, it provides guidelines for the design of experimental work, and the marriage of a good theoretical analysis with reliable experimental data is certainly a winning union which promises some healthy and continuously productive offsprings. This is the challenge which this gathering of cardiac clinicians, physiologists, engineers, biophysicists and mathematicians is called to face.

Hoffman: One point that I would like to make concerns the uniqueness of models. They should fit the relevant data. But the main point that I would like to make is that models should be used to predict and evaluate potential situations rather than just fit and describe available data. Hence, the collaboration and cooperation of theoretical and clinical people is a must.

Bassingthwaighte: Responding to Dr Hoffman's argumentation on modeling, I think that we were challenged on a couple of points. One is a point of agreement that if you have more free parameters you can probably get a better fit. If you take a linear regression, a y on x regression, and you make it parbolic, the odds are that you can get a slightly better fit, by making another coefficient available for the fitting. That does not mean that either model is correct. The y on x regression is a perfectly explicit model, a fact that is seldom appreciated; a noisy y-variable is dependent on a noise-free x-variable and the minimization is the sum of squares of the y-distances of the points from the line. One has to be very careful when one uses any model fitting such as a y on x regression, as to whether the model is meaningful or not, or whether it is simply a descriptor. But I do not buy in general the idea that models with more parameters give more freedom or improvement in fitting. The name of the game is to circumscribe the parameters with the data; the key is a surfeit of data, and by so constraining the parameters you can be predictive. I want to pick up on Dr Hoffman's idea that there should be 'unique' values of parameters. Relating to the y on x regression, is the answer that you get on that regression line unique? Clearly not! If you added one other data point you may have a different line. So there is never uniqueness in any model fitting to any data, unless they are absolutely perfect. I oppose the idea that one should seek uniqueness in modeling. The best you can do is to get the best resolution of the data tested against a variety of hypotheses. You can then compare hypotheses, but none of them can be anything but the best fit. The word 'unique' is misleading.

Arts: When you are thinking about a model, you have to be able to compare it to reality. The model of Dr Perl, for instance, shows how ischemia affects mechanics. There are quite a number of experimental possibilities to check it. You can measure deformations of the heart. You can measure local coronary blood flow, with the microsphere method. You can even measure deformation in relation to fiber orientation, if you can detect fiber orientation. There can be some matching you can calculate. As the constitutive behavior of the material is known from isolated muscle experiments, the theory and experiment can be merged into each other.

Sideman: The point that Dr Hoffman made is very well taken but very hard to perform. His point is that models should not only describe or fit data but should predict, should be a tool which allows to check new assumptions or a new concept and introduce new questions into the field. I do not think, though, that reviewers appreciate this kind of speculation game. The point made concerning the prediction capacity of a model, rather than its uniqueness, is however the road we should follow.

Spaan: We made a distinction here between making models and doing experiments. I would like to stress that if one interprets an experiment, one uses a model either explicitly or implicitly. A nice example is an end-diastolic resistance index. Some say 'I do not use a model', but then they apply an index to interpretate vasoconstriction. One ignores that there is a theoretical model behind the index and that the data is interpreted accordingly. Hence, the 'end-diastolic resistance index' is interpreted as the real ED resistance, which is a meaningless concept. The distinction between models and experiments is artificial. It is very important for experimental people that they make their thoughts explicit in a model. Then, at least, one can evaluate the experiment and extrapolate the conclusions to a different set of conditions.

Hoffman: I agree. Everything you do is obviously a model, whether it is explicit or not. Clearly, the more explicit you make it the better off you are likely to be. I was just saying that because of the enormous complexity of the heart there can be a tendency to go off into technicalities of the model.

Arts: Dr Hoffman remarked that models should be predictive and that we should do experiment to check ideas. We had ideas about torsion before doing any experiments. Our model predicted a value for the ratio of torsion divided by the amount of shortening. Then we did the experiments and the value we got was 10% off the predicted value with a standard deviation of 10%. We repeated the experiments with 2-D echocardiography and the same value came out. This parameter ratio of torsion to shortening reflects an equilibrium of stresses in the wall and that makes this parameter meaningful. If you are interested in transmural differences of stresses in the cardiac wall, I suggest that you look at the ratio of shortening to torsion.

Sideman: I would like to relate to the Technion simulation program. The Technion's three dimensional simulator includes mechanical aspects, hemodynamics and flow, metabolic and energetic aspects, electrophysiology, imaging and control. The latter is a subject which we have not applied ourself to as yet and needs great attention.

Needless to say that an ambitious task of this magnitude requires close cooperation and collaboration between the clinitians, experimentalists and the theoreticians so as to make this simulator meaningful.

Today's discussion brought into focus many old and new problems which are really at the heart of the cardiac system, and give us all food for thought and some ideas concerning the interactions affecting cardiac performance. We have heard suggestions and advice concerning the theoretical approach, and I would like to address a few remarks to the forgotten experimentalists. Obviously, they should be very careful when they take data, and use the correct equipment and the exact gages. However, they should also use the right model and use this equipment correctly. I have just seen a paper which came from Holland where they showed very clearly that if you do not place your gage in the correct direction and in the right place, the data can be quite misleading and one can erroneously develop a new physiology of the ventricle just because one did not place the gages properly. The fact is that the gages are usually good in all experiments, but the knowledge of where to put them comes from theory and helps get correct measurements. Also, experimentally accurate data does not make the interpretation correct. Another request that I have to the experimentalists is to record seemingly simple 'unrelated' data, like heart beat, blood pressure, etc., because eventually we try to use this data ...

To conclude, we have started something important, a dialogue between theory and practice. Now we can attempt to tackle pathology quantitatively. We have seen a beginning at this meeting. We should go about it carefully and this will eventually lead us to a better understanding of the cardiac system.

Concluding remarks

Sideman: In closing this meeting, we thank all the participants for presenting excellent studies and for their active participation in the discussions. Personal thanks go to the scientific advisory committee headed by Dr Sonnenblick and particularly to Dr Beyar and Dr Bassingthwaighte for their continued help and productive suggestions. Also, the members of the organizing committee and particularly Dr Welkowitz, gave their help and support. I am sure you will all join me in thanking Mr Henry Goldberg, again, for his generosity and vision in making this workshop possible. With his support and our ingenuity and persistence we should, by working together, achieve our goals of better understanding of cardiac performance and of developing the quantitative analytical tools for predicting cardiac operation under various constraints.
Welkowitz: I would like to thank everybody here on behalf of Rutgers University and Rutgers Medical School and invite you all to come back and visit us more extensively. Also, since I am now at the Technion on sabbatical leave, I thank you on behalf of the Technion as well for this wonderful meeting. Finally, I am sure you will all join me in thanking Dr Sideman for making this meeting a most efficient and very enjoyable experience.

Index